W9-CNC-291

Pediatric Nuclear Medicine/PET

Third Edition

S.T. Treves, MD

Editor

Pediatric Nuclear Medicine/PET

Third Edition

With a Foreword by George A. Taylor, MD

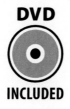

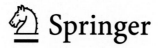

S.T. Treves, MD
Chief
Division of Nuclear Medicine
Children's Hospital Boston
Professor of Radiology
Harvard Medical School
Boston, MA 02115
USA

Library of Congress Control Number: 200690202

ISBN-10: 0-387-32321-X   e-ISBN-10: 0-387-32322-8
ISBN-13: 978-0387-32321-3   e-ISBN-13: 978-0387-32322-0

Printed on acid-free paper.

© 2007 Springer Science+Business Media, LLC
All rights reserved. This work may not be translated or copied in whole or in part
without the written permission of the publisher (Springer Science+Business Media,
LLC, 233 Spring Street, New York, NY 10013, USA), except for brief excerpts in
connection with reviews or scholarly analysis. Use in connection with any form of
information storage and retrieval, electronic adaptation, computer software, or by
similar or dissimilar methodology now known or hereafter developed is forbidden.
The use in this publication of trade names, trademarks, service marks, and similar
terms, even if they are not identified as such, is not to be taken as an expression of
opinion as to whether or not they are subject to proprietary rights.
While the advice and information in this book are believed to be true and accurate
at the date of going to press, neither the authors nor the editors nor the publisher
can accept any legal responsibility for any errors or omissions that may be made.
The publisher makes no warranty, express or implied, with respect to the material
contained herein.

9 8 7 6 5 4 3 2 1

springer.com

To my wife, Nancy,
my children, Erik, Alex, Blake,
and Olivia
and my parents, Catherine and Elias

Foreword

This third edition of *Pediatric Nuclear Medicine/PET* comes at a very propitious time. In the decade since the last edition was published, we have had major successes in decoding the human genome, technological developments in image processing, image quantification, and a new understanding of the molecular events triggering normal and abnormal cellular processes. These advances have resulted in a revolution in medical imaging. We are well into the transformation from a qualitative, descriptive discipline involved in imaging anatomic structures to one that is more quantitative and much more capable of imaging physiologic and cellular processes and displaying them in four dimensions (three-dimensional images over time).

The field of nuclear medicine has benefited from these transformational changes, and its role remains quite strong in pediatric imaging. Technical innovations have increased our ability to visualize functional, physiologic processes more quickly, more specifically, and with more anatomic certainty than ever before. The impact of this new knowledge on the clinical practice of pediatric nuclear medicine has been substantial. Some imaging studies performed commonly in the recent past are no longer used clinically, such as dacryoscintigraphy and scrotal scintigraphy. Despite the high degree of accuracy for distinguishing between inflammatory and ischemic conditions, scrotal scintigraphy has been essentially replaced by color Doppler sonography. As some techniques have faded, others have been added to the nuclear medicine armamentarium. Single photon emission computed tomography (SPECT) has become much more prevalent, and tissue-specific imaging with metaiodobenzylguanidine (MIBG) for neuroblastoma and sestamibi for myocardial perfusion studies have been some of the major improvements in the traditional practice of nuclear medicine. These have been incremental changes in existing technology. The most significant development has been the dissemination of positron emission tomography (PET) into pediatric practice. At the time of the last edition, probably only one PET scanner had any major pediatric use in the United States. As of this writing, several pediatric centers, including ours, have installed PET scanners dedicated primarily to imaging children.

As a pediatric radiologist, I have seen the impact of PET on the clinical care of children with solid tumors. It is very humbling to interpret ill-defined nodules on a contrast-enhanced computed tomography (CT) of the abdomen as unopacified loops of bowel, only to have them practically jump off the monitor screen as PET-avid lesions. Our imaging practice has had to change to accommodate the powerful nature of these new images.

This third edition of *Pediatric Nuclear Medicine/PET* incorporates the major advances that have been made in nuclear medicine in the recent past. The book is streamlined, up to date, and very readable. Chapters on brain and cerebrospinal fluid imaging have been combined; chapters on bone scintigraphy, Legg-Calvé-Perthes syndrome, evaluation of growth centers, and mandibular asymmetry have been consolidated into an excellent chapter on bone disorders; and chapters on scrotal scintigraphy and dacryoscintigraphy have been replaced with new, more focused chapters on PET and oncologic imaging. Each chapter is organized around the concepts of applicable radionuclides, imaging techniques, clinical applications, and specific disease entities. There is a significant effort to include correlative imaging in many of the chapters, and image fusion is displayed liberally throughout the book.

Pediatric Nuclear Medicine/PET will continue to be the bible of nuclear imaging in children. It will serve as the standard reference for medical students, residents, nuclear medicine physicians, technologists, and referring clinicians on how to perform and use radioactive tracer studies in the optimal care of sick children.

George A. Taylor, MD
John A. Kirkpatrick Professor of Radiology (Pediatrics)
Radiologist-in-Chief, Children's Hospital
Boston, MA

Preface

The second edition of *Pediatric Nuclear Medicine* was published just over 10 years ago. This third edition is entitled *Pediatric Nuclear Medicine/PET*. This book reflects advances in the technology and applications of classic pediatric nuclear medicine that have occurred during the past decade or so. Early pediatric experience with positron emission tomography (PET) has been included in the appropriate chapters, and there is a new chapter covering the physics and technical aspects of PET as they apply to pediatric patients. With very few exceptions, many of the chapters in *Pediatric Nuclear Medicine/PET* have been either significantly updated or rewritten entirely.

This book largely reflects the experience at Children's Hospital Boston. In addition, I am very fortunate that the work includes contributions from several outstanding colleagues from other institutions.

Following the first chapter that covers general aspects of pediatric nuclear medicine, the work is organized according to organs and systems including the brain and cerebrospinal fluid, thyroid, calculations of I-131 therapy doses, pulmonary system, cardiovascular system, gastroesophageal reflux and aspiration, gastrointestinal bleeding, liver and spleen, kidneys, vesicoureteral reflux, glomerular filtration rate, bone, oncology, infection and inflammation, magnification, single photon emission computed tomography (SPECT), PET, radiation risk, and internal dosimetry.

As in the prior editions, this book concentrates specifically on pediatric aspects of nuclear medicine; it is not intended to provide a multimodality review of pediatric imaging. For that type of perspective, the reader is directed to textbooks that cover all aspects of pediatric imaging. However, because of the relatively recent introduction of hybrid systems [PET/computed tomography (CT), SPECT/CT] and the significant improvements in image registration and fusion, several clinical examples in this text include image correlations.

This book includes an accompanying DVD, which allows the reader to review over 130 pediatric nuclear medicine cases. These cases are from the Division of Nuclear Medicine, Children's Hospital Boston.

Each case is logically organized to illustrate specific applications, techniques, and teaching points that nuclear medicine physicians are likely to encounter in daily practice, including multimodality image fusion in pediatric patients.

The DVD provides physicians who would like to become familiar with a view of the full scope of pediatric nuclear medicine applications, but who are not able to spend much time in a pediatric nuclear medicine unit.

I hope that this book will be helpful to physicians, technologists, and students involved in the care of pediatric patients.

S.T. Treves, MD

Acknowledgments

I would like to thank many friends and colleagues who in one way or another have contributed to make this third edition of *Pediatric Nuclear Medicine/PET* a reality.

I would like to thank Chris Durall for his great help in the preparation of the manuscript through its many drafts and revisions, and for helping organize the work and communications among the contributors, the editor, and the publisher. His meticulous and consistent attention to detail and commitment to this project has made my work more bearable. Jennifer Duane assisted with various communications with authors. Royal Davis, (CNMT), provided personnel and organizational leadership and ensured the smooth technical operations of the Division of Nuclear Medicine. Many technologists contributed expert technical assistance, excellent imaging, and computer application skills. Their dedication, care, patience, and compassion in dealing with our pediatric patients cannot be acknowledged enough. These included Diane Itrato, Tracy Tetrault, Vicky Kourmouzi, Erin Kistler, Joanne Olofson, and Steven Laffin. Our nurses, Valerie Dinan, Maura Heckmann, and Dell Spangler, have provided expert care, comfort, and compassion to many children being examined in our division. Our child life specialist, Tricia Ashe, participated in the preparation of patients and parents by providing explanations, educational materials, appropriate toys and other materials to help make their experience a positive one. Karl Mitchell provided excellent clinical computer software programs for display and analysis of several clinical applications, as well as an excellent systems integration environment. He also provided invaluable assistance in clinical database research, image registration, and fusion. Fred Fahey, DSc, provided excellent nuclear medicine and positron emission tomography (PET) physics support and served as reviewer of chapters in the book as well. Alan Packard, PhD, contributed to the text and reviewed chapters. Miriam Geller and Allison Clapp provided expert literature research support. I would like to thank my colleagues, the referring physicians, for trusting us with their patients. I would like to thank all the members of the Department of Radiology at Children's Hospital Boston for their collegiality and support. I would like to give special thanks to S.J. Adelstein, MD, PhD, for his support, advice, and encouragement over the past 35 years.

I would like to thank Rob Albano from Springer for his encouragement and support to make the third edition of this book possible.

Last, but not least, I would like to thank my wife, Nancy, and my children, Erik, Alex, Blake, and Olivia, for their immense patience and constant support, without which this book would not have been possible.

S.T. Treves, MD

Contents

Contributors

S. James Adelstein, MD, PhD, Paul C. Cabot Professor of Medical Biophysics, Harvard Medical School, Boston, MA 02115, USA

Laurie Armsby, MD, Assistant Professor of Cardiology, Children's Hospital Boston, Assistant Professor of Pediatrics, Harvard Medical School, Boston, MA 02115, USA

Ramsey D. Badawi, PhD, Assistant Professor of Radiology, University of California Davis Medical Center, Sacramento, CA 95817, USA

Zvi Bar-Sever, MD, Director, Division of Nuclear Medicine, Schneider Children's Medical Center, Petach-Tikva 49202 Israel

Elizabeth D. Blume, MD, Medical Director, Heart Failure/ Transplant Program, Associate in Cardiology, Children's Hospital Boston, Assistant Professor of Pediatrics, Harvard Medical School, Boston, MA 02115, USA

Blaise F.D. Bourgeois, MD, Director, Division of Epilepsy and Clinical Neurophysiology, Department of Neurology, Children's Hospital Boston, Professor of Neurology, Harvard Medical School, Boston, MA 02115, USA

Harry T. Chugani, MD, Chief, Department of Pediatric Neurology, Co-Director, Positron Emission Tomography Center, Children's Hospital of Michigan, Rosalie and Bruce Rosen Professor of Neurology, Professor of Pediatrics and Radiology, Wayne State University Medical Center, Detroit, MI 48201, USA

Leonard P. Connolly, MD, Staff Nuclear Medicine Physician, Children's Hospital Boston, Assistant Professor of Radiology, Harvard Medical School, Boston, MA 02115, USA

Susan A. Connolly, MD, Assistant Professor of Radiology, Children's Hospital Boston, Harvard Medical School, Boston, MA 02115, USA

Royal T. Davis, CNMT, RT(N), Technical Director, Division of Nuclear Medicine, Children's Hospital Boston, Boston, MA 02115, USA

Laura A. Drubach, MD, Staff Nuclear Medicine Physician, Children's Hospital Boston, Instructor in Radiology, Harvard Medical School, Boston, MA 02115, USA

Frederic H. Fahey, DSc, Director of Nuclear Medicine/PET Physics, Children's Hospital Boston, Associate Professor of Radiology, Harvard Medical School, Boston, MA 02115, USA

Richard J. Grand, MD, Program Director, General Clinical Research Center, Department of Medicine, Children's Hospital Boston, Professor of Pediatrics, Harvard Medical School, Boston, MA 02115, USA

Beth A. Harkness, MS, Nuclear Medicine Physicist, Department of Diagnostic Radiology, Henry Ford Health System, Detroit, MI 48202, USA

William E. Harmon, MD, Professor of Pediatrics, Harvard Medical School, Director of Pediatric Nephology, Children's Hospital Boston, Boston, MA, 02115, USA

Stephen A. Huang, MD, Director, Thyroid Program, Children's Hospital Boston, Assistant Professor of Pediatrics, Harvard Medical School, Boston, MA 02115, USA

Hossein Jadvar, MD, PhD, MPH, Associate Professor of Radiology and Biomedical Engineering, Director of Research, Department of Radiology, Keck School of Medicine, University of Southern California, Los Angeles, CA 90033, USA

A.G. Jones, PhD, Professor of Radiology, Harvard Medical School, Boston, MA 02115, USA

Alvin Kuruc, MD, PhD, Director, Credit Suisse First Boston, New York, NY 10010, USA

Charito Love, MD, Research Scientist, Nuclear Medicine, Long Island Jewish Medical Center, New Hyde Park, NY 11040, USA

Karl Mitchell, Nuclear Medicine Information Systems Manager, Children's Hospital Boston, Boston, MA 02115, USA

Jane W. Newburger, MD, MPH, Associate Cardiologist-in-Chief, Department of Cardiology, Children's Hospital Boston, Professor of Pediatrics, Harvard Medical School, Boston, MA 02115, USA

Alan B. Packard, PhD, Senior Research Associate, Division of Nuclear Medicine, Children's Hospital Boston, Assistant Professor of Radiology (Nuclear Medicine), Harvard Medical School, Boston, MA 02115, USA

Christopher J. Palestro, MD, Chief, Division of Nuclear Medicine, Long Island Jewish Medical Center, Professor of Nuclear Medicine and Radiology, Albert Einstein College of Medicine, New Hyde Park, NY 11040, USA

Barry L. Shulkin, MD, Chief, Division of Nuclear Medicine, Professor of Radiology, St. Jude's Children's Research Hospital, Memphis, TN 38105, USA

Michael G. Stabin, PhD, CHP, Assistant Professor of Radiology and Radiological Sciences, Vanderbilt University, Nashville, TN 37232, USA

Maria B. Tomas, MD, Attending Physician in Nuclear Medicine, Long Island Jewish Medical Center, Assistant Professor of Nuclear Medicine and Radiology, Albert Einstein College of Medicine, New Hyde Park, NY 11040, USA

S. T. Treves, MD, Chief, Division of Nuclear Medicine, Children's Hospital Boston, Professor of Radiology, Harvard Medical School, Boston, MA 02115, USA

Ulrich V. Willi, MD, Professor of Pediatric Radiology, University of Zurich, Switzerland

Robert E. Zimmerman, MSEE, Director of Physics and Engineering, Joint Program in Nuclear Medicine, Principal Associate of Radiology (Physics), Harvard Medical School, Boston, MA 02115, USA

1
Introduction

S.T. Treves

The fundamental difference between adult nuclear medicine and pediatric nuclear medicine is the child. The child makes pediatric nuclear medicine a very interesting, dynamic, and exciting field. Pediatric nuclear medicine includes the application of diagnos-tic, therapeutic, and investigational aspects of nuclear medicine to pediatric patients. Because they are sensitive, minimally invasive, and safe, diagnostic nuclear medicine procedures are well suited for the evaluation of pediatric patients. Nuclear medicine provides qualitative and quantitative information about the function of organs, systems, and lesions in the body. Research in pediatric nuclear medicine is full of potential, but clinical investigation in pediatric patients presents practical and ethical challenges.

During the 1960s, the application of radionuclide techniques in children was very limited. An important reason for this early limitation was that available radiopharmaceuticals were tagged with radioisotopes with relatively long physical half-lives, which resulted in high patient radiation doses. Early imaging devices consisted principally of rectilinear scanners that permitted only static imaging at relatively low spatial resolution. In addition, concern about patient radiation exposure limited the amount of radiotracer activity that could be administered, which in turn resulted in very lengthy examination times. In these early days, nuclear medicine examinations could be performed only on patients with a known malignancy. Radionuclide imaging of brain tumors and liver using planar scintigraphy accounted for most pediatric studies performed in the 1960s and early 1970s. Therefore, there was no significant role for nuclear medicine in the early diagnosis of disease or in the assessment of nonmalignant disorders. Advances in radiopharmaceuticals and imaging devices have increased the capability of nuclear medicine to achieve earlier and better diagnosis.

During the past three decades, these advances have resulted in an increase in the number, scope, and variety of pediatric nuclear medicine examinations. The growth of pediatric nuclear medicine is due in great part to its proven ability to provide information about many pediatric disorders that could not be obtained, or could not be obtained easily, with other diagnostic imaging technology. Pediatric nuclear medicine is now well established and is widely used in the diagnosis and follow-up of many pediatric disorders. Underscoring the physiologic nature of the field, nuclear medicine is ideally suited for assessment of organ function, for monitoring the progress of a number of pediatric disorders, and to evaluate the effect of therapies. During the past decades the greatest number of patients examined by nuclear medicine have been those affected by benign disorders. Radionuclide studies are increasingly valuable in the early diagnosis, staging, and evolution of oncologic disorders, as well as in the monitoring of therapy. In 2005, oncology studies accounted for <20% of the total nuclear medicine examinations at Children's Hospital Boston.

This chapter provides a broad overview of the practice of pediatric nuclear medicine, including consultation, interaction with patients and families, use of radiopharmaceuticals, radionuclide therapy, instrumentation and equipment, image fusion and systems integration, and the physical facility.

The Consultation

The goal for every pediatric nuclear medicine study is to obtain the best diagnostic information employing the highest quality standards, in the shortest period of time, and with the lowest patient radiation exposure. The importance of specially trained, dedicated personnel in the pediatric nuclear medicine practice cannot be emphasized enough. It is important to obtain sufficient clinical information in each case and to determine the clinical appropriateness of each indication before proceeding with the study. A patient's clinical history, knowledge of previous surgery or other therapy, and results of previous imaging studies are all valuable pieces of information that enable the nuclear medicine team to select the best approach. Whenever possible, the patients' medical records should accompany them. Knowledge of potentially conflicting imaging tests already scheduled is essential when planning the study. It is important to determine if the patient had been given radiographic contrast during the past few days. It is also important to determine, in advance, if the patient may require sedation and if there are any special precautions.

Pediatric studies are often adapted to individual patients. Obtaining a clear description of the clinical question being asked is of utmost importance in guiding the procedure. If the nuclear medicine consultant determines that the examination requested is not appropriate to the problem in question or that another type of examination is indicated, he or she should communicate such concern to the referring physician in order to select a more appropriate examination or to avoid an unnecessary examination. Questioning parents and patients (when possible) about the clinical history and symptoms and an appropriately directed physical examination should be considered integral parts of the nuclear medicine study. Often, the nuclear medicine physician obtains key information from the patient or the parent that is helpful in tailoring the examination and to produce a better interpretation of findings within the clinical context. The physician and the technologist should review and consult in order to determine if any aspect of the examination requires special attention. Female patients should be asked about the possibility of pregnancy (see below). The technologist should examine patients for metallic objects that can shield gamma radiation (e.g., keys, belt buckles, coins, jewelry). Once the first images are obtained, any diapers, clothing, or gauze contaminated with radionuclides should be removed and the area reimaged. Contaminated skin should be thoroughly washed, monitored, and reimaged. Once the examination is completed, the physician and the technologist should review and evaluate the quality and adequacy of the study and determine if additional imaging is necessary. Depending on the initial result, the physician may need to reexamine the patient and the clinical data before the patient is discharged. When appropriate, the physician may recommend additional diagnostic imaging to clarify an abnormal finding or to try to increase the specificity of a scintigraphic finding.

In the modern era, nuclear medicine results should be reported promptly to the referring physician. Results of image analysis should be available immediately after the studies are completed so results can be reported rapidly and within a clinically useful time. It is highly desirable that previous studies be easily accessible, as many pediatric patients come back for follow-up examination. The report should be clear and concise, and it must address the clinical question(s) being asked. Easy and rapid electronic access to nuclear medicine reports and images facilitates communication with referring physicians and often helps improve patient care.

Interaction with Patients and Families

The practice of pediatric nuclear medicine includes patients ranging from premature infants to adolescents and young adults. The wide range of disorders, body sizes, and stages of development often requires individualized approaches and adjustments of imaging methodology, dosimetry, and interpretation. Physicians and technologists working in pediatric nuclear medicine should be familiar with children, their varied behavior, and the disorders that affect them. Certain procedures that in an adult setting can be conducted adequately by a single technologist may require two technologists (or a technologist and an aide) in the case of a child. More time and patience is necessary when dealing with children than with adults. Despite the best efforts of staff, procedures in children usually take longer than in adults (sometimes as much as twice as long).

Communication with Patients and Parents

The importance of good communication with patients and parents about nuclear medicine procedures cannot be emphasized enough. Under most optimal conditions, patients and families should be given information about what the anticipated nuclear medicine procedure will entail. If possible, the patient's family should be contacted by a member of the nuclear medicine staff a day or two in advance to confirm the appointment and to discuss the test. It is important to let parents know in advance approximately how long the examination will take and if it will be necessary to return later the same day or on a later day so that they can plan their day accordingly. It is also helpful to provide referring physician's offices with brochures for parents or patients explaining the nuclear medicine tests. Information about nuclear medicine tests should be available in the department's waiting room. Also, it is useful to post information about the tests and preparation instructions on the department's Web site.

The first contact, whether by phone or in person, is important and should include a clear and honest explanation of the procedure. Physicians and technologists should make a concerted effort to inform patients (whenever possible) and parents personally about the examination. Every pediatric patient must be treated as an individual with individual emotional and physical needs. Pediatric nuclear medicine procedures are "people-intensive." Children who are prepared can be more cooperative, often facilitating the examination for everyone involved. Patients should be told what they will see, hear, feel, and most important, what they will be expected to do. For example, they should be informed of an impending injection, the injection site, if there will be any pain, and any other appropriate explanations, all of which should help to reduce anxiety. Children have highly developed imaginations, and their fantasies can be anxiety provoking. It is important to keep in mind a child's developmental level when giving information and defining expectations during the procedure. Explanations and words should be chosen accordingly to ensure proper understanding of the information being given. It is sometimes helpful to explain the procedure to the child at least twice, first outside the imaging room where the child may feel less threatened and then in the imaging room. Throughout the examination, the technologist should provide reassurance and positive verbal reinforcement to enhance the child's sense of mastery. Parents are naturally concerned about what is going to happen to their child. To some parents and patients, the word *nuclear* elicits concern. It is important that the nuclear medicine physician be available to parents and patients to explain the low radiation exposures of nuclear medicine examinations and the physiologic nature of the field.

Should the patient's parents/family be allowed in the examining rooms? Children from about 8 months to approximately 3 years of age may suffer from separation anxiety and generally fare better with the parent(s) in the room. In most instances, children of all ages benefit from having a parent, relative, or a familiar staff person in the imaging room. This tends to have a calming effect on the patient and facilitates examination. In some instances, however, the presence of parents in the examination room has the opposite effect, in which case they should be asked to leave. Some children can cope better with the examination when they are alone rather than with their parents, and adolescents may prefer privacy and independence. Young children may be comforted by having a favorite toy or stuffed animal with them during the examination. This should be permitted so long as it does not interfere with the test.

Before proceeding with a nuclear medicine study, a female adolescent or young adult, should be asked if she might possibly be pregnant. If the postmenarcheal patient does not know if she is pregnant, it is prudent to wait until the next menstrual period or to perform a pregnancy test. If the patient is pregnant, it is advisable to consult with the referring physicians about the need for the test at this time and to evaluate the potential risk and benefit balance of having the test or not. Asking a young woman if she is pregnant however, can be a very delicate matter, and it needs to be handled with extreme care and sensitivity. This can be difficult, and it can be worse if the mother does not know that the young woman is sexually active. Sometimes it is necessary to consult with the referring physicians about the best way to handle the situation given each individual family situation. If the mother of the patient having an examination is pregnant, she should be instructed on how to avoid or reduce her radiation exposure.

Positioning and Immobilization During Imaging

Proper patient positioning is essential for a good examination. Because most nuclear medicine imaging requires the patient to remain still for a relatively long period, immobilization techniques are commonly used. Sandbags, adhesive tape, a papoose wrap with blanket, Velcro straps, and contoured pillows may be employed, depending on the size, age, condition, and activity of the patient. Newborns usually find swaddling comforting. In addition

to these immobilization techniques, it is sometimes necessary that a technologist or an aide hold a patient in position during imaging. Difficult cases may require two or even three technologists in attendance. Imaging artifacts resulting from holding patients by hand should be anticipated, recognized on the image, and, if possible, avoided. Technologists often need to talk, support, encourage, and distract the child while ensuring that the gamma camera is set up and functioning correctly. With a quiet environment, dim lights, and care, some children fall asleep during long examinations. Watching television can be an effective "sedative." Viewing television often helps to distract and relax some patients (and parents) during the examination. Small television monitors mounted on flexible arms, which enable positioning for easy viewing by the patient, are helpful. In addition, a program of interest to the child can be played using a videocassette recorder or DVD player. In some cases, immobilization alone is not successful, and sedation is required.

From time to time, pediatric nuclear medicine specialists are presented with inadequate pediatric studies performed at institutions not familiar with the examination of children. Technical problems observed include, but are not limited to, radiopharmaceutical overdose, poor patient positioning, body motion, inadequate selection or use of instrumentation (e.g., collimators, etc.), and inadequate display. Some of these factors can contribute to problems with interpretation. Nuclear medicine training programs for physicians and technologists should include training in pediatric aspects of nuclear medicine. Additional practical experience in a pediatric institution with a good nuclear medicine unit is recommended for those interested in the practice this field.

Sedation and General Anesthesia

With the increased use of single photon emission computed tomography (SPECT) and positron emission tomography (PET) in children, the need for sedation has become more frequent. Sedation or general anesthesia should be planned in advance of the patient's visit to nuclear medicine. It is important to assess the candidacy of the patient for sedation or general anesthesia in advance. Proper advance instructions about eating, diet, and any other preparation should also be clearly communicated to the patient or family. Similarly, outpatients need to be informed about the need for the patient to meet discharge criteria after sedation or general anesthesia and the time commitment that may be needed. The type and dose of sedation drug must be individualized and should be decided in consultation with the referring physician. Some institutions have specialized imaging sedation guidelines, and teams of specialized nurses and anesthesiologists that manage all sedation and anesthesia for imaging procedures. When administering sedatives to patients, potential side effects such as aspiration and respiratory arrest should be anticipated and appropriate means of treatment made available. A physician or nurse must monitor patients from the time of sedation until they have fully recovered. It is essential to ensure that the sedated outpatient is fully recovered from the sedation before discharge. The nuclear medicine department must be equipped with a cart containing all appropriate medications and equipment needed in case of emergency. This cart must be checked regularly and replenished as necessary. Sphygmomanometers and stethoscopes for various ages should be available and within easy reach. Oxygen and suction must be available in each examination room. All related equipment and facilities mentioned above must be checked regularly to ensure their proper functioning. Telephones (with emergency numbers posted visibly) should be available in each room. Even when not sedated, patients must never be left alone in the imaging room. One should anticipate that children might fall off the examination table, choke on a small toy, or remove an intravenous line or a nasogastric tube.

Some patients can only be examined properly while under general anesthesia. General anesthesia should be arranged with a pediatric anesthesiologist. When contemplating sedation or general anesthesia, one should be aware that sedation can affect several functions, such as cerebrospinal fluid flow, cardiovascular shunt flow, cardiac function, renal function, and brain function and consider these effects on image interpretation.

Radiopharmaceuticals

Radiopharmaceuticals are physiologically innocuous and do not produce toxic or pharmacologic effects or allergic reactions; nor do they result in hemodynamic or osmotic overload. To date, there have been no indications or reports of deleterious effects secondary to the administration of diagnostic radiopharmaceuticals in children.

Major improvements in radiopharmaceutical research over the past three decades have resulted in the introduction of a variety of agents labeled with short-lived radionuclides. These radiopharmaceuticals have enabled shorter examinations times and have allowed rapid dynamic studies, while resulting in low patient radiation exposures. Examples of radiopharmaceuticals applicable to pediatrics that have been introduced during the past several years include technetium-99m-disodium [N-[N-N-(mercaptoacetyl)glycyl]-glycinato(2-)-N,N',N'',S]oxotechnetate(2-) (^{99m}Tc-MAG$_3$), technetium-99m-bicisate (^{99m}Tc-ECD), and hexakis (2-methoxy-isobutylisonitrile) technetium, sestamibi (^{99m}Tc-MIBI). These agents have resulted in improved evaluation of the kidneys, the brain, and the myocardium using planar scintigraphy and SPECT. The introduction of iodine-123 metaiodobenzylguanidine (^{123}I-MIBG), with its high affinity for neuroendocrine tumors, has demonstrated the possibility that other disease-specific radiopharmaceuticals could be developed. Along with the recent impressive growth of PET, fluorine-18 fluorodeoxyglucose (^{18}F-FDG) and ^{18}F-fluoride have now become widely available, and FDG is being used to assist in the diagnosis, staging, and follow-up of several pediatric malignancies (Fig. 1.1). Also ^{18}F-FDG has shown promise in the assessment of inflammation and infection (Fig. 1.2). ^{18}F-fluoride is being used to obtain skeletal PET. Skeletal PET can be obtained rapidly and at high resolution (Fig. 1.3). Newer radiopharmaceuticals of potential use in pediatrics are

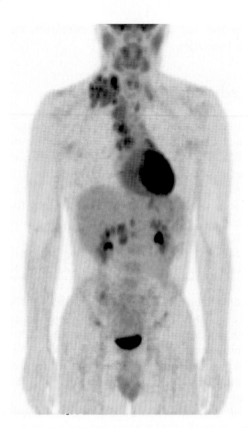

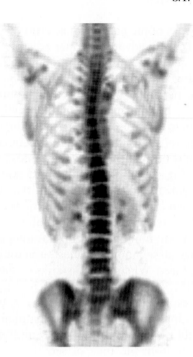

FIGURE 1.3. ¹⁸F-sodium fluoride bone PET. The image shows the detail that can be obtained with this technique.

FIGURE 1.1. Fluorine-18 fluorodeoxyglucose (¹⁸F-FDG) positron emission tomography (PET) in a patient with Hodgkin's lymphoma at presentation. Several regions of increased tracer uptake can be identified within the mediastinum, the right clavicular region, and the abdomen.

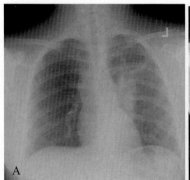 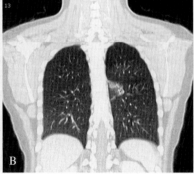 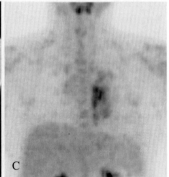

FIGURE 1.2. ¹⁸F-FDG uptake in pneumonia. A 13-year-old girl following chemotherapy and radiation therapy for Hodgkin's lymphoma presented with 5 days of fever and cough. A: The chest x-ray revealed left lower lobe pneumonia. B: A selected coronal computed tomography (CT) slice also reveals a lesion in the left thorax. C: The ¹⁸F-FDG-PET reveals increased tracer uptake in the same region, indicating active inflammatory disease extending beyond the visible CT lesion.

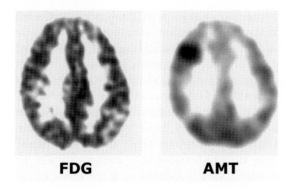

FDG   **AMT**

FIGURE 1.4. Transverse sections of PET from a 3-year-old boy with infantile spasms and a right frontal electroencephalograph (EEG) focus. On the left, an ^{18}F-FDG-PET is within normal limits. A corresponding α-[^{11}C]-methyl-L-tryptophan (AMT) PET reveals a well-defined region of increased tracer uptake corresponding to the epileptogenic zone. (*Source:* Courtesy of Harry Chugani, M.D.)

Growth, Development, and Radiopharmaceutical Kinetics

While growth and development are occurring during the neonatal and infant periods, radiopharmaceutical biokinetics are often different from those in the older child or the adult. For example, newborns and infants have a lower glomerular filtration rate, faster washout of radioactive gases from the lungs, and faster circulation times than adult patients. As growth and maturation take place, physiologic processes in children reach adult levels. Another example of differences in radiopharmaceutical biodistribution occurs in the developing brain. As the brain undergoes maturation, regional cerebral blood flow and metabolic patterns change with age. These changes are reflected on ^{99m}Tc-ECD perfusion brain SPECT and ^{18}F-FDG PET. In the newborn, regional cerebral perfusion and metabolism are initially more intense in the sensorimotor cortex, thalamus, brainstem, and cerebellar vermis; later the parietal, temporal, and occipital cortex, basal ganglia, cerebellar cortex, and, finally, the frontal cortex are involved (see Chapter 2). Similarly, in children, the concentration of ^{99m}Tc-methylene diphosphonate (MDP) in growth centers is relatively high. As growth centers close, the biodistribution of ^{99m}Tc-MDP gradually reaches the adult pattern.

being evaluated. One example is α-[^{11}C]-methyl-L-tryptophan (AMT), an agent that has been shown to concentrate in epileptogenic zones in the brain, which can be imaged with PET (Fig. 1.4). Another example is ^{18}F-dihydroxyphenylalanine (^{18}F-DOPA) for the localization of insulinomas in patients with hyperinsulinemia (Fig. 1.5).

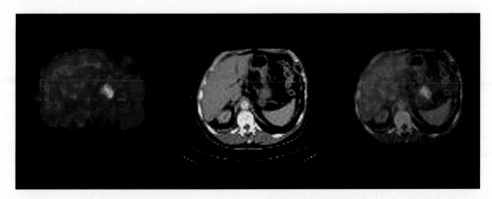

FIGURE 1.5. ^{18}F-dihydroxyphenylalanine (^{18}F-DOPA) PET from a very young patient with hyperinsulinism. The focal region of increased tracer uptake corresponds to an insulinoma that was surgically excised later. (*Source:* Courtesy of Abass Alavi, M.D.)

Administered Radiopharmaceutical Doses: Concept of Minimal Dose

Pediatric radiopharmaceutical doses should be determined by the minimal amount necessary to ensure satisfactory examination. Administered doses in pediatric nuclear medicine have been developed by experience, taking into account the body mass absorbed radiation dose, type of examination, available photon flux, instrumentation, and examination time. High doses (which do not result in improved diagnostic sensitivity or accuracy) or low doses (which do not permit adequate examination) should be considered unnecessary radiation exposures. Dose estimations for pediatric patients based on adult dose corrected for body weight or body surface area are generally good guides for children over 1 year of age. Premature infants and newborns require special consideration, and the concept of minimal total dose should be applied. *Minimal total dose* can be defined as the minimal dose of radiopharmaceutical below which the study will be inadequate regardless of the patient's body weight or surface area. The minimal dosage is determined by the type of study: dynamic or static. As a general rule, dynamic studies require a higher dose of tracer than do static studies. For example, the usual pediatric dose of ^{99m}Tc-pertechnetate for radionuclide angiography is 0.2 mCi/kg (7.4 MBq/kg) of body weight. However, a radionuclide angiogram obtained on a premature baby who weighs 900 g requires a minimal total does of 2 mCi (74 MBq). Lack of information on pediatric administered doses and absorbed doses, and the desire of some physicians or technologists to obtain a study in the shortest possible time, combined with inexperience in handling pediatric patients, are factors that can contribute to radiopharmaceutical overdose in children. For specific guidelines and recommendations on radiopharmaceutical administered doses, consult the individual chapters.

Radiopharmaceutical Administration

Routes of radiopharmaceutical administration include intravenous, oral, inhalation, subcutaneous, intradermal, instillation, and intrathecal. Intravenous injection is the most frequent route of radiopharmaceutical administration and warrants special attention. In advance of tracer administration, a tray lined with absorbent paper should be prepared for each patient dose. This tray should contain disposable gloves, skin antiseptic, needles, gauze, the radiopharmaceutical dose, adhesive tape, and a tourniquet. The radiopharmaceutical syringe should be shielded, clearly labeled with the name of the patient, the name of the tracer, the dose, the date and time of calibration, and the volume. Injection technique varies somewhat for static and dynamic studies. Dynamic studies require high temporal resolution, and a rapid, compact intravenous bolus of tracer. Volume and site of injection are important. A 23- to 25-gauge needle of the butterfly type can be used. A disposable T-type connector with a one-way valve permits rapid injection of the tracer followed by a saline flush. The radiopharmaceutical should be in 0.2 to 0.5 mL of solution. Premature and newborn infants require smaller volumes (0.1 to 0.2 mL). A large proximal vein, such as an antecubital vein, is usually adequate to permit rapid administration of the radiopharmaceutical and the saline flush. As long as they can tolerate the rapid bolus and the saline flush, other veins may be used. Patients usually lie supine for the injection. The site of injection should not overlap the area of interest. Once an appropriate vein is identified, a tourniquet is applied and the skin is cleaned with an antiseptic. The tubing is filled with sterile saline. The extremity is immobilized or held by an aide if necessary, and the vein is entered. As soon as blood return occurs, the tourniquet is released. If there is no free retrograde venous flow into the tube of the butterfly needle, no attempt should be made to inject the radiopharmaceutical, and another injection site should be identified. When dealing with venous access in small infants, there is no substitute for an experienced nuclear medicine technologist or physician. After successful venous entry, the needle is secured in place with adhesive tape. One should check once more to make sure that there is free flow into the vein. It is good practice to flush the tubing with a small volume (1 to 3 mL) of normal saline before injecting the tracer. The radiopharmaceutical should then be injected and the tubing flushed with normal saline.

The injection technique for static studies is easier than that for dynamic studies, as the volume of radiopharmaceutical solution, injection site, and the speed of injection are not as critical as for dynamic studies.

Absorbed Radiation Doses

Absorbed doses vary with age and weight, as well as with the physiologic or pathologic condition of the patient. Chapter 20 discusses pediatric internal dosimetry of currently available radiopharmaceuticals.

Instrumentation and Equipment

Advances in nuclear medicine imaging equipment, as well as in detector and computer technology, continue to occur with amazing frequency. When evaluating pediatric patients, it is important to employ the most modern imaging equipment whenever possible. New gamma camera systems allow faster imaging and are capable of higher spatial resolution, better field uniformity, and improved spatial and count linearity than previous versions. Single photon emission computed tomography has become an indispensable technique in pediatric nuclear medicine. Positron emission tomography is also becoming a very important tool in the assessment of pediatric patients. Newer PET devices offer rapid imaging at very high spatial resolution. Hybrid systems such as PET/computed tomography (CT) scanners are becoming widely available. At the time of this writing, most major manufacturers are also marketing SPECT/CT devices. These hybrid devices help obtain rapid attenuation correction maps and anatomic localization. Computed tomography devices associated with hybrid PET/CT systems vary from two slices to 36 or even 64, all capable of high-resolution imaging. A conventional gamma camera with SPECT capabilities can be used to perform many types of examinations on pediatric patients ranging from babies to young adults.

Dual, large area-detector cameras can perform whole-body planar and pinhole magnification scintigraphy as well as SPECT. Their rapid imaging capability is an obvious advantage for small children, as immobilization time can be reduced. Collimator selection for individual types of examinations is important. Awareness of the characteristics of various collimators helps optimize imaging. Collimation in pediatric nuclear medicine should favor ultrahigh-resolution–type collimators. Magnification scintigraphy provides the highest spatial resolution with gamma cameras, and it is an indispensable technique to image small body parts in children (discussed in Chapter 16). Mobile cameras can be used for the evaluation of patients in intensive care units, recovery rooms, catheterization laboratories, and operating rooms.

Image Fusion and Systems Integration

As stated before, nuclear medicine studies focus on functional aspects, early diagnosis, and diagnostic specificity. Anatomic and functional imaging methodologies are increasingly regarded as complementary and not competitive. Understanding the relationships between anatomic or structural imaging and functional imaging is increasingly valued. In the past, physicians relied on spatial sense to mentally reorient and superimpose one type of image with respect to the other. Such an approach was subjective and varied among observers. Image fusion methods overlay two or more three-dimensional (3D) image sets of the same or different imaging modalities in the same orientation in the same space. Image fusion enables the direct comparison of function and structure [SPECT and magnetic resonance imaging (MRI)], function and function (gallium SPECT and FDG-PET), or structure and structure (MRI and CT). With advances in electronic communications, computer processing power, high-capacity networks, and the wider acceptance of imaging standards, image registration and fusion are easier to obtain and are now within the reach of routine practice, and more advances are anticipated. Electronic imaging and nonimaging information can now

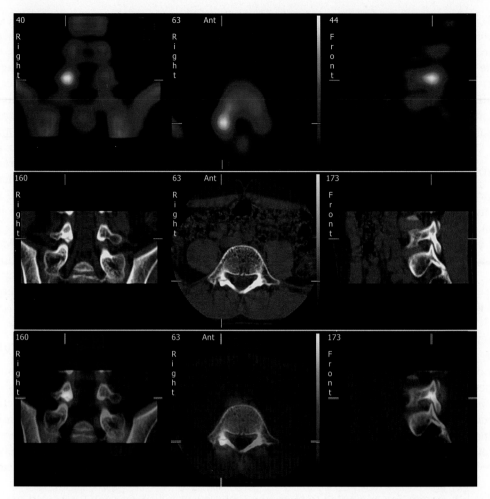

FIGURE 1.6. ^{18}F-fluoride PET and CT fusion. Selected fused slices reveal intense fluoride uptake in the region of the right L5 pars. On CT there was a linear defect through the right L5 pars interarticularis.

be easily accessed within local and wide area networks. With the increasing sophistication of picture archiving and communication systems (PACSs), all imaging modalities can be viewed on workstations. Archiving and retrieving of multimodality 3D image sets is now possible with relatively little effort. Several imaging equipment manufacturers offer image fusion technology as part of their systems. The introduction of PET/CT scanners has sparked tremendous interest in image fusion. This hardware approach to image fusion often needs to be complemented by software adjustments on the images when patients move between the PET and the CT. The PET/CT scanners limit image fusion to two modalities. Although manufacturers are introducing SPECT/CT devices, it is desirable not to limit image fusion solely based on hardware approaches. Software methods expand the application of image fusion to other 3D image sets including PET, SPECT, CT, and MRI (Figs. 1.6 to 1.12).

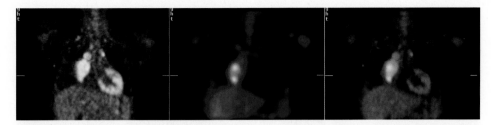

FIGURE 1.7. ^{18}F-FDG-PET and gallium-67 (^{67}Ga) single photon emission computed tomography (SPECT) fusion in a 17-year-old boy with Hodgkin's lymphoma. Left: ^{18}F-FDG-PET. Middle: ^{67}Ga SPECT. Right: Image fusion. These studies were obtained 5 days apart. Although there is a general concordance on the tracer uptake between the two tracers, the superior aspect of the right paramedial mass seems to be more FDG avid than Ga avid.

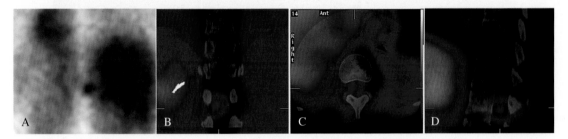

FIGURE 1.8. Iodine-123 metaiodobenzylguanidine (^{123}I-MIBG) scan from a 16-year-old girl with recurrent neuroblastoma shows a focal region of increased tracer uptake in the midline (A). Coronal (B), transverse (C), and sagittal (D) slices of a fused MIBG SPECT and CT clearly reveal the anatomic localization of this lesion.

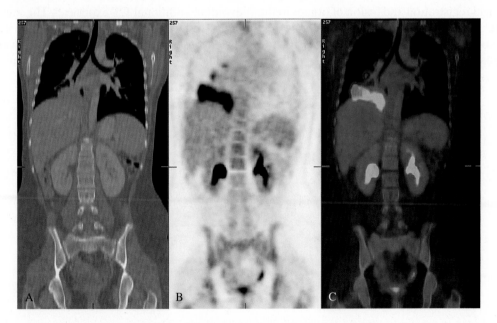

FIGURE 1.9. Lymphoma. ^{18}F-FDG (B) with CT (A) fusion. This patient shows a large right suprahepatic lesion as well as pericardial nodes that are FDG avid. Image fusion with CT (C) reveals the anatomic localization of these lesions.

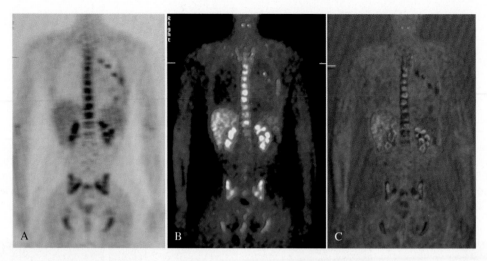

FIGURE 1.10. ^{18}F-FDG/^{18}F-FDG fusion. Two ^{18}F-FDG-PET studies of a patient with lymphoma obtained at presentation (A) and following chemotherapy (B). The fused image (C) permits the identification of lesions that have responded to treatment and those that have not.

Advances in image fusion methods now allow rapid and automated processing of the image sets. Current methods allow so-called rigid organ registration such as the brain, and even nonrigid registration and fusion of organs in the chest and abdomen. Most methods now rely on voxel matching or mutual information approaches. It is common that pediatric patients referred for PET or SPECT have had a CT study already. In these cases it is advantageous to use the CT already obtained and fuse it with the PET or the SPECT, thus avoiding additional CT exposures. The increasingly widely available multimodality image fusion poses interesting advantages as well as challenges for technologists and physicians.

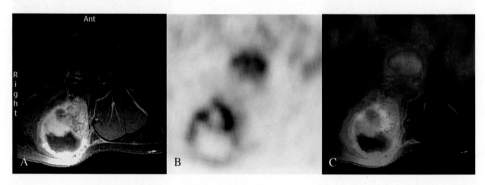

FIGURE 1.11. ^{18}F-FDG-PET (B) and magnetic resonance imaging (MRI) (A) fusion. Selected fused images (C) from a 14-year-old boy with a paraspinal Ewing's sarcoma. The active areas are evident on the ^{18}F-FDG-PET.

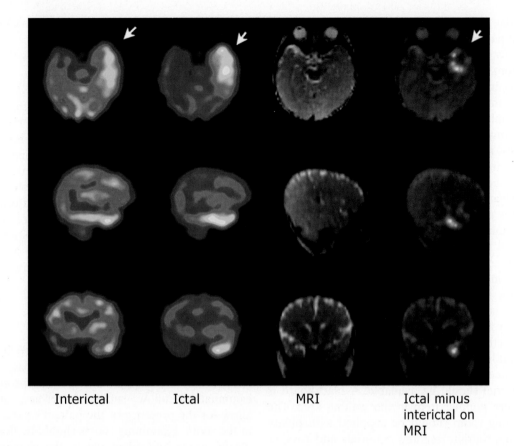

Interictal   Ictal   MRI   Ictal minus
                                                    interictal on
                                                    MRI

FIGURE 1.12. Interictal and ictal SPECT and MRI. Images have been registered: the registered ictal SPECT was subtracted from the interictal SPECT and the results fused with the MRI. The arrows show the epileptogenic zone.

Radionuclide Therapy

Therapy with internally administered radionuclides is employed less often in children than in adults. The most frequently performed radionuclide therapy in children is with iodine-131, for the treatment of patients with metastatic papillary carcinoma of the thyroid, patients suffering from hyperthyroidism refractory to medical treatment, and those who refuse surgery (see Chapter 3).

Physical Facility

The physical facility of the nuclear medicine department should help support patient comfort, safety, and efficient work flow. Space is needed for reception, patient waiting, imaging rooms, computers, personnel offices, injection/examination room, radiopharmacy, technologist's processing room, and a consultation/reading room. The radiopharmacy, injection/examination room, and the imaging rooms should be adjacent to one another. The waiting room and reception area should be located away from the examination rooms. The consultation/reading room and the technologist's processing rooms should be easily accessible to nuclear medicine personnel and referring physicians. Emergency supplies should be readily accessible.

Waiting Room

Currently, the majority of patients undergoing nuclear medicine examinations are outpatients (>85% of the total). Careful scheduling of studies can reduce waiting time for patients and parents. However, in practice, parents and family almost always experience some waiting before, during, and after an examination. Certain nuclear medicine examinations require that the patient wait in the department for a few minutes after administration of the radiopharmaceutical, before imaging (e.g., examinations using FDG-PET and SPECT). Other examinations require that, following radioisotope administration, the patient return to the nuclear medicine department one or more times after initial imaging [e.g., bone, kidney, gallium-67, indium-111 (^{111}In), ^{99m}Tc–white blood cells, thyroid, hepatobiliary system]. Similarly, parents and other family members who may accompany the patient may wait for a few minutes to several hours while the patient is undergoing an examination. The waiting room should be spacious, comfortable, attractively decorated, and well lit, and seating should be sufficient to accomodate family members. Toys, games, and writing and reading material should be available. A blackboard is a very popular item in the waiting area. The waiting room should be supplied with plenty of appropriate reading materials and toys, as well as information about parking, nuclear medicine, and other subjects appropriate for patients and their families. The reception desk should be at a writing height so children can see the receptionist and are not intimidated by a tall counter.

Radiopharmacy

The radiopharmacy should be well equipped with lead-shielded cabinets (for SPECT and PET radiopharmaceuticals), hood, sufficient counter space, and appropriate safety equipment and exhaust for volatile or gaseous materials (and a laminar flow hood). The room itself should be under negative air pressure. Data entry tools for radiopharmaceuticals and other pharmaceuticals (e.g., sedatives, furosemide, pentagastrin) should be provided in this area. The radiopharmacy should have sufficient space for supplies and for storage and disposal of radioactive materials. In addition, space should be allowed for nonradioactive supplies.

Injection/Examination Room

Busy pediatric nuclear medicine departments should have a room for administration of radiopharmaceuticals so that the examining rooms are free for imaging. The injection/examination room should be adjacent to the radiopharmacy. This room could be useful for administering sedation, EEG monitoring, and monitoring patients after sedation, before they are discharged. Oxygen, suction, sphygmomanometer, and other safety equipment should be available. In addition, the room should have an emergency call button.

Imaging Rooms

Examining rooms should be designed so that they are attractive and sufficiently spacious to contain the equipment, permit proper examination, allow sufficient privacy, and allow for the presence of the patient's parents in the room. Examining rooms should be flexible in design and adaptable to the changing technology in nuclear medicine. Some useful attributes of a nuclear medicine exam room include:

1. Sufficient general ambient light as well as dimmers in order to be able to provide a soothing effect (some children fall asleep during the examination)
2. Ceiling-mounted spotlight for illuminating the injection or catheterization fields
3. Ceiling-mounted hooks or hangers to hold bottles or containers for intravenous infusion
4. Ceiling-mounted heating lamps
5. Telephone with a cancelable bell; emergency numbers must be posted clearly on the telephone
6. Oxygen and vacuum outlets, preferably wall-mounted and within easy reach from the patient's head on the examination table
7. Facilities for safe disposal of radioactive gases (xenon-133 for ventilation studies)

8. Small television set mounted over the examining table within easy view of the patient; DVD player to play appropriate programming for the patient

9. Sufficient space to house associated electronic equipment, such as electrocardiographs, electroencephalograph (EEG), monitoring anesthesia, and external detectors

10. Doors wide enough to permit safe access to regular and special patient beds

11. Room designed to permit safe maneuvering of the patient's bed in relation to the examining equipment

2
Central Nervous System

Part 1 Brain
S.T. Treves, Harry T. Chugani, and
Blaise F.D. Bourgeois

The brain is a highly complex organ, composed
of billions of neurons, linked into vast networks.
The brain utilizes electrical and neurochemical
signals to process information and control
behavior. Brain function consumes and produces a great deal of metabolic energy, and it is
served by a rich, well-regulated blood supply
system.[1,2]

Although great advances in the fields of
neurosciences, physiology, physiopathology,
neurology, psychiatry, and neuroimaging have
been made, our understanding of the brain is
still in its infancy. Many imaging tools have
been developed to explore the structure and
functions of the brain, including computed
tomography (CT), structural and functional
magnetic resonance imaging (MRI and fMRI),
MR spectroscopy (MRS), diffusion weighted
imaging, perfusion weighted imaging, single
photon emission tomography (SPECT),
positron emission tomography (PET), and
magnetic source localization using magnetoen-
cephalography (MEG).[3] These powerful tools
have opened the door for the development
of new methods for the exploration of the
brain in vivo. Changes in local metabolism
and activity are often inferred from changes
in perfusion. However, although metabolism
and perfusion are usually closely linked, this is
not always the case. Activity detected by receptor ligands may not relate to either perfusion or
metabolism.

Single photon emission computed tomography and positron emission tomography play an
important role in the evaluation of the pediatric
brain. These methods can depict regional
cerebral perfusion and glucose metabolism and
provide maps of the location, quantification,
and biokinetics of specific receptors. In addition, these techniques can detect rapid changes
due to normal brain activity in different functional conditions or those caused by pharmacologic or cognitive stimulation. During the
early 1960s, xenon-133 (^{133}Xe) was used to
measure regional cerebral blood flow (rCBF).[4]
Because of its relative complexity, this method
was limited to a small number of research institutes and therefore did not become widely
used. From the late 1960s to the mid-1970s,
scintigraphy with technetium-99m (^{99m}Tc) as
pertechnetate was extensively used for the
diagnosis of brain tumors, brain abscess and
infections, subdural hematomas, and the assessment of brain death. When CT and MRI
became widely available during the 1970s and
1980s, respectively, the use of radionuclide
techniques for brain imaging declined dramatically. However, during the past decade or so,
SPECT has experienced significant improvements and has naturally found its place in
routine practice. Although PET technology
existed for many years, its use in the past three
decades was largely limited to very few
research centers. Over the past few years,
however, dramatic improvements in radiophar-

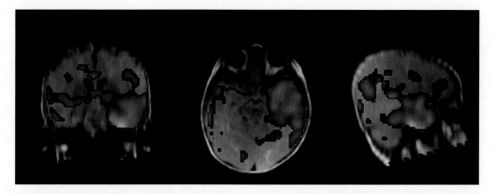

FIGURE 2.1. Single photon emission computed tomography (SPECT) and magnetic resonance imaging (MRI) image fusion in a patient with intractable seizures. Ictal minus interictal perfusion SPECT superposed on a brain MRI. The image reflects ictal increase of cerebral blood flow in the left temporal region.

maceuticals (including distribution), instrumentation, and clinical applications have made PET a practical tool in routine clinical practice. Advances in instrumentation and data processing in SPECT and PET have resulted in systems that are simpler to operate and that can yield three-dimensional (3D) images of high functional and anatomic resolution.

Each imaging technique has its own strengths and limitations, and it is natural that physicians and scientists want to combine them in order to take full advantage of the different and often complementary information they provide. Several methods for image registration and fusion are now available in many commercial systems. These methods enable more detailed assessment of functional and anatomic relationships that assist in the interpretation of the images. Current methods enable registration and fusion of two or more 3D image sets. Although the current proliferation of PET/CT scanners is impressive, CT image registration is not as useful in brain imaging as registration of functional images to MRI and among themselves (SPECT/SPECT, SPECT/MRI, SPECT/PET, PET/MRI, etc.) (Fig. 2.1).[5]

Fused images can be helpful to improve the selection of biopsy sites in order to ensure the highest yield of abnormal tissue to be evaluated. Also, image fusion can assist in guiding surgery and optimizing the targeting of radiotherapy and radiosurgery. Along with improvements in SPECT scanners, the availability of single photon emitting radiopharmaceuticals labeled with ^{99m}Tc, such as those that are trapped intracellularly in proportion to rCBF, are being used extensively. For example, ^{99m}Tc-bicisate and ^{99m}Tc–hexamethylpropyleneamine oxime (HMPAO) are extensively used for brain SPECT in pediatric patients such as those affected with epilepsy, cerebrovascular disorders (e.g., moyamoya, stroke), etc. Technetium-99m hexakis (2-methoxy-isobutylisonitrile) sestamibi (^{99m}Tc-MIBI) and thallium-201 (^{201}Tl)-chloride have been found useful in the assessment of brain tumors following surgery and in radiation therapy to differentiate fibrosis or necrosis from residual tumor or tumor recurrence. The relatively recent approval for the use of ^{18}F-FDG has created renewed interest in PET scanning of the brain in a variety of pediatric disorders such as epilepsy, brain tumors, cerebrovascular disorders, and stroke, to name a few.

The future holds almost infinite potential for the development of radiolabeled molecules of relevance to the study of the brain with SPECT and PET. The potential availability of radiopharmaceuticals that bind to neurotransmitter receptors will open further diagnostic opportunities. An impressive number of radiolabeled ligands have been developed, the number and type of such ligands are quite large, and a detailed discussion of this topic is well beyond the scope of this chapter. It is anticipated that in the near future, neuroreceptor imaging will be used principally in basic research to define patient populations for clinical trials in neurology, and for basic neuropharmacology research. New ligands are being developed all the time, and it is tempting to speculate that in the future, neuroreceptor imaging may find its way to join other neuroimaging modalities.

Ongoing developments in radiopharmaceutical research, imaging methodology, computer science, and clinical research will likely expand the use of nuclear medicine techniques for the investigation of regional brain function in pediatric patients.

Clinical Applications

Clinical applications of brain SPECT and PET in pediatric patients are expected to evolve as new methodology is developed. Table 2.1 lists the indications for radionuclide brain imaging at Children's Hospital Boston during the past 10 years. The most frequent indications included seizure disorders, cerebrovascular diseases, and brain tumors.

Normal Brain Development

When evaluating pediatric perfusion brain with SPECT or FDG-PET, it is important to keep in mind the normal development of the brain in terms of regional perfusion and metabolism. Ethical considerations, however, make study of normal children with SPECT or PET difficult or almost impossible. Therefore, data on the normal distribution of cerebral perfusion and metabolism in children is scarce. The evolution of cerebral glucose utilization in infants during

TABLE 2.1. Indications for radionuclide brain imaging

Epilepsy
Cerebrovascular disease
Infantile spasms
Alternating hemiplegia
Attention deficit/hyperactivity disorder (ADHD)
Complications of extracorporeal membrane oxygenation
Effect of hypothermia and hypoxia
Brain death
Tumors
Rasmussen encephalitis

different stages of development was described by Chugani et al.[6] using PET (Fig. 2.2).

Metabolic activity is initially more intense in the sensorimotor cortex, thalamus, brainstem, and cerebellar vermis; later it involves the parietal, temporal, and occipital cortex, basal ganglia, and cerebellar cortex, and finally the frontal cortex. More recent studies using higher resolution PET scanners have found that a number of limbic structures (i.e., amygdala, hippocampus, cingulated cortex) also show relatively high glucose metabolism in the newborn period.[7] The development of normal brain in children has also been studied with SPECT using iodine-123 iodoamphetamine[8] (IMP) and xenon-133 (^{133}Xe),[9] and in general the studies confirmed the findings of Chugani and colleagues.[6,10–12]

Childhood Epilepsy

Epilepsy in children is treated with considerable success by medical means. A significant number (20% to 30%) of epileptic patients, however, do not respond to drug therapy or remain refractory to this or other medical interventions. Patients with medically refractory partial seizures are referred for surgical resection of epileptogenic tissue. Epilepsy surgery has become a specialized field, and surgical removal or disconnection of a portion of brain believed to contain the epileptogenic focus may control seizures.[13,14] Patients with refractory seizures may be evaluated for epilepsy surgery, including those with seizures secondary to structural lesions of the brain as well as those with nonlesional epilepsy. Seizure types that may be treated by epilepsy surgery are simple partial seizures, complex partial seizures, and some types of generalized seizures. The largest group of surgical candidates comprises patients with complex partial seizures of temporal lobe origin. Preoperative evaluation identifies t hose patients with dysplasias, migrational disorders, tumors, or vascular malformations and can determine whether the epileptic focus is deep (for example, in the amygdala or hippocampus) or superficial (convexity cortex). When a single epileptogenic focus can be identified, its surgical resection is often followed by cessation of seizures or by a

Level   A   B   C   D   E   F   G   H

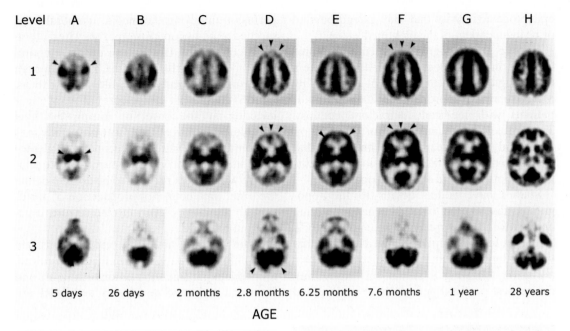

        5 days   26 days   2 months 2.8 months 6.25 months 7.6 months 1 year   28 years

AGE

FIGURE 2.2. Normal brain development. Fluorodeoxyglucose positron emission tomography (FDG-PET) images illustrating developmental changes in local cerebral metabolic rates for glucose (lCMRGlc) in the normal human infant with increasing age compared to that of the adult (image sizes not on the same scale). Gray scale is proportional to lCMRGlc, with black being highest. In each image the anterior brain is at the top and the left brain is at the left. A: At 5 days lCMRGlc is highest in sensorimotor cortex, thalamus, cerebellar vermis (arrowheads), and brainstem (not shown). B–D: lCMRGlc gradually increases in parietal, temporal, and calcarine cortices, basal ganglia, and cerebellar cortex (arrowheads). E: In the frontal cortex lCMRGlc increases first in the lateral prefrontal regions (arrowheads) at around 6 months. F: At around 8 months lCMRGlc increases in the medial aspects of the front cortex (arrowheads) and in the dorsolateral occipital cortex. G: By 1 year the lCMRGlc pattern resembles that of adults (H). (From Chugani et al.,[6] with permission of the *Annals of Neurology*.)

reduction of seizure frequency accompanied by an improvement for the quality of life for many patients.

The postsurgical success is dependent on accurate presurgical localization of epileptogenic foci. It would be catastrophic to operate on the wrong site or to overlook a second active focus. Appropriately directed, surgical resection of epileptogenic tissue has resulted in success rates of 55% to 80% of patients. Success has been defined as no seizures (some auras may be present) for 2 years after surgery, sometimes with some patients still taking anticonvulsant medication. Partial seizures of frontal origin and from other extratemporal sites may also be treated surgically when the clinical manifestations and diagnostic studies indicate an epileptic region in a resectable area.[15]

Imaging in Epilepsy

A battery of tests is employed to verify seizure zone localization. Subdural or depth electroencephalograph (EEG) recordings and intraoperative or chronic subdural EEG, SPECT, and PET are among the diagnostic aids that can be employed to help in this regard. Localization of temporal and extratemporal epileptogenic foci in these patients can be quite challenging. Electroencephalography provides an initial noninvasive approach, but it may not localize the foci and could even be misleading. Brain MRI is the best structural imaging study and can demonstrate mesial temporal sclerosis. However, in some cases MRI may not reveal anatomic lesions. Furthermore, even if an anatomic lesion is detected on MRI, it cannot detect epileptogenic activity that may extend beyond or be independent of the identified lesion.[16]

Despite great progress in structural neuro-imaging, in most specialized epilepsy centers the epileptogenic focus cannot be localized by MRI scanning in approximately 20% to 50% of patients with medically refractory epilepsy. This problem has stimulated efforts to develop functional neuroimaging techniques that can demonstrate transient physiologic disturbances, not just static structural ones.

Studies have added details to the topographic distribution of rCBF changes during and following a seizure. Perfusion brain SPECT studies in temporal epilepsy reveal characteristic time-dependent changes in regional cerebral perfusion following a partial seizure. During the earliest postictal period, there is increased

perfusion involving the medial temporal lobe, succeeded by hypoperfusion of the lateral temporal cortex, and later of the entire temporal lobe.[17,18] Ictal perfusion SPECT provides an opportunity to localize an epileptogenic focus. Ictal SPECT must be performed with tracer injection at the onset or during the ictal episode. Injections of the tracer postictally may demonstrate activation of secondary epileptogenic tissue and may lead to erroneous conclusions.[19] Much work remains to be done to define the exact time course of propagation of perfusion abnormalities following the seizure, especially in children.

Brain SPECT and PET can demonstrate focal changes in patients with medically refractory epilepsy. Image subtraction techniques and fusion of radionuclide studies and MRI are

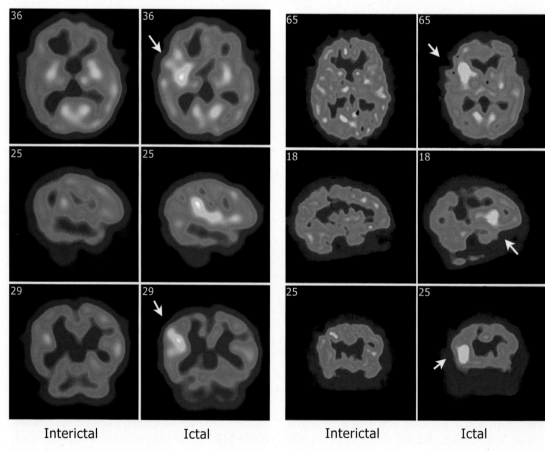

Interictal	Ictal		Interictal	Ictal

FIGURE 2.3. Eight-month-old with intractable seizures. Ictal ^{99m}Tc-ECD SPECT reveals increased brain flow in the epileptogenic zone (arrows).

FIGURE 2.4. Interictal and ictal ^{99m}Tc-ECD SPECT reveals focal ictal hyperperfusion in the right parietal region (arrows).

important to assist in the localization and interpretation of these findings (Figs. 2.3 to 2.10).

These functional abnormalities are frequently accompanied by normal or almost normal CT or MRI scans. In other instances the perfusion abnormalities are seen to extend far beyond the limits of structural lesions. These findings have been demonstrated by several authors using ^{99m}Tc-HMPAO, ^{99m}Tc-ECD, or ^{133}Xe-SPECT.[20–26]

For localization of epileptogenic foci, it is generally agreed that ictal SPECT is better than interictal PET and that interictal PET is better than interictal SPECT. In addition to its widespread availability, ictal perfusion brain SPECT has one unique advantage over all other methods. The ^{99m}Tc brain ligands (^{99m}Tc-ECD and ^{99m}Tc-HMPAO) are extracted and trapped intracellularly following its first pass according to rCBF. The tracer remains fixed in the brain for several hours after intravenous administration, permitting imaging at a convenient time following cerebral stimulation. At the moment of injection, the child need not be near the camera. It is possible to inject the material through an established intravenous line in a comfortable room while the child's behavior, task performance, and EEG are recorded. Changes in rCBF during predictable or unpredictable events, such as seizures, can be captured when the subject is far from the imaging room. Single photon emission computed tomography can be obtained under controlled conditions at 0.5 to 2 or 3 hours following tracer administration. Therefore a "snapshot" of rCBF during specific events can be obtained.

These advantages are of considerable practical value. Unpredictable events cannot be captured by perfusion studies using CT, PET, or MRI unless they occur while the child's head is in the gantry of the machine. This positioning often provokes anxiety, which may itself alter

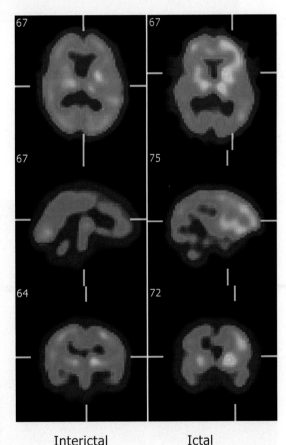

FIGURE 2.5. Interictal and ictal ^{99m}Tc-ECD perfusion brain SPECT. A rather large region of hyperperfusion on the left involves the frontal, parietal, and temporal regions. Increased perfusion is also seen in the central structures in the same side.

Interictal   Ictal

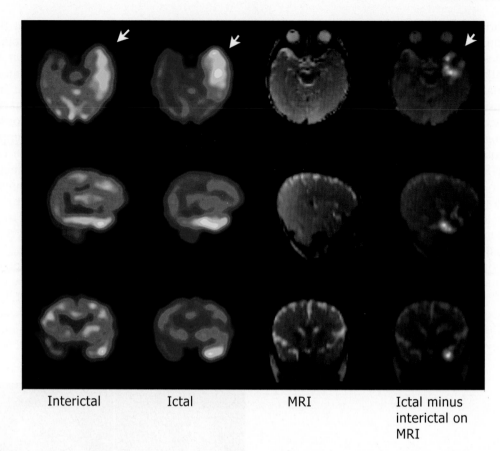

Interictal   Ictal   MRI   Ictal minus
                                                                  interictal on
                                                                  MRI

FIGURE 2.6. Young child with infantile spasms. The interictal ^{99m}Tc-ECD SPECT reveals relatively increased perfusion in the left temporal lobe, probably indicating activity in this region. The ictal SPECT shows a dramatic increase in perfusion to the left temporal lobe. Note the relative lower intensity in the rest of the brain. Ictal SPECT was subtracted from the interictal SPECT, and the resultant image was superposed ("fused") with the MRI.

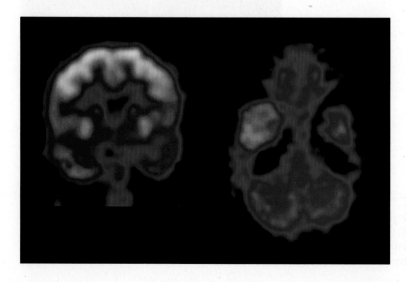

FIGURE 2.7. Interictal ^{18}F-FDG-PET in a patient with intractable seizures. There is less tracer uptake in the left temporal lobe.

FIGURE 2.8. Six-week-old infant with seizures. Patient had recurrent convulsions with the head turning left and stiffening of the right side of the body. A computed tomography (CT) scan at 10 days of age showed evidence of hemorrhage in the left frontal periventricular white matter as well as prominent cortical sulci. Magnetic resonance imaging (MRI) showed subacute hemorrhage in the left caudothalamic groove. An ictal perfusion SPECT reveals high blood flow to almost the entire left hemisphere. An interictal FDG-PET reveals marked decrease of tracer uptake in the same regions.

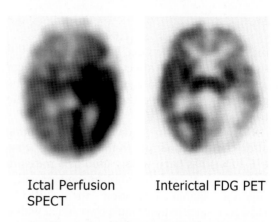

Ictal Perfusion SPECT   Interictal FDG PET

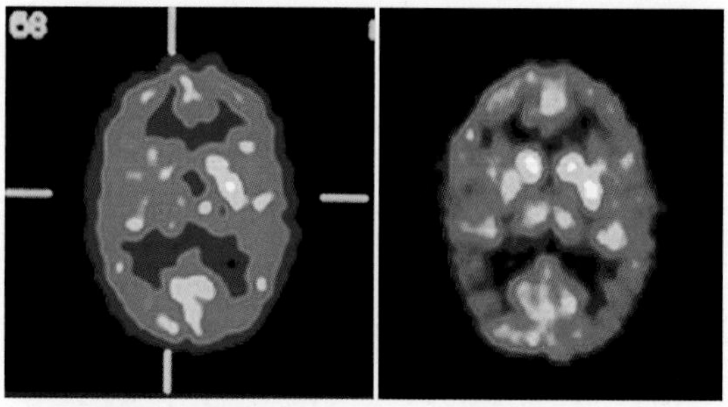

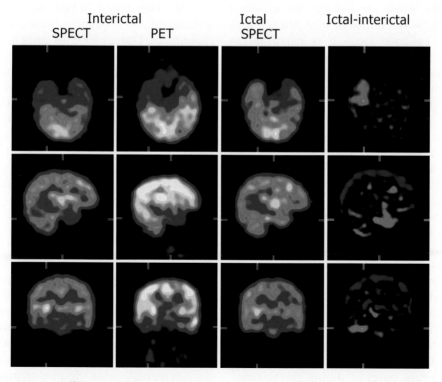

FIGURE 2.9. Interictal ^{99m}Tc-ECD SPECT and ^{18}F-FDG-PET in the same patient. The asymmetry in tracer uptake is more pronounced on the SPECT.

^{99m}Tc-ECD SPECT ^{18}F-FDG PET

Interictal SPECT   PET   Ictal SPECT   Ictal-interictal

FIGURE 2.10. Interictal ^{18}F-FDG-PET reveals significant decrease of tracer in the right temporal lobe. This is not as dramatic as on the interictal SPECT. The ictal SPECT clearly demonstrates high perfusion to the right temporal lobe. On the right panel are the ictal-minus-interictal SPECT subtraction images.

regional brain function. Administration of sedatives also may affect rCBF. After tracer injection of perfusion agents, sedation may be given without altering the distribution of the tracer in the brain.

Positron emission tomography scanning after the injection of 18-fluorodeoxyglucose (^{18}F-FDG) has been widely used as a measure of cerebral glucose metabolism and provides superior spatial resolution than SPECT. However, since patients must be scanned within minutes of ^{18}F-FDG administration (due to the half-life of ^{18}F), this technique is impractical for ictal studies. Comparison of interictal PET to ictal/interictal SPECT indicates that PET has a slightly lower sensitivity (60% versus 87%) in patients with no structural MRI abnormalities.

New computer techniques allow us to define the differences between ictal and interictal perfusion brain SPECT. These can be superimposed onto the patient's MRI to help pinpoint the seizure focus. This technique is most helpful when MRI scans do not show a structural abnormality within or outside the temporal lobe.[27–29] However, although ictal SPECT may show the epileptic focus, it is important to define the "epileptogenic zone" (e.g., an area of microdysgenesis), which is typically larger than the epileptic focus and is better delineated on interictal FDG-PET (Fig. 2.11).

In our institution, patients with intractable seizures are admitted for up to a week into the neurosciences unit and monitored clinically and by video and surface EEG. The yield of true successful ictal SPECT requires the coordination of several groups. In our setting ictal SPECT requires the coordination of nuclear medicine, neuroscience unit, nurses, and radiation safety personnel. During that time, the patient has an ictal and interictal perfusion SPECT, and an interictal PET to assist in the presurgical evaluation. Ictal injections are the most difficult to achieve as they depend ideally on the availability of a qualified health care professional to be at the patient's bedside and be ready to administer the radiotracer at the time of seizure onset or during the seizure.[30] Unfortunately, due to practical considerations, it is not always possible to ensure that a staff

member is available to sit next to the patient awaiting a seizure. Therefore, using a special acoustic signal, specialized nurses are called to the patient's room as soon as a seizure occurs and the tracer is injected as quickly as possible following the onset of the seizure. This limitation makes the yield of true ictal injections lower than it could be. In practice, a number of perfusion brain SPECTs that are obtained do not reflect true ictal distribution but rather immediate postictal distribution of the tracer. When this takes place, it is not uncommon to see secondary hyperperfused regions in the brain that may extend beyond the initial focus or may be remote from the initial ictal focus. Therefore, it would be desirable to free up personnel who could ensure that true ictal injections and therefore true ictal brain SPECTs are possible. An alternative to ensure a higher yield of ictal injections would be to utilize the EEG signal at seizure onset to trigger the automatic injection of the tracer. In this scenario one would utilize a small automatic pump appropriately attached to the patient. This pump would contain a small volume of appropriately time-precalibrated radiotracer. Our division of nuclear medicine in collaboration with the epilepsy department and colleagues at Massachusetts Institute of Technology are looking into the development of patient-specific automatic EEG seizure onset detection and into the possibility that such seizure onset detection could trigger the injection of the radiotracer into the patient via small automatic injector pumps. Initial work reveals that the signal-processing portion of the research shows promise.[31]

Infantile Spasms

Both SPECT and PET have been helpful in the assessment of patients with infantile spasms. Both have shown that in patients with infantile spasms several patterns of focal altered distribution of perfusion and glucose uptake can be found. With this entity a characteristic pattern of seizures is followed frequently by profound developmental delay, despite treatment with anticonvulsants and corticosteroids.[32] Chugani et al.[33,34] have identified a subgroup of children

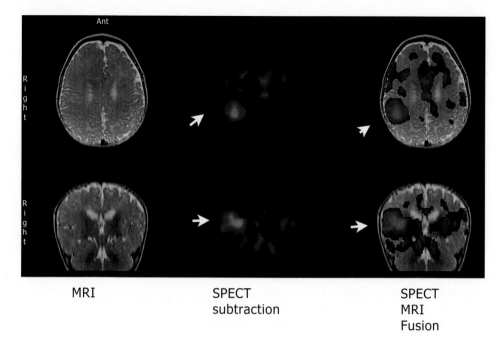

MRI　　　　　　SPECT　　　　　　SPECT
　　　　　　　subtraction　　　　　MRI
　　　　　　　　　　　　　　　　　Fusion

FIGURE 2.11. Six-month-old boy with one to two spells/day since birth. More recently he developed five to six seizures in a row over a 2- to 5-minute period, up to five to seven times per day. The electroencephalograph (EEG) was quite active during sleep. The MRI revealed an abnormal gyral pattern in the right frontal and parasylvian regions suggestive of "neuronal migration disorder." An interictal ^{18}F-FDG-PET revealed generally decreased tracer uptake in the entire right hemisphere. An interictal ^{99m}Tc-ECD SPECT also revealed generalized decreased perfusion in the entire right hemisphere. An ictal perfusion SPECT showed focal increased perfusion in the right temporoparietal region. Subtraction of ictal and interictal SPECT reveals the regional changes in cerebral perfusion in the right parietal region that are fused with the MRI.

with infantile spasms who harbor focal cortical malformative or dysplastic lesions. Positron emission tomography in these patients reveals marked, focal areas of cortical hypometabolism. These areas of functional abnormality, not seen on structural imaging, concur with electrographic abnormalities and can be treated by focal cortical resection.

Perfusion brain SPECT also show striking focal cerebral perfusion abnormalities in infantile spasms. Abnormalities involve the temporal or parietal lobe but can involve the entire supratentorial cortex. These changes can be single or multiple, and unilateral or bilateral. The extent and intensity of these abnormalities appear greater than is noted in most patients with other forms of partial epilepsy. In infantile spasms the SPECT findings, when taken in conjunction with clinical and electrographic data, are suggestive of but not specific for the diagnosis.[35] Patients can reveal definite focal cortical ictal hyperperfusion. Activation of subcortical structures can be found in some cases. A diffuse pattern can be present on ictal SPECT. In several such patients, surgical resection is followed by marked improvement in seizure frequency and in some a normal developmental course. Thus functional imaging has revealed a previously unsuspected abnormality in these children and has influenced the development of a therapy with the possibility of alleviating the otherwise dismal developmental outcome (Fig. 2.6).[34,36–39]

Tuberous Sclerosis

Multiple cortical tubers are characteristic of tuberous sclerosis complex. Seizures often originate from a single tuber, making excisional surgery a therapeutic option for intractable patients. In certain cases these regions can be removed surgically in the hope of providing better seizure control and improving developmental outcome. Ictal and interictal perfusion SPECT can help to identify an area of the brain from which seizures are originating. A SPECT may reveal regions consisting of comma-shaped areas surrounding hypoperfused areas in the candidate tuber. A PET or SPECT can be superimposed over corresponding MRI of the brain. In this way the brain's structure or specific tubers can be identified in terms of metabolic activity. This aids the neurologist and surgeon in determining who might benefit from seizure surgery.[40] Studies using the PET tracer α-[^{11}C]methyl-L-tryptophan have found that epileptogenic tubers show increased uptake while nonepileptogenic tubers show decreased uptake (Fig. 2.12). These PET scans are per-

formed in the interictal state and are very helpful to the epilepsy surgery team in selecting suitable candidates for surgery.[41,42]

Cerebrovascular Disease of Childhood

Although more common than previously realized, cerebrovascular disease in children is relatively much rarer than in adults and tends to occur in the context of an underlying anatomic abnormality (e.g., congenital heart disease) or systemic disease (e.g., sickle cell hemoglobinopathy).[43] Perfusion brain SPECT is making contributions to our understanding of pathogenic mechanisms in a variety of the childhood cerebrovascular disorders.

Moyamoya Disease

Moyamoya is a rare disorder of uncertain etiology that leads to irreversible blockage of the

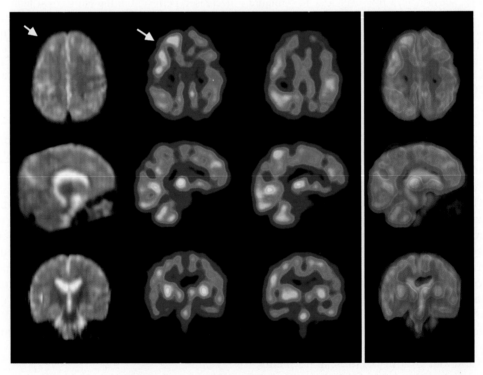

FIGURE 2.12. Three-year-old boy with tuberous sclerosis and intractable seizure disorder. The MRI shows multiple tubers. The interictal ^{99m}Tc-ECD perfusion SPECT reveals grossly irregular tracer distribution with apparent reduction within the tubers. The ictal SPECT reveals increased perfusion surrounding the tubers (arrow).

main blood vessels to the brain as they enter into the skull. This disorder occurs predominantly in children and in adults during the third to fourth decades of life. Moyamoya is characterized by an angiographic pattern of supraclinoid internal carotid artery stenosis, followed ultimately by a luxuriant pattern of collateral vascularization. This angiographic appearance has been likened to a puff of cigarette smoke (from the Japanese translation).[44] Moyamoya tends to cause strokes or seizures. Once the process of vascular occlusion begins, it tends to continue despite medical management. Repeated strokes can lead to severe functional impairment or even death. Surgery can produce good results. Therefore, it is important to recognize these lesions and treat them early. Serial cerebral perfusion studies using iodine-123-iodoamphetamine (^{123}I-IMP) were found to document accurately the changes in cerebral blood flow that occur during the course of the disorder.[45] The SPECT abnormalities were partly congruent with MRI and CT findings but showed larger perfusion defects than those revealed by the other modalities. Hence brain SPECT offers an effective way of following the natural history of moyamoya disease, and its noninvasive nature may offer an attractive alternative to serial arteriography. Single photon emission computed tomography may play an important role in evaluating the success of proposed treatments for the disorder, such as superficial temporal artery–middle cerebral artery bypass.[46]

Once a diagnosis is suspected by CT or MRI, the next step is usually an angiogram to confirm the diagnosis and to see the anatomy of the vessels involved. Often nuclear medicine studies such as SPECT are used to demonstrate the decreased blood and oxygen supply to areas of the brain involved with moyamoya disease. The neurosurgeon would decide what type of operation is best suited for the patient. Several operations have been developed to treat moyamoya. They have in common the objective of bringing blood to the brain by bypassing the areas of vascular obstruction. The moyamoya vessels and the involved brain are very sensitive to changes in blood pressure, blood volume, and the relative amount of carbon dioxide in the

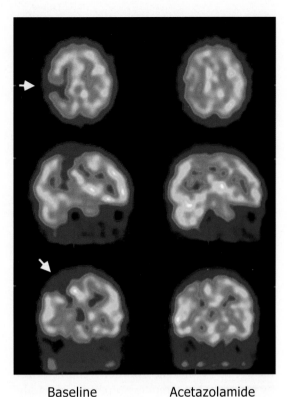

Baseline   Acetazolamide

FIGURE 2.13. Patient with moyamoya. The baseline ^{99m}Tc-ECD SPECT reveals markedly focal decreased perfusion (arrows). A repeat SPECT following the administration of acetazolamide reveals improved perfusion in the affected regions. This patient was considered a good candidate for revascularization.

blood. Studies using acetazolamide (Diamox) a vasodilator that increases cerebral blood flow (by 50% to 100% within 20 to 30 minutes) are helpful in identifying the vascular reserve of involved territories before surgery. The lack of flow augmentation indicates a loss of autoregulation and inadequate vascular reserves (Fig. 2.13).

Other Forms of Childhood Cerebrovascular Disease

Using ^{99m}Tc-HMPAO SPECT, Shahar et al.[47] described the scintigraphic findings in 15 infants and children presenting with a variety of cerebrovascular disorders. They correlated these findings with clinical, EEG, and radiologic abnormalities. Focal rCBF changes were found

FIGURE 2.14. ⁹⁹ᵐTc-ECD SPECT in a child following a stroke.

in all patients. In some patients, SPECT abnormalities occurred in the absence, or before the detection, of radiologic changes. This experience is an example of the importance of SPECT as a sensitive, early detector of functional brain abnormality in pediatric cerebrovascular disease (Figs. 2.14 and 2.15).

Alternating Hemiplegia

Alternating hemiplegia is a rare neurologic disorder that develops in childhood, usually before the age of 4 years. The disorder is characterized by recurrent but temporary episodes of paralysis on one side of the body as well as other transient neurologic symptoms affecting eye movements, limbs, or facial muscles. One form of the disorder, identified very recently, has a favorable outlook. It occurs primarily at night, when a child awakens, and is apparently related to migraine. These children have no other mental or neurologic impairments. In more serious cases symptoms may include mental impairment, balance and gait difficulties, excessive sweating, and changes in body temperature. Seizures can occur. Sleep helps in the recovery from the periods of paralysis, but the paralysis can recur upon waking. The cause of the disorder is unknown but is suspected to be channelopathy. There is frequently relief

in response to the calcium-entry blocker flunarizine.[48]

Perhaps reflecting the temporally fluctuating quality of the symptoms, brain SPECT findings by different groups of investigators in this entity have been variable and at times contradictory. Perfusion brain SPECT[49] showed ictal hypoperfusion of the relevant hemisphere with interictal normalization. Mikati et al.[50] defined the familial occurrence and apparent autosomal dominant inheritance of this entity. In this initial paper by Mikati et al., SPECT and EEG failed to show abnormalities of cortical perfusion during hemiplegia compared to non-hemiplegic periods. More recently, however, several patients with alternating hemiplegia have shown striking abnormalities in regional cerebral perfusion at both the cortical and subcortical levels.

No characteristic distribution in the perfusion abnormality is evident so far in these patients, however.

Attention Deficit Hyperactivity Disorder

Attention deficit/hyperactivity disorder (ADHD) is the most common neurobehavioral disorder in children, estimated to affect between 4% and 12% of all school-aged children. The chief features of ADHD are inattention, hyperactivity, and impulsiveness, and this disorder is often associated with substantial impairments, including low self-esteem, poor family and peer relationships, school difficulties, and academic underachievement.[51]

A series of studies by Lou et al.[52,53] using ^{133}Xe suggested a pattern of hypoperfusion of striate and periventricular structures, with sensorimotor cortical hyperperfusion. This pattern tended to reverse after administration of methylphenidate, a commonly prescribed medication that improves attention and academic performance in some ADHD youngsters. This pattern is consistent with some neurophysiologic models of the disorder and with ^{18}F-FDG-PET studies in adult ADHD.[54] This study noted that four regions, primarily in the premotor and sensorimotor cortex, showed a significant decrease in local cerebral metabolic

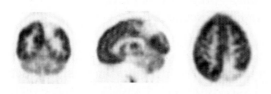

FIGURE 2.15. ¹⁸F-FDG-PET appearance in a patient with a rupture of an arteriovenous malformation.

utilization of glucose, suggesting a corresponding regional dysfunction. In a later study in ADHD adolescents, glucose metabolism was significantly reduced in six brain regions, including the left anterior frontal lobe.[54,55]

Single photon emission computed tomography in children and adolescents with ADHD have shown regions of hypoperfusion in the temporal lobes, frontal lobes, and basal ganglia. These findings can be bilateral.[56]

There are problems inherent in obtaining consistent imaging results in patients during rest, which may range from extreme stress in a hyperactive child to another in somnolence. Effective treatment of ADHD may be associated with increases in perfusion in the prefrontal cortex and caudate nucleus. In addition, it is difficult to obtain optimal controls,[57] or the experimental groups are too small to yield statistically valid results.[58-60] A lot of work remains to be done in the investigation of changes in the brain with ADHD. The lack of a sufficient number of observations, and studies with inadequate controls can yield contradicting or confusing results.[59,61,62]

Functional MRI holds promise for future study of rCBF.[58] Infrared spectroscopy may be useful alternatives in some investigations.[63,64] Both PET and SPECT will remain important primary means of evaluating the neuropharmacology of the brain.[65,66] The focus of these techniques may be in the study and exploration of central catecholamines and dopamine receptors and dopamine release.[65,67-74]

Other conditions that have been studied with SPECT and PET include childhood dysphasias,[35,75] cerebral palsy,[76] autism,[77-84] schizophrenia,[85-88] and depression.[89,90]

Complications of Extracorporeal Membrane Oxygenation

In newborns undergoing extracorporeal membrane oxygenation (ECMO) for refractory respiratory failure, perfusion brain SPECT has been used to investigate the status of cerebral perfusion following the surgical interventions associated with ECMO, involving permanent or temporary occlusion of the right common carotid artery or the major cervical veins. In seven of 13 children, significant perfusion defects in either the ipsilateral or contralateral hemisphere were documented, whereas only two patients showed abnormalities on ultrasonography, CT, or MRI. Single photon emission computed tomography can demonstrate rCBF deficits not detectable by structural imaging modalities that may be of major importance to the neurodevelopmental outcome of such infants.[91] However, although a normal SPECT scan is more likely to predict a normal neurodevelopmental outcome, an abnormal SPECT scan does not predict an abnormal outcome in these infants.[92]

Effect of Hypothermia and Hypoxia

Surgical repair of complex congenital heart disease in very small children is possible today because of advances in anesthesia and techniques of hypothermia with hypoxia. This method, however, carries a risk of brain damage. A known complication of hypothermia with hypoxia is the choreoathetosis syndrome (CAS).[93] We studied eight patients suffering from CAS following deep (<20°C) hypothermic circulatory arrest or low-flow bypass during cardiac surgery during the neonatal period. Single photon emission computed tomography showed striking focal rCBF abnormalities at both the cortical (frontal, parietal, and temporal cortex) and subcortical (anterior basal ganglia) levels, in seven of these eight patients. The distribution of the perfusion abnormalities was not predictable from clinical examination. In these patients, CT and MRI were normal or showed only generalized nonspecific abnormalities. These cerebral perfusion abnormalities may have important implications for developmental outcome in these children (Fig. 2.16).[94]

Developmental and Neuropsychiatric Disorders

Behavioral function studies with SPECT have been done predominantly using perfusion radiopharmaceuticals such as ^{133}Xe[52,53,57] and ^{99m}Tc-HMPAO. Oxygen-15 PET and ^{133}Xe SPECT can both allow multiple measurements

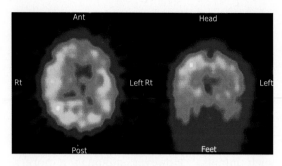

FIGURE 2.16. Effect of hypothermia on regional cerebral blood flow. The ^{99m}Tc-HMPAO SPECT reveals marked hypoperfusion of the left frontal, temporal, and parietal regions.

in the same patient. A serious drawback of these methods, however, is that the patient must be in the field of view of the detectors while the tracer is administered. In this circumstance, multiple affective states, such as anxiety and anger, may exist at the moment of radiopharmaceutical injection, so "baseline" behavioral states cannot be achieved. As mentioned above, the unique advantage of ^{99m}Tc-ECD and ^{99m}Tc-HMPAO is that once they are taken up there is lack of significant redistribution within the brain.

Brain Tumors

In the United States, approximately 2000 brain tumors are diagnosed every year in patients under the age of 20 years. Malignant brain tumors are the leading cause of cancer death in children. Brain tumors are the second most common type of pediatric cancers after leukemia. The distribution of childhood brain tumors (CBTs) is as follows: astrocytomas, 52%; primitive neuroectodermal tumors (PNETs) or medulloblastoma/embryonal tumors, 21%; ependymomas, 9%; and other gliomas, 15%. The number of central nervous system (CNS) tumors during childhood and adolescence has been steadily increasing. The proportion of cancer deaths due to CNS tumors has nearly doubled during the past 25 years.[95–97] Worldwide, approximately 30,000 to 40,000 children develop CNS tumors each year, and

the majority do not survive. In many countries, CNS tumors are the greatest challenge in pediatric oncology.[98] The promise of new approaches to treatment of childhood brain tumor increases the importance of developing accurate methods for the accurate assessment of the viability and extent of the tumors and for the assessment of residual disease after therapy.

Both MRI and CT have high sensitivity and specificity in the diagnosis of brain tumors in children. These techniques frequently cannot differentiate radiation effect from residual or recurrent brain tumor.[99,100] Functional imaging (SPECT or PET), on the other hand, can detect the presence of active tumor. In combination with MRI, this ability is useful for diagnosing residual brain tumor following therapy and differentiating between recurrent tumor and radiation necrosis.

The roles of nuclear medicine in the evaluation of brain tumors include diagnosis, localization, detection of local extent and metastatic disease, assistance with therapy planning, and follow-up and assessment of the effect(s) of therapy. The techniques available include SPECT, and PET. Three-dimensional multimodality image co-registration and fusion are important complements to these techniques.

Image fusion of CT, MRI, PET, and SPECT images provides more accurate and precise target volume, more exact localization of catheters and isotope seeds (verification fusion), and differentiation between the localization and amount of the necrotic and proliferating parts of the tumors and shows the volume changes relating to interstitial irradiation. Image fusion should help to improve the accuracy and minimize the perifocal morbidity of interstitial irradiation.[101]

Several routinely available radiopharmaceuticals have been used in the assessment of brain tumors. Of these commonly available radiopharmaceuticals, some agents actually concentrate in brain tumors and are excluded from the brain tissue, including ^{201}Tl, ^{99m}Tc-MIBI, and carbon-11 (^{11}C)-methionine (proximity to a cyclotron is needed for ^{11}C). Other agents such as ^{99m}Tc–ECD and ^{99m}Tc-HMPAO localize in brain tumors as well as in normal brain tissue. Fluorine-18-FDG localizes in normal brain tissue and in some tumors.

Work by Kaplan and his colleagues in 1987 using ^{201}Tl planar scintigraphy demonstrated that uptake of this tracer in brain tumors correlated closely with biologic extent.[102]

Technetium-99m-MIBI SPECT has been used to assess the viability of brain tumors in children.[103,104] Early experience with ^{99m}Tc-MIBI SPECT for the assessment of brain tumor viability showed consistent uptake of this agent in brain tumors.[104] The tumor-to–normal brain ratio for tracer uptake of ^{201}Tl and ^{99m}Tc-MIBI exceed those reported for the most tumor-avid PET agent, ^{11}C-L-methionine, or for the SPECT amino acid analogue ^{123}I-α-methyl-paratyrosine.[105] ^{99m}Tc-MIBI also localizes in the normal choroid plexus. This characteristic may prevent diagnosis of adjacent tumor activity. Choroidal plexus uptake of ^{99m}Tc-MIBI cannot be blocked by perchlorate (Figs. 2.17 to 2.22).[106–109]

Brain Death

Cerebral radionuclide angiography followed by planar scintigraphy with ^{99m}Tc-pertechnetate is frequently used in patients with an equivocal clinical diagnosis of brain death. Experienced observers can make a satisfactory determination as to the presence or absence of cerebral perfusion (Figs. 2.23 to 2.25).

Single photon emission computed tomography using ^{99m}Tc-ECD or ^{99m}Tc-HMPAO or radioiodinated amphetamine has been used as an adjunct in the assessment of brain death.[110] It is probable that these radiopharmaceuticals allow superior definition of posterior fossa or subtler supratentorial perfusion abnormalities.

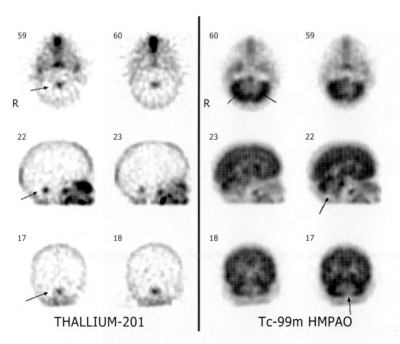

THALLIUM-201   Tc-99m HMPAO

FIGURE 2.17. Ependymoma in the posterior fossa in a 4-year-old boy. He was evaluated for the possibility of residual or recurrent tumor following a course of radiation therapy. Thallium-201 SPECT shows intense uptake of tracer in the tumor (arrows) (left). ^{99m}Tc-HMPAO SPECT reveals a well-defined region of decreased perfusion corresponding to the field of radiation therapy (right).

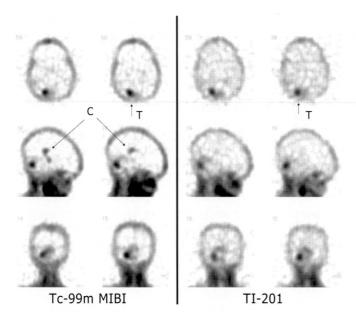

C   ↑T   ↑T

Tc-99m MIBI   TI-201

FIGURE 2.18. Posterior fossa tumor. This 4-year-old girl had a partially resected cerebellar astrocytoma. Left: ^{99m}Tc-MIBI brain SPECT reveals an intense focus of increased tracer uptake in the posterior fossa corresponding to active tumor. In addition, there is normal ^{99m}Tc-MIBI uptake in the choroid plexus (C). Right: ^{201}Tl SPECT defines the region of active tumor. Unlike ^{99m}Tc-MIBI, however, ^{201}Tl does not concentrate in the choroid plexus.

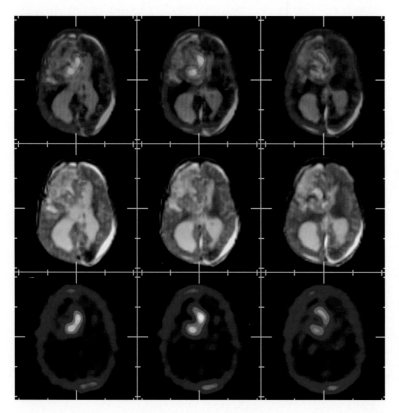

FIGURE 2.19. Metastatic neuroblastoma in the brain. Top row: MRI/^{201}Tl fusion showing anatomic-functional relations. Middle row: Selected MRI slices depicting extensive abnormality in the right frontoparietal region. Bottom row: Selected ^{201}Tl brain SPECT revealing tracer uptake in the tumor. (Images obtained with the assistance of I. Haboush and K. Mitchell.)

FIGURE 2.20. Large
brain tumor well seen
on the MRI. Within
the large tumor, there
are two distinct foci
of ^{18}F-FDG uptake
that may indicate
active residual tumor.

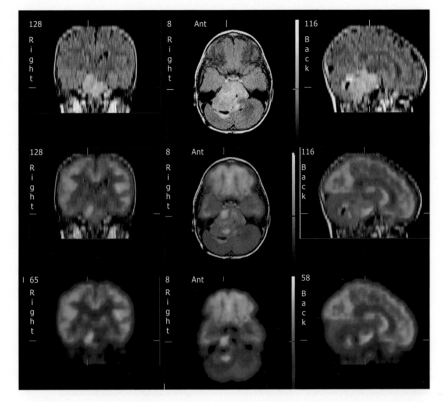

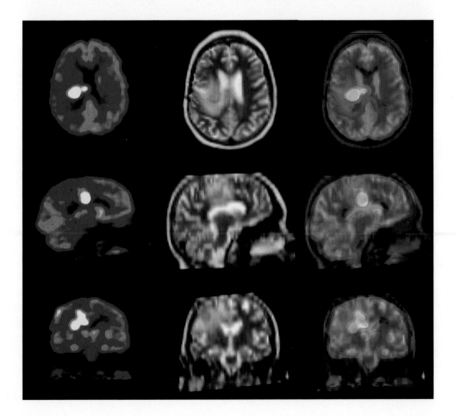

FIGURE 2.21. Brain
tumor showing
intense uptake of
^{18}F-FDG. The tumor
uptake is more
intense than normal
gray matter.

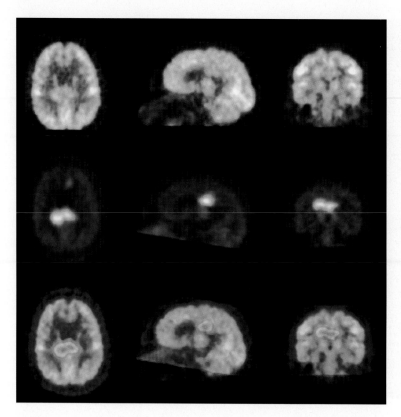

FIGURE 2.22. Brain tumor: carbon-11 (^{11}C) methionine versus ^{18}F-FDG. Top: ^{18}F-FDG brain PET that faintly outlines tumor uptake. Tracer within the normal brain matter tends to make diagnosis of active tumor difficult. Center: ^{11}C-methionine brain PET shows the region of tumor activity quite clearly. Bottom: Fused ^{18}F-FDG and ^{11}C-methionine PET. (*Source:* Courtesy of Dr. Alan Fischman, M.D., Ph.D., Massachusetts General Hospital, Boston.).

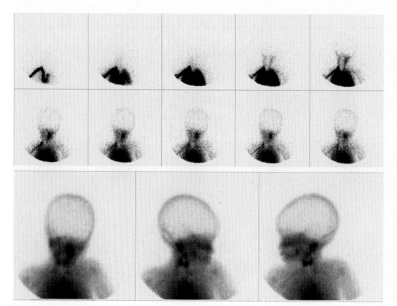

FIGURE 2.23. Top: A ^{99m}Tc-pertechnetate cerebral radionuclide angiogram reveals no evidence of intracranial blood flow. Bottom: Anterior and lateral images of the head confirm the absence of intracranial blood flow.

Brain perfusion agents can be used for cerebral radionuclide angiography followed by planar scintigraphy or brain SPECT. In addition to the characteristic of perfusion agents for the assessment of the brain and the cerebellum, with them one may obviate the need to repeat a study should there be equipment or other technical failure. It remains to be shown, however, whether this additional information can provide assistance to the clinician faced with the need to reach decisions about life support, in contrast to what can be gleaned from conventional planar scintigraphy.[111–113]

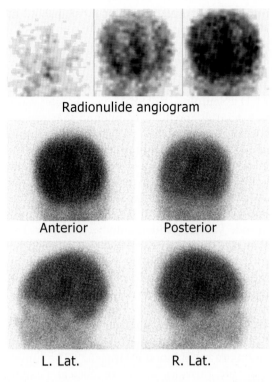

Radionulide angiogram

Anterior   Posterior

L. Lat.   R. Lat.

FIGURE 2.25. This patient was being evaluated for the possibility of brain death. A ⁹⁹ᵐTc-ECD study reveals evidence of intracranial flow in the regions of the anterior and middle cerebral artery territories (angiogram, top). Four static images obtained soon after tracer injection reveal evidence of intracranial blood flow (bottom).

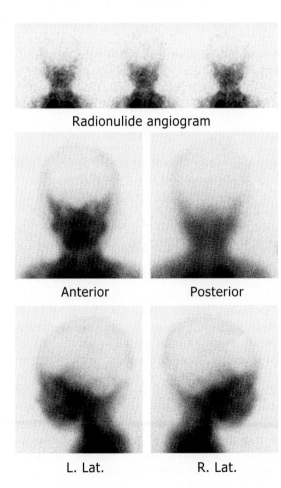

Radionulide angiogram

Anterior   Posterior

L. Lat.   R. Lat.

FIGURE 2.24. Selected images from a ⁹⁹ᵐTc-ECD cerebral radionuclide angiogram (top) reveal no evidence of intracranial flow. Static images obtained following administration of the tracer reveal no evidence of tracer uptake in the brain substance. A SPECT confirmed this finding. The patient was considered brain dead.

Radiopharmaceuticals

The development of SPECT and PET radiopharmaceuticals for imaging different aspects of brain function has been and continues to be the focus of considerable effort. But despite this effort, very few compounds have been approved for human use at this time.[3,114–116]

Perfusion Radiopharmaceuticals

Two ⁹⁹ᵐTc radiopharmaceuticals are used for the assessment of regional cerebral perfusion. The distribution of both of these compounds within the brain reflects rCBF. Tracer distribution is essentially fixed after uptake, and there is very little redistribution or efflux over a period of several hours. This combination of properties is important because it allows the tracers to be used to obtain a "snapshot" of rCBF at the time of injection.

Technetium-99m ECD

Technetium-99m-bicisate, also known as ^{99m}Tc-ECD (Neurolite, Bristol-Meyers-Squibb Co.), is a neutral, lipophilic, compound that rapidly concentrates in the brain following intravenous injection, with a total brain uptake of approximately 6% of the administered dose. The activity washes out of the brain quite slowly over time, which allows static imaging. The major organs of retention other than the brain include the gallbladder, kidneys, and liver. The primary route of excretion is the urinary tract, and approximately 50% is cleared by the kidneys within the first 2 hours after administration. Approximately 11% of the tracer is eliminated via the gastrointestinal tract over 48 hours. This agent has two advantages over ^{99m}Tc-HMPAO: a longer (6-hour) shelf life and more rapid blood clearance.[117] The longer shelf life provides for more clinical flexibility because the dose can be prepared ahead of time without concern about decomposition. For example, ^{99m}Tc-ECD can be used to obtain ictal images of regional cerebral perfusion.[25,118,119] Other paroxysmal disorders in which this technique might also be used include migraine or transient cerebral ischemic episodes.

Technetium-99m-HMPAO

Technetium-99m-exametazine, also known as ^{99m}Tc-HMPAO (Ceretec, Amersham Co., Arlington Heights, IL), is also a neutral lipophilic compound that is rapidly cleared from the blood after intravenous injection.[120] Brain uptake is 3.5% to 7.0% of the injected dose within 1 minute after administration. Approximately 15% of the initial cerebral uptake is cleared within 2 minutes, and the rest is retained for 24 hours. The remainder of the dose is distributed throughout the body, particularly in the muscles and soft tissues. Approximately 30% of the administered tracer activity is found in the gastrointestinal tract a few minutes after injection, and approximately 50% is eliminated by this route in 24 hours. Approxi-

mately 40% of the tracer activity is eliminated in the urine within 48 hours. The original formulation of ^{99m}Tc-HMPAO was subject to radiolytic decomposition,[121] which limited its shelf life to 30 minutes, but the current, stabilized, version has a longer shelf life.[122]

Iodine-123-Iodoamphetamine

In the past, the radiolabeled amine N-isopropyl-p-^{123}I-iodoamphetamine (^{123}I-IMP, Spectamine) was used to evaluate cerebral perfusion during pediatric onset seizures. In contrast to ^{99m}Tc-HMPAO and ^{99m}Tc-ECD, ^{123}I-IMP undergoes substantial redistribution within brain tissue over time, which makes it less useful than the [99m]Tc rCBF agents for localizing seizure foci.[123] This radiopharmaceutical is currently not commercially available in the United States.

Xenon-133

Xenon-133 has been used for the characterization of rCBF, but it has fallen into disuse since the introduction of the ^{99m}Tc agents.[124–126]

Tumor-Avid Radiopharmaceuticals

Fluoro-2-Deoxyglucose

The use of ^{18}F-labeled 2-deoxyglucose (^{18}F-FDG) has greatly expanded in recent years with the development of a nationwide distribution network that provides this agent to sites that do not have access to on-site cyclotrons. Fluorine-18 FDG accumulates in the brain (and elsewhere) as a function of glucose metabolism, which is typically increased in malignant tissues. It is, however, less than optimal for imaging brain tumors because its high uptake in the normal brain complicates the differentiation of tumor from normal brain.[114] It also accumulates in inflammatory lesions, which may complicate interpretation of posttherapy image.[127]

Usual administered dose: 150 µCi/kg (5.5 MBq/kg) with a minimum dose of 1 mCi (37 MBq) and a maximum dose of 10 mCi (370 MBq).

Thallium-201

Thallium-201 (^{201}Tl), although primarily used as a myocardial perfusion agent (see Chapter 6), has also been used for imaging tumors, including those in the brain, where its low uptake in normal brain provides high contrast between the lesion and the normal brain.[102,128] The tracer accumulates in active tumor tissue within a few minutes after intravenous injection and remains within the tumor for some time, allowing static imaging.

Thallium-201 accumulates in gliomas, medulloblastomas, and oligodendrogliomas, and may be useful in evaluating the histologic grade of astrocytomas.[129] An important caveat to the use of ^{201}Tl for tumor imaging is that uptake may also occur in nonneoplastic lesions within the brain.[130]

Usual administered dose: 0.03 to 0.05 mCi (1.11–1.85 MBq)/kg body weight; minimum dose 0.5 mCi (18.5 MBq), maximum dose 2.0 mCi (74 MBq).

Technetium-99m-MIBI and 99mTc-Tetrofosmin

Technetium-99m-MIBI (Sestamibi, Cardiolite, Bristol-Myers Squibb, N. Billerica, MA) and ^{99m}Tc-tetrofosmin (Myoview, GE Healthcare, Boston, MA) are lipophilic, cationic, ^{99m}Tc complexes that were developed as myocardial perfusion agents (see Chapter 6). As is the case the myocardial perfusion agent ^{201}Tl, ^{99m}Tc-MIBI was found to accumulate in brain tumors,[131] and similar behavior has been observed for ^{99m}Tc-tetrofosmin.[132,133] The ^{99m}Tc agents typically provide higher tumor-to–normal brain ratios and better definition of tumor margins than ^{201}Tl. Both tracers accumulate in the (normal) choroid plexus, which may complicate interpretation of paraventricular lesions.[104,133] This uptake is not seen with ^{201}Tl.

Usual administered dose: 0.3 mCi (11.1 MBq)/kg body weight; minimum dose 1 mCi (37 MBq), maximum dose 20 mCi (740 MBq).

Carbon-11-Labeled Methionine

A promising radiopharmaceutical for imaging neurologic tumors is ^{11}C-labeled L-methionine (^{11}C-MET).[116,129] Its use, however, is limited to sites with on-site cyclotrons because of the short half-life of ^{11}C (20 minutes). Radiation absorbed doses for these radiopharmaceuticals are given in Chapter 20.

Receptor-Specific Radiopharmaceuticals

The evaluation of receptor distribution within the brain is proving to be a valuable research tool, with a large number of studies targeting a variety of receptors and their functional response to various disease states. Virtually all of these are a PET studies carried out in the research setting, primarily with ^{11}C-labeled analogues of known receptor agonists and antagonists. The success of the ^{18}F-FDG distribution network has prompted efforts to develop ^{18}F-labeled versions of several of these tracers, but none of these are commercially available at this time.

Iodinated agents (^{123}I) have been developed that target several different neuroreceptors including γ-aminobutyric acid (GABA) and dopamine.[134] At the present time, however, none of these compounds is commercially available in the United States.

Developing ^{99m}Tc receptor-specific radiopharmaceuticals is even more challenging because of the need to incorporate a chelating agent into the molecule without disrupting receptor binding. A ^{99m}Tc-labeled dopamine transporter (DAT) agent has been developed,[135,136] but it is not commercially available at this point.

Radiopharmaceuticals Normally Excluded from the Brain

^{99m}Tc-pertechnetate, ^{99m}Tc–diethylenetriamine pentaacetic acid (DTPA), and ^{99m}Tc-glucoheptonate were used extensively in the past for cerebral radionuclide angiography (CRA) and planar brain imaging. However, these agents are seldom used now for this purpose.

Usual administered doses: 0.2 mCi/kg (7.4 MBq/kg); minimum dose 10 mCi (370 MBq), maximum dose 20 mCi (740 MBq).

Imaging Methods

Perfusion Single Photon Emission Computed Tomography

Image quality is dependent on meticulous attention to detail. It is especially important to ensure that the detectors are positioned as close to the head as possible and that patient movement is minimized. Care is taken to reduce patient anxiety about the intravenous injection of the tracer. Injection of perfusion tracers should be done in a quiet environment to minimize anxiety and distractions. A butterfly-type needle should be inserted intravenously and secured with tape. The intravenous line is kept open with normal saline. After a few minutes, when the patient is more relaxed, intravenous injection of the tracer should proceed. A few minutes after intravenous injection of the tracer, the patient is positioned supine on the imaging table. The patient's head should be positioned and firmly secured. Imaging preference is for a multi-detector gamma camera system or a dedicated system, and it should be equipped with ultrahigh-resolution collimators. An example of SPECT recording is as follows: Using a multi-detector system, each detector rotates 360 degrees around the patient's head. Each detector acquires 128 × 128 images. Total imaging time is approximately 20 minutes.

Very young children and children who are unable or unwilling to cooperate may require sedation. Sedation may affect brain activity and is usually given after injection of the tracer.

Methods

There are four methods for perfusion brain SPECT: (1) a single controlled baseline study, (2) an ictal study, (3) an activation study, and (4) a split-dose study.

1. *Single controlled baseline study.* To facilitate interpretation of results, it is highly desirable to attempt uniformity of conditions at the time of tracer injection. Care is taken to reduce to a practical minimum patient anxiety, sensory stimulation, and motor activity, as these factors alter the rCBF and therefore the perfusion patterns on brain SPECT. Thus it is essential to ensure that the procedure is explained and the intravenous access established in advance. From a few minutes before until at least 5 minutes after tracer injection, the patient should be encouraged to engage in a simple task, such as staring at a spot on the wall of a quiet, dimly lit room. Image recording may proceed thereafter.

2. *Ictal study.* This study is best performed in collaboration with a specialized epilepsy unit offering EEG videotelemetry. Intravenous access is established. As soon as possible after the onset of seizure activity, an appropriate dose of tracer is given. Preferably, the tracer is administered during the actual ictal event. SPECT may begin a few minutes later, or it may be delayed until seizures are under control. The availability of stable radiopharmaceuticals (^{99m}Tc-ECD) enhances the yield of ictal examinations.

3. *Activation study.* This type of study is conducted in the same way as the controlled baseline study, except that the patient is instructed to perform a specific task from a few minutes before until approximately 5 minutes after tracer injection. The task may involve repetitive visual, auditory, or somatosensory stimulation, a repetitive motor task, or a psychological test depending on the issue of interest. Such a study is exemplified by the work of Woods et al.,[137] and a useful general review has been provided by George et al.[83]

4. *Split-dose study.* It is possible to perform two perfusion brain SPECT studies during the same day. The total dose is split such that one third is given for the first study, and two-thirds of the dose is given for the second study. The second injection may be given immediately after the first SPECT, or it may be delayed for a few minutes or a few hours. Residual tracer activity from the first injection is present on the second SPECT, but it is overwhelmed to some extent. It is possible to subtract residual tracer activity, which requires decay correction, image reorientation, and co-registration. Final image and comparison may be enhanced by normalization and subtraction of co-registered images.

Radiopharmaceutical Dosimetry
(⁹⁹ᵐTc-HMPAO, ⁹⁹ᵐTc-ECD)

1. Single-dose studies
   a. Dose: 0.2 to 0.3 mCi (7.4–11.1 MBq)/kg body weight
   b. Minimum dose 1.0 mCi (37 MBq)
   c. Maximum total dose 10 to 20 mCi (370–740 MBq)
2. Split-dose studies
   a. First study: 0.2 mCi (7.4 MBq)/kg body weight
      (1) Minimum dose 1.0 mCi (37 MBq)
      (2) Maximum dose 10 mCi (370 MBq)
   b. Second study: 0.4 mCi (14.8 MBq)/kg body weight
      (1) Minimum dose 2.0 mCi (74 MBq)
      (2) Maximum dose 20 mCi (740 MBq)

Tumor Perfusion Single Photon Emission Computed Tomography

Approximately 5 minutes after intravenous injection of ^{201}Tl or ^{99m}Tc-MIBI, the patient is positioned supine on the SPECT imaging table with the detector(s) placed as close to the patient's head as possible. The patient's head is positioned with the aid of laser guides and secured firmly, and then imaging continues exactly as for perfusion SPECT. To repeat, imaging preference is for a triple-detection gamma camera system or a dedicated system, and it should be equipped with a high-resolution collimator. An example of acquisition is as follows: Using a triple-detector system, each detector rotates 360 degrees around the patient's head. Each detector stops 40 times and acquires a 128 × 128 image for 30 seconds per stop. A total of 120 images are obtained.

Cerebral Radionuclide Angiography and Planar Scintigraphy

For cerebral radionuclide angiography (CRA), the patient is given oral potassium perchlorate 6 mg/kg 30 minutes prior to tracer injection. Alternatively, sodium perchlorate is given at the time of injection when ^{99m}Tc-sodium pertechnetate is used. Perchlorate is not necessary if ^{99m}Tc-DTPA or ^{99m}Tc-glucoheptonate are used. The radiotracer is administered as a rapid intravenous bolus. The study is usually recorded in the anterior projection, with the gamma camera fitted with a high sensitivity parallel hole collimator. The CRA is recorded at one frame per second for 60 seconds using a 128 × 128 matrix. Immediately after the CRA, planar scintigraphic static images, including anterior and lateral views, are obtained for 300,000 to 500,000 counts on a 256 × 256 matrix format.

Part 2 Cerebrospinal Fluid*
S.T. Treves and Alvin Kuruc

Sensitive, elegant assessments of normal and abnormal cerebrospinal fluid (CSF) dynamics can be obtained with relatively straightforward planar scintigraphy; it is used as a diagnostic tool for disorders affecting the CSF. The introduction of CT and MRI[138] has resulted in a significant reduction in the use of radionuclide cisternography. The method continues to be used in conjunction with clinical examination, structural imaging, and other neurologic procedures in children to aid in the evaluation of selected clinical problems, such as evaluation of shunt function, assessment of the delivery of chemotherapeutic agents, localization of leaks, and in evaluation of the hydrocephalic patient. Radionuclide cisternography provides accurate quantification of CSF dynamics.

Normal Cerebrospinal Fluid Physiology

Radionuclide cisternography permits observation of the flow, mixing, and absorption of

---

*Some of the concepts and portions of the wording in this part of the chapter were contributed by K. Welch, M.D., formerly professor of surgery at Harvard Medical School and chairman of the Department of Neurosurgery at Children's Hospital, and by L.A. O'Tuama, M.D., who was coauthor of this chapter in the second edition of *Pediatric Nuclear Medicine*.

CSF. Cerebrospinal fluid is produced primarily by the choroid plexus (CP), which is located within the lateral third and fourth ventricles. From here the fluid courses into the basal cisterns; it passes along discrete spinal and cranial subarachnoid pathways to its eventual destination over the convexities of the cerebral and cerebellar hemispheres. Resorption into the systemic venous circulation occurs through the arachnoid villi and granulations.[139,140]

Although the transvenous pathway is thought to be the major route of CSF absorption, several studies suggest that lymphatic vessels associated with cranial and spinal nerves within the subarachnoid spaces provide an alternative pathway of CSF absorption.[141,142] These accessory routes may also be important when the usual routes of CSF egress are compromised. Winston et al.[143] reported that the surgical correction of orthopedic abnormalities in a child with congenital dysfunction of the spinal cord was followed by acute elevation of the intracranial pressure, perhaps reflecting interference with the spinal accessory pathway for CSF circulation.

The rate of CSF turnover is faster in children than in adults when judged by scintigraphic criteria (as detailed below). As measured by ventriculocisternal perfusion, however, no significant difference has been noted between CSF formation in adults $(0.37 \, mL/minute)$[144] and children up to 13 years of age $(0.35 \, mL/minute)$.[145] Lorenzo et al.[139] and Page et al.[146] did note lower formation rates in newborns and younger children.

It is firmly established that CSF is formed by a secretory process,[140,147] as shown, inter alia, by the difference in electrolyte concentration between CSF and plasma ultrafiltrates.[148] Several discrete enzyme systems play a role in the formation process, primarily Na^+/K^+-activated adenosine triphosphatase (ATPase)[149,150] but also adenylate cyclase[139] and carbonic anhydrase.[151] For comprehensive reviews of these topics, the reader is referred to authoritative reviews by Cserr,[152] Netsky and Samruay,[153] Milhorat,[154] Wright,[155] Davson et al.,[140] and Spector and Johanson.[156]

Abnormal Cerebrospinal Fluid Physiology

An imbalance between the normal rates of production and removal of CSF results in a progressive increase in the total volume of CSF, known generically as hydrocephalus. Hydrocephalus is caused by a relative obstruction of CSF absorption and, rarely, by overproduction.

Diminished Absorption

The most common cause of hydrocephalus in the neonate is congenital malformation. In infants and older children, hydrocephalus is caused by trauma, inflammation, bleeding, or intracranial tumor. In most cases, CT or MRI of the brain distinguishes extraventricular from intraventricular obstructive hydrocephalus. Difficult cases may be solved by radionuclide cisternography.

With hydrocephalus, there is an active, progressive increase in the size of spaces containing CSF. In infants, open sutures allow for an increase in the volume of the ventricles initially with little increase in intracranial pressure. A persistent increase in intracranial pressure ultimately results in atrophy of the brain. This condition is due to a reduction in cerebral blood flow, which results in cerebral hypoxia.

Various animal models of hydrocephalus have been used to study the pathophysiologic sequelae of CSF obstruction. For example, in adult dogs, chronic communicating hydrocephalus was produced by injection of kaolin into the subarachnoid space.[157] Most cases of hydrocephalus are due to a mechanism of impaired absorption. They may be further grouped as intraventricular ("obstructive") or extraventricular ("communicating obstructive"). With extraventricular hydrocephalus, there is a functional block to the circulation of CSF, and this mechanism is by far the commonest encountered in children.

Overproduction

The rarest cause of hydrocephalus is an increase in CSF formation rates, associated with a tumor of the choroid plexus, either benign (papilloma) or malignant (carcinoma).[158] A specific diagnosis of this condition can be provided preoperatively, as the choroidal transport of anions can be imaged as a prominent uptake of ^{99m}Tc-pertechnetate. It can be prevented by prior treatment with potassium perchlorate, a specific inhibitor of the anion uptake mechanism.[106]

Method

Tracers used for radionuclide cisternography are confined to the CSF space and are quickly eliminated through the arachnoid plexus without being metabolized. Either (^{111}In-DTPA or ^{99m}Tc-DTPA is given in the subarachnoid space. Usual administered doses for ^{99m}Tc-DTPA are 0.3 to 1.0 mCi (11.1–37.0 MBq) and ^{111}In-DTPA 0.05 to 0.20 mCi (1.85–74.0 MBq). For routine cisternography in children, we prefer ^{99m}Tc-DTPA for its higher photon flux and lower radiation dose. The relatively short physical half-life of ^{99m}Tc is not an obstacle to the evaluation of CSF in children because it is distributed quickly.[159] In older children and adults, ^{111}In-DTPA is preferable. The radiation dose to the spinal cord and the surface of the brain with ^{99m}Tc-DTPA is about 1.0 rad per millicurie administered. The radiation absorbed dose with ^{111}In-DTPA is approximately 2.5 rad/mCi.

Careful technique is essential. The tracer is usually administered into the lumbar subarachnoid space. Other sites of injection include the cisterna magna or a lateral ventricle. Reported success rates for lumbar puncture vary considerably and clearly are highest with the most experienced operator. For this reason, we routinely request that the referring staff neurosurgeon inject the radiotracer in our department, with a nuclear medicine physician in attendance.

Following the subarachnoid administration of the tracer, an image of the injection site is obtained to establish the adequacy of the injection. Epidural injections typically produce a "Christmas tree" or a "railroad" appearance on the scintigraph, resulting in an unsatisfactory examination. Routinely, a series of images with the gamma camera are obtained in the anterior, posterior, and lateral projections at 2, 6, and 24 hours after administration of the tracer. Because the turnover of CSF in children is more rapid than in adults, more frequent imaging may be necessary. A high-resolution, low-energy collimator is used.

For the evaluation of CSF leaks, more frequent images are obtained soon after administration of the tracer. This point is important in order to increase the chances of localizing the leakage. It is important that the patient be studied while there is active CSF leak in the position in which the leak is most profuse; otherwise, visualization of the leak by this method may not be possible. For this purpose, the patient is maintained in the position in which he or she may be known to leak most profusely, and images are obtained sequentially in the appropriate projection in an attempt to localize any extracranial activity. If extracranial activity due to a CSF leak is detected, the patient is imaged in other projections to allow for localization in three dimensions. The timing of the lateral and the anterior views is critical, as the CSF leak may be transient.[159]

Small CSF leaks may not be detectable by scintigraphy. In some instances, it may be useful to place cotton pledgets in the nasal orifices; these pledgets should be changed and carefully labeled every 2 to 4 hours and counted for activity. In some instances, it may be necessary to place small cotton pledgets in selected locations deeper inside the nasal cavity (e.g., over the orifices of drainage of the nasal sinuses) to determine the site of the leak. A CSF leak can be stopped with cotton pledgets.[159] Placement and maintenance of nasal cotton pledgets in children is difficult and in many cases impossible. An additional problem with pledgets is that tracers used for cisternography diffuse into the blood and may appear in nasal secretions. The pledgets should be weighed and counted and the activity in the plasma measured. This practice helps to account for normal nasal activity and to facilitate recognition of differences in absorption. Nose/serum activity ratios of less than 1.5 should not be considered indicative of CSF leak.[160] In some children, cotton pledgets were placed and maintained under general anesthesia in an attempt to localize a CSF leak. General anesthesia, however, tends to decrease or stop leakage of CSF.[159]

Clinical Applications

Normal Radionuclide Cisternogram

On images at 2 and 6 hours, the tracer can be seen as it migrates upward into the interhemispheric fissure and the sylvian fissure. By 24 hours, the tracer can be seen over the convexity (Fig. 2.26).

Hydrocephalus

With communicating hydrocephalus (extraventricular obstructive hydrocephalus), the radiotracer circulates into the ventricular system and does not appear in the cerebral fissures and on the convexity. Persistence of the tracer within

ventricles for more than 24 hours is thought to indicate a progressive form of hydrocephalus that eventually needs shunting. In other instances of communicating hydrocephalus, a mixed pattern is seen; some tracer appears in the ventricular system and some in the fissures and over the convexity (Fig. 2.27).[142,151,161–163] This pattern may indicate a partially compensated form of hydrocephalus, and these patients probably do not need CSF shunting immediately but must be followed carefully to detect any worsening. Radionuclide cisternography, however, has not been found to be a reliable test for determining the need for shunting in adults, and there is not enough experience with it in children.[164–167] It has been proposed that the pattern of turnover of tracer in CSF is a reflection of ventricular size and the increased volume of distribution of CSF.[168] This idea is in keeping with the poor correlations found by earlier investigators. In the preterm infant, Donn et al.[169] used ^{111}In-DTPA radionuclide cis-

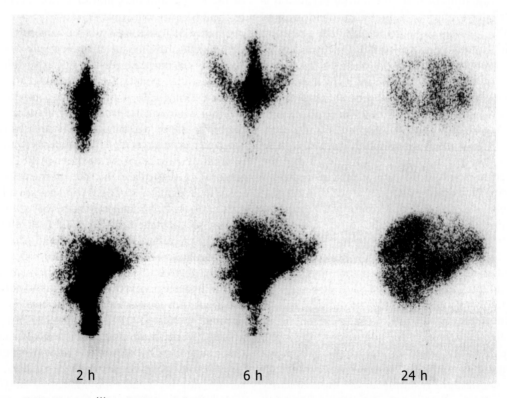

2 h   6 h   24 h

FIGURE 2.26. Normal ^{111}In–diethylenetriamine pentaacetic acid (DTPA) cisternography. Anterior (top) and right lateral (bottom) images were obtained 2, 6, and 24 hours after injection of the tracer into the lumbar subarachnoid space.[159]

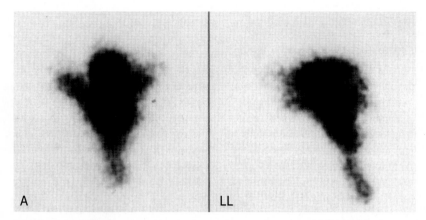

FIGURE 2.27. Communicating hydrocephalus with intra- and extraventricular diffusion of tracer: ^{111}In-DTPA cisternography 2 hours after injection. A, anterior view; LL, left lateral view.[159]

ternography to delineate CSF dynamic abnormalities associated with posthemorrhagic, "ex vacuo," and postmalformational types of hydrocephalus. Obstructive hydrocephalus is equated with intraventricular obstructive hydrocephalus. If intraventricular obstructive hydrocephalus is considered, the tracer is injected into a lateral ventricle. Hydrocephalus due to oversecretion of CSF is in most cases caused by a papilloma of the choroid plexus.[158,170–173] Cerebrospinal fluid production rates of 0.75 to 1.45 mL/minute in patients with papilloma of the choroid plexus have been measured.[158,174]

Cerebrospinal Fluid Liquorrhea

Cerebrospinal fluid liquorrhea is generally manifested by dripping from the nose or ear (Figs. 2.28 and 2.29). Profuse leakage suggests communication with a large cistern. If rhinorrhea is invariably unilateral, an opening into the nose or a paranasal sinus is suggested. If the

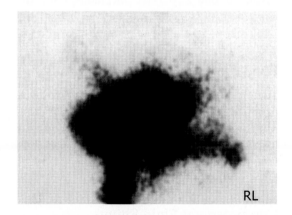

FIGURE 2.28. Cerebrospinal fluid (CSF) leak, shown by ^{99m}Tc-DTPA cisternography. This right lateral view was obtained 4 hours after injecting the tracer into the lumbar subarachnoid space. It is one of several images obtained every 15 minutes. Activity in the oropharynx due to a CSF leak is obvious. It was a posttraumatic leak through the fossa of Rosenmüller.[180]

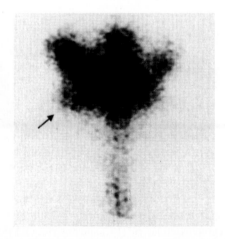

FIGURE 2.29. Otorrhea, shown by ^{111}In-DTPA cisternography. This anterior view was obtained 4 hours after injecting the tracer into the lumbar subarachnoid space. Extracranial tracer activity in the region of the right ear is visualized (arrow).[159]

side that drips alternates with position, a nasopharyngeal site, either directly or from the ear, is suggested. With CSF leaks, radionuclide cisternography reveals extracranial activity due to leak of the tracer outside the cranial cavity. Cerebrospinal fluid leak complicates up to one third of fractures of the base of the skull. Most of these leaks cease spontaneously within a week. Meningitis occurs in about one fourth of the patients if they are not treated with antibiotics.[170] Both rhinorrhea and otorrhea are amenable to investigation with radionuclide cisternography (Figs. 2.28 and 2.29).[161,175–178] Contrast-enhanced CT cisternography has been found less sensitive than radionuclide cisternography for the detection of intermittent rhinoliquorrhea in children.[179]

Loculations of Cerebrospinal Fluid

It is possible to have loculations of CSF in free communication with the subarachnoid pathways without loss of fluid to the external environment. Loculations of CSF appear on radionuclide cisternography as areas of accumulation and retention of the tracer over a relatively long period, for example, a nasal encephalocele or a subconjunctival loculation of CSF (Figs. 2.30 and 2.31).[180,181]

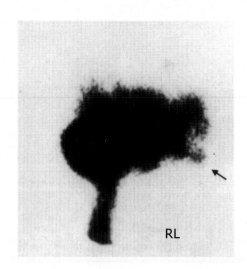

FIGURE 2.31. Subconjunctival CSF loculation, shown by a right lateral view of an ^{111}In-DTPA cisternogram. There is focal extracranial tracer activity corresponding to a massive subconjunctival CSF loculation (arrow).[159]

Porencephalic Cyst

Porencephalic cysts are caused by infection, trauma, or vascular problems that result in localized atrophy of the brain. These cysts have a pia-arachnoid lining, and communicate with a ventricle. Such abnormalities lead to stasis of the tracer on radionuclide cisternography, suggesting a one-way valve mechanism for the movement of CSF.[182,183]

Block of Spinal Cerebrospinal Fluid Flow

Tumors or other lesions in the spine, meninges, or spinal cord may cause blockage of CSF flow. They are seen on radionuclide cisternography as filling defects in which the radiotracer does not circulate or accumulate (Fig. 2.32), or as abrupt termination of CSF flow.

Cerebrospinal Fluid Shunts

Method of Assessment

Assessment of patency and quantitation of flow through CSF shunts can be made with radionuclide techniques in a rapid, safe, and accurate way. Technetium-99m as pertechnetate in a

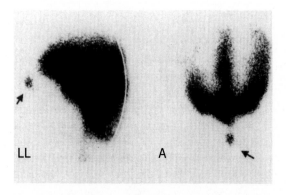

FIGURE 2.30. Nasal encephalocele. ^{99m}Tc-DTPA cisternography, left lateral (LL) and anterior (A) views, obtained 4 hours after injecting the tracer into the lumbar subarachnoid space. A pool of extracranial activity is visualized anteriorly, corresponding to a nasal encephalocele (arrows).[159]

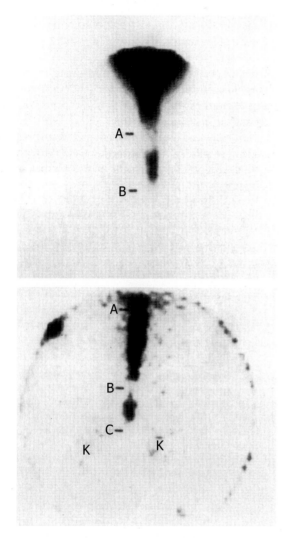

FIGURE 2.32. Block of CSF diffusion due to metastatic medulloblastomas in the spine. ^{99m}Tc-DTPA was injected into a lateral ventricle. Top: Posterior view of the cervical and thoracic spine 1 hour after injection of the tracer. There are two "filling defects" corresponding to a tumor mass (A and B). Bottom: View of the lower thoracic and lumbar spine reveals another block of tracer movement in the CSF (C). Renal activity is visualized bilaterally (K).[159]

dose of 0.25 to 0.50 mCi (9.25–18.50 MBq) in a volume of 0.01 to 0.02 mL is used.

The patient should rest in a horizontal position for 30 to 60 minutes before the study so as to enable the measurement of shunt flow at baseline CSF pressures. The patient is positioned under the gamma camera equipped with a col-limator of high sensitivity. The patient must remain immobile for the duration of the study.

The radiotracer is injected into the valve reservoir of the shunt, and its disappearance is monitored with the gamma camera and the computer at a rate of one frame every 5 seconds for 5 minutes. At the end of this time a series of images is obtained along the course of the shunt to detect any interruption of the flow of CSF. These images are evaluated visually (Figs. 2.33 and 2.34).[159]

Meticulous attention to technical detail is essential when conducting this examination. Before injecting the radiotracer, one must ensure that the needle is within the lumen of the shunt. When it is not, the tracer can be accidentally injected outside the shunt. Pertechnetate is then absorbed slowly, and it is taken up by the salivary glands, thyroid, and stomach. It is then slowly eliminated by the kidneys (Fig. 2.35).

A time-activity curve is calculated from a region over the valve of the shunt. As discussed further below, the CSF shunt flow can be calculated from this curve (Fig. 2.36).[184–186]

Alternatively, the radionuclide can be injected into the ventricle in order to follow its flow through the shunt. This method allows only qualitative estimation of shunt flow.

Clinical Applications

Ventriculoperitoneal and ventriculoatrial shunts are used in hydrocephalic patients to divert CSF into a body space so it can be absorbed. Mechanical failure, occlusion, and the development of loculated spaces around the ventricular or distal end of the shunt are causes of malfunction of a shunt. Such malfunction can usually be determined on clinical grounds, but in doubtful cases special measures may be indicated. Radionuclide studies can measure the shunt flow, determine the presence of an obstruction, and diagnose loculation of CSF at the distal end of the shunt.[159,186]

Rarely, CSF collections exist in free communication with the subarachnoid pathway, but without connecting with the exterior, as with nasoethmoidal encephaloceles.[187] With intracranial arachnoid cysts in children, radionuclide cisternography has proven useful

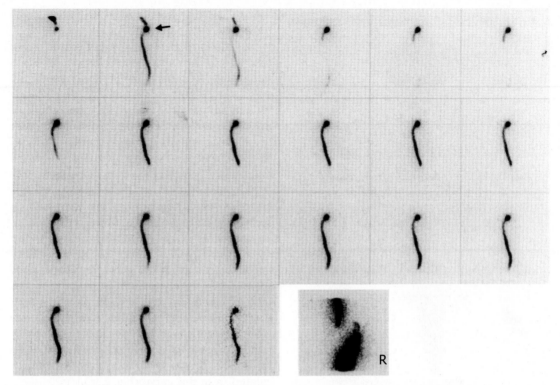

FIGURE 2.33. Patent ventriculoperitoneal shunt. Series of 10-second images with the administration of 0.30 mCi of ^{99m}Tc-pertechnetate in a volume of 0.1 mL in the valve (arrow). The tracer can be seen as it rapidly circulated through the shunt. An image obtained at 6 minutes after radiotracer administration reveals tracer within the shunt loops in the abdomen (single image, bottom right).

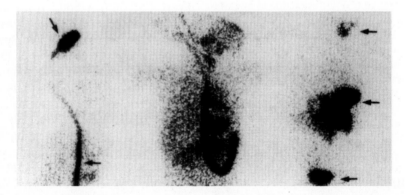

FIGURE 2.34. Patent ventriculoperitoneal shunt. Left: Image obtained almost immediately after tracer administration in the shunt. Activity in the valve and in the tubing is visualized (arrows). Center: Image 5 minutes later shows the trajectory of the tube and the activity in the stomach, thyroid, salivary glands, and soft tissues indicating rapid absorption of the tracer. Right: At 2.5 hours most of the activity is concentrated in the bladder, gastrointestinal tract, and thyroid (arrows).

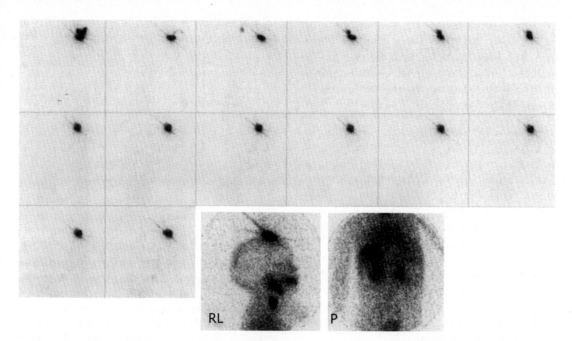

FIGURE 2.35. Extravasation of pertechnetate. Serial imaging (1 frame = 20 seconds) reveals that the tracer remains largely at the site of injection outside the shunt. There is no tracer activity detected distally within the shunt or proximally within the ventricular system. Static planar images obtained at 10 minutes after injection reveal pertechnetate uptake in the salivary glands, thyroid, stomach, kidneys, and bladder, indicating systemic absorption of tracer from the injection site.

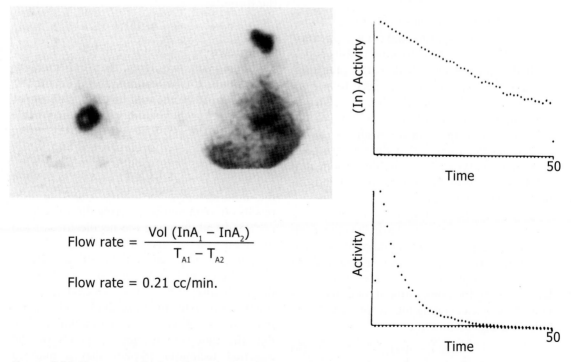

$$\text{Flow rate} = \frac{\text{Vol } (\text{InA}_1 - \text{InA}_2)}{T_{A1} - T_{A2}}$$

Flow rate = 0.21 cc/min.

FIGURE 2.36. Patent ventriculoperitoneal shunt. Top left: Anterior views of the chest and abdomen 10 minutes after injection of ^{99m}Tc-pertechnetate into the valve of the shunt. Both images show widespread distribution of the tracer in the body, indicating patency of the shunt. Right: Logarithmic (top) and linear (bottom) time-activity curves from the valve obtained from images at one frame every 5 seconds. Calculation of CSF shunt flow is shown.[159]

in establishing the communication of the cyst with the ventricular or subarachnoid compartment[149,188] and can aid in the assessment of associated hydrocephalus.[189]

Quantification of Cerebrospinal Fluid Shunt Flow

Cerebrospinal fluid shunt flow may be estimated from the time-activity curve obtained from the valve of the shunt (Fig. 2.36).

In one approach, the valve is modeled as a single, well-mixed compartment. The term *well-mixed* means that the tracer becomes equilibrated with the entire volume of the compartment immediately after its introduction and remains so for the duration of the experiment. In such a system, the disappearance curve is of the form

$$A(t) = A(0)e^{-t/k}, \qquad (1)$$

where t is time, and k is the time constant of the system. The time constant is equal to the mean time the tracer remains in the valve. Flow (F) is calculated using the formula

$$F = V/k, \qquad (2)$$

where V is the volume of distribution.[184]

There is much experimental evidence at variance with the well-mixed compartment model. With the method described in the preceding paragraph, it was found necessary to use an experimentally determined volume of distribution rather than the physical volume of the valve to obtain quantitative results.[184] Moreover, it has been found that the observed disappearance curve differs from the exponential curve predicted by the model and depends on the injection technique.[185]

As the well-mixed compartment assumption appears to be invalid, we have developed an alternative approach for estimating flow. If the radiotracer is instantaneously introduced, so the tracer is uniformly distributed across the fluid entering the compartment, one may estimate flow by calculating the mean transit time (MTT) using the formula

$$MTT = A/H, \qquad (3)$$

where A is the total area under the disappearance curve, and H is the initial height of the dis-

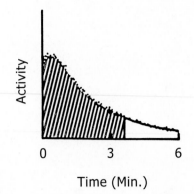

FIGURE 2.37. Cerebrospinal fluid flow may be estimated from the area under the valve disappearance curve using Eq. 3. Because the curve may not have reached zero before the end of the recording period, the curve is extrapolated by fitting an exponential function to its final portion. The fit starts when the activity is 25% of the maximum activity or when 75% of the recording period has expired, whichever comes first. The total area is computed by numerically integrating the initial portion and adding the area under the exponential fit.[159]

appearance curve. Flow is then calculated using the formula

$$F = V/MTT. \qquad (4)$$

This method is illustrated in (Fig. 2.37). The method, which we term the A/H method, was found to be more precise than the method based on the well-mixed compartment model.[185] It has the additional advantage that it works with the physical volume of the valve, obviating the need for experimentally determined volumes of distribution.

The idea behind the A/H method is to label the fluid entering the value. Thus the best results are obtained by entering the valve at its proximal end, pointing the needle toward the proximal end of the valve, or both. If this maneuver is not feasible, the method overestimates the shunt flow to some degree. As mentioned before, the volume injected must be small in order to minimize fluid displacement from the injection. The experimental finding that the time-activity curve depends on the injection technique implies that a uniform injection technique is essential to obtain reproducible results.

References

1. Isacson O. On neuronal health. Trends Neurosci 1993;16(8):306–8.
2. Kavdel ER, Schwartz JH. Principles of Neural Science. New York: Elsevier Science, 1991.
3. Gallen CC, Sobel DF, Lewine JD, et al. Neuromagnetic mapping of brain function. Radiology 1993;187(3):863–7.
4. Ingvar DH, Lassen NA. Quantitative determination of regional cerebral blood flow in man. Lancet 1961;2:806–7.
5. Habboush IH, Mitchell KD, Mulkern RV, Barnes PD, Treves ST. Registration and alignment of three-dimensional images: an interactive visual approach. Radiology 1996;199(2):573–8.
6. Chugani HT, Phelps ME, Mazziotta JC. Positron emission tomography study of human brain functional development. Ann Neurol 1987;22(4):487–97.
7. Chugani HT. Metabolic imaging: a window on brain development and plasticity. Neuroscientist 1999;5:29–40.
8. Rubinstein M, Denays R, Ham HR, et al. Functional imaging of brain maturation in humans using iodine-123 iodoamphetamine and SPECT. J Nucl Med 1989;30(12):1982–5.
9. Chiron C, Raynaud C, Maziere B, et al. Changes in regional cerebral blood flow during brain maturation in children and adolescents. J Nucl Med 1992;33(5):696–703.
10. Chugani HT, Phelps ME. Maturational changes in cerebral function in infants determined by 18FDG positron emission tomography. Science 1986;231(4740):840–3.
11. Chugani HT. A critical period of brain development: studies of cerebral glucose utilization with PET. Prev Med 1998;27(2):184–8.
12. Chugani HT, Muller RA, Chugani DC. Functional brain reorganization in children. Brain Dev 1996;18(5):347–56.
13. Wyllie E, Rothner AD, Luders H. Partial seizures in children: clinical features, medical treatment, and surgical considerations. Pediatr Clin North Am 1989;36(2):343–64.
14. Epilepsy surgery. eMedicine.com, 2004. http://www.emedicine.com/med/topic3177.htm.
15. Health NIo. National Institutes of Health Consensus Conference. Surgery for epilepsy. JAMA 1990;264(6):729–33.
16. Koo CW, Devinsky O, Hari K, Balasny J, Noz ME, Kramer EL. Stratifying differences on ictal/interictal subtraction SPECT images. Epilepsia 2003;44(3):379–86.
17. Rowe CC, Berkovic SF, Austin MC, McKay WJ, Bladin PF. Patterns of postictal cerebral blood flow in temporal lobe epilepsy: qualitative and quantitative analysis. Neurology 1991;41(7):1096–103.
18. Rowe CC, Berkovic SF, Sia ST, et al. Localization of epileptic foci with postictal single photon emission computed tomography. Ann Neurol 1989;26(5):660–8.
19. Kuzniecky R, Mountz JM, Wheatley G, Morawetz R. Ictal single-photon emission computed tomography demonstrates localized epileptogenesis in cortical dysplasia. Ann Neurol 1993;34(4):627–31.
20. Adams C, Hwang PA, Gilday DL, Armstrong DC, Becker LE, Hoffman HJ. Comparison of SPECT, EEG, CT, MRI, and pathology in partial epilepsy. Pediatr Neurol 1992;8(2):97–103.
21. Chiron C, Raynaud C, Dulac O, Tzourio N, Plouin P, Tran-Dinh S. Study of the cerebral blood flow in partial epilepsy of childhood using the SPECT method. J Neuroradiol 1989;16(4):317–24.
22. Miles D, Holmes G, Pearl P, et al. Comparison of CT, MRI, SPECT and BEAM in evaluation of pediatric epilepsy candidates in focal surgical resection. Epilepsia 1990;31:672.
23. Uvebrant P, Bjure J, Hedstrom A, Ekholm S. Brain single photon emission computed tomography (SPECT) in neuropediatrics. Neuropediatrics 1991;22(1):3–9.
24. Vles JS, Demandt E, Ceulemans B, de Roo M, Casaer PJ. Single photon emission computed tomography (SPECT) in seizure disorders in childhood. Brain Dev 1990;12(4):385–9.
25. Packard AB, Roach PJ, Davis RT, et al. Ictal and interictal technetium-99m-bicisate brain SPECT in children with refractory epilepsy. J Nucl Med 1996;37(7):1101–6.
26. Kaminska A, Chiron C, Ville D, et al. Ictal SPECT in children with epilepsy: comparison with intracranial EEG and relation to postsurgical outcome. Brain 2003;126(pt 1):248–60.
27. O'Brien TJ, So EL, Mullan BP, et al. Subtraction peri-ictal SPECT is predictive of extratemporal epilepsy surgery outcome. Neurology 2000;55(11):1668–77.
28. Buchhalter JR, So EL. Advances in computer-assisted single-photon emission computed tomography (SPECT) for epilepsy surgery in children. Acta Paediatr Suppl 2004;93(445):32–5; discussion 6–7.
29. O'Brien TJ, So EL, Mullan BP, et al. Subtraction ictal SPECT co-registered to MRI

improves clinical usefulness of SPECT in localizing the surgical seizure focus. Neurology 1998;50(2):445–54.

30. Davis RT, Treves ST, Zurakowski D, Bauer SB. Ictal perfusion brain SPECT in pediatric patients with intractable epilepsy: a multidisciplinary approach. J Nucl Med Technol 1996; 24:219–22.

31. Shoeb A, Edwards H, Connolly J, Bourgeois B, Treves ST, Guttag J. Patient-specific seizure onset detection. Epilepsy Behav 2004;5(4):483–98.

32. Hrachovy RA, Frost JD Jr. Infantile spasms. Pediatr Clin North Am 1989;36(2):311–29.

33. Chugani HT, Shewmon DA, Shields WD, et al. Surgery for intractable infantile spasms: neuroimaging perspectives. Epilepsia 1993;34(4): 764–71.

34. Chugani HT, Shields WD, Shewmon DA, Olson DM, Phelps ME, Peacock WJ. Infantile spasms: I. PET identifies focal cortical dysgenesis in cryptogenic cases for surgical treatment. Ann Neurol 1990;27(4):406–13.

35. O'Tuama LA, Urion DK, Janicek MJ, Treves ST, Bjornson B, Moriarty JM. Regional cerebral perfusion in Landau-Kleffner syndrome and related childhood aphasias. J Nucl Med 1992;33(10):1758–65.

36. Chiron C, Dulac O, Bulteau C, et al. Study of regional cerebral blood flow in West syndrome. Epilepsia 1993;34(4):707–15.

37. Otsubo H, Hwang PA, Jay V, et al. Focal cortical dysplasia in children with localization-related epilepsy: EEG, MRI, and SPECT findings. Pediatr Neurol 1993;9(2):101–7.

38. Miyazaki M, Hashimoto T, Fujii E, Tayama M, Kuroda Y. Infantile spasms: localized cerebral lesions on SPECT. Epilepsia 1994;35(5):988–92.

39. Haginoya K, Munakata M, Yokoyama H, et al. Mechanism of tonic spasms in West syndrome viewed from ictal SPECT findings. Brain Dev 2001;23(7):496–501.

40. Koh S, Jayakar P, Resnick T, Alvarez L, Liit RE, Duchowny M. The localizing value of ictal SPECT in children with tuberous sclerosis complex and refractory partial epilepsy. Epileptic Disord 1999;1(1):41–6.

41. Chugani DC, Chugani HT, Muzik O, et al. Imaging epileptogenic tubers in children with tuberous sclerosis complex using alpha-[11C]methyl-L-tryptophan positron emission tomography. Ann Neurol 1998;44(6):858–66.

42. Kagawa K, Chugani DC, Asano E, et al. Epilepsy surgery outcome in children with tuberous sclerosis complex evaluated with alpha [11C] methyl-L-tryptophan positron emission tomography (PET). J Child Neurol 2005;20(5):429–38.

43. Roach ES, Garcia JC, McLean WT Jr. Cerebrovascular disease in children. Am Fam Physician 1984;30(5):215–27.

44. Yamashiro Y, Takahashi H, Takahashi K. Cerebrovascular moyamoya disease. Eur J Pediatr 1984;142(1):44–50.

45. Feole JB, Ali A, Fordham EW, Huckman M, Shenker DM. Serial SPECT imaging in moyamoya using I-123 IMP. A method of noninvasive evaluation and follow-up. Clin Nucl Med 1993;18(1):43–5.

46. Kobayashi H, Hayashi M, Handa Y, Kabuto M, Noguchi Y, Aradachi H. EC-IC bypass for adult patients with moyamoya disease. Neurol Res 1991;13(2):113–6.

47. Shahar E, Gilday DL, Hwang PA, Cohen EK, Lambert R. Pediatric cerebrovascular disease. Alterations of regional cerebral blood flow detected by TC 99m-HMPAO SPECT. Arch Neurol 1990;47(5):578–84.

48. Bourgeois M, Aicardi J, Goutieres F. Alternating hemiplegia of childhood. J Pediatr 1993; 122(5 pt 1):673–9.

49. Zupanc ML, Dobkin JA, Perlman SB. 123I-iodoamphetamine SPECT brain imaging in alternating hemiplegia. Pediatr Neurol 1991; 7(1):35–8.

50. Mikati MA, Maguire H, Barlow CF, et al. A syndrome of autosomal dominant alternating hemiplegia: clinical presentation mimicking intractable epilepsy; chromosomal studies; and physiologic investigations. Neurology 1992; 42(12):2251–7.

51. Clinical practice guideline: diagnosis and evaluation of the child with attention-deficit/hyperactivity disorder. American Academy of Pediatrics. Pediatrics 2000;105(5):1158–70.

52. Lou HC, Henriksen L, Bruhn P. Focal cerebral hypoperfusion in children with dysphasia and/or attention deficit disorder. Arch Neurol 1984;41(8):825–9.

53. Lou HC, Henriksen L, Bruhn P, Borner H, Nielsen JB. Striatal dysfunction in attention deficit and hyperkinetic disorder. Arch Neurol 1989;46(1):48–52.

54. Zametkin AJ, Nordahl TE, Gross M, et al. Cerebral glucose metabolism in adults with hyperactivity of childhood onset. N Engl J Med 1990;323(20):1361–6.

55. Zametkin AJ, Liebenauer LL, Fitzgerald GA, et al. Brain metabolism in teenagers with

attention-deficit hyperactivity disorder. Arch Gen Psychiatry 1993;50(5):333–40.

56. Lorberboym M, Watemberg N, Nissenkorn A, Nir B, Lerman-Sagie T. Technetium-99m ethyl-cysteinate dimer single-photon emission computed tomography (SPECT) during intellectual stress test in children and adolescents with pure versus comorbid attention-deficit hyperactivity disorder (ADHD). J Child Neurol 2004; 19(2):91–6.

57. Lou HC, Henriksen L, Bruhn P. Focal cerebral dysfunction in developmental learning disabilities. Lancet 1990;335(8680):8–11.

58. Langleben DD, Acton PD, Austin G, et al. Effects of methylphenidate discontinuation on cerebral blood flow in prepubescent boys with attention deficit hyperactivity disorder. J Nucl Med 2002;43(12):1624–9.

59. Langleben DD, Austin G, Krikorian G, Ridlehuber HW, Goris ML, Strauss HW. Interhemispheric asymmetry of regional cerebral blood flow in prepubescent boys with attention deficit hyperactivity disorder. Nucl Med Commun 2001;22(12):1333–40.

60. Kim BN, Lee JS, Cho SC, Lee DS. Methylphenidate increased regional cerebral blood flow in subjects with attention deficit/hyperactivity disorder. Yonsei Med J 2001; 42(1):19–29.

61. Gustafsson P, Thernlund G, Ryding E, Rosen I, Cederblad M. Associations between cerebral blood-flow measured by single photon emission computed tomography (SPECT), electro-encephalogram (EEG), behaviour symptoms, cognition and neurological soft signs in children with attention-deficit hyperactivity disorder (ADHD). Acta Paediatr 2000;89(7): 830–5.

62. Arndt S, Cohen G, Alliger RJ, Swayze VW 2nd, Andreasen NC. Problems with ratio and proportion measures of imaged cerebral structures. Psychiatry Res 1991;40(1):79–89.

63. Barbour RL, Graber HL, Pei Y, Zhong S, Schmitz CH. Optical tomographic imaging of dynamic features of dense-scattering media. J Opt Soc Am A Opt Image Sci Vis 2001;18(12):3018–36.

64. Franceschini MA, Toronov V, Fillaci ME, Gratton E, Fantini S. On-line optical imaging of the human brain with 160–ms temporal resolution. Optics Express 2000;6:49–57.

65. Volkow ND, Wang GJ, Fowler JS, et al. Effects of methylphenidate on regional brain glucose metabolism in humans: relationship to dopamine D2 receptors. Am J Psychiatry 1997;154(1):50–5.

66. Volkow ND, Wang G, Fowler JS, et al. Therapeutic doses of oral methylphenidate significantly increase extracellular dopamine in the human brain. J Neurosci 2001;21(2): RC121.

67. Dougherty DD, Bonab AA, Spencer TJ, Rauch SL, Madras BK, Fischman AJ. Dopamine transporter density in patients with attention deficit hyperactivity disorder. Lancet 1999; 354(9196):2132–3.

68. Krause KH, Dresel SH, Krause J, Kung HF, Tatsch K. Increased striatal dopamine transporter in adult patients with attention deficit hyperactivity disorder: effects of methylphenidate as measured by single photon emission computed tomography. Neurosci Lett 2000;285(2):107–10.

69. van Dyck CH, Quinlan DM, Cretella LM, et al. Unaltered dopamine transporter availability in adult attention deficit hyperactivity disorder. Am J Psychiatry 2002;159(2):309–12.

70. Ilgin N, Senol S, Gucuyener K, Gokcora N, Sener S. Is increased D2 receptor availability associated with response to stimulant medication in ADHD. Dev Med Child Neurol 2001;43(11):755–60.

71. Koepp MJ, Gunn RN, Lawrence AD, et al. Evidence for striatal dopamine release during a video game. Nature 1998;393(6682):266–8.

72. Strafella AP, Paus T, Barrett J, Dagher A. Repetitive transcranial magnetic stimulation of the human prefrontal cortex induces dopamine release in the caudate nucleus. J Neurosci 2001;21(15):RC157.

73. Volkow ND, Wang GJ, Fowler JS, et al. Relationship between blockade of dopamine transporters by oral methylphenidate and the increases in extracellular dopamine: therapeutic implications. Synapse 2002;43(3):181–7.

74. Castellanos FX. Proceed, with caution: SPECT cerebral blood flow studies of children and adolescents with attention deficit hyperactivity disorder. J Nucl Med 2002;43(12): 1630–3.

75. Denays R, Tondeur M, Foulon M, et al. Regional brain blood flow in congenital dysphasia: studies with technetium-99m HM-PAO SPECT. J Nucl Med 1989;30(11):1825–9.

76. Denays R, Tondeur M, Toppet V, et al. Cerebral palsy: initial experience with Tc-99m HMPAO SPECT of the brain. Radiology 1990;175(1): 111–6.

77. Mauk JE. Autism and pervasive developmental disorders. Pediatr Clin North Am 1993;40(3): 567–78.

78. Rumsey JM, Duara R, Grady C, et al. Brain metabolism in autism. Resting cerebral glucose utilization rates as measured with positron emission tomography. Arch Gen Psychiatry 1985;42(5):448–55.

79. Heh CW, Smith R, Wu J, et al. Positron emission tomography of the cerebellum in autism. Am J Psychiatry 1989;146(2):242–5.

80. De Volder AG, Bol A, Michel C, Cogneau M, Goffinet AM. [Cerebral glucose metabolism in autistic children. Study and positron emission tomography.] Acta Neurol Belg 1988;88(2):75–90.

81. Horwitz B, Rumsey JM, Grady CL, Rapoport SI. The cerebral metabolic landscape in autism. Intercorrelations of regional glucose utilization. Arch Neurol 1988;45(7):749–55.

82. Zilbovicius M, Garreau B, Tzourio N, et al. Regional cerebral blood flow in childhood autism: a SPECT study. Am J Psychiatry 1992;149(7):924–30.

83. George M, Ring H, Costa D, et al. Neuroactivation and Neuroimaging with SPET. London: Springer-Verlag, 1991.

84. Chugani DC, Muzik O, Behen M, et al. Developmental changes in brain serotonin synthesis capacity in autistic and nonautistic children. Ann Neurol 1999;45(3):287–95.

85. Ingvar DH. Measurements of regional cerebral blood flow and metabolism in psychopathological states. Eur Neurol 1981;20(3):294–6.

86. Weinberger DR, Berman KF, Zec RF. Physiologic dysfunction of dorsolateral prefrontal cortex in schizophrenia. I. Regional cerebral blood flow evidence. Arch Gen Psychiatry 1986;43(2):114–24.

87. Andreasen NC, Rezai K, Alliger R, et al. Hypofrontality in neuroleptic-naive patients and in patients with chronic schizophrenia. Assessment with xenon-133 single-photon emission computed tomography and the Tower of London. Arch Gen Psychiatry 1992; 49(12):943–58.

88. Wolkin A, Sanfilipo M, Wolf AP, Angrist B, Brodie JD, Rotrosen J. Negative symptoms and hypofrontality in chronic schizophrenia. Arch Gen Psychiatry 1992;49(12):959–65.

89. Drevets WC, Videen TO, Price JL, Preskorn SH, Carmichael ST, Raichle ME. A functional anatomical study of unipolar depression. J Neurosci 1992;12(9):3628–41.

90. Addario D. Developmental considerations in the concept of affective illness. J Clin Psychiatry 1985;46(10 pt 2):46–56.

91. Park CH, Spitzer AR, Desai HJ, Zhang JJ, Graziani LJ. Brain SPECT in neonates following extracorporeal membrane oxygenation: evaluation of technique and preliminary results. J Nucl Med 1992;33(11):1943–8.

92. Kumar P, Bedard MP, Shankaran S, Delaney-Black V. Post extracorporeal membrane oxygenation single photon emission computed tomography (SPECT) as a predictor of neurodevelopmental outcome. Pediatrics 1994;93(6 pt 1):951–5.

93. Wong PC, Barlow CF, Hickey PR, et al. Factors associated with choreoathetosis after cardiopulmonary bypass in children with congenital heart disease. Circulation 1992;86(5 suppl):II118–26.

94. du Plessis AJ, Treves ST, Hickey PR, et al. Regional cerebral perfusion abnormalities after cardiac operations: single photon emission computed tomography (SPECT) findings in children with postoperative movement disorders. J Thorac Cardiovasc Surg 1994;107: 1036–43.

95. Cancer Facts and Figures 2003. Atlanta, GA: American Cancer Society, Surveillance Research, 2003.

96. Gurney JG, Smith MA, Bunin GR. CNS and miscellaneous intracranial and intraspinal neoplasms. In: Ries LA, Smith MA, Gurney JG, et al., eds. Cancer Incidence and Survival Among Children and Adolescents: United States Seer Program 1975–1995. Bethesda, MD: National Cancer Institute, Seer Program, 1999:51–63.

97. Baldwin RT, Preston-Martin S. Epidemiology of brain tumors in childhood—a review. Toxicol Appl Pharmacol 2004;199(2):118–31.

98. Bleyer WA. Epidemiologic impact of children with brain tumors. Childs Nerv Syst 1999; 15(11–12):758–63.

99. Kingsley DP, Kendall BE. CT of the adverse effects of therapeutic radiation of the central nervous system. AJNR 1981;2(5):453–60.

100. van Dellen JR, Danziger A. Failure of computerized tomography to differentiate between radiation necrosis and cerebral tumour. S Afr Med J 1978;53(5):171–2.

101. Julow J, Major T, Emri M, et al. The application of image fusion in stereotactic brachytherapy of brain tumours. Acta Neurochir (Wien) 2000;142(11):1253–8.

102. Kaplan WD, Takvorian T, Morris JH, Rumbaugh CL, Connolly BT, Atkins HL. Thallium-201 brain tumor imaging: a comparative study with pathologic correlation. J Nucl Med 1987;28(1):47–52.

103. O'Tuama LA, Phillips PC, Strauss LC, et al. Two-phase [11C]L-methionine PET in childhood brain tumors. Pediatr Neurol 1990;6(3): 163–70.

104. O'Tuama LA, Treves ST, Larar JN, et al. Thallium-201 versus technetium-99m-MIBI SPECT in evaluation of childhood brain tumors: a within-subject comparison. J Nucl Med 1993;34(7):1045–51.

105. Biersack HJ, Coenen HH, Stocklin G, et al. Imaging of brain tumors with L-3–[123I]iodo-alpha-methyl tyrosine and SPECT. J Nucl Med 1989;30(1):110–2.

106. Kaplan WD, McComb JG, Strand RD, Treves S. Suppression of 99mTc-pertechnetate uptake in a choroid plexus papilloma. Radiology 1973;109(2):395–6.

107. Kim KT, Black KL, Marciano D, et al. Thallium-201 SPECT imaging of brain tumors: methods and results. J Nucl Med 1990;31(6): 965–9.

108. Coleman RE, Hoffman JM, Hanson MW, Sostman HD, Schold SC. Clinical application of PET for the evaluation of brain tumors. J Nucl Med 1991;32(4):616–22.

109. Maria BL, Drane WE, Mastin ST, Jimenez LA. Comparative value of thallium and glucose SPECT imaging in childhood brain tumors. Pediatr Neurol 1998;19(5):351–7.

110. Galaske RG, Schober O, Heyer R. Determination of brain death in children with 123I-IMP and Tc-99m HMPAO. Psychiatry Res 1989; 29(3):343–5.

111. Donohoe KJ, Frey KA, Gerbaudo VH, Mariani G, Nagel JS, Shulkin B. Procedure guideline for brain death scintigraphy. J Nucl Med 2003; 44(5):846–51.

112. Spieth M, Abella E, Sutter C, Vasinrapee P, Wall L, Ortiz M. Importance of the lateral view in the evaluation of suspected brain death. Clin Nucl Med 1995;20(11):965–8.

113. Spieth ME, Ansari AN, Kawada TK, Kimura RL, Siegel ME. Direct comparison of Tc-99m DTPA and Tc-99m HMPAO for evaluating brain death. Clin Nucl Med 1994;19(10):867–72.

114. Jacobs AH, Dittmar C, Winkeler A, Garlip G, Heiss WD. Molecular imaging of gliomas. Mol Imaging 2002;1(4):309–35.

115. Camargo EE. Brain SPECT in neurology and psychiatry. J Nucl Med 2001;42(4):611–23.

116. Del Sole A, Falini A, Ravasi L, et al. Anatomical and biochemical investigation of primary brain tumours. Eur J Nucl Med 2001; 28(12):1851–72.

117. Leveille J, Demonceau G, De Roo M, et al. Characterization of technetium-99m-L,L-ECD for brain perfusion imaging, Part 2: Biodistribution and brain imaging in humans. J Nucl Med 1989;30(11):1902–10.

118. Hertz-Pannier L, Chiron C, Vera P, et al. Functional imaging in the work-up of childhood epilepsy. Childs Nerv Syst 2001;17(4–5):223–8.

119. Van Paesschen W. Ictal SPECT. Epilepsia 2004;45(suppl 4):35–40.

120. Sharp PF, Smith FW, Gemmell HG, et al. Technetium-99m HM-PAO stereoisomers as potential agents for imaging regional cerebral blood flow: human volunteer studies. J Nucl Med 1986;27:171–7.

121. Tubergen K, Corlija M, Volkert WA, Holmes RA. Sensitivity of technetium-99m-d,1–HMPAO to radiolysis in aqueous solutions. J Nucl Med 1991;32(1):111–5.

122. Weisner PS, Bower GR, Dollimore LA, Forster AM, Higley B, Storey AE. A method for stabilising technetium-99m exametazime prepared from a commercial kit. Eur J Nucl Med 1993;20(8):661–6.

123. Greenberg JH, Kushner M, Rango M, Alavi A, Reivich M. Validation studies of iodine-123–iodoamphetamine as a cerebral blood flow tracer using emission tomography. J Nucl Med 1990;31(8):1364–9.

124. Devous MD Sr, Payne JK, Lowe JL, Leroy RF. Comparison of technetium-99m-ECD to Xenon-133 SPECT in normal controls and in patients with mild to moderate regional cerebral blood flow abnormalities. J Nucl Med 1993;34(5):754–61.

125. Saha GB, MacIntyre WJ, Go RT. Radiopharmaceuticals for brain imaging. Semin Nucl Med 1994;24(4):324–49.

126. Payne JK, Trivedi MH, Devous MD, Sr. Comparison of technetium-99m-HMPAO and xenon-133 measurements of regional cerebral blood flow by SPECT. J Nucl Med 1996;37(10):1735–40.

127. Leskinen-Kallio S. Positron emission tomography in oncology. Clin Physiol 1994;14(3): 329–35.

128. Black KL, Hawkins RA, Kim KT, Becker DP, Lerner C, Marciano D. Use of thallium-201

SPECT to quantitate malignancy grade of glioma. J Neurosurg 1989;71:342.

129. Sasaki M, Kuwabara Y, Yoshida T, et al. A comparative study of thallium-201 SPET, carbon-11 methionine PET and fluorine-18 fluorodeoxyglucose PET for the differentiation of astrocytic tumours. Eur J Nucl Med 1998;25(9):1261–9.

130. Krishna L, Slizofski WJ, Katsetos CD, et al. Abnormal intracerebral thallium localization in a bacterial brain abscess. J Nucl Med 1992;33(11):2017–9.

131. O'Tuama LA, Packard AB, Treves ST. SPECT imaging of pediatric brain tumor with hexakis (methoxyisobutylisonitrile) technetium (I). J Nucl Med 1990;31(12):2040–1.

132. Soricelli A, Cuocolo A, Varrone A, et al. Technetium-99m-tetrofosmin uptake in brain tumors by SPECT: comparison with thallium-201 imaging. J Nucl Med 1998;39(5):802–6.

133. Choi JY, Kim SE, Shin HJ, Kim BT, Kim JH. Brain tumor imaging with 99mTc-tetrofosmin: comparison with 201Tl, 99mTc-MIBI, and 18F-fluorodeoxyglucose. J Neuro-Oncol 2000; 46(1):63–70.

134. Kung HF, Kung MP, Choi SR. Radiopharmaceuticals for single-photon emission computed tomography brain imaging. Semin Nucl Med 2003;33(1):2–13.

135. Meegalla SK, Plossl K, Kung MP, et al. Synthesis and characterization of technetium-99m-labeled tropanes as dopamine transporter-imaging agents. J Med Chem 1997;40(1):9–17.

136. Dresel S, Krause J, Krause KH, et al. Attention deficit hyperactivity disorder: binding of [99mTc]TRODAT-1 to the dopamine transporter before and after methylphenidate treatment. Eur J Nucl Med 2000;27(10):1518–24.

137. Woods SW, Hegeman IM, Zubal IG, et al. Visual stimulation increases technetium-99m-HMPAO distribution in human visual cortex. J Nucl Med 1991;32(2):210–5.

138. Stehling MK, Firth JL, Worthington BS, et al. Observation of cerebrospinal fluid flow with echo-planar magnetic resonance imaging. Br J Radiol 1991;64(758):89–97.

139. Lorenzo AV, Page LK, Watters GV. Relationship between cerebrospinal fluid formation, absorption and pressure in human hydrocephalus. Brain 1970;93(4):679–92.

140. Davson H, Welch K, Segal MB, Davson H. Physiology and Pathophysiology of the Cerebrospinal Fluid. Edinburgh, New York: Churchill Livingstone, 1987.

141. Jackson RT, Tigges J, Arnold W. Subarachnoid space of the CNS, nasal mucosa, and lymphatic system. Arch Otolaryngol 1979;105(4):180–4.

142. McComb JG, Hyman S, Weiss MH. Lymphatic drainage of cerebrospinal fluid in the cat. In: Shapiro K, Marmarou A, Portnoy H, eds. Hydrocephalus. New York: Raven Press, 1984.

143. Winston K, Hall J, Johnson D, Micheli L. Acute elevation of intracranial pressure following transection of non-functional spinal cord. Clin Orthop Rel Res 1977(128):41–4.

144. Rubin RC, Henderson ES, Ommaya AK, Walker MD, Rall DP. The production of cerebrospinal fluid in man and its modification by acetazolamide. J Neurosurg 1966;25(4):430–6.

145. Cutler RW, Page L, Galicich J, Watters GV. Formation and absorption of cerebrospinal fluid in man. Brain 1968;91(4):707–20.

146. Page LK, Bresnan MJ, Lorenzo AV. Cerebrospinal fluid perfusion studies in childhood hydrocephalus. Surg Neurol 1973;1(6):317–20.

147. Welch K. Secretion of cerebrospinal fluid by choroid plexus of the rabbit. Am J Physiol 1963;205:617–24.

148. de Rougemont J, Ames AI, Nesbett FB, Hofmann HF. Fluid formed by choroid plexus; a technique for its collection and a comparison of its electrolyte composition with serum and cisternal fluids. J Neurophysiol 1960;23:485–95.

149. Bonting SL, Simon KA, Hawkins NM. Studies on sodium-potassium-activated adenosine triphosphatase. I. Quantitative distribution in several tissues of the cat. Arch Biochem Biophys 1961;95:416–23.

150. Vates TS Jr, Bonting SL, Oppelt WW. Na-K activated adenosine triphosphatase formation of cerebrospinal fluid in the cat. Am J Physiol 1964;206:1165–72.

151. Johanson CE. The choroid plexus-arachnoid membrane-cerebrospinal fluid system. In: Boulton AA, Baker GB, Walz W, eds. Neuromethods: The Neuronal Microenvironment. Clifton, NJ: Humana Press; 1988:xxvi, 732.

152. Cserr HF. Physiology of the choroid plexus. Physiol Rev 1971;51(2):273–311.

153. Netsky MG, Samruay S. The Choroid Plexus in Health and Disease. Charlottesville, VA: University Press of Virginia, 1975.

154. Milhorat TH. Structure and function of the choroid plexus and other sites of cerebrospinal fluid formation. Int Rev Cytol 1976;47:225–88.

155. Wright EM. Transport processes in the formation of the cerebrospinal fluid. Rev Physiol Biochem Pharmacol 1978;83:3–34.

156. Spector R, Johanson CE. The mammalian choroid plexus. Sci Am 1989;261(5):68–74.

157. Price DL, James AE Jr, Sperber E, Strecker EP. Communicating hydrocephalus. Cisternographic and neuropathologic studies. Arch Neurol 1976;33(1):15–20.

158. Eisenberg HM, McComb JG, Lorenzo AV. Cerebrospinal fluid overproduction and hydrocephalus associated with choroid plexus papilloma. J Neurosurg 1974;40(3):381–5.

159. Treves ST, Welch K, Kuruc A. Cerebrospinal fluid. In: Treves ST, ed. Pediatric Nuclear Medicine. New York: Springer-Verlag, 1985: 223–31.

160. Dichiro G. Movement of the cerebrospinal fluid in human beings. Nature 1964;204:290–1.

161. Bannister R, Gilford E, Kocen R. Isotope encephalography in the diagnosis of dementia due to communicating hydrocephalus. Lancet 1967;2(7524):1014–7.

162. Benson DF, LeMay M, Patten DH, Rubens AB. Diagnosis of normal-pressure hydrocephalus. N Engl J Med 1970;283(12):609–15.

163. Glasauer FE, Alker GJ, Leslie EV, Nicol CF. Isotope cisternography in hydrocephalus with normal pressure: case report and technical note. J Neurosurg 1968;29:555–61.

164. Greitz T, Grepe A. Encephalography in the diagnosis of convexity block hydrocephalus. Acta Radiol Diagn 1971;11(3):232–42.

165. Rau H, Fas A, Horst W, Baumgartner G. [Clinical observations on communicating hydrocephalus of unknown etiology (author's transl).] J Neurol 1974;207(4):279–87.

166. Shenkin HA, Crowley JN. Hydrocephalus complicating pituitary adenoma. J Neurol Neurosurg Psychiatry 1973;36(6):1063–8.

167. Tator CH, Murray S. A clinical, pneumoencephalographic and radioisotopic study of normal-pressure communicating hydrocephalus. Can Med Assoc J 1971;105(6):573–9.

168. O'Brien MD, Haggith JW, Appleton D. Cerebro-spinal fluid dynamics in dementia. Exp Brain Res 1982;suppl 5:196–200.

169. Donn SM, Roloff DW, Keyes JW Jr. Lumbar cisternography in evaluation of hydrocephalus in the preterm infant. Pediatrics 1983;72(5): 670–6.

170. Khan EA, Luros JT. Hydrocephalus from overproduction of cerebrospinal fluid. J Neurosurg 1952;9:59–67.

171. Matson DD. Hydrocephalus in a premature infant caused by papilloma of the choroid plexus; with report of surgical treatment. J Neurosurg 1953;10(4):416–20.

172. Matson DD, Crofton FD. Papilloma of the choroid plexus in childhood. J Neurosurg 1960;17:1002–27.

173. Ray BS, Peck FC Jr. Papilloma of the choroid plexus of the lateral ventricles causing hydrocephalus in an infant. J Neurosurg 1956;13(4): 317–22.

174. Johnson RT. Clinicopathological aspects of the cerebrospinal fluid circulation. In: Wolstenholme GEW, O'Connor CM, eds. Ciba Foundation Symposium on the Cerebrospinal Fluid; Production, Circulation and Absorption. Boston: Little, Brown, 1958:265–78.

175. Caldicott WJ, North JB, Simpson DA. Traumatic cerebrospinal fluid fistulas in children. J Neurosurg 1973;38(1):1–9.

176. Cowan RJ, Maynard CD. Trauma to the brain and extracranial structures. Semin Nucl Med 1974;4(4):319–38.

177. Harwood-Nash DC. Fractures of the petrous and tympanic parts of the temporal bone in children: a tomographic study of 35 cases. AJR Radium Ther Nucl Med 1970;110(3):598–607.

178. Lantz EJ, Forbes GS, Brown ML, Laws ER, Jr. Radiology of cerebrospinal fluid rhinorrhea. AJR 1980;135(5):1023–30.

179. Wocjan J, Klisiewicz R, Krolicki L. Overpressure radionuclide cisternography and metrizamide computed tomographic cisternography in the detection of intermittent rhinoliquorrheas in children. Childs Nerv System 1989;5(4): 238–40.

180. Jaffe B, Welch K, Strand R, Treves S. Cerebrospinal fluid rhinorrhea via the fossa of Rosenmuller. Laryngoscope 1976;86(7): 903–7.

181. McLennan JE, Mickle JP, Treves S. Radionuclide cisternographic evaluation and follow-up of posttraumatic subconjunctival CSF loculation. Case report. J Neurosurg 1976;44(4):496–9.

182. Ferreira S, Jhingran SG, Johnson PC. Radionuclide cisternography for the study of arachnoid cysts: a case report. Neuroradiology 1980;19(3): 167–9.

183. Front D, Minderhoud JM, Beks JW, Penning L. Leptomeningeal cysts diagnosed by isotope cisternography. J Neurol Neurosurg Psychiatry 1973;36(6):1018–23.

184. Harbert J, Haddad D, McCullough D. Quantitation of cerebrospinal fluid shunt flow. Radiology 1974;112(2):379–87.

185. Kuruc A, Treves S, Welch K, Merlino D. Radionuclide estimation of cerebrospinal fluid shunt flow. Evidence supporting an alternative theoretical model. J Neurosurg 1984;60(2): 361–4.

186. Rudd TG, Shurtleff DB, Loeser JD, Nelp WB. Radionuclide assessment of cerebrospinal fluid shunt function in children. J Nucl Med 1973; 14(9):683–6.

187. Gelfand MJ, Walus M, Tomsick T, Benton C, McLaurin R. Nasoethmoidal encephalomeningocele demonstrated by cisternography: case report. J Nucl Med 1977;18(7):706–8.

188. Lusins J, Nakagawa H, Sorek M, Goldsmith S. Cisternography and CT scanning with 111In-DTPA in evaluation of posterior fossa arachnoid cysts. Clin Nucl Med 1979;4(4):161–3.

189. Marinov M, Undjian S, Wetzka P. An evaluation of the surgical treatment of intracranial arachnoid cysts in children. Childs Nerv System 1989;5(3):177–83.

3
Thyroid

Stephen A. Huang

Thyroid scintigraphy plays an important role in the evaluation of the thyroid gland owing to the functional and anatomic information it provides. Ultrasound-guided fine-needle aspiration (FNA), as well as the increased availability of sensitive serum assays for thyrotropin (thyroid-stimulating hormone, TSH) and thyroglobulin (Tg), play an important role in the routine evaluation of thyroid disease. However, measurement of radioactive iodine uptake remains the only direct test of thyroid function and, when complemented by studies that permit anatomic correlation, scintigraphy is a powerful tool in the investigation of both benign and malignant thyroid disorders. This chapter focuses on the role of radioiodine in the diagnosis and therapy of hyperthyroidism and in the treatment and surveillance of children with differentiated thyroid cancer (DTC). The rarity of these diseases in children has precluded the generation of consensus guidelines, but approaches for the evaluation of thyroid nodules and for the preparation of patients prior to iodine-131 (^{131}I) therapy are suggested.

Method

Radiopharmaceuticals

This chapter focuses on the three radiopharmaceuticals routinely employed in clinical thyroid practice: ^{131}I, ^{123}I, and technetium-99m (^{99m}Tc)O$_4$. Several noniodine radiopharmaceuticals have been used for thyroid scintigraphy, including thallium-201 (^{201}Tl), technetium-99m-methoxyisobutylisotitrile (^{99m}Tc-sestamibi), ^{99m}Tc–tetrafosmin, and fluorine-18-fluorodeoxyglucose (^{18}F-FDG).[1] The utility of these radionuclides in the imaging of differentiated thyroid cancer patients who have measurable serum Tg but negative radioiodine scans is an area of active investigation. However, their clinical application is controversial and their role in pediatrics has yet to be established.

Iodine-131 (^{131}I)

Radioactive isotopes of iodine are physiologically indistinguishable from the naturally occurring iodine-127 (^{127}I). Iodine-131 (^{131}I) (physical half-life 8.1 days; gamma emission 364 keV) has been used in thyroid scintigraphy for decades. Its advantages include wide availability and relatively low cost. Its major disadvantage is its high radiation absorbed dose due to its long physical half-life and beta-particle emission. These features make ^{131}I inappropriate for routine scintigraphy in pediatric patients but useful for the therapeutic ablation of benign or malignant thyroid follicular cells.

Iodine-123 (^{123}I)

For pediatric thyroid scintigraphy, ^{123}I (physical half-life 0.55 days; gamma emission 159 keV) is the ideal isotope. Due to its short half-life and the absence of beta radiation, compared to ^{131}I, ^{123}I delivers only 1% of radiation to the thyroid per millicurie administered. The energy of its main gamma ray is ideal for detection by gamma cameras, and so it is routinely used for thyroid uptake and scans. Recent data suggest that it is also superior to ^{131}I for diagnostic whole-body scans in patients with differentiated thyroid cancer. Disadvantages include more limited availability and high expense.[2] A tracer quantity of inorganic radioiodine (^{123}I or ^{131}I) is administered orally and then rapidly equilibrates with the endogenous [127]I in the extracellular fluid. Plasma levels of radioiodine fall exponentially with more than 90% of the administered dose removed by the thyroid and kidneys at the end of 24 hours.[3] However, the thyroid iodine concentration increases to a plateau [radioactive iodine uptake (RAIU) at plateau $= C_t/(C_t + C_k)$] defined by the relative clearance of iodide by the thyroid (C_t) and the kidneys (C_k).

Technetium-99m Pertechnetate ($^{99m}Tc\text{-}NaO_4^-$)

^{99m}Tc-pertechnetate (Tc-NaO4) (physical half-life 6 hours; gamma emission 140 keV) is a monovalent anion that, like iodine, is actively transported by the sodium-iodine symporter (NaIS) and can therefore be used to measure thyroid uptake. Unlike iodine, it undergoes negligible organic binding and rapidly diffuses out of the thyroid as its plasma concentration falls. ^{99m}Tc-pertechnetate is administered by intravenous injection with scintigraphy performed within 30 minutes of administration during peak thyroid activity. Advantages include its wide availability, low cost, low radiation exposure, and the short interval required for scintigraphy. Also, as ^{99m}Tc-pertechnetate only measures uptake, scans can be performed during antithyroid treatment with thionamides. Disadvantages include its relatively low thyroid uptake (4.0% 20 minutes after administration), its susceptibility to background artifact from salivary and vascular activity, and its low sensitivity in the detection of hypofunctioning thyroid nodules. Salivary and vascular activity can obscure uptake in the lateral neck and thorax; therefore, ^{99m}Tc-pertechnetate is not appropriate for the assessment of substernal/intrathoracic goiters or metastatic DTC. For scintigraphy that is performed to evaluate possible thyroid ectopy, patients should be instructed to drink water before imaging to reduce background activity from saliva; early images (5 minutes after administration) before salivary uptake is high are helpful. Approximately 5% to 10% of thyroid tumors that are hypofunctioning on radioiodine scintigraphy appear to be functioning with ^{99m}Tc-pertechnetate, presumably because these nodules can trap but not organify iodine.[4] This can lead to the false conclusion that a thyroid nodule is functioning and therefore benign. Accordingly ^{99m}Tc-pertechnetate scintigraphy is not appropriate to evaluate the malignant potential of thyroid nodules.

Thyroid Scintigraphy

Thyroid follicular cells concentrate iodine under the regulation of thyrotropin (TSH) via the NaIS. Thyroid scintigraphy should be interpreted in the context of anatomic and biochemical data. This information should be obtained prior to scintigraphy to evaluate thyroid dysfunction or a palpable thyroid mass.[5] Before scintigraphy, full thyroid function tests [TSH, thyroxine (T_4), THBR] should be obtained and the physician should palpate the thyroid gland to document thyroid size and the location of any discrete mass. The normal thyroid gland is bilobed and connected by an isthmus that overlies the second through fourth tracheal cartilages. The main lobes of the thyroid are usually equal in size, but the right lobe is frequently a little larger and tends to enlarge to a greater degree that the left in patients with diffuse thyromegaly. Assessment of goiter should take into account the normal thyroid size for age. Several pediatric norms have been published. The equation of $T = 1.48 + 0.054A$, where T is the weight of the thyroid in grams and A is the age in months, describes the average thyroid weight from birth to 20 years.[6] In North America, the normal adult thyroid weighs approximately 14 to 20 g (average weight 14.4 g for females 20 to 69 years of age; 16.4 g for males 20 to 29 years of age; 18.5 g for males 30 to 69 years of age).[7,8] If a thyroid ultrasound has been obtained prior to scintigraphy, the mass of the gland in grams can

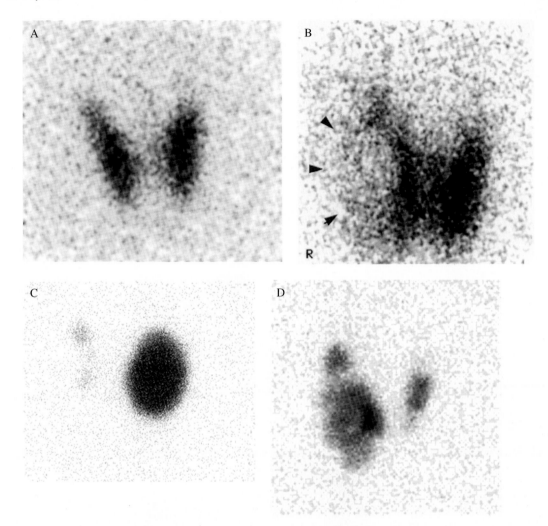

FIGURE 3.1. Iodine-123 (^{123}I) thyroid scans in the evaluation of nodular disease. A: Normal bilobed thyroid gland. B: Hypofunctioning nodule replacing most of the right thyroid lobe. C: Hyperfunctioning thyroid nodule in an 18-year-old woman who presented with hyperthyroidism [serum thyroid-stimulating hormone (TSH) 0.008 μU/mL] and a 3.4-cm palpable nodule in the left lobe. An ^{123}I thyroid scan revealed a corresponding focus of uptake with minimal activity in the contralateral lobe due to TSH suppression. D: Toxic multinodular goiter in a 15-year-old girl who presented with subclinical hyperthyroidism (serum TSH 0.11 μU/mL) and a 3-cm nodule palpable in the right lobe. An ^{123}I thyroid scan revealed several areas of uptake, and comparison of multiple scintigraphy images (anterior, lateral, and oblique) with thyroid ultrasound permitted correlation of each foci to a thyroid nodule.

be estimated using the formula for a rotational ellipsoid (length (cm) × width (cm) × depth (cm) × π/6 for each lobe).[9,10]

Most nuclear medicine departments use a gamma camera equipped with a pin-hole collimator (aperture <3 mm) for routine thyroid scintigraphy. Images are obtained for 25,000 to 150,000 counts with imaging times ranging from 5 to 15 minutes. Thyroid scintigraphy of the normal gland reveals the thyroid silhouette (Fig. 3.1A). Depending on thyroid size and function, the isthmus may not be visualized. Oblique images may clarify the location of thyroid nodules, and anatomic correlation may

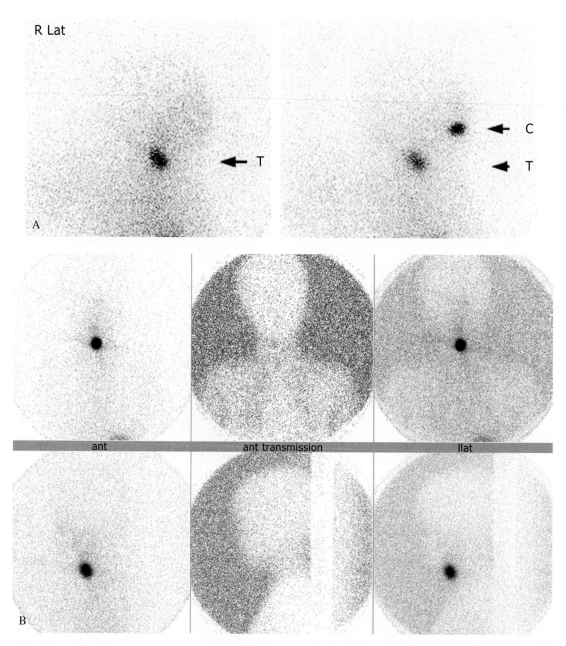

Figure 3.2. [123]I thyroid scans in the evaluation of thyroid dysgenesis. A: [123]I uptake by an ectopic sublingual thyroid gland (T) in a patient with congenital hypothyroidism. Localization was facilitated by using a radioactive marker at the level of the chin (C). B: Thyroglossal duct cyst with ectopic thyroid tissue. This patient was diagnosed with congenital hypothyroidism by newborn screening and presented later at the age of 7 years with a midline neck mass that moved with tongue protrusion. A preoperative ^{123}I scan revealed uptake that localized to the palpable mass. Localization was facilitated by transmission images.

be further improved through the use of markers or by using a transmission scan to outline body margins (Fig. 3.2).

Patients are scanned in the supine position with the neck extended. Thyroid uptake measurements and scintigraphy are typically performed 4 hours and 24 hours after the administration of radioiodine as this approximates the achievement of this plateau. In some patients with severe hyperthyroidism, the release of hormone from the gland is so rapid that RAIU has returned to normal range by 24 hours; therefore, the early uptake measurement at 4 hours can be helpful. Images of the patient's thigh and of the imaging table without the patient present are used to correct for body and room background activity, respectively. Radioactive iodine uptake indicates the rate of thyroid hormone synthesis and, indirectly, the rate of thyroid hormone secretion. In general, the normal values for RAIU in North America range from 5% to 25% and vary inversely with dietary iodine intake. In our laboratory, normal values of pediatric RAIU range from 5% to 12% at 4 hours and 10% to 30% at 24 hours after radiotracer administration. Dietary iodine and exposure to excessive iodine are important causes of a low RAIU. Iodinated radiographic contrast media, amiodarone, and solutions of inorganic iodide administered in the initial therapy of hyperthyroidism are common sources, and iodinated antiseptics such as povidone, certain vaginal/rectal suppositories, and dietary sources such as kelp can also be contributors. Such exposures can impair the interpretation of RAIU for months or, in the case of amiodarone, even longer due to its storage in fat. A brief medication and dietary history should be obtained prior RAIU to determine if any of these sources are relevant. If in question, iodine status can be estimated by a random simultaneous measurement of urinary iodine (I_U) and urine creatinine (Cr_U). Assuming that the I_U/Cr_U ratio is grossly constant and that approximately 20 mg of creatinine is excreted daily per kg of ideal body weight (IBW) in a child, the following formula can be used to estimate daily urinary excretion where I_U is the urinary iodine concentration in μg/L and Cr_U is the urinary creatinine concentration in mg/dL

(μg of iodine excreted per day = [IBW × I_U × 20 mg creatinine/kg] ÷ [Cr_U × 10]). If estimated daily urinary iodine excretion exceeds 1000 μg, deferring scintigraphy and initiating a low-iodine diet should be considered.

Clinical Applications

Primary Hypothyroidism

Congenital hypothyroidism occurs with a frequency of 1 per 3000 to 4000 births. Approximately 15% of cases are hereditary (autosomal recessive inheritance), and the remaining 85% are sporadic and usually due to thyroid dysgenesis.[11] Thyroid hormone is critical to infantile neurodevelopment, and the etiology of hypothyroidism does not affect initial therapy. As genetic testing for most hereditary forms of congenital hypothyroidism is not clinically available and newborn screening is mandatory in the United States, the indications for thyroid imaging are controversial. In the newborn period, ultrasound offers the potential to diagnose thyroid dysgenesis. Another approach is to attempt a trial of decreased levothyroxine therapy in all patients after 3 years of age when hypothyroidism carries a lower risk of neurologic injury. Patients who remain euthyroid without exogenous replacement can be assumed to have transient congenital hypothyroidism as has been described from the transplacental transfer of maternal thyroid antibodies. For those children who become hypothyroid, thyroid scintigraphy with ^{123}I or ^{99m}Tc-pertechnetate (TcO$_4$) can be performed (Fig. 3.2). Outside of the newborn period, most acquired hypothyroidism is due to autoimmune thyroiditis. The presence of circulating antithyroid antibodies is sufficient to diagnosis this and, because as many as 90% of patients with autoimmune hypothyroidism have detectable circulating anti-TPO antibodies, scintigraphy adds little further diagnostic benefit.[12]

Hyperthyroidism

The term *thyrotoxicosis* refers to the manifestations of excessive quantities of circulating thyroid hormone. In contrast, hyperthyroidism refers only to the subset of thyrotoxic diseases that are caused by the overproduction of hormone by the thyroid itself. Hyperthyroidism is relatively rare in children (yearly incidence of 8 per 1,000,000 children less than 15 years old and 1 per 1,000,000 children less than 4 years old), but the ability to accurately diagnose it is critical as antithyroid drugs have no role in the treatment of thyrotoxicosis without hyperthyroidism.[13] Biochemical thyrotoxicosis, recognized by an elevation of serum free T_4 (or FT_4I) with a decreased serum TSH (typically less than $0.1\,\mu U/mL$), should be confirmed by laboratory studies prior to considering scintigraphy. A determination of the FT_3I should be added only if TSH is suppressed and the serum free T_4 is normal. Once biochemical derangement has been documented, it is helpful to address the duration of thyrotoxicosis to facilitate the differentiation of Graves' disease from painless thyroiditis. Onset may be documented by prior laboratory studies or inferred from the review of symptoms. If thyrotoxicosis has been present for less than 8 weeks, transient thyrotoxicosis secondary to subacute thyroiditis or the thyrotoxic phase of autoimmune/silent thyroiditis should be considered. These forms of thyroiditis are self-limited and refractory to therapy with thionamides. Thyrotoxicosis that has been present for more than 8 weeks suggests true hyperthyroidism with Graves' as the most likely etiology. In the majority of these cases, the palpation of a symmetrically enlarged thyroid coupled with the chronicity of symptoms is adequate to allow a clinical diagnosis of Graves' diseases without additional laboratory tests or imaging studies. However, if thyromegaly is subtle and eye changes are absent, an ^{123}I uptake, with or without a scan, should be performed.

The differential diagnosis of thyrotoxicosis includes Graves' hyperthyroidism, hyperfunctioning nodule(s), transient thyroiditis, and thyrotoxicosis factitia (Table 3.1).[14] Radioactive iodine uptake is high in hyperthyroidism. In contrast, RAIU is low during the thyrotoxic phase of transient thyroiditis. Radioiodine uptake is diffusely increased in Graves' hyperthyroidism. In patients with a toxic nodule, ^{123}I

TABLE 3.1. Differential diagnosis of thyrotoxicosis in children

Thyrotoxicosis associated with sustained hormone overproduction (hyperthyroidism) (high RAIU)
Graves' disease
Toxic multinodular goiter
Toxic adenoma
Increased TSH secretion

Thyrotoxicosis without associated hyperthyroidism (low RAIU)
Thyrotoxicosis factitia
Subacute thyroiditis
Chronic thyroiditis with transient thyroiditis (painless thyroiditis, silent thyroiditis, postpartum thyroiditis)
Ectopic thyroid tissue (struma ovarii, functioning metastatic thyroid cancer)

RAIU, radioactive iodine uptake.
Source: Adapted from *William's Textbook of Endocrinology*, 10th ed., with permission from Elsevier.[14]

uptake localizes to the nodule and the signal in the surrounding tissue will be low secondary to TSH suppression (Fig. 3.1C,D). Autonomous nodules must be large to cause hyperthyroidism (typically 2.5 cm or more in diameter), so, with careful physical examination by an experienced clinician, radioiodine scanning can be reserved for patients in whom a discrete nodule(s) is palpable. Thyrotoxicosis factitia can be recognized by a low RAIU and serum thyroglobulin in the presence of thyrotoxicosis and a suppressed TSH.

Radioiodine Ablation for Hyperthyroidism

The treatment of Graves' hyperthyroidism may be divided into two categories: antithyroid medications and definitive therapy. The thionamide derivatives Tapazole (methimazole, MMI) and propylthiouracil (PTU) are the most commonly used antithyroid drugs.[15] For severe hyperthyroidism, inorganic iodine is used to speed the fall in circulating thyroid hormones. Reports of long-term remission rates in children treated with antithyroid drug are variable, ranging from 30% to 60%.[16,17] The two options for the definitive treatment of Graves' disease are ^{131}I and thyroidectomy. Both are likely to result in lifelong hypothyroidism, and there is disagreement in the literature as to their indications. Some centers consider these modalities as options for the initial treatment of pediatric hyperthyroidism.[18-20] However, as a remission of Graves' disease occurs in a significant percentage of children, we recommend the long-term use of antithyroid medications until young adulthood. If patient noncompliance prevents the successful treatment of thyrotoxicosis or both antithyroid medications must be discontinued secondary to serious drug reactions, definitive therapy is appropriate.

Therapeutic administration of ^{131}I is the definitive treatment of choice in adults. Concerns over the potential long-term complications of pediatric radiation exposure have traditionally made endocrinologists cautious in applying this approach to children, but ^{131}I is experiencing wider acceptance within pediatrics.[21] It is estimated that more than 1000 children have received ^{131}I for the treatment of Graves' disease.[17] To date, there are no reports of an increase in the incidence of thyroid carcinoma or leukemia in this population.[21-24] Despite the reassurances found in this literature, experience with x-rays and the Chernobyl nuclear power plant accident indicate that the carcinogenic effects of radiation to the thyroid are highest in young children.[25-27] This argues for continued surveillance and, for children who fail antithyroid medication, the provision of an ^{131}I dose adequate to destroy all thyroid follicular cells. Some institutions administer an empiric dose of 3 to 15 mCi (111 to 555 MBq) or a dose based on the estimated weight of the gland (50 to 200 microcuries per gram of thyroid tissue).[17,23,24] An analysis of radioiodine therapy at the Brigham and Women's Hospital included 261 Graves' patients.[28] Successful outcome, defined as hypothyroidism after a single dose of radioiodine, was associated with significantly higher doses of [131]I (178.1 μCi/g (6.6 MBq/g) compared to 141.3 μCi/g (5.2 MBq/g) in the treatment failure group, $p < .01$). Patients who failed single-dose treatment tended to be young with biochemically more severe hyperthyroidism and a history of pretreatment with antithyroid medications. Efficacy is dependent on both thyroid uptake and mass, so we perform an ^{123}I RAIU prior to treatment and prescribe a dose that provides approximately 200 μCi/g (7.4 MBq/g) estimated weight in the gland at 24 hours. We limit the dose to a maximum of 11 mCi (407 MBq) total into the gland at 24 hours (corrected for uptake).

Dose [131]I = (200 μCi/g (7.4 MBq/g) × estimated weight of thyroid in grams × 100)/ (% uptake at 24 hours)

Radioiodine therapy is also used to treat adults with thyrotoxicosis secondary to hyperfunctioning "hot" thyroid nodule(s). When TSH is suppressed, the normal thyroid parenchyma is theoretically protected from radioiodine uptake, and euthyroidism without exogenous levothyroxine has been described in patients several years after ^{131}I therapy.[29,30] Radioiodine therapy is not recommended, however, for children with hyperfunctioning nodules because of the greater sensitivity of the pediatric thyroid to radiation and the theoretical concern that the rim of normal parenchyma surrounding the nodule will receive a subcytotoxic dose of radiation that will predispose to the development of thyroid cancer. Children with thyrotoxicosis from hyperfunctioning nodule(s) are frequently treated with surgical resection or, alternatively, maintained with antithyroid medication until they are young adults and ^{131}I can be administered.

Practical Aspects of [131]I Therapy for Hyperthyroidism

All therapeutic options should be discussed with the family prior to their consent for treatment. Radioiodine is contraindicated in pregnant or lactating women, and so, for postmenarchal females, a negative serum human chorionic gonadotropin (hCG) measurement should be documented prior to its administration and pregnancy avoided for at least 6 months after [131]I. For children who are unable to swallow a capsule, a liquid preparation of ^{131}I is available. In severely hyperthyroid patients, inorganic iodine [saturated solution of potassium iodide (SSKI) three drops po b.i.d. for 5 to 10 days] can be used to rapidly restore euthyroidism, but its use should be avoided until 3 days post-^{131}I to avoid competition with therapeutic uptake. Similarly, thionamides should be discontinued for at least 3 days prior to ^{131}I administration and resumed no sooner than 7 days posttreatment. As in adults, the frequency of acute side effects is low, but nausea and vomiting occur in a significant minority of children, and so antiemetic medications such as ondansetron and lorazepam should be available for pro re nata (prn, as needed) use.[20] Patients should be informed that the response to ^{131}I therapy typically takes months, and clinicians should wait 6 months before concluding that a treatment has failed and offering a second ^{131}I dose. Patients should be counseled that definitive therapy does not eliminate circulating TSH-receptor antibodies, and so Graves' orbitopathy and fetal thyroid dysfunction due to transplacental antibody transfer can occur even after successful ablation.[31,32]

The transition to adulthood should prompt a repeated discussion of therapy. For young adults with persistent hyperthyroidism, ^{131}I is the current treatment of choice. An RAIU is performed prior to treatment, with the goal of delivering approximately 8 mCi (296 MBq) of ^{131}I into the gland at 24 hours. For glands larger than three times normal size, about 11 mCi (407 MBq) is required.[28] Definitive therapy typically results in permanent hypothyroidism, but it allows for a simpler regimen of medication and laboratory monitoring (daily levothyroxine and a yearly TSH measurement). Definitive therapy simplifies the management of female patients during pregnancy.

Nodular Thyroid Disease

The frequency of nodular thyroid disease increases with age. Thyroid nodules are rare in children (estimated frequency of 0.05% to 1.8%)[33–35] and more common in adults (present in up to 50% of adults after the sixth decade of life). In comparison to the 5% to 10% cancer prevalence cited for adults, early pediatric series reported a 40% to 60% prevalence of thyroid cancer in children with thyroid nodules.[4,34,35] More recent studies estimate the cancer prevalence of pediatric thyroid nodules to be 5% to 33%.[36–45] The reason for this discrepancy is

not clear, although differences in cohort size, geographic variation, improvements in thyroid screening, and the discontinuation of the practice of neck irradiation for benign conditions are speculated to be contributors. As thyroid cancer prognosis depends in part on tumor size, the early identification of differentiated thyroid cancer is the primary goal in the evaluation of nodular thyroid disease.[46]

Upon referral, the medical history should include inquiry into prior neck irradiation, family history of thyroid cancer or multiple endocrine neoplasia type II (MEN-II), and any extrathyroidal manifestations suspicious of other syndromes associated with nodular thyroid disease (Cowden's syndrome, Bannayan-Riley-Ruvalcaba syndrome, familial adenomatous polyposis, gigantism, etc.).[47–49] A complete review of systems should include symptoms of thyroid dysfunction and neck compression (dysphagia, hoarseness, pain, etc.). Physical examination should include palpation of both the thyroid gland and the cervical lymph nodes, and the initial laboratory evaluation should include thyroid function testing (measurement of serum TSH concentration) to screen for autonomous/hyperfunctioning nodule(s). Almost all malignant nodules are hypofunctioning by scintigraphy, but more than 80% of benign nodules are also hypofunctioning (Fig. 3.1B).[4] Therefore, the author recommends that ^{123}I scintigraphy be reserved for patients with suppressed serum TSH concentrations. For all others, ultrasound is the most cost-effective imaging modality to confirm the presence of a thyroid nodule.

In a retrospective review of 223 adults referred for suspected nodular thyroid disease, ultrasound altered clinical management in 63% due to the detection of nonpalpable nodules or the determination that no nodules met the criteria for biopsy.[50] This illustrates the limitations of physical examination alone. We recommend that thyroid ultrasonography be performed in all children with suspected thyroid nodules prior to any attempt at biopsy. Ultrasound-guided FNA is the procedure of choice for the cytologic evaluation of thyroid nodules, as it improves the diagnostic accuracy of FNA guided by palpation alone and reduces the likelihood of accidental penetration into the trachea or the great vessels.[51–55] Furthermore, ultrasound guidance is necessary to successfully biopsy nodules that are primarily cystic or non-palpable due to their location in the posterior aspect of the gland. Papillary thyroid cancer is the most common malignant tumor of the thyroid (85% to 90% of pediatric thyroid cancers) and is characterized by nuclear abnormalities that are readily identifiable by cytology.[56] However, even under optimal conditions, cytology alone cannot accurately differentiate follicular adenomas from follicular carcinoma, as the latter diagnosis requires the documentation of capsular or vascular invasion. Despite this limitation, cytology should be obtained in all patients prior to considering surgery. Benign cytology obviates surgical resection. Conversely, in patients with atypical cytology, the degree and type of cytologic abnormality allows a more specific assignment of cancer risk and facilitates the discussion of surgical options with the family.

Suggested Approach for Evaluation of Pediatric Thyroid Nodules

A serum TSH measurement should be obtained prior to endocrine consultation for nodular thyroid disease. If the patient's serum TSH concentration is suppressed, an ^{123}I scan is obtained to address the possibility of a hyperfunctioning nodule. Children with normal to elevated serum TSH concentrations are sent to ultra-sonography and any thyroid nodule ≥1 cm in diameter is biopsied by ultrasound-guided FNA. Classification of biopsy interpretations into cytologic risk categories facilitates the decision of surgical approach, based on the likelihood of malignancy associated with the patient's specific category and an individual assessment of the child's operative risks. Children with thyroid nodules <1 cm or with benign cytology should have long-term follow-up by serial ultrasonography every 6 to 12 months, and ultrasound-guided FNA should be repeated if significant interval growth or other concerning sonographic features develop.

Differentiated Thyroid Cancer

Follicular cell–derived cancers (FCDCs) are by far the most common thyroid malignancies; it is divided into three categories: papillary thyroid cancer (PTC), follicular thyroid cancer (FTC), and anaplastic thyroid cancer. In North America, PTC is the most common FCDC, comprising 75% to 80% of adult thyroid cancers and 85% to 90% of pediatric thyroid cancers.[46,57] Like PTC and FTC, anaplastic thyroid cancers originate from follicular cells and stain for thyroglobulin by immunohisto-chemistry. However, anaplastic cancers are relatively poorly differentiated and characterized by aggressive growth and poor prognosis. For this reason, the terms *differentiated thyroid cancer* (DTC) and *well-differentiated thyroid cancer* (WDTC) are generally used to refer to PTC and FTC. The endocrine management of DTC is predicated on the principle that these tumors retain some properties of normal differentiated thyroid follicular cells, such as responsiveness to TSH, Tg secretion, and the ability to concentrate iodine. While endocrinologists may also participate in the diagnosis and management of patients with other thyroid tumors, it is important to recognize that the interventions of TSH suppression and radioiodine ablation are specific to DTC and have no established role in the treatment of thyroid tumors of nonfollicular origin.

Epidemiology

Thyroid cancer comprises 90% of all endocrine cancers with approximately 18,000 new diagnoses and 1200 thyroid cancer-related deaths annually in the United States.[58] In comparison to those in adults, pediatric thyroid cancers are rare (incidence of 0.3 to 0.5 per 100,000 population annually) and are characterized by high rates of regional lymph node (74%) and distant (25%) metastases.[59,60] Rates of recurrence (13% to 42%) are also higher in children, illustrated in one series of 50 children where 28% developed distant metastases, 8% upon initial presentation and 20% as recurrences.[58–61] The relative rarity of pediatric thyroid cancer has prevented the publication of many large series, and reports of cause-specific mortality (CSM) vary widely from 0% to 18%.[60,62–74] As this is superior to the survival rates of many other pediatric cancers and similar to general adult DTC statistics (25-year CSM of 5% for PTC and 34% for FTC), the outcome of pediatric DTC is generally referred to in the literature as favorable.[3] However, the direct comparison of pediatric and adult DTC statistics is problematic due to the shorter duration of follow-up in most pediatric series and the fact that the majority of CSM in adult DTC occurs in a minority of patients with high-risk factors. Approximately 84% of adult PTC patients present with favorable risk factors (MACIS score <6) and are predicted to have a 20-year CSM of <0.6%.[75] Therefore, when controlled for duration of follow-up and staging, most published pediatric CSM rates are actually higher than for the vast majority of adult DTC patients.

Primary Therapy (Surgery)

Cytologic abnormalities that suggest malignancy warrant surgical resection with either unilateral (lobectomy) or bilateral (total) thyroidectomy. In practice, bilateral thyroidectomy is the most common operation performed for both adults (77.4%) and children (79%) with DTC, but debate persists among experts as to the optimal degree of resection for patients with "minimal" DTC that appears on imaging to be confined to one lobe.[59,60,76–78] As reduction of the thyroid remnant facilitates radioiodine ablation and subsequent disease surveillance, the author recommends bilateral thyroidectomy as the default procedure for children with DTC. For the rare low-risk patient with a solitary microfocus of PTC or minimally invasive FTC, the literature suggests that prognosis is excellent regardless of the specific surgical treatment, so the necessity of completion thyroidectomy in this limited subpopulation is unproven. Regardless of the degree of resection, referral to a surgeon with extensive experience in pediatric thyroidectomy and a low complication rate is paramount, as the individual surgeon's experience has been shown to be the primary determinant of operative complications.[79]

Adjunctive Therapy (Thyroid-Stimulating Hormone Suppression)

Thyrotropin stimulates thyroid follicular cell growth. The suppression of endogenous TSH secretion reduces DTC recurrence and, in some series, decreases cancer-related death.[46] Modern serum TSH assays permit the precise titration of levothyroxine therapy and, with isolated TSH suppression, most patients are clinically euthyroid. Pediatric DTC is characterized by high rates of recurrence, and lesser degrees of TSH suppression are associated with an increased incidence of relapse.[80] Accordingly, serum TSH concentrations should be monitored every 3 to 6 months in children with DTC and levothyroxine therapy titrated to a goal serum TSH concentration of 0.1 μU/mL. Thyroid-stimulating hormone suppression should be interrupted only for stimulated radionuclide imaging or treatment as described below.

Adjunctive Therapy (Radioactive Iodine)

Even after total thyroidectomy, radioiodine uptake usually persists in the thyroid bed due to residual normal thyroid tissue. Ablation of this thyroid remnant with radioactive iodine (RAI) has been shown to lower recurrence rates and, in some series, to reduce cancer mortality, presumably due to the destruction of malignant or premalignant thyrocytes within the macroscopically normal remnant.[58] Similar to completion thyroidectomy, radioiodine remnant ablation (RRA) also facilitates disease surveillance by increasing the specificity of Tg measurements and the sensitivity of diagnostic whole body scans (dxWBS). Radioiodine remnant ablation is defined as "the destruction of residual macroscopically normal thyroid tissue after surgical thyroidectomy" and should be distinguished from the term *RAI therapy*, which describes the use of higher ^{131}I doses to destroy local or distant DTC.

Several groups have published dosimetric guidelines for effective RRA [30,000 rads (300 Gy) to remnant] and the RAI therapy of nodal metastases [10,000 rads (100 Gy)].[81,82] Administered ^{131}I doses should be calculated to deliver these therapeutic activities without exceeding safe radiation exposures to normal tissues such as the bone marrow and gonads. [131]I doses may be calculated by formal quantitative dosimetry or by using standardized empiric, fixed dose methods (see Chapter 4). Both of these approaches have been employed in children. Formulas for the estimation of relative pediatric doses have been generated based on average pediatric anthropometrics and the International Commission of Radiological Protection (ICRP) model of absorbed dose estimation.[83-85] As rule of thumb, individual ^{131}I doses should not exceed 200 mCi (7400 MBq) and total cumulative doses should be limited to 1000 mCi (37,000) MBq). The absorbed dose to the red marrow should be limited to 200 rad (2 Gy), and 48-hour whole-body retention should be limited to 120 mCi (4440 MBq) [or below 80 mCi (2960 MBq) in the setting of pulmonary metastases] to limit the risks of secondary acute myelogenous leukemia (AML) or pulmonary fibrosis, respectively.[86] If necessary, formal dosimetry should be performed in children with avid pulmonary metastases to ensure adherence to these thresholds. Tumor avidity and sensitivity to radioiodine can vary significantly between children with DTC and even within the same patient over time (Fig. 3.3). Accordingly, the diagnostic and therapeutic role of radioiodine must be individualized to each child through collaboration between the patient's endocrinologist and the nuclear medicine physician. An interval of at least 12 months between ^{131}I treatments is recommended to minimize the risk of secondary AML.[87]

Monitoring and Surveillance

Pediatric DTC can recur more than 30 years after initial surgery, so all children with DTC warrant long-term surveillance.[88] Radioactive iodine efficacy is inversely proportional to metastatic focus size, so the successful outcome of recurrent or metastatic thyroid cancer is dependent on early diagnosis and treatment.[86] Serum Tg is routinely employed as a tumor marker, but, as Tg is also produced by normal thyroid tissue, its greatest utility is realized only after thyroidectomy and remnant ablation. Based on data in adults, 68% of DTC recurrences are local (cervical or mediastinal).[58] Accordingly, surveillance should include annual neck imaging. Thyroid ultrasonography (US) is a sensitive and, when coupled with US-guided FNA, a specific method to screen for local recurrence. As the sensitivity of US is operator dependent, institutions with less experience may consider CT or MRI, remembering to avoid iodinated contrast. Local recurrences that are palpable or easily visualized with US or CT should be excised surgically rather than treated with [131]I.[89] Hyperthyrotropinemia increases the sensitivity of serum Tg and radionuclide scanning. Therefore, levothyroxine withdrawals should be performed through childhood with serum Tg measurements and diagnostic whole-body scanning performed during TSH elevation (Figs. 3.3 and 3.4). [123]I is the preferred agent for diagnostic whole-body scanning as it is a pure gamma emitter, which minimizes the patient's radiation exposure and avoids the theoretical concern of "stunning."[58] In general, withdrawals should be performed no more frequently than annually, as the ^{131}I treatments of any avid metastases detected by dxWBS should be separated by an interval of 12 months to minimize the risk of secondary AML.

Practical Considerations for Patients with Differentiated Thyroid Cancer

Clinical interventions can impact [131]I's biologic half-life within tissues. [131]I uptake into follicular thyrocytes is increased by hyperthyrotropinemia and the reduction of dietary iodine uptake.[90] Levothyroxine withdrawal is the standard method of achieving hyperthyrotropinemia. The traditional method of thyroid hormone withdrawal for the preparation of radioiodine administration is a 6-week protocol that includes the transient administration of triiodothyronine. However, in our experience, adequate hyperthyrotropinemia ($\geq 25\,\mu U/mL$) onsets 2 to 3 weeks after the simple discontinuation of levothyroxine. Recombinant human

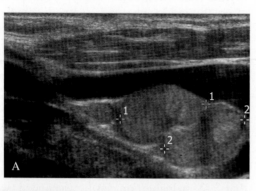

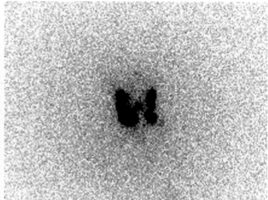

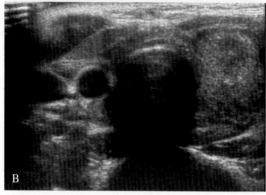

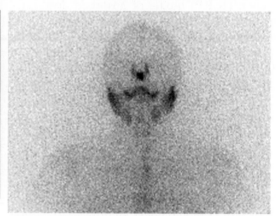

Figure 3.3. Variable iodine avidity in two patients with papillary thyroid cancer. A: A 7-year-old girl referred for treatment after two thyroid surgeries at an outside hospital had palpable bilateral lymphadenopathy and multiple enlarged/abnormal lymph nodes by ultrasonography (left panel, sagittal view of two enlarged right-sided cervical lymph nodes). An ^{123}I scan confirmed residual lymph node metastases by demonstrating corresponding uptake (right panel). These 12 metastatic lymph nodes were removed by a third surgery prior to treatment with

[131]I. B: A 15-year-old girl with a history of papillary thyroid cancer treated at the age of 13 years presented to the emergency department with a palpable mass in the thyroid bed. Thyroid ultrasonography revealed a 4.2 × 2.7 × 2.1 cm mass (left panel, transverse slice) that was confirmed to be papillary thyroid cancer recurrence by ultrasound-guided fine-needle aspiration. A scan performed after a low-iodine diet revealed no corresponding ^{123}I uptake in the mass.

TSH (rhTSH) has been increasingly studied in the adult DTC population as an alternative to withdrawal for radionuclide imaging and remnant ablation, but similar studies in children have not yet been published, and rhTSH is currently not approved for use in patients under 16 years of age (Genzyme Corp., Cambridge, MA).[91,92]

Adherence to a low-iodine diet for 1 week will further increase the absorbed radiation dose to follicular cells.[93] A printable version of instructions for a low iodine diet, as well as recipes, is available on the Web site of the Thyroid Cancer Survivor's Association (www.thyca.org). Prepubertal children are more likely to experience nausea and vomiting with ^{131}I therapy, so antiemetic medications such as ondansetron and lorazepam should be available for prn use or administered prophylactically before ^{131}I in children who have vomited with prior RAI therapy.[20] Oral hydration, frequent urination, regular stooling, and

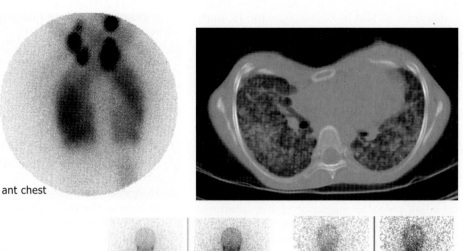

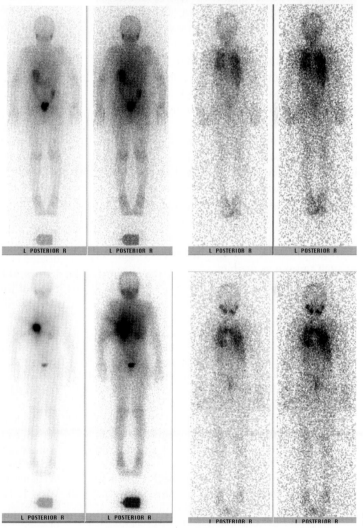

FIGURE 3.4. Whole-body scanning in differentiated thyroid cancer. A: A diagnostic whole-body scan performed in a teenage girl with papillary thyroid cancer revealed diffuse pulmonary uptake as well as the presence of residual post-operative cervical disease (left panel). Chest computed tomography (CT) confirmed the presence of multiple nodules in all lung fields, consistent with the typical pattern of pulmonary metastases from differentiated thyroid cancer (DTC). B: Serial scintigraphy performed in two patients with papillary thyroid cancer (a 7-year-old boy and a 9-year-old boy) illustrate the increased sensitivity of posttherapy whole-body scans (WBSs) performed 4 to 7 days after ^{131}I treatment (right panels) compared to even optimally performed diagnostic WBSs (left panels). Pulmonary metastases are visible only on the posttherapy scans.

sialagogues should be encouraged for 48 hours after ^{131}I administration to minimize radiation exposure to the intestinal tract, bladder, gonads, and the salivary glands. Levothyroxine therapy and normal diet can be reinstituted 2 days after ^{131}I administration.

As the diagnostic sensitivity of radioiodine scanning is proportional to the specific activity of the tracer, posttreatment scans are optimally sensitive and should be performed after all ^{131}I treatments (Fig. 3.4B).[94] If scintigraphy reveals a region of abnormal uptake without a corresponding palpable mass, correlative anatomic imaging should be performed, US for neck uptake, and CT or MRI for thoracic or central nervous system (CNS) uptake (Figs. 3.3A and 3.4A). In addition to the thyroid, iodine is also trapped by mammary tissue, the choroid plexus, and the salivary glands.[1] Radioiodine has also been reported to localize to the normal thymus prior to its involution.[95] Without proper care, uptake in these normal tissues and in the urinary and gastrointestinal tract as radioiodine is cleared can be misinterpreted as metastatic disease. Additional imaging and wash-ins over suspicious areas are helpful in these cases. An understanding of the pattern of DTC metastasis together with the measurement of serum thyroglobulin will often permit the recognition of such uptake as artifact.

References

1. Mc Dougall IR. In vivo radionuclide tests and imaging. In: Braverman LE, ed. Werner & Ingbar's The Thyroid. A Fundamental and Clinical Text. New York: Lippincott Williams & Wilkins, 2005:309–28.
2. Mandel SJ, Shankar LK, Benard F, Yamamoto A, Alavi A. Superiority of iodine-123 compared with iodine-131 scanning for thyroid remnants in patients with differentiated thyroid cancer. Clin Nucl Med 2001;26:6–9.
3. Berson SA, Yalow RS, Sorrentino J, Roswit B. The determination of thyroidal and renal plasma I131 clearance rates as a routine diagnostic test of thyroid dysfunction. J Clin Invest 1952;31: 141–58.
4. Schlumberger M, Filetti S, Hay ID. Nontoxic goiter and thyroid neoplasia. In: Larsen PR, Kronenberg HM, Melmed S, Polonsky KS, eds.
5. Williams Textbook of Endocrinology. Philadelphia: Saunders, 2002:457–90.
5. Paltiel HJ, Summerville DA, Treves ST. Iodine-123 scintigraphy in the evaluation of pediatric thyroid disorders: a ten year experience. Pediatr Radiol 1992;22:251–6.
6. Kay C, Abrahams S, McClain P. The weight of normal thyroid glands in children. Arch Pathol 1966;82:349–52.
7. Pankow BG, Michalak J, McGee MK. Adult human thyroid weight. Health Phys 1985;49: 1097–1103.
8. Mochizuki Y, Mowafy R, Pasternack B. Weights of Human Thyroids in New York City. Health Phys 1963;65:1299–1301.
9. Brunn J, Block U, Ruf G, Bos I, Kunze WP, Scriba PC. [Volumetric analysis of thyroid lobes by real-time ultrasound (author's transl).] Dtsch Med Wochenschr 1981;106:1338–40.
10. Tannahill AJ, Hooper MJ, England M, Ferriss JB, Wilson GM. Measurement of thyroid size by ultrasound, palpation and scintiscan. Clin Endocrinol (Oxf) 1978;8:483–6.
11. LaFranchi S. Congenital hypothyroidism: etiologies, diagnosis, and management. Thyroid 1999; 9:735–40.
12. Saravanan P, Dayan CM. Thyroid autoantibodies. Endocrinol Metab Clin North Am 2001;30: 315–37, viii.
13. Segni M, Leonardi E, Mazzoncini B, Pucarelli I, Pasquino AM. Special features of Graves' disease in early childhood. Thyroid 1999;9:871–7.
14. Davies TFLP. Thyrotoxicosis. In: Williams Textbook of Endocrinology. Philadelphia: Saunders. 2003:372–421.
15. Franklyn JA. The management of hyperthyroidism. N Engl J Med 1994;330:1731–8.
16. Rivkees SA, Sklar C, Freemark M. Clinical review 99: The management of Graves' disease in children, with special emphasis on radioiodine treatment. J Clin Endocrinol Metab 1998;83: 3767–76.
17. Lafranchi SHC. Graves' disease in the neonatal period and childhood. In Braverman LE, ed. Werner & Ingbar's The Thyroid. A Fundamental and Clinical Text. Philadelphia: Lippincott Williams & Wilkins, 2000:989–97.
18. Ward L, Huot C, Lambert R, Deal C, Collu R, Van Vliet G. Outcome of pediatric Graves' disease after treatment with antithyroid medication and radioiodine. Clin Invest Med 1999;22: 132–9.
19. Moll GW Jr, Patel BR. Pediatric Graves' disease: therapeutic options and experience with radio-

iodine at the University of Mississippi Medical Center. South Med J 1997;90:1017–22.

20. Clark JD, Gelfand MJ, Elgazzar AH. Iodine-131 therapy of hyperthyroidism in pediatric patients. J Nucl Med 1995;36:442–5.

21. Read CH Jr, Tansey MJ, Menda Y. A 36–year retrospective analysis of the efficacy and safety of radioactive iodine in treating young Graves' patients. J Clin Endocrinol Metab 2004;89: 4229–33.

22. Safa AM, Schneider AB, Stachura ME, et al. Long term follow-up results in children and adolescents treated with radioactive iodine (^{131}I) for hyperthyroidism. N Engl J Med 1975;292:167–71.

23. Foley TP Jr, Charron M. Radioiodine treatment of juvenile Graves disease. Exp Clin Endocrinol Diabetes 1997;105:61–5.

24. Cheetham TD, Wraight P, Hughes IA, Barnes ND. Radioiodine treatment of Graves' disease in young people. Horm Res 1998;49:258–62.

25. Refetoff S, Harrison J, Karanfilski BT, Kaplan EL, De Groot LJ, Bekerman C. Continuing occurrence of thyroid carcinoma after irradiation to the neck in infancy and childhood. N Engl J Med 1975;292:171–5.

26. Baverstock K, Egloff B, Pinchera A, Ruchti C, Williams D. Thyroid cancer after Chernobyl. Nature 1992;359:21–2.

27. Nikiforov Y, Gnepp DR, Fagin JA. Thyroid lesions in children and adolescents after the Chernobyl disaster: implications for the study of radiation tumorigenesis. J Clin Endocrinol Metab 1996;81:9–14.

28. Alexander EK, Larsen PR. High dose of (131)I therapy for the treatment of hyperthyroidism caused by Graves' disease. J Clin Endocrinol Metab 2002;87:1073–7.

29. Ross DS, Ridgway EC, Daniels GH. Successful treatment of solitary toxic thyroid nodules with relatively low-dose iodine-131, with low prevalence of hypothyroidism. Ann Intern Med 1984;101:488–90.

30. Goldstein R, Hart IR. Follow-up of solitary autonomous thyroid nodules treated with 131I. N Engl J Med 1983;309:1473–6.

31. Alexander EK, Marqusee E, Lawrence J, Jarolim P, Fischer GA, Larsen PR. Timing and magnitude of increases in levothyroxine requirements during pregnancy in women with hypothyroidism. N Engl J Med 2004;351:241–9.

32. Zimmerman D. Fetal and neonatal hyperthyroidism. Thyroid 1999;9:727–33.

33. Mazzaferri EL. Management of a solitary thyroid nodule. N Engl J Med 1993;328:553–9.

34. Rallison ML, Dobyns BM, Keating FR Jr, Rall JE, Tyler FH. Thyroid nodularity in children. JAMA 1975;233:1069–72.

35. Trowbridge FL, Matovinovic J, McLaren GD, Nichaman MZ. Iodine and goiter in children. Pediatrics 1975;56:82–90.

36. Burch HB. Evaluation and management of the solid thyroid nodule. Endocrinol Metab Clin North Am 1995;24:663–710.

37. Belfiore A, Giuffrida D, La Rosa GL, et al. High frequency of cancer in cold thyroid nodules occurring at young age. Acta Endocrinol (Copenh) 1989;121:197–202.

38. Hung W, August GP, Randolph JG, Schisgall RM, Chandra R. Solitary thyroid nodules in children and adolescents. J Pediatr Surg 1982;17:225–9.

39. Silverman SH, Nussbaum M, Rausen AR. Thyroid nodules in children: a ten year experience at one institution. Mt Sinai J Med 1979;46:460–3.

40. Hung W, Anderson KD, Chandra RS, et al. Solitary thyroid nodules in 71 children and adolescents. J Pediatr Surg 1992;27:1407–9.

41. Degnan BM, McClellan DR, Francis GL. An analysis of fine-needle aspiration biopsy of the thyroid in children and adolescents. J Pediatr Surg 1996;31:903–7.

42. Lafferty AR, Batch JA. Thyroid nodules in childhood and adolescence—thirty years of experience. J Pediatr Endocrinol Metab 1997;10: 479–86.

43. Al-Shaikh A, Ngan B, Daneman A, Daneman D. Fine-needle aspiration biopsy in the management of thyroid nodules in children and adolescents. J Pediatr 2001;138:140–2.

44. Khurana KK, Labrador E, Izquierdo R, Mesonero CE, Pisharodi LR. The role of fine-needle aspiration biopsy in the management of thyroid nodules in children, adolescents, and young adults: a multi-institutional study. Thyroid 1999;9:383–6.

45. Arda IS, Yildirim S, Demirhan B, Firat S. Fine needle aspiration biopsy of thyroid nodules. Arch Dis Child 2001;85:313–7.

46. AACE/AAES medical/surgical guidelines for clinical practice: management of thyroid carcinoma. American Association of Clinical Endocrinologists. American College of Endocrinology. Endocr Pract 2001;7:202–20.

47. Schneider AB, Ron E. Carcinoma of follicular epithelium. In: Braverman LE, Utiger RD, eds. Werner & Ingbar's The Thyroid: A Fundamental and Clinical Text. Philadelphia: Lippincott Williams & Wilkins, 2000:875–929.

48. Kameyama K, Takami H, Miyajima K, Mimura T, Hosoda Y, Ito K. Papillary carcinoma occurring within an adenomatous goiter of the thyroid gland in Cowden's disease. Endocr Pathol 2001; 12:73–6.

49. Perriard J, Saurat JH, Harms M. An overlap of Cowden's disease and Bannayan-Riley-Ruvalcaba syndrome in the same family. J Am Acad Dermatol 2000;42:348–50.

50. Marqusee E, Benson CB, Frates MC, et al. Usefulness of ultrasonography in the management of nodular thyroid disease. Ann Intern Med 2000;133:696–700.

51. Bennedbaek FN, Hegedus L. Management of the solitary thyroid nodule: results of a North American survey. J Clin Endocrinol Metab 2000;85:2493–8.

52. Danese D, Sciacchitano S, Farsetti A, Andreoli M, Pontecorvi A. Diagnostic accuracy of conventional versus sonography-guided fine-needle aspiration biopsy of thyroid nodules. Thyroid 1998;8:15–21.

53. Cochand-Priollet B, Guillausseau PJ, Chagnon S, et al. The diagnostic value of fine-needle aspiration biopsy under ultrasonography in nonfunctional thyroid nodules: a prospective study comparing cytologic and histologic findings. Am J Med 1994;97:152–7.

54. Rosen IB, Azadian A, Walfish PG, Salem S, Lansdown E, Bedard YC. Ultrasound-guided fine-needle aspiration biopsy in the management of thyroid disease. Am J Surg 1993;166:346–9.

55. Hatada T, Okada K, Ishii H, Ichii S, Utsunomiya J. Evaluation of ultrasound-guided fine-needle aspiration biopsy for thyroid nodules. Am J Surg 1998;175:133–6.

56. LiVolsi VA. Pathology of pediatric thyroid cancer. In: Robbins J, ed. Treatment of Thyroid Cancer in Childhood. Bethesda, MD: National Institutes of Health, 1994:11–22.

57. LaVolsi V. Pathology of pediatric thyroid cancer. In: Robbins J, ed. Treatment of Thyroid Cancer in Childhood. Springfield, VA: National Technical Information Service, 1992:11–22.

58. Mazzaferri EL, Kloos RT. Clinical review 128: Current approaches to primary therapy for papillary and follicular thyroid cancer. J Clin Endocrinol Metab 2001;86:1447–63.

59. La Quaglia MP, Corbally MT, Heller G, Exelby PR, Brennan MF. Recurrence and morbidity in differentiated thyroid carcinoma in children. Surgery 1988;104:1149–56.

60. Newman KD, Black T, Heller G, et al. Differentiated thyroid cancer: determinants of disease progression in patients <21 years of age at diagnosis: a report from the Surgical Discipline Committee of the Children's Cancer Group. Ann Surg 1998;227:533–41.

61. Hung W, Sarlis NJ. Current controversies in the management of pediatric patients with well-differentiated nonmedullary thyroid cancer: a review. Thyroid 2002;12:683–702.

62. Vassilopoulou-Sellin R, Goepfert H, Raney B, Schultz PN. Differentiated thyroid cancer in children and adolescents: clinical outcome and mortality after long-term follow-up. Head Neck 1998;20:549–55.

63. Winship T, Rosvoll RV. Childhood thyroid carcinoma. Cancer 1961;14:734–43.

64. Schweisguth O. Differentiated thyroid carcinoma in childhood: long-term evolution. Ann Radiol (Paris) 1977;20:859–60.

65. Doci R, Pilotti S, Costa A, Semeraro G, Cascinelli N. Thyroid cancer in childhood. Tumori 1978;64: 649–57.

66. Uchino J, Hata Y, Kasai Y. Thyroid cancer in childhood. Jpn J Surg 1978;8:19–27.

67. Zimmerman D. Papillary thyroid carcinoma in children. In: Robbins J, ed. Treatment of Thyroid Cancer in Childhood. Springfield, VA: National Technical Information Service, 1994:3–10.

68. Welch Dinauer CA, Tuttle RM, Robie DK, et al. Clinical features associated with metastasis and recurrence of differentiated thyroid cancer in children, adolescents and young adults. Clin Endocrinol (Oxf) 1998;49:619–28.

69. Segal K, Shvero J, Stern Y, Mechlis S, Feinmesser R. Surgery of thyroid cancer in children and adolescents. Head Neck 1998;20:293–7.

70. Landau D, Vini L, A'Hern R, Harmer C. Thyroid cancer in children: the Royal Marsden Hospital experience. Eur J Cancer 2000;36:214–20.

71. Jarzab B, Handkiewicz Junak D, Wloch J, et al. Multivariate analysis of prognostic factors for differentiated thyroid carcinoma in children. Eur J Nucl Med 2000;27:833–41.

72. Storm HH, Plesko I. Survival of children with thyroid cancer in Europe 1978–1989. Eur J Cancer 2001;37:775–9.

73. Kowalski LP, Goncalves Filho J, Pinto CA, Carvalho AL, de Camargo B. Long-term survival rates in young patients with thyroid carcinoma. Arch Otolaryngol Head Neck Surg 2003;129: 746–9.

74. Thompson GB, Hay ID. Current strategies for surgical management and adjuvant treatment of childhood papillary thyroid carcinoma. World J Surg 2004;28:1187–98.

75. Hay ID, McConahey WM, Goellner JR. Managing patients with papillary thyroid carcinoma: insights gained from the Mayo Clinic's experience of treating 2,512 consecutive patients during 1940 through 2000. Trans Am Clin Climatol Assoc 2002;113:241–60.

76. Hundahl SA, Cady B, Cunningham MP, et al. Initial results from a prospective cohort study of 5583 cases of thyroid carcinoma treated in the United States during 1996. U.S. and German Thyroid Cancer Study Group. An American College of Surgeons Commission on Cancer Patient Care Evaluation study. Cancer 2000;89: 202–17.

77. Danese D, Gardini A, Farsetti A, Sciacchitano S, Andreoli M, Pontecorvi A. Thyroid carcinoma in children and adolescents. Eur J Pediatr 1997; 156:190–4.

78. Miccoli P, Antonelli A, Spinelli C, Ferdeghini M, Fallahi P, Baschieri L. Completion total thyroidectomy in children with thyroid cancer secondary to the Chernobyl accident. Arch Surg 1998;133:89–93.

79. Sosa JA, Bowman HM, Tielsch JM, Powe NR, Gordon TA, Udelsman R. The importance of surgeon experience for clinical and economic outcomes from thyroidectomy. Ann Surg 1998; 228:320–30.

80. Pujol P, Daures JP, Nsakala N, Baldet L, Bringer J, Jaffiol C. Degree of thyrotropin suppression as a prognostic determinant in differentiated thyroid cancer. J Clin Endocrinol Metab 1996; 81:4318–23.

81. Maxon HR, Thomas SR, Hertzberg VS, et al. Relation between effective radiation dose and outcome of radioiodine therapy for thyroid cancer. N Engl J Med 1983;309:937–41.

82. Benua RS, Cicale NR, Sonenberg M, Rawson RW. The relation of radioiodine dosimetry to results and complications in the treatment of metastatic thyroid cancer. AJR Radium Ther Nucl Med 1962;87:171–82.

83. Becker DV. Radioiodine Therapy in Children. In: Robbins J, ed. Treatment of Thyroid Cancer in Childhood. Springfield, VA: National Technical Information Service, 1994:117–25.

84. Maxon HR. The role of radioiodine in the treatment of childhood thyroid cancer—a dosimetric approach. In: Robbins J, ed. Treatment of Thyroid Cancer in Childhood. Springfield, VA: National Technical information Service, 1994: 109–16.

85. Reynolds JC. Comparison of I-131 absorbed radiation doses in children and adults: a tool for estimating therapeutic I-131 doses in children. In: Robbins J, ed. Treatment of Thyroid Cancer in Childhood. Springfield, VA: National Technical Information Service, 1994: 127–35.

86. Maxon HR. The role of 131I in the treatment of thyroid cancer. Thyroid Today 1993;16:1–10.

87. Maxon HR, Smith HS. Radioiodine-131 in the diagnosis and treatment of metastatic well differentiated thyroid cancer. Endocrinol Metab Clin North Am 1990;19:685–718.

88. Viswanathan K, Gierlowski TC, Schneider AB. Radiation-induced thyroid cancer in children. In: Robbins J, ed. Treatment of Thyroid Cancer in Childhood. Springfield, VA: National Technical Information Service, 1994:23–6.

89. Schlumberger MJ. Papillary and follicular thyroid carcinoma. N Engl J Med 1998;338:297–306.

90. Sweeney DC, Johnston GS. Radioiodine therapy for thyroid cancer. Endocrinol Metab Clin North Am 1995;24:803–39.

91. Robbins RJ, Robbins AK. Clinical review 156: Recombinant human thyrotropin and thyroid cancer management. J Clin Endocrinol Metab 2003;88:1933–8.

92. Barbaro D, Boni G, Meucci G, et al. Radioiodine treatment with 30 mCi after recombinant human thyrotropin stimulation in thyroid cancer: effectiveness for postsurgical remnants ablation and possible role of iodine content in L-thyroxine in the outcome of ablation. J Clin Endocrinol Metab 2003;88:4110–5.

93. Maxon HR, Thomas SR, Boehringer A, et al. Low iodine diet in I-131 ablation of thyroid remnants. Clin Nucl Med 1983;8:123–6.

94. Sherman SI, Tielens ET, Sostre S, Wharam MD Jr, Ladenson PW. Clinical utility of posttreatment radioiodine scans in the management of patients with thyroid carcinoma. J Clin Endocrinol Metab 1994;78:629–34.

95. Connolly LP, Connolly SA. Thymic uptake of radiopharmaceuticals. Clin Nucl Med 2003;28: 648–51.

4

Calculation of Administered Doses of Iodine-131 in the Treatment of Thyroid Disease

Robert E. Zimmerman

In some instances patients present with thyroid cancer that does not seem to fit the usual treatment guidelines as set forth in conventional texts. For example, there may be an unusual distribution of thyroid remnants or metastases or there sometimes are extensive metastases to the lung or other organs. In these cases knowledge about regional uptake of therapeutic iodine-131 (^{131}I) is useful.

The properly collimated gamma camera with attached computer is well suited to serve as a probe to determine regional quantitative ^{131}I distribution using a tracer dose prior to administration of the therapeutic dose. Benua et al.,[1] Thomas et al.,[2] and Maxon et al.[3,4] discuss the use of quantitative thyroid counting, and their methods can be adapted to gamma camera measurements of tissues that may take up the tracer iodine. Described below are the methods used at Children's Hospital Boston and Brigham and Women's Hospital Boston.

Quantitative Thyroid Counting

There are two clinical situations where quantitative counting is indicated. The first is the simpler case in which multiple discrete thyroid remnants or metastases are present. It is desirable to know the uptake of the remnants and the metastases, which can be accomplished with a rather simple quantitative uptake study using the gamma camera.

A more difficult case arises when there are extensive metastases that, if treated without proper consideration given to dosimetry, could cause a significant dose to be delivered to lung tissue or bone marrow. In these relatively rare cases, a full dosimetry study can be performed using the gamma camera.

Quantitative Estimate of ^{131}I in Isolated Metastases or Thyroid Remnants

Imaging

Iodine-131 is administered in a 37-MBq (1-mCi) dose on day 0, and measurements are usually made at 24 hours, with similar measurements sometimes made on subsequent days. A 1% to 5% fraction of the administered dose must be available as an imaging standard. It should be placed in a vial or tissue culture flask approximately 3 to 6 cm in extent. Imaging is performed with a gamma camera with a high-energy collimator and a computer. The imaging protocol is shown in Table 4.1.

Analysis

The analysis assumes that the isotope is ^{131}I and that tissue attenuation can be neglected. Scatter and background contributions are minimized by using tight (50% threshold) regions of interest (ROIs) around the lesion(s). The analysis protocol is shown in Table 4.2. The data sheet for recording the counts from the ROI analysis is shown in Figure 4.1 and the worksheet for calculation of the uptake for each focus of activity in Figure 4.2.

TABLE 4.1. Imaging protocol for quantitative estimate of ^{131}I in isolated metastases or thyroid remnants

1. High-energy collimator; computer matrix of at least 64×64; 128×128 is better; keep track of times on computer images.
2. Imaging times are ideally 24, 48, and 72 hours to establish the washout rates for the lesions and tissues that may be treated.
3. Take anterior images of all areas suspected of having ^{131}I using both camera images and computer images. Counting time should be such that significant number of counts (50,000+) are obtained for each lesion. Ensure that pixel overflow does not occur.
4. If posterior lesions exist they should be imaged with a posterior view.
5. Image the standard at the same time as the patient, in a separate view. Source should be 0 to 2 cm from the collimator.

TABLE 4.2. Analysis protocol for quantitative estimate of ^{131}I in isolated metastases or thyroid remnants

1. A nine-point smooth of the images is usually helpful but not necessary.
2. Draw a region of interest (ROI) at the 50% contour level. If there is tissue background activity, it should be corrected for so the ROI is at the 50% level for the lesion.
3. Draw a background ROI in an unaffected area of the patient. The counts in the background region should be subtracted from the counts in the lesion region.
4. Obtain the counts per second (cps) for each lesion as described in steps 2 and 3.
5. Obtain the counts per second (cps) for the standard using exactly the same procedures as for the lesion (e.g., smoothing, 50% ROI).
6. Calculate the percent uptake for each lesion using the known information about the standard:

$$\text{Lesion uptake} = \frac{\text{lesion cps} \times F}{\text{standard cps}}$$

where F is the fraction of administered activity in the standard.

Example

Patient S.R. was administered 37 MBq (1.0 mCi) of ^{131}I on March 1, 1993. A standard with 3.626 MBq (98 µCi) was also prepared. The quantitative thyroid scan of the neck on March 2, 1993 revealed five foci of increased tracer uptake (Fig. 4.3). No other sites of abnormal uptake were noted on the whole-body survey. The ROIs were drawn on the five hot spots and for a representative background in the shoulder region (Fig. 4.3). The standard was imaged and an ROI drawn for that also (Fig. 4.3). All data were recorded on the data sheet reproduced in Figure 4.4. Calculations related to the

QUANTITATIVE THYROID UPTAKE

Patient name: _____

Patient number: _____

Date of scan: _____

Dose administered: _____ µCi on Date: _____

Dose standard: _____ µCi on Date: _____

Number of hot foci:

    Draw tight irregular ROI around each focus.

    If uptake is very low draw a background ROI in soft tissue region.

Location	Time (sec)	Counts	Pixels	Mean counts/pixel
Focus 1: thyroid				
Focus 2:				
Focus 3:				
Focus 4:				
Background				
Standard				

Consult physicist for problem cases.

FIGURE 4.1. Data sheet for quantitative estimate of iodine 131 (^{131}I) in isolated metastases or thyroid remnants.

QUANTITATIVE THYROID UPTAKE

Patient name: _____   Patient number: _____   Date of scan: _____

Definition

$$\% \text{ Uptake} = \frac{100 \times \text{activity in thyroid}}{\text{activity administered}} \text{ at day 0}$$

Calculations

<u>Focus 1</u> (thyroid)   *Correction factor*

Bkg corr cts = (mean cts/pix − bkg mean cts/pix) × pixels   1 day = 1.090

Bkg corr cts = (−   ) ×   =   2 day = 1.188

3 day = 1.295

$$\% \text{ Uptake} = 100 \times \frac{\text{bkg corr cts}}{\text{std counts}} \times \frac{\text{dose std}}{\text{dose adm}} \times \text{corr factor}$$ 4 day = 1.412

5 day = 1.539

% Uptake = 100 ×   ×   ×   =   6 day = 1.677

7 day = 1.828

<u>Focus 2</u>

Bkg corr cts = (mean cts/pix − bkg mean cts/pix) × pixels

Bkg corr cts = (−   ) ×   =

% Uptake = 100 ×   ×   ×   =

<u>Focus 3</u>

Bkg corr cts = (mean cts/pix − bkg mean cts/pix) × pixels

Bkg corr cts = (−   ) ×   =

% Uptake = 100 ×   ×   ×   =

<u>Focus 4</u>

Bkg corr cts = (mean cts/pix − bkg mean cts/pix) × pixels

Bkg corr cts = (−   ) ×   =

% Uptake = 100 ×   ×   ×   =

Notes

1. If counting time is not the same for lesion and standard, use counts per second for background correction counts and standard counts.
2. If standard counts are obtained on the same day as the patient scan, do not use a correction factor.

FIGURE 4.2. Worksheet for quantitative estimate of ^{131}I in isolated metastases or thyroid remnants.

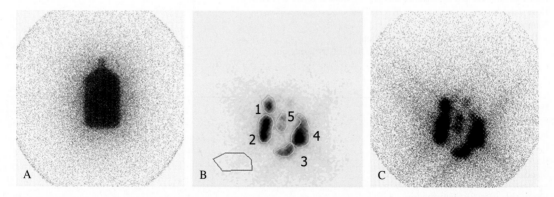

FIGURE 4.3. A: [131]I standard counted during the same imaging session as the patient with the range of interest (ROI) drawn. B,C: Patient S.R.'s neck scan with (B) and without (C) ROIs. Note the five hot foci and the background region, which was chosen to be in the shoulder.

QUANTITATIVE THYROID UPTAKE

Patient name: ___SR___
Patient number: _123456789_
Date of scan: __3/2/93__
Dose administered: ___1000 µCi__ on Date: ___3/1/93___
Dose standard: __98 µCi__ on Date: __3/1/93__
Number of hot foci: 5
  Draw tight irregular ROI around each focus.
  If uptake is low draw a background ROI in soft tissue region.

Location	Time (sec)	Counts	Pixels	Mean counts/pixel
Focus 1: thyroid	175	4925	417	11.81
Focus 2	175	16778	927	18.10
Focus 3	175	6089	486	12.53
Focus 4	175	16707	1091	15.31
Background: soft tissue shoulder	1433	679	847	0.80
Standard	677	60541	5643	10.73
Focus 5	175	3026	394	7.68

Consult physicist for problem cases.

FIGURE 4.4. Data sheet for patient S.R.

data sheet are shown on the worksheet (Fig. 4.5). The same calculations can be done using a computer spreadsheet (Fig. 4.6). The report that is provided to the therapy decision makers consists of the images showing the ROIs and the report on the percent uptakes.

The accuracy of this procedure has not been determined with quantitative phantom experiments or tissue counting. Iodine-131 is relatively penetrating, and thyroid lesions are often shallow. For these reasons, the decision was made not to obtain anterior and posterior views with geometric means and attenuation correction or to use an anthropomorphic phantom for the standard. Accuracy is estimated to be in the neighborhood of 10% to 20% based on experiments described in the literature.[2]

It may be possible to use ^{123}I for these measurements, but there are quantification problems that make it less desirable. The lower photon energy of the principal gamma ray from ^{123}I leads to more scattered radiation being detected. Furthermore, the significant number of high-energy photons associated with ^{123}I leads to excess penetration of the collimator introducing yet more potential for errors. Iodine-131 remains the preferred isotope when quantifying lesions remaining in the neck area.

Future work may perfect techniques for using [123]I.

Quantitative Determination of [131]I Distribution with Widely Disseminated Metastases

In patients who have widely disseminated metastases, as in the case of gross lung involvement, it is advantageous to estimate the dose to the lung parenchyma and the bone marrow. In such cases a more extensive dosimetry process is justified.

Quantitative methods used to determine the biodistribution of the ^{131}I are those as generally described by Thomas et al.[2] using the gamma camera as a whole-body counter. Iodine-131 in a dose of 37 MBq (1 mCi) in saline is administered orally to the patient. Anterior and posterior images of the entire body are performed as soon as possible after tracer administration (before the patient voids) and again at 4, 24, 48, 72, and 96 hours. Ideally a dual-detector gamma camera capable of anterior and posterior whole-body sweeps is employed. Single camera images (100,000 counts) of the significant body parts can also be obtained if whole-body sweeps are not feasible. Regions of interest are

QUANTITATIVE THYROID UPTAKE

Patient name: _____ S.R. _____   Patient number: ___123456789___   Date of scan: ____3/2/93____

Definition

$$\% \text{ Uptake} = \frac{100 \times \text{activity in thyroid}}{\text{activity administered}} \text{ at day 0}$$

Calculations

Focus 1 thyroid

Bkg corr cts = (mean cts/pix − bkg mean cts/pix) × pixels

Bkg corr cts =   (11.81 − 0.80)   × 417 = 4591

$$\% \text{ Uptake} = 100 \times \frac{\text{bkg corr cts}}{\text{std counts}} \times \frac{\text{dose std}}{\text{dose adm}} \times \text{corr factor}$$

$$\% \text{ Uptake} = 100 \times \frac{4591/175}{60541/677} \times \frac{98}{1000} \times 1 = 2.87\%$$

Focus 2

Bkg corr cts = (mean cts/pix − bkg mean cts/pix) × pixels

Bkg corr cts =   (18.10 − 0.80)   × 927 = 16035

$$\% \text{ Uptake} = 100 \times \frac{16035/175}{60541/677} \times \frac{98}{1000} \times 1 = 10.04\%$$

Focus 3

Bkg corr cts = (mean cts/pix − bkg mean cts/pix) × pixels

Bkg corr cts =   (12.53 − 0.80)   × 486 = 5699

$$\% \text{ Uptake} = 100 \times \frac{5699/175}{60541/677} \times \frac{98}{1000} \times 1 = 3.57\%$$

Focus 4

Bkg corr cts = (mean cts/pix − bkg mean cts/pix) × pixels

Bkg corr cts =   (15.31 − 0.80)   × 1091 = 15832

$$\% \text{ Uptake} = 100 \times \frac{15832/175}{60541/677} \times \frac{98}{1000} \times 1 = 9.91\%$$

Correction factor
1 day = 1.090
2 day = 1.188
3 day = 1.295
4 day = 1.412
5 day = 1.539
6 day = 1.677
7 day = 1.828

Notes

1. If counting time is not the same for the lesion and the standard, use counts per seconds for background correction counts and standard counts.
2. If standard counts are taken on the same day as the patient scan, do not use a correction factor.

FIGURE 4.5. Worksheet for quantitative estimate of ^{131}I in isolated metastases or thyroid remnants.

drawn on important body parts. The geometric mean of the counts for each part is calculated and the organ uptake is obtained. A sample protocol is shown in Table 4.3.

The ROI data form the basis of the calculation of the biological distribution vs. time data. Using standard medical internal radiation dose (MIRD) techniques, the residence time is calculated. The residence time is the input to the MIRD dosimetry calculation that is performed using PC-compatible software available from Vanderbilt University.[6] Other software can be used such as NucliDose distributed for Siemens ICON computer systems.[7] This software has the significant advantage of integrating the drawing of ROI, geometric mean calculation, attenuation correction, and MIRD dose calculations. The dose to the bone marrow is calculated using the method of Benua et al.[1] The quantity of ^{131}I to be administered for therapy is chosen based on limiting the dose to the bone marrow or lung (see example below).

Imaging

Figure 4.7A shows the set of whole-body images taken over a 72-hour period. Also shown are the transmission image and the

Patient SR
Patient Number 123456789
Date March 15, 1993
   Injected dose (ID) 1000 μCi March 1, 1993
   Standard dose   98 μCi March 1, 1993

March 2, 1993 ANT

Focus	Time (sec)	Counts	Pixels	Avg/pixel	Avg/pixel/sec	Net count	% ID
Focus 1	175	4925	417	11.81	0.067	4884	3.06
Focus 2	175	16778	927	18.10	0.103	16687	10.45
Focus 3	175	6089	486	12.53	0.072	6041	3.78
Focus 4	175	16707	1091	15.31	0.088	16600	10.40
Focus 5	175	3026	394	7.68	0.044	2987	1.87
Background	1433	679	847	0.80	0.001		
Standard	677	60541	5643	10.73	0.016		
Total uptake:							29.6%

FIGURE 4.6. Spreadsheet showing worksheet calculations for patient S.R.

blank scan used to derive attenuation correction for each ROI. The ROIs are drawn for the lung (Fig. 4.7B), whole body (Fig. 4.7C), and thyroid remnant (Fig. 4.7D), and the associated background ROIs are also shown.

Analysis

After the images are obtained and ROIs are defined, biodistribution analysis is performed. Data from the ROI analysis of each time point are entered into a spreadsheet (Fig. 4.8) that is used to correct for decay, to calculate geometric means, and to calculate the percent injected dose for the selected organs. The percent injected dose is then summarized on a spreadsheet (Table 4.4). These data are then fit to a one- or two-compartment model using standard techniques. The residence times are then calculated using the biologic half-life and the

TABLE 4.3. Protocol for determination of whole-body distribution, clearance, and dosimetry of [131]I

1. Use large field of view camera with high-energy collimator and computer for all studies. Whole-body scanning mode is preferred but not absolutely necessary. Spot views of known areas of nodal uptake should be performed.
2. Calibrate the camera with a 100-mL tissue culture flask filled with a known fraction of the patient dose (1.85–3.7 MBq [50–100 μCi] of ^{131}I in water). This calibration should be repeated before *every* acquisition. When doing whole-body images, place the phantom at the patient feet.
3. Perform transmission study before isotope is injected:
   a. Scan the table using a flood phantom filled with 18.5–37 MBq (500–1000 μCi) of [131]I. Setup should be exactly as with a patient, but patient is not to be on the scanning table. The flood phantom should be 2 to 4 cm below the scanning table. This is the blank scan.
   b. Bring patient to the scanning table and repeat to obtain the transmission scan.
4. Scan the patient at 0 to 1 hr before voiding or elimination. Perform an anterior scan followed immediately by a posterior scan (or simultaneous anterior-posterior scans). Patient should not be moved between views. Draw 2 cc of blood at time of imaging.
5. Repeat anterior and posterior scans and draw 2 cc blood samples at 4 hr, 1 day, 2 day, 3 day, and up to 4 days.

Analysis:
1. Use ROI analysis to determine anterior and posterior counts in whole body, lungs, thyroid, nodal regions, and other sites of uptake if present.
2. Determine the uptake of each of the above regions using the geometric mean corrected for patient attenuation.
3. Correct for physical half-life and plot as a function of time; determine the biologic washout.
4. Calculate blood, organ, and node dosimetry using medical internal radiation dose (MIRD) formulation and procedure outlined in Appendix E of Harbert and Rocha.[5] It is the Sloan-Kettering protocol of Benua et al.[1]

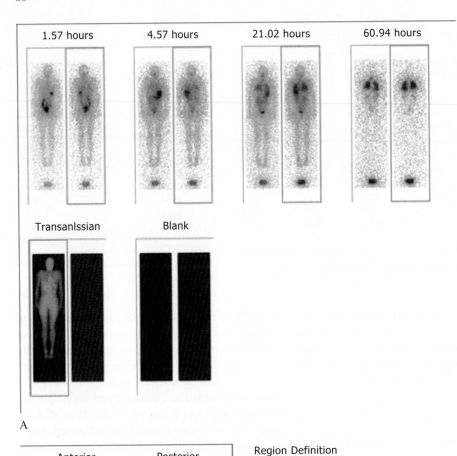

| 1.57 hours | 4.57 hours | 21.02 hours | 60.94 hours |

Transanlssian   Blank

A

Anterior   Posterior

Region Definition

◉ Organ/Tumor
○ Background
○ Standard Source
☒ Mirror

ROI Statistics

ANTERIOR

Cts:	59967
Pixels:	6280
Bkgd Pixels:	717
BKgd Cts/Pix:	1.75593
Std Cts:	32758
Std Pixels:	3650

POSTERIOR

Cts:	72037
Pixels:	6285
Bkgd Pixels:	718
BKgd Cts/Pix:	1.66992
Std Cts:	35642
Std Pixels:	3657

FIGURE 4.7. A: Images for patient obtained over a period of 72 hours. B: The ROIs for the lungs and background region associated with the lungs. The ROIs for the standard are also shown. These ROIs will be applied to each image shown in A. C: The ROIs for the whole body and background region associated with the whole body. The ROIs for the standard are also shown. These ROIs will be applied to each image shown in A. D: The ROIs for the thyroid bed and background region associated with the thyroid. The ROIs for the standard are also shown. These ROIs will be applied to each image shown in A.

B

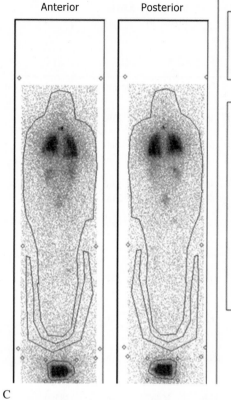

C

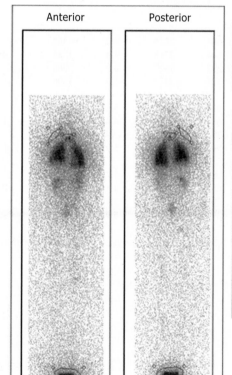

Figure 4.7. *Continued*   D

Biodistribution for K.K.   Injection time: 10:45
Inj dose: 1.10 mCi   Isotope $T_{1/2}$: 8.04 hr
Inj dose: 1524 counts/sec   Hours: 24
Std dose: 0.110 mCi

December 2, 1992

Region	Time clock	Time (sec)	Raw count	Decay corr. ct. rt	No. of pixels	Norm bkg ct rt	Net ct rt	Geo. mean	% ID	Count dens. × 100
Standard	10:45	466	67762	159	6360	*	*	*	*	*
Head & neck										
Ant	10:45	684	27887	44	15759		44	51	3.34	0.32
Post	10:45	397	21264	58	15116		58			
Thorax										
Ant	10:45	301	65089	236	24452		236	227	14.89	0.93
Post	10:45	303	60701	218	21592		218			
Stomach & intestine										
Ant	10:45	362	30868	93	17119		93	97	6.40	0.57
Post	10:45	331	31045	102	16196		102			
Legs, upper										
Ant	10:45									
Post	10:45	487	23779	53	13405		53	53	3.49	0.40
Knees										
Ant	10:45									
Post	10:45	834	8231	11	8097		11	11	0.71	0.13
Legs, lower										
Ant	10:45									
Post	10:45	959	14102	16	12798		16	16	1.05	0.13
Feet										
Ant	10:45									
Post	10:45	1136	16267	16	18599		16	16	1.02	
Total									30.90	
Region 1										
Ant	10:45	684	2515	4.0	368		3.1	3.1	0.21	0.85
Bkg ant	10:45	684	2768	4.4	1584	0.9				
Post	10:45	397	1537	4.2	366		3.2			
Bkg post	10:45	397	2131	5.9	1896	1.0				
Region 2										
Ant	10:45	684	2440	3.9	585		2.4	2.1	0.14	0.36
Bkg ant	10:45	684	2768	4.4	1584	1.5				
Post	10:45	397	1048	2.9	378		1.8			
Bkg post	10:45	397	2131	5.9	1896	1.1				
Region 3										
Ant	10:45	684	1073	1.7	265		1.0	1.4	0.09	0.55
Bkg ant	10:45	684	2768	4.4	1584	0.7				
Post	10:45	397	1195	3.3	445		2.0			
Bkg post	10:45	397	2131	5.9	1896	1.3				

FIGURE 4.8. Spreadsheet for analysis of biodistribution at 24 hours for patient K.K.

Region	Time clock	Time (sec)	Raw count	Decay corr. ct. rt	No. of pixels	Norm bkg ct rt	Net ct rt	Geo. mean	% ID	Count dens. × 100
Region 4										
Ant	10:45	684	2284	3.6	435		2.5	3.0	0.19	0.68
Bkg ant	10:45	684	2768	4.4	1584	1.1				
Post	10:45	397	1785	4.9	510		3.5			
Bkg post	10:45	397	2131	5.9	1896	1.4				
Lungs										
Ant	10:45	301	46324	168	12599		136	130	8.51	1.03
Bkg ant	10:45	684	2768	4	1584	32				
Post	10:45	303	44762	161	13033		124			
Bkg post	10:45	397	2131	6	1896	37				
Bladder										
Ant	10:45	362	14110	42	2876		42	58	3.83	2.03
Post	10:45	331	24406	80	4307		80			

FIGURE 4.8. *Continued*

TABLE 4.4. Summary of percent injected dose for patient K.K.

	% Injected dose					
	4 hr	24 hr	48 hr	72 hr	Attenuation	Corr. factor
No attenuation correction						
Head and neck	6.22	3.34	1.64	1.26	0.38	0.61
Thorax	18.82	14.89	11.41	9.34	0.42	0.65
Stomach and intestine	23.57	6.40	2.94	2.04	0.41	0.64
Legs	11.13	6.27	0.00	0.00	0.37	0.61
Total	59.74	30.90	15.99	12.64		
R 1 l-superior	0.25	0.21	0.10	0.12	0.40	0.63
R 2 r-superior	0.12	0.14	0.06	0.04	0.40	0.63
R 3 r-inferior	0.16	0.09	0.08	0.06	0.40	0.63
R 4 l-inferior	0.21	0.19	0.14	0.07	0.40	0.63
Lungs	7.68	8.51	6.65	6.02	0.44	0.66
With attenuation correction						
Head and neck	10.14	5.45	2.67	2.05		
Thorax	28.90	22.87	17.52	14.34		
Stomach and intestine	36.63	9.95	4.57	3.17		
Legs	18.30	10.31	0.00	0.00		
Total	93.98	48.57	24.77	19.57		
Node 1	0.39	0.33	0.16	0.19		
Node 2	0.19	0.22	0.09	0.06		
Node 3	0.25	0.14	0.13	0.09		
Node 4	0.33	0.30	0.22	0.11		
Lungs	11.62	12.87	10.06	9.11		
Remainder of body calculation						
Total	93.98	48.57	24.77	19.57		
Head and neck	10.14	5.45	2.67	2.05		
Stomach and intestine	28.90	22.87	17.52	14.34		
Lungs	11.62	12.87	10.06	9.11		
Remainder of body	43.31	7.38	−5.49	−5.94		

TABLE. 4.5. Spreadsheet for calculation of residence time for the various organs

Organ	f	T_b day	T_p day	Residence time	
				Day	Hour
Lung	0.127	6.578	8.04	0.46	11.03
Stomach and intestine	0.346	0.704	8.04	0.22	5.377
Head and neck, thyroid	0.101	1.2	8.04	0.11	2.531
Marrow	0.003	0.913	8.04	0.00	0.055
Remainder of body	0.617	0.325	8.04	0.19	4.626
Blood	0.047	0.913	8.04	0.04	0.924
Urine (TB)	0.918	1.233	8.04	0.98	23.56

Marrow is 0.06 of blood based on 600 g of marrow containing 60 g of blood.
f, the fractional uptake for the organ; T_b, the biological half-life; T_p, the physical half-life of the isotope.

concentrations resulting from the fits, shown in Table 4.5. Once the residence time has been calculated, the dosimetry calculations can be performed using the MIRD software. The bone marrow dose is calculated using the method of Benua et al.[1] as shown in Table 4.6. The summary of the dosimetry for a patient is shown in Table 4.7, which shows the relationship between the absorbed dose to the critical organs as a function of the dose administered. The therapist can then make an informed judgment on the quantity of ^{131}I to be administered. This analysis can be greatly simplified using special purpose software such as NucliDose[7] or OLINDA.[6]

Comment

Again, the accuracy of this method has not been documented except that it follows methods reported in the literature. It probably has an accuracy within 20% to 40%. The amount of camera time, technician time, physician time, and physicist time is considerable. It is hoped that this extra information can prevent complications while allowing the maximum dose to be given to the patient.

TABLE 4.6. Bone marrow calculation per method of Benua et al.[1]

Blood dose: must be less than 2 Gy (200 rad)
Patient weight: 25 kg
Fit for blood samples gives:
    Intercept: 4.7% ID/L
    T-biol. 21.9 hr
    Area of blood curve: 6.19% dose-day/L
    D-beta: 0.160 mGy/MBq (0.592 rad/mCi)
    Area—body retention curve
Fit to total body retention curve:
    Intercept: 91.8% ID
    T-biol: 29.6 hr
    Area—total body curve: 163% dose-days
    D-gamma: 0.10 mGy/MBq (0.376 rad/mCi)
    Total blood dose: 0.26 mGy/MBq (0.968 rad/mCi)
Retained dose at 48 hours must be <4.4 GBq (120 mCi) or
    3 GBq (80 mCi) if there are diffuse lung metastases
At 48 hours in body: 29.8%
Retained dose = GBq (mCi) admin. × 0.298

ID, injected dose; T-biol, the biological half-life.

TABLE 4.7. Dose summary for patient K.K.

Organ	rad/mCi	Administered dose (mCi)															
		150	160	170	180	190	200	210	220	230	240	250	260	270	280	290	300
MIRD																	
Lungs	11	1650	1760	1870	1980	2090	2200	2310	2420	2530	2640	2750	2860	2970	3080	3190	3300
Ovaries	0.52	78	83	88	94	99	104	109	114	120	125	130	135	140	146	151	156
Red marrow	0.24	36	38	41	43	46	48	50	53	55	58	60	62	65	67	70	72
T. body	0.47	71	75	80	85	89	94	99	103	108	113	118	122	127	132	136	141
Bladder	5	750	800	850	900	950	1000	1050	1100	1150	1200	1250	1300	1350	1400	1450	1500
Benua et al.[1]																	
Blood (marrow)	0.96	144	154	163	173	182	192	202	211	221	230	240	250	259	269	278	288
Retained at 48hr (mCi)*		38	40	43	45	48	50	53	55	58	60	63	65	68	70	73	75

*The amount retained at 48 hours should be less than 80 mCi.
MIRD, medical internal radiation dose.

Radiation Precautions During Thyroid Treatment

The United States Nuclear Regulatory Commission has specific requirements regarding safe use and administration of therapeutic quantities of ^{131}I, and they must be followed. The precautions noted here are not detailed. Consult your radiation safety officer.

There must be a quality management program as indicated in Title 10, Chapter 1, Code of Federal Regulations, Part 35.32 (10 CFR 35.32). This written program lists procedures and review actions to ensure that prescribed doses are given to the correct patient, error checking is in place, and follow-up actions ensure continuing compliance with written procedures.

Patients given more than 1110 MBq (30 mCi) of ^{131}I must be hospitalized or their release justified (10 CFR 35.75) and various safety precautions must be followed. Private rooms with private toilets are required. Frequent monitoring for uncontrolled radiation must be done. Special instruction must be given to personnel caring for the patient. The door must be posted with radiation warning signs, and survey meters must be in possession of the licensee (10 CFR 35.315).

References

1. Benua RS, Cicale NR, Sonenberg M, et al. The relation of radioiodine dosimetry to results and complications in the treatment of metastatic thyroid cancer. AJRRadium Ther Nucl Med 1962;87:171–82.
2. Thomas SR, Maxon HR, Kereiakes JG, et al. Quantitative external counting techniques enabling improved diagnostic and therapeutic decisions in patients with well-differentiated thyroid cancer. Radiology 1977;122(3):731–7.
3. Maxon HR 3rd, Englaro EE, Thomas SR, et al. Radioiodine-131 therapy for well-differentiated thyroid cancer—a quantitative radiation dosimetric approach: outcome and validation in 85 patients. J Nucl Med 1992;33(6):1132–6.
4. Maxon HR, Thomas SR, Hertzberg VS, et al. Relation between effective radiation dose and outcome of radioiodine therapy for thyroid cancer. N Engl J Med 1983;309(16):937–41.
5. Harbert JC, Rocha AFG. Textbook of Nuclear Medicine, 2nd ed. Philadelphia: Lea & Febiger, 1984.
6. Stabin MG. The OLINDA/EXM personal computer code. http://www.doseinfo-radar.com/OLINDA.html.
7. Erwin W, Groch MW. NucliDose—quantitative radionuclide imaging and MIRD dosimetry. http://www.nuclear.uhrad.com/nuclidos.htm.

5
Lungs

S.T. Treves and Alan B. Packard

Nuclear medicine offers imaging methods to assess regional pulmonary blood flow as well as ventilation, gas and fluid transport across the alveolar-capillary membrane, mucociliary clearance, pulmonary aspiration, and parenchymal diseases.

Regional ventilation can be best assessed with radioactive gases such as xenon-133 (^{133}Xe) or krypton-81m (^{81m}Kr). Other radiopharmaceuticals, such as aerosolized technetium-99m (^{99m}Tc)–sulfur colloid, ^{99m}Tc-diethylenetriamine pentaacetic acid (DTPA), and ^{99m}Tc-Technegas (a fine aerosol of carbonized technetium particles), can be utilized to obtain images that reflect the regional distribution of these particles after inhalation.

Regional pulmonary blood flow can be assessed with ^{99m}Tc macroaggregated albumin (^{99m}Tc-MAA) or intravenous ^{133}Xe dissolved in saline.

Gas transport from the blood across the alveolar-capillary membrane into the alveolar space can be studied with intravenous ^{133}Xe. *Fluid transport* from the alveolar space into the blood can be assessed following inhalation of aerosolized ^{99m}Tc-DTPA.

Mucociliary clearance can be evaluated following inhalation of aerosolized ^{99m}Tc–sulfur colloid.

Pulmonary aspiration can be evaluated in two ways: oral administration of ^{99m}Tc–sulfur colloid to diagnose gastroesophageal reflux and subsequent aspiration, and sublingual administration of ^{99m}Tc–sulfur colloid to detect aspiration of saliva (see Chapter 7).

Pulmonary parenchymal diseases (inflammation, infection, and tumors) can be assessed with gallium-67 (^{67}Ga) citrate, thallium-201 (^{201}Tl) chloride, technetium-99m sestamibi (^{99m}Tc-MIBI), and radioiodine (^{131}I or ^{123}I).

Indications for pulmonary scintigraphy in pediatric patients are listed in Table 5.1.

Methods

Regional Ventilation

Ventilation is defined as the process of exchange of air between the lungs and the ambient air. Regional ventilation can be elegantly assessed using radioactive gases such as ^{133}Xe or ^{81m}Kr. Aerosolized particles (e.g., ^{99m}Tc-sulfur colloid) are not exhaled and cannot therefore, completely assess ventilation. The pulmonary distribution of some aerosolized materials does, however, appear to follow the distribution of inhaled gas.

Assessment of Regional Ventilation Using Radioactive Gases

Xenon-133

For simplicity, the methods of ventilation and perfusion using ^{133}Xe are described together. Xenon-133 is the most widely used radioactive gas for the evaluation of regional lung function. Xenon is an inert gas with low solubility in body fluids. The solubility of ^{133}Xe in fat is considerably higher than in blood. The partition

TABLE 5.1. Indications for pulmonary scintigraphy in children

---

Cystic fibrosis
Pneumonia, inflammation, infection
Cyanosis
Lobar emphysema
Assessment of pulmonary artery angioplasty or surgery
Congenital diaphragmatic hernia and repair
Bronchopulmonary dysplasia
Foreign body
Aspiration
Asthma
Pulmonary hypoplasia, stenosis, aplasia, agenesis
Pulmonary sequestration
Pulmonary embolism
Pulmonary valve stenosis
Arteriovenous malformation
HIV-related pathology
Pectus excavatum
Sarcoidosis
Evaluation of pulmonary transplants
Effects of irradiation

---

coefficients are 8 for fat/blood, approximately 1 for brain/blood, and lower for other tissues. Xenon-133 has a physical half-life of 5.2 days, and it decays by β emission. The principal photon energy is 80 keV (37% abundance). Using the suggested administered doses (see below) for a 1-year-old patient, one can estimate the radiation absorbed dose to the lungs at 0.6 to 0.8 rad (6–8 mGy) and the gonadal dose at 0.005 to 0.015 rad (0.05–0.15 mGy). For a 15-year-old patient, the estimated radiation absorbed dose is 0.1 to 0.3 rad (1–3 mGy) to the lung and 0.004 to 0.008 rad (0.04–0.08 mGy) to the gonads.[1]

Xenon-133 can be administered by inhalation (ventilation) or intravenous injection (pulmonary blood flow and ventilation). When ^{133}Xe gas is inhaled in a single breath, its distribution within the lungs reflects regional ventilation. When a patient without airway obstruction breathes an oxygen-air-^{133}Xe mixture from a closed system during several respiratory cycles (and the volume of the gas reservoir is kept at a constant volume by replenishment with oxygen), the concentration of ^{133}Xe in the lungs reaches a equilibrium with that in the reservoir. Xenon-133 distribution in the lungs during this rebreathing is more

uniform than after a single breath of the gas. This uniform concentration allows calculation of the distribution of aerated lung volume. After equilibration, when the patient breathes room air in an open system, the amount of ^{133}Xe in the lungs normally decreases rapidly (washout), with a half-time of 5 to 30 seconds in children. The younger the patient, the shorter is the washout half-time. The rate of ^{133}Xe removal from the lungs depends primarily on alveolar ventilation. Estimates of regional ventilation obtained by inhalation permit assessment of the aerated lung tissue only.

Although ^{133}Xe is poorly soluble in water, under appropriate partial pressure it dissolves in various liquids, including saline. When ^{133}Xe dissolved in saline is exposed to room air, it rapidly comes out of solution. Similarly, ^{133}Xe dissolved in saline injected intravenously comes out of solution as it reaches the alveolar-capillary membrane. If a small (0.5–1.5 mL), rapid (<3 seconds) bolus of ^{133}Xe in saline is given intravenously, its initial distribution in the capillaries of the lungs (peak activity) is directly proportional to regional pulmonary blood flow. As ^{133}Xe reaches the alveolar-capillary membrane, most (approximately 95%) comes out of solution rapidly and enters the alveolar space. Removal of intravenously injected ^{133}Xe from the lungs depends on alveolar ventilation. Therefore, after intravenous injection of ^{133}Xe in saline it is possible to assess both regional pulmonary blood flow and ventilation. Estimates of regional ventilation obtained in this manner primarily reflect ventilation of perfused lung tissue. When assessing regional pulmonary blood flow with ^{133}Xe, the effect of intrapulmonary diffusion and rebreathing of this gas must be kept in mind. Because passage of intravenously injected ^{133}Xe into the alveolar air is instantaneous, delivery of a single small, rapid bolus is essential to obtain adequate assessment of regional pulmonary blood flow. If the injection of tracer is prolonged (>3 seconds), the bolus is fragmented, or the volume of the injectate is large, the results will be poor temporal resolution which will prevent clear separation of the perfusion from the ventilation phases of the study.

It should be noted that estimation of regional pulmonary ventilation and blood flow using ^{133}Xe requires more than one staff member in attendance, meticulous attention to technical detail, and adequate facilities for the safe handling and disposal of [133]Xe.

There are two principal methods for the study of ventilation and perfusion in children using [133]Xe. One method, called radiospirometry, requires patient cooperation for several respiratory maneuvers (e.g., breath-holding, deep inspiration, forced expiration).[2] The other method does not require patient cooperation and can be used in patients of all ages, including premature infants.[3] The method for radiospirometry has been described in detail elsewhere[4]; because it is not widely used in routine clinical practice, it is not discussed here.

Examination of Small Children and Uncooperative Patients Using [133]Xe. The procedure[3] is explained to the parents and, if possible, to the child. The patient is taken to the examination room and shown the equipment and the mask to be used for the ventilation study. A practice run without ^{133}Xe is often helpful for reducing patient anxiety and promoting cooperation. The study consists of a ventilation phase and a perfusion phase.

The study is recorded at a rate of one frame per 5 seconds for its entire duration using a 128×128 matrix format. The patient lies supine with the camera equipped with a low-energy parallel-hole collimator viewing the posterior thorax. In preparation for the perfusion phase, intravenous access is established using a butterfly-type needle (gauge 23 to 25) or a short intravenous catheter, which is securely fastened to the skin with tape and connected to a syringe containing 10 mL of normal saline. Intravenous access is maintained by frequently injecting small amounts of normal saline. In preparation for the ventilation phase, ^{133}Xe is introduced into an 800-mL plastic bag previously filled with oxygen. The bag is connected to a mask of appropriate size for the patient (Non-Conductive Single Use Face Mask, Vital Signs, Totowa, NJ) and its outlet closed with a surgi-cal clamp (Fig. 5.1). The concentration of ^{133}Xe in the bag is approximately 0.02 mCi/mL (0.74 MBq/mL).

For the ventilation phase of the study, the face mask is placed gently and firmly over the patient's face and the clamp is released simultaneously; the patient is encouraged to breathe as normally as possible (Fig. 5.1). The patient's crying is not generally an obstacle to the examination, as it promotes deep breathing. As the patient breathes the oxygen-xenon mixture, one can observe a period of wash-in on the time-activity curve followed by a "plateau" when a similar concentration of tracer is reached in the bag and the patient's lungs (equilibrium). The mask is withdrawn and the patient is allowed to breathe room air. Xenon-133 is then rapidly released (washout) in the air (exhaust system) by ventilation.

For the perfusion phase of the study, ^{133}Xe in saline is rapidly injected intravenously as a single, compact (<3 second) bolus using a special one-way valve mechanism (Injection Unit Bolus, International Medicine Industries, Watertown, MA) and is immediately flushed with 2 to 10 mL of normal saline. The usual dose of ^{133}Xe in saline is 0.3 mCi/kg body weight (11.1 MBq/kg) with a minimum total dose of 3 mCi (111 MBq).[3] The concentration of tracer in the solution should be 10 to 40 mCi/mL (370–1480 MBq/mL). Estimates of regional pulmonary blood flow using intravenous ^{133}Xe in saline during breath-holding and normal breathing are very similar, and either is therefore adequate for clinical work.[5]

In small children, recording the entire study usually takes 2.0 to 3.0 minutes. In patients with obstructive airway disease, ^{133}Xe almost never reaches equilibrium throughout the lungs because its pulmonary distribution is governed by many irregular regional flow rates. In fact, ever-increasing levels of activity in the lung during ^{133}Xe rebreathing is diagnostic of obstructive airway disease.

The study is displayed as shown in (Fig. 5.2). Images are evaluated visually (as multiple frames or as a movie), and this evaluation is complemented by quantitative assessment of regional ventilation and perfusion.

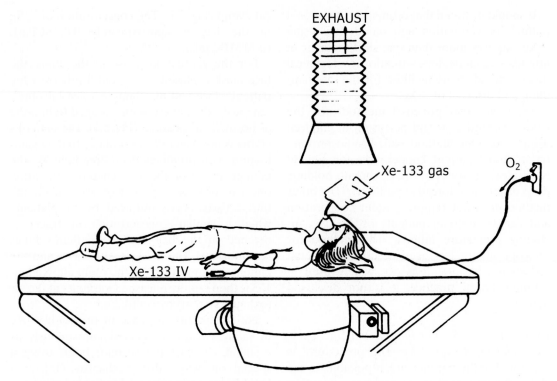

FIGURE 5.1. Method for examination of ventilation and perfusion in children and uncooperative patients using xenon-133. The patient is supine, and the gamma camera is underneath the examination table to view the posterior aspect of the chest. Xenon-133 is introduced into a plastic bag (shielding not shown) connected to a pediatric anesthesia mask. External oxygen is added into the mask if needed. The mask is withdrawn, and xenon is allowed to wash out of the lungs into the exhaust system. Next, a rapid intravenous bolus of ^{133}Xe in saline is given to assess regional perfusion and washout. During the time of examination, the patient is asked to breathe normally.

For quantitative analysis, an image of lung activity during the equilibrium phase is displayed on the monitor of the computer. A region of interest (ROI) is marked over the lung away from the superior vena cava and heart in order to calculate a reference time-activity curve (reference ROI) (Fig. 5.3).

Using an interactive computer program, the operator selects various points on the time-reference curve, including equilibrium, start of washout after equilibrium, background prior to perfusion, perfusion peak, and perfusion washout. Identical points in time are automatically marked by the computer on time-activity curves corresponding to other lung regions. These curves are then analyzed to determine regional distribution of activity representing ventilation, perfusion, and volume (Fig. 5.4).

Regional distribution of equilibrium and perfusion are calculated with the following formula:

$$D_i(\%) = \frac{A_i \times 100}{\sum\limits_{i-1}^{N} A_i}$$

where D_i is the regional distribution expressed as a percentage of total equilibrium and perfusion, A_i is the regional activity measured at peak perfusion, and N is the number of regions of interest (exclusive of the reference ROI). Regional distribution of ventilation is calculated from washout of equilibrated ^{133}Xe in lung and washout of perfused lung according to the following extension of the mean clearance rate formula[6]:

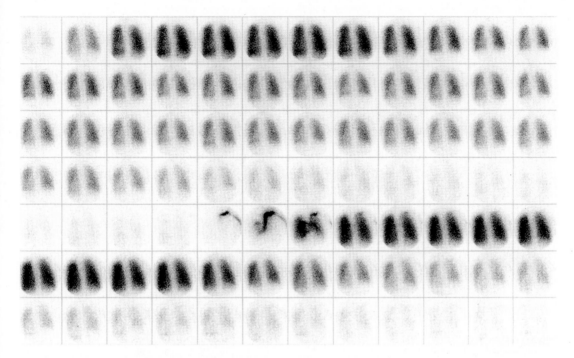

FIGURE 5.2. Normal xenon-133 ventilation and perfusion study, series of 3-second images. At the top of the image, inhaled ^{133}Xe is distributed throughout the lungs where it reaches a steady level, followed by washout. The lower portion of the figure reveals intravenous ^{133}Xe that was injected in a vein of the right arm; it circulated into the superior vena cava, right side of the heart, and pulmonary artery, and distributed according to regional pulmonary blood flow (rPBF). Xenon-133 immediately washes out of the lungs without trapping.

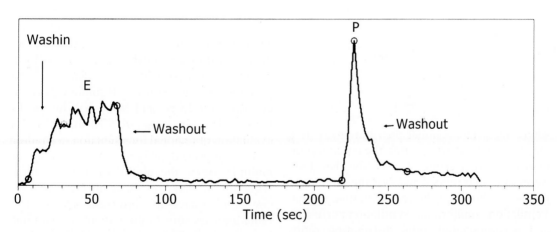

FIGURE 5.3. Xenon-133 reference time-activity curve. This curve is from a region of interest from a lung region and shows in sequence the wash-in, equilibrium (E), washout, perfusion (P) and washout phases of the study.

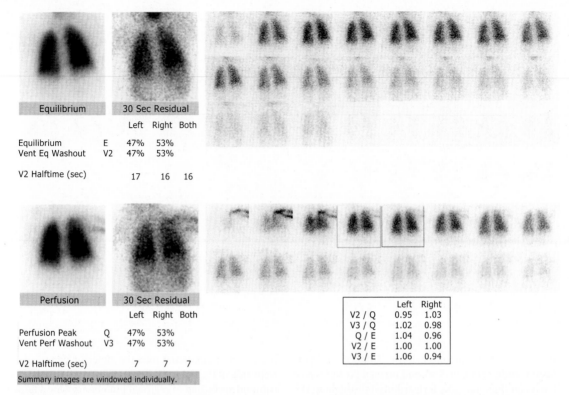

		Left	Right	Both
Equilibrium	E	47%	53%	
Vent Eq Washout	V2	47%	53%	
V2 Halftime (sec)		17	16	16

Equilibrium — 30 Sec Residual

Perfusion — 30 Sec Residual

		Left	Right	Both
Perfusion Peak	Q	47%	53%	
Vent Perf Washout	V3	47%	53%	
V2 Halftime (sec)		7	7	7

Summary images are windowed individually.

	Left	Right
V2 / Q	0.95	1.03
V3 / Q	1.02	0.98
Q / E	1.04	0.96
V2 / E	1.00	1.00
V3 / E	1.06	0.94

FIGURE 5.4. Normal xenon-133 ventilation and perfusion study. The ventilation and perfusion portions of the study are represented on the top and bottom half of the image, respectively. Note that the summary images on the left are windowed individually. (V2/Q, ventilation/perfusion, ventilation calculated from inhaled ^{133}Xe; Q/E, perfusion/equilibrium; V2/E, ventilation/equilibrium; V3/E, ventilation from perfusion washout/equilibrium).

$$D_i(\%) = \frac{\dfrac{A_i}{T_{1/2}} \times 100}{\displaystyle\sum_{i-1}^{N} \dfrac{A_i}{T_{1/2}}}$$

where D_i is the regional distribution; A_i is a mean regional activity during the equilibration plateau or perfusion; $T_{1/2}$ is the half-time washout in that region; and N is the number of regions exclusive of the representative region. Ventilation/equilibrium, ventilation/perfusion, and perfusion/equilibrium distribution ratios are calculated.

Krypton-81m

Krypton-81m has a physical half-life of 13 seconds and during its decay emits a 190 keV gamma ray (66%), which is excellent for imaging with gamma cameras. Krypton-81m is produced by a rubidium-81 (^{81}Ru) → ^{81m}Kr radionuclide generator. Rubidium-81m is cyclotron produced and has a half-life of 4.7 hours.[7–9] The advantages of ^{81m}Kr over ^{133}Xe for evaluation of regional lung function in children include improved imaging, ease of obtaining multiple views, the ability to perform rapid sequential studies to evaluate the effect of exercise or pharmacologic interventions, and low radiation exposure to the patient. In addition, because of its ultrashort physical half-life, handling of ^{81m}Kr does not require special exhaust systems, and it may be used at the patient's bedside or in intensive care units (Figs. 5.5 to 5.7). Unfortunately, ^{81m}Kr generators are expensive and have a short shelf life. Krypton-81m is

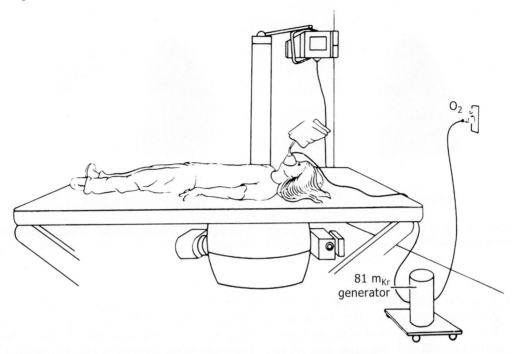

FIGURE 5.5. Krypton-81m delivery apparatus.

eluted from the generator with humidified oxygen at a flow rate of approximately 1 L per minute. From a typical generator, absorbed radiation dose to the lung from [81m]Kr for a 1-year-old is approximately 0.075 rad (0.75 mGy) and the gonadal dose 4 mrad (0.04 mGy). For a 15-year-old, the dose to the lungs is 0.015 rad (0.15 mGy) and to the gonads 0.78 mrad (0.0078 mGy). The estimated whole-body absorbed doses for 1- and 15-year-olds are 0.96 mrad (0.0096 mGy) and 0.91 mrad (0.0091 mGy), respectively.[8]

Methods Using Inhalation of Aerosolized Particles

Three methods rely on inhalation of aerosolized materials to produce images reflecting regional ventilation.

Aerosolized ^{99m}Tc-Sulfur Colloid

Aerosolized ^{99m}Tc–sulfur colloid can be administered by inhalation through a face mask connected to a nebulizer containing a solution of the radiopharmaceutical. Technetium-99m–sulfur colloid is an inert agent that is not absorbed through the alveolar-capillary membrane or in the gastrointestinal tract. Tracer is visible within the stomach in some patients from the swallowing of saliva-^{99m}Tc–sulfur

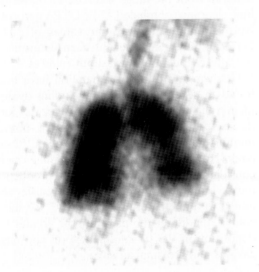

FIGURE 5.6. Krypton-81m ventilation study performed in a premature infant with respiratory difficulty. Anterior image reveals decreased ventilation in the left mid-lung field. This study was conducted in the neonatal intensive care unit.

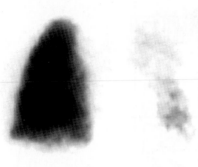

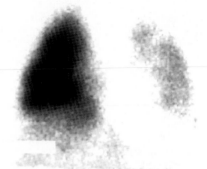

Krypton-81m   Technetium-99m MAA

FIGURE 5.7. Evaluation of a lung transplant. Krypton-81m and [99m]Tc—macroaggregated albumin (^{99m}Tc-MAA) studies from a recipient of a left lung transplant. Anterior images reveal significantly decreased ventilation and perfusion in the transplant.

colloid mixture that occurs during radiopharmaceutical administration. The method of aerosolization is critical. Most of the material is left in the aerosolizing apparatus and tubing, and only a small proportion of material within the apparatus reaches the lungs. Careful technique is essential to avoid contamination of the environment around the patient during aerosolization. The larger the aerosol particles, the more material is deposited in the tubing coming from the aerosolizing apparatus, nasal and oral cavities, and proximal airways. When such deposition occurs, it interferes with the assessment of distal aerosol distribution. The aerosol particles that reach the alveolar spaces clear slowly, whereas aerosol that deposits in the lined airways is rapidly cleared by mucociliary motion. On serial imaging, material can be seen migrating toward the proximal airways. Aerosolized ^{99m}Tc–sulfur colloid can therefore be used to evaluate mucociliary clearance. This has been used in clinical investigation, but use in routine pediatric practice is limited.

Technetium-99m-DTPA Aerosol

Inhalation of ^{99m}Tc-DTPA aerosol is accomplished in a similar manner to that for aerosolized ^{99m}Tc–sulfur colloid. Once deposited in the alveolar space, however, ^{99m}Tc-DTPA is absorbed through the alveolar-capillary membrane into the bloodstream. There, it is distributed into the extracellular space and excreted by the kidneys.[10] Serial imaging reveals a gradual disappearance of the agent from the lungs (Fig. 5.8). As with aerosolized sulfur colloid, especially in small children, material mixed with saliva during the inhalation is swallowed and appears in the stomach. This gastric deposition should not be confused with radioaerosol trapped in the left lower lung field. Increased permeability of the alveolar-capillary membrane results in accelerated washout of the material from the lungs. Exercise increases the lung clearance of inhaled ^{99m}Tc-DTPA aerosol.[11] Normal pulmonary washout values of ^{99m}Tc-DTPA in children have not been determined, but altered pulmonary washout rates of ^{99m}Tc-DTPA aerosol following inhalation have been found in several conditions including hyaline membrane disease,[10,12,13] cystic fibrosis lung disease, pulmonary complications of human immunodeficiency virus (HIV) infection,[14,15] sarcoidosis,[16] and lung transplants. The same considerations regarding aerosol production method and particle sizes mentioned earlier also apply to this material. As with ^{99m}Tc-sulfur colloid, the larger the particles, the greater the deposition in the tubing, mask, oral and nasal cavities, and proximal airways.

Technetium-99m-Pseudogas (Technegas)

Technetium-99m-pseudogas (Technegas) is produced by evaporation of sodium ^{99m}Tc pertechnetate at approximately 2500°C in a

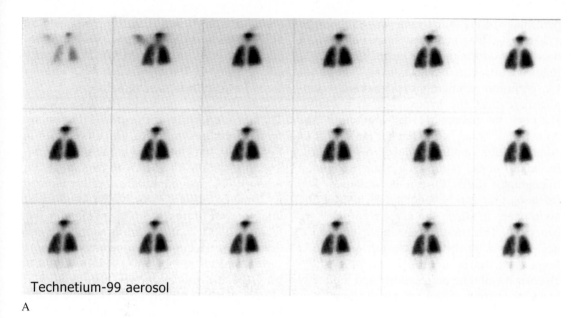

Technetium-99 aerosol

A

FIGURE 5.8. Aerosol ^{99m}Tc—diethylenetriamine pentaacetic acid (^{99m}Tc-DTPA) study. A: Series of posterior images (1 frame = 0.5 minute) show gradual accumulation of tracer in the lung fields and gradual washout. In the later images, renal elimination of tracer is seen. Tracer is visualized in the oropharynx. B: Time-activity curve represents washout of ^{99m}Tc-DTPA from the lungs.

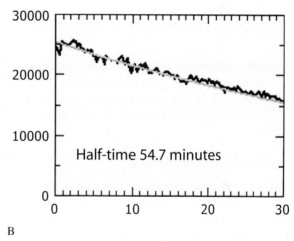

B

graphite crucible in a stream of argon gas. The material generated consists of an ultrafine aerosol of ^{99m}Tc-labeled carbon clusters. The exact size of the particles is the subject of some discussion, but the material is most likely comprised of 30-60 nm particles which aggregate into clusters with a median diameter of approximately 150 nm.[17-20] This radiopharmaceutical is said to combine characteristics of an aerosol and a gas and to be superior to radiopharmaceuticals produced by ultrasonic and jet nebulizers. The "pseudogas" is inhaled via a face mask, and the radioactive particles adhere to the walls of the respiratory bronchioles and

alveolar epithelium. If the airflow is not laminar or there is technical failure, the particles also deposit in the bronchial passages. High-quality images of the distribution of these particles in the lungs have been reported following a few breaths in adults and children.[21] The distribution of Technegas in the lung appears to be similar to that of ^{81m}Kr and ^{133}Xe.[22-25]

One drawback of Technegas use is that administration may lead to hypoxia. James et al.[26] measured a decrease in oxygen saturation in patients undergoing Technegas ventilation studies and observed a decrease in oxygen saturation in 87% of the patients.[26] The mean change, as a percentage of the initial value was 83% (range 1% to 24%. These investigators also observed a decrease in saturation in the range of 2% to 11% following intravenous injection of ^{99m}Tc-MAA for perfusion scintigraphy. With each radiopharmaceutical, the hypoxia was temporary). Because the pulmonary distribution of the "pseudogas" does not change rapidly after administration, multiple images of the lungs, including single photon emission computed tomography (SPECT), can be obtained. The retention time can be modified by altering the atmosphere in which the carbon particles are generated. This modified Technegas (pertechnegas) has a much faster clearance from the lungs[27] and can be used to assess pulmonary-alveolar membrane permeability and indirectly to identify hypoperfused areas in the lung.[28]

Regional Pulmonary Blood Flow

Regional pulmonary blood flow (rPBF) can be determined by two principal methods. One employs ^{99m}Tc-MAA, and the other, described above, employs intravenous ^{133}Xe dissolved in saline.

Technetium-99m-MAA

After intravenous injection, macroaggregated albumin particles temporarily embolize arterioles in the lungs in a distribution proportional to regional arterial pulmonary blood flow. Interrupted or decreased pulmonary arterial blood flow is reflected on scintigraphy as a region or regions of absent or reduced tracer concentration. The number of arterioles occluded with one typical intravenous injection of ^{99m}Tc-MAA is relatively small and under normal conditions, these obstructions are without physiologic significance. Approximately 90% of ^{99m}Tc-MAA particles range in

diameter from 10 to 40 μm. Approximately 280 million pulmonary arterioles in adults are small enough to trap the ^{99m}Tc-MAA, and typically only 200,000 to 700,000 particles are administered for pulmonary scintigraphy.

Once lodged in the pulmonary arterioles, the ^{99m}Tc-MAA particles are degraded into smaller particles and polypeptides, which are taken up by the liver and eliminated in the bile. The biologic half-life of ^{99m}Tc-MAA in the lungs is 6 to 8 hours. The minimum toxic dose for albumin is 20 mg/kg, which exceeds the usual adult imaging dose of less than 10 μg of albumin by a factor of 1000.[29,30] In newborns and young children whose pulmonary vasculature is immature, a smaller number of particles should be used. In the human infant, the number of alveoli increases rapidly during the first year of life and gradually reaches adult levels at approximately 8 years of age.[30,31] Although the precise age at which alveolar multiplication ceases is not known with certainty, one study shows a rapid increase from approximately one tenth to one third of adult values during the first year of life and to one half the adult number by 3 years of age.[32] If injection of 500,000 ^{99m}Tc-MAA particles is considered safe in the adult, the number of injected particles should not exceed 50,000 in the newborn or 165,000 at 1 year of age.[33] We recommend that a small number of particles (<10,000) be used in neonates and patients with severe pulmonary disease. For quantitation of right-to-left shunting, <10,000 is sufficient. To attain images with an apparent uniform distribution of activity in the mature lung, at least 60,000 particles should be injected. Table 5.2 lists suggested number of injected particles and usual administered doses for patients at various ages.

The ^{99m}Tc-MAA is usually injected with the patient in the supine position. If possible, the patient should be instructed to breathe normally while the tracer is injected slowly over 5

TABLE 5.2. Usual administered doses of ^{99m}Tc–macroaggregated albumin (^{99m}Tc-MAA)

Parameter	Newborn	1 Year	5 Years	10 Years	15 Years	Adult
Body weight (kg)	3.5	12.1	20.3	33.5	55.0	70.0
Administered dose (mCi)	0.2	0.5	1.0	1.5	2.5	3.0
Range of particles administered (×100)	10–50	50–150	200–300	200–300	200–700	200–700

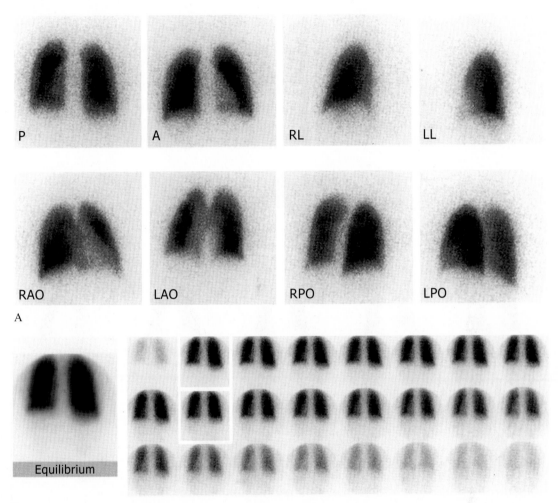

P

A

RL

LL

RAO

LAO

RPO

LPO

A

Equilibrium

B

FIGURE 5.9. Normal pulmonary scintigraphy. A: These normal images are from an 18-year-old man with deep venous thrombosis who presented with

to 10 seconds.* In the supine position, the distribution of ⁹⁹ᵐTc-MAA reflects the ventral-to-dorsal perfusion gradient so that relatively more particles localize in the dependent portions of the lung. The vertical perfusion gradient (apex to base) is not as prominent on scintigra-

tachypnea and diaphoresis. There is normal distribution of pulmonary blood flow by ⁹⁹ᵐTc-MAA. B: Corresponding normal ¹³³Xe ventilation study.

phy obtained after injection of ⁹⁹ᵐTc-MAA in the supine position as in the upright position. For the intravenous injection, we recommend a butterfly-type needle previously filled with normal saline. Once venous access has been gained, a few milliliters of normal saline are injected to verify patency; then ⁹⁹ᵐTc-MAA is injected slowly and flushed with saline. Imaging can begin immediately after the tracer injection.

After intravenous administration of ⁹⁹ᵐTc-MAA, anterior, posterior, both lateral, and four oblique projections are obtained. A gamma camera with a high-resolution collimator is recommended with each view recorded for 300,000 to 500,000 counts (Fig. 5.9). Single

---

*Some practitioners prefer to inject the MAA while the patient is breathing deeply. Others prefer to inject the patient in the sitting position. *Warning*: It is important to avoid drawing blood into the syringe containing ⁹⁹ᵐTc-MAA, as it could result in the rapid formation of large clots within the syringe, which if injected into the patient could cause massive pulmonary embolism.

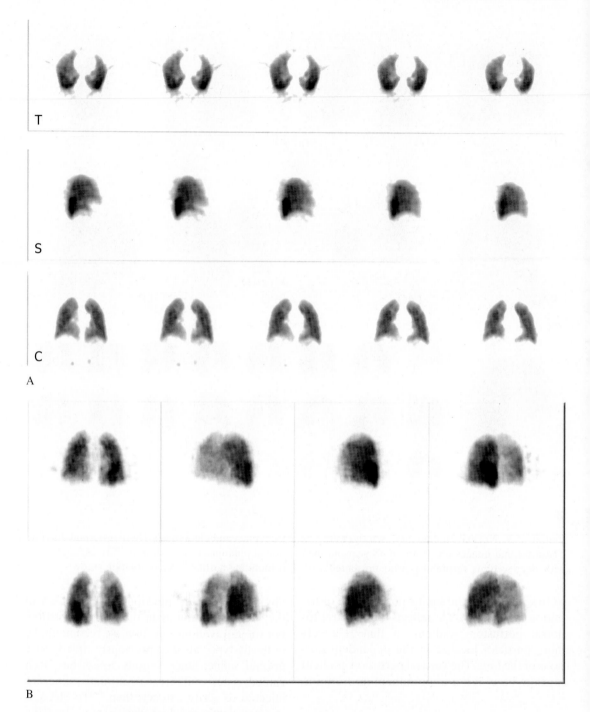

T

S

C

A

B

FIGURE 5.10. Normal ^{99m}Tc-MAA pulmonary single photon emission computed tomography (SPECT). A: Normal selected transverse (T), sagittal (S), and coronal (C) slices. B: Selected images from a volume rendered set.

photon emission computed tomography should perhaps be considered as the standard imaging method for the assessment of pulmonary perfusion instead of multiple planar projections. It can be performed in about the same time as planar imaging and is more advantageous (Fig. 5.10).

Clinical Applications

Cystic Fibrosis

Cystic fibrosis (CF) is a systemic disorder that involves almost all organ systems including the lungs, pancreas, liver, intestine, and genitalia. It is hereditary and is transmitted as an autosomal recessive trait. This disease causes most of the chronic progressive pulmonary disease encountered in children. The incidence of CF in the United States is 1:1600 to 1:2000 live Caucasian births. Approximately 5% of the general population are carriers of the gene. More than 99% of patients with CF have an elevated sweat electrolyte concentration.[34–36] During the past decade, the typical clinical course of CF has improved significantly due to more accurate and earlier diagnosis, better understanding of the pathophysiology of this disorder, and improved therapy.

In the lungs of CF patients, excessive mucus is produced that is thick and sticky. The cilia cannot move this mucus effectively; it accumulates in the bronchi and bronchioles, causing obstruction. Stagnation of secretions favors the development of infection; *Staphylococcus aureus* and *Pseudomonas aeruginosa* are common pathogens found in the lungs of these patients. Obstruction and infection lead to hyperaeration or atelectasis depending on whether the obstruction is partial or total. One problem compounds another in this disease. Accumulation of thick mucus interferes with ventilation, mucociliary clearance, and the normal mechanism of cough, resulting in further accumulation of mucus. Moreover, the inflammatory reaction and infection destroy the ciliated epithelium, and bronchiectasis develops after the loss of integrity of the bronchial walls. Purulent secretions are accumulated in peribronchial pools. These regions become chronic sources of local infection and seed infection to other parts of the lung. The course of the disease leads to complications, such as abscess, hemoptysis, and spontaneous pneumothorax. As the disease progresses, it leads to respiratory insufficiency, cor pulmonale, and finally death.

With early mild involvement, ^{133}Xe studies reveal nearly normal regional distribution of inhaled gas and perfusion. However, diffuse, minimal to moderate delay of ^{133}Xe washout (trapping) can be detected in this stage. In our laboratory, we have investigated the early pulmonary manifestations of CF in a group of infants with positive sweat chloride tests and good clinical condition. Xenon-133 studies in these patients detected early changes by demonstrating trapping even in the presence of normal chest radiographs. In addition, some of these patients showed evidence of increased permeability of the alveolar capillary membrane evidenced by high systemic penetration of ^{133}Xe after both inhalation of the gas and intravenous administration of ^{133}Xe in saline. The liver concentrates relatively higher amounts of tracer, which may be due to the increased permeability of the alveolar-capillary membrane and/or pulmonary right-to-left shunting.

As the disease progresses, irregular abnormalities in regional ventilation and perfusion set in, along with more severe trapping of ^{133}Xe. The lungs are involved globally, although the upper lung zones are usually more affected than the lower zones (Figs. 5.11 and 5.12). With more advanced disease, distribution of ^{133}Xe during inhalation is irregular throughout the lungs, and it is difficult if not impossible to reach an equilibrium of ^{133}Xe in the lung during rebreathing. Some regions of the lung accumulate ^{133}Xe, but the gas does not penetrate obstructed air spaces. During the early stages of the disease, the distribution of pulmonary blood flow as assessed with ^{133}Xe matches the abnormal distribution of ventilation. With advanced disease, however, the distribution of pulmonary blood flow, though abnormal, appears more uniform than ventilation. Some regions of the lung that do not receive ^{133}Xe by

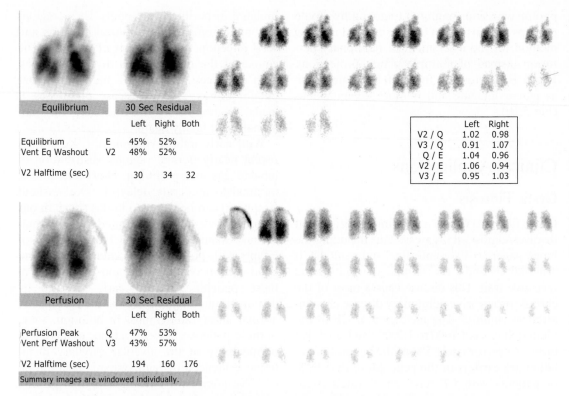

		Left	Right	Both
Equilibrium	E	45%	52%	
Vent Eq Washout	V2	48%	52%	
V2 Halftime (sec)		30	34	32

	Left	Right
V2 / Q	1.02	0.98
V3 / Q	0.91	1.07
Q / E	1.04	0.96
V2 / E	1.06	0.94
V3 / E	0.95	1.03

		Left	Right	Both
Perfusion Peak	Q	47%	53%	
Vent Perf Washout	V3	43%	57%	
V2 Halftime (sec)		194	160	176

Summary images are windowed individually.

FIGURE 5.11. Cystic fibrosis. Xenon-133 ventilation and perfusion study from a 12-year-old girl with advanced disease. There is very poor overall lung function with diffuse and focal air trapping. The upper lung zones reveal the poorest ventilation. The distribution of pulmonary blood flow is also abnormal, but it is relatively more uniformly distributed than ventilation.

inhalation are reached by pulmonary blood flow. Marked air trapping is evident throughout the lung fields.

During the remission phase, perfusion abnormalities correlate with the severity of disease. During the acute phase, striking transient alterations develop.[37] With hemoptysis, the region of the lung involved may show further reduction in ventilation with or without apparent reduction of regional blood flow. In CF, the ventilation-perfusion gradient is reversed from normal, and the regional ventilation/perfusion ratios are unevenly distributed.[38] Good correlation between perfusion and ventilation abnormalities and the severity of CF has been demonstrated. The superior sensitivity of perfusion scintigraphy (^{99m}Tc-MAA) over chest radiographs for detecting the presence and extent of early pulmonary involvement has also been shown.[39]

Scintigraphy has been used to assess the effects of physical therapy of the chest on ciliary clearance and ventilation. A study using 5-μm polystyrene particles labeled with ^{99m}Tc found that chest physiotherapy increases clearance of excessive bronchial secretions in patients with chronic airway obstruction.[40] Using serial ^{81m}Kr scintigraphy, we evaluated the effect of bronchial drainage with percussion and vibration on peripheral ventilation in patients with CF. There were no changes in the distribution of ventilation in patients with mild disease. The ventilatory pattern in patients with moderate disease was variable and seemingly independent of treatment. The patients with severe lung disease exhibited some apparent

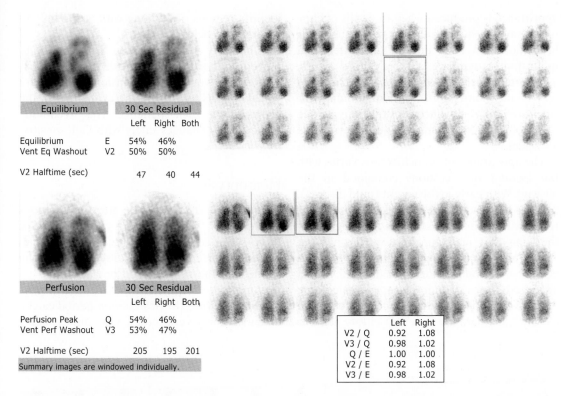

		Left	Right	Both
Equilibrium	E	54%	46%	
Vent Eq Washout	V2	50%	50%	
V2 Halftime (sec)		47	40	44

		Left	Right	Both
Perfusion Peak	Q	54%	46%	
Vent Perf Washout	V3	53%	47%	
V2 Halftime (sec)		205	195	201

Summary images are windowed individually.

	Left	Right
V2 / Q	0.92	1.08
V3 / Q	0.98	1.02
Q / E	1.00	1.00
V2 / E	0.92	1.08
V3 / E	0.98	1.02

FIGURE 5.12. Cystic fibrosis. Xenon-133 ventilation and perfusion study from a 23-year-old woman with advanced cystic fibrosis lung disease. The distribution of inhaled ^{133}Xe is irregular, particularly in the upper lung zones (the right upper lung is worse than the left), and there is severe air trapping. Pulmonary blood flow is more regularly distributed than ventilation, and washout is significantly delayed from all lung zones.

improvement in regional aeration of the lungs. As expected, there was a relationship between ventilatory changes and the amount of sputum produced. Because the distribution of regional ventilation in patients with CF is highly variable from time to time even without treatment, all changes in regional ventilation in these patients could not be attributed to chest physical therapy alone.[41]

In practice, most patients with CF referred for ^{133}Xe ventilation-perfusion studies are those with established or advanced lung disease. Although early pulmonary involvement can be detected with ^{133}Xe studies (even in the presence of a normal chest radiograph and normal pulmonary function tests), radionuclide studies have not been routinely utilized to make the diagnosis of early lung disease. Radionuclide assessment of lung disease is more frequently left to rather late stages of the disease, which are appreciable by other means. It is tempting

to speculate that if lung involvement were identified earlier, therapeutic intervention might improve the clinical course of patients affected with CF. Xenon-133 ventilation-perfusion studies in patients with CF have been used to assess regional lung function before surgery to ensure that removal of a lobe would not further compromise a patient with already severe pulmonary disease.

Early radiologic manifestations include diffuse bronchial thickening, hyperinflation, and evidence of retained secretions. Later, peribronchial fibrosis, involvement of the hilar nodes, bronchiectasis, and enlargement of the pulmonary artery occur. Increased interstitial markings or cyst-like structures are apparent. Haziness of the bronchovascular shadows and irregular areas of hyperinflation are seen predominantly in the upper lobes. Interstitial markings tend to become more and more irregular and reticulonodular. A honeycomb appearance is produced when the walls of clustered, small cyst-like areas (ectatic bronchi or bronchioles on end) thicken and interstitial infiltration progresses. With advanced stages, a distorted picture suggesting Swiss cheese is seen on the radiographs. Transient nodular densities are replaced by lucencies that may be due to endobronchial collections and peribronchial abscesses.

The appearance of bronchiectasis varies with the amount of secretions contained in the airways. With early involvement (mild disease), findings on radiographs of the chest do not correlate with pulmonary scintigraphy. Regions of the lung that may appear normal on chest radiographs may show ventilation-perfusion abnormalities on pulmonary scintigraphy. With advanced stages of lung disease, scintigraphic and radiographic findings correlate more closely.[38] Scintigraphy with ^{67}Ga-citrate helps to identify regions of the lung with active inflammation (see below).

Pulmonary transplantation has been employed to treat patients with advanced CF. Xenon-133 ventilation-perfusion studies are valuable tools to assist in the evaluation of the progress of such patients. This technique depicts early changes safely with high sensitivity (Fig. 5.13).

Hemoptysis

Scintigraphy of the lungs after intravenous injection of ^{99m}Tc–red blood cells (RBCs) or ^{99m}Tc–sulfur colloid may be useful for the localization of bleeding.[42,43] Because of their long residence time in the blood pool, ^{99m}Tc-RBCs may increase the possibility of localizing intermittent bleeding; the observation period can be extended for several hours. One disadvantage

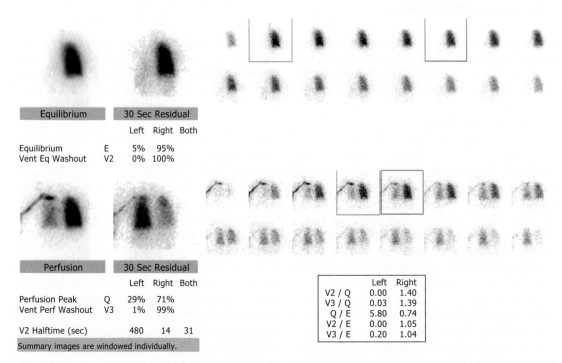

		Left	Right	Both
Equilibrium	E	5%	95%	
Vent Eq Washout	V2	0%	100%	

		Left	Right	Both
Perfusion Peak	Q	29%	71%	
Vent Perf Washout	V3	1%	99%	
V2 Halftime (sec)		480	14	31

Summary images are windowed individually.

	Left	Right
V2 / Q	0.00	1.40
V3 / Q	0.03	1.39
Q / E	5.80	0.74
V2 / E	0.00	1.05
V3 / E	0.20	1.04

FIGURE 5.13. Bilateral lung transplant. Xenon-133 ventilation and perfusion study from a recipient of a lung transplant. This patient had a stenosis of the left main bronchus that had been dilated twice. The patient did not seem to improve, and this study reveals no ventilation of the entire left lung (top). The perfusion study, however, demonstrates that approximately 30% of the total pulmonary blood flow reaches the left lung. Left lung washout is prolonged. These findings are strongly compatible with obstruction of the left main stem bronchus.

of labeled RBCs is that the bleeding/background ratio and the bleeding/cardiac blood pool ratio are lower than with ^{99m}Tc–sulfur colloid, preventing detection of small volumes of bleeding. Our limited experience with ^{99m}Tc-RBCs suggests that it has good potential for localizing pulmonary bleeding.

After intravenous injection, ^{99m}Tc–sulfur colloid is extracted rapidly from the blood by cells of the reticuloendothelial system. If bleeding occurs during its brief presence in the blood pool, the tracer extravasates in the area of active bleeding. Because of the high bleeding/background activity ratio achievable with this tracer, small amounts of bleeding may be detected. In the gastrointestinal tract, this technique has detected bleeding at rates as low as 0.1 mL/minute.[29,44] Bleeding rates of 0.1 to 0.2 mL/minute have been detected in dogs.[45]

An important source of error in detecting pulmonary bleeding in animals and humans has been attributed to diffuse distribution of the radiotracer related to bleeding into a large bronchus.[45,46] Unfortunately, many patients have intermittent pulmonary bleeding, as in CF, and in our limited experience we have not been successful in localizing bleeding with ^{99m}Tc–sulfur colloid in these individuals. Presumably, this failure occurred because bleeding did not coincide in time with the brief presence of radiocolloid in blood.

Congenital and Acquired Anomalies of Heart and Great Vessels

At the time of this writing, the most frequent indication for pulmonary scintigraphy with ^{99m}Tc-MAA in our institution is assessment of regional pulmonary blood flow in patients with congenital or acquired (surgically induced) abnormalities of pulmonary blood flow. The technique is rapid, safe, and easy to perform, and it provides useful information about the regional distribution of total pulmonary blood flow. Pulmonary scintigraphy is the only quantitative way of assessing the results of interventional procedures designed to relieve obstruction to pulmonary blood flow. Although echocardiography has assumed an increasingly prominent role in assessment of congenital anomalies of the heart, the distal pulmonary arteries remain inaccessible to investigation because of the overlying lungs. Pulmonary perfusion scintigraphy is therefore essential for overall assessment of patients before and after catheter or surgical arterioplasty, intravascular stent placement, and coil occlusion of unwanted vascular communications (Figs. 5.14 and 5.15).

As a relatively large proportion of patients in this group have right-to-left shunting, we routinely employ fewer than 10,000 particles for pulmonary scintigraphy. Localization of ^{99m}Tc-MAA in the kidneys after its intravenous injection indicates the presence of a right-to-left shunt of at least 15% (Fig. 5.16).[47] Radionuclide detection and quantitation of shunts is discussed in Chapter 6. The purpose of the ^{99m}Tc-MAA lung study in most of these patients is to establish the percent distribution of total pulmonary blood flow in the right and left lungs, which can be accomplished well with a small number of particles. Use of such a low number of particles frequently results in an apparent inhomogeneity of activity distribution in the lungs. Interpreters must be careful to recognize this expected pattern of inhomogeneous distribution and not confuse it with pulmonary disease. Only significant abnormalities in regional pulmonary blood flow can be confidently identified when evaluating pulmonary scintigraphy obtained with such small numbers of particles.

Peripheral Pulmonary Stenosis

Stenosis of the major branches of the pulmonary arterial tree can occur congenitally (especially in patients with tetralogy of Fallot and pulmonary atresia) or be acquired because of surgically created shunts (e.g., Blalock-Taussig, Waterston shunts, etc.). Asymmetric distribution of pulmonary blood flow can result in abnormal angiogenesis and alveologenesis and can lead to pulmonary hypertension in the contralateral lung without stenoses. Balloon angioplasty, with or without placement of an intravascular stent, has become the procedure of choice in our institution for the relief of these obstructions. Lung perfusion scintigraphy is

Anterior   Posterior

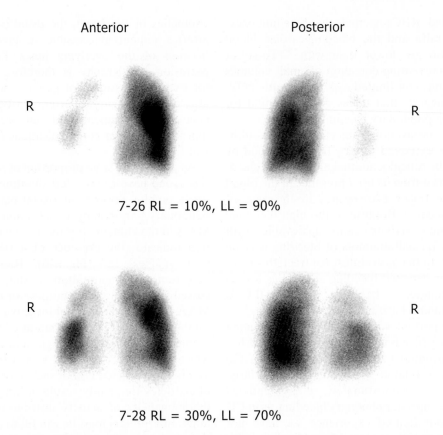

7-26 RL = 10%, LL = 90%

7-28 RL = 30%, LL = 70%

FIGURE 5.14. Pulmonary blood flow before and after right pulmonary artery dilation. Two ^{99m}Tc-MAA studies are from a 9-year-old boy with surgically repaired tetralogy of Fallot. The first study (top) reveals poor perfusion to the right lung (10%). The second study, following balloon dilation of the right pulmonary artery, reveals an improvement of left pulmonary artery blood flow to 28% of the total.

frequently used before and after these procedures to assess results.

Pulmonary Vein Stenosis

Obstruction to pulmonary venous outflow from the lungs can also lead to asymmetric pulmonary blood flow and pulmonary hypertension. Unilateral pulmonary vein stenosis may be associated with complex congenital heart disease; left pulmonary vein stenosis has been rarely reported in patients with transposition of the great arteries. Pulmonary artery stenosis may be difficult to detect echocardiographically and angiocardiographically but may be identified by pulmonary scintigraphy by demonstrating regions of low perfusion in the lung in the absence of pulmonary artery stenoses.

Pulmonary Artery Stenosis

Infants with *pulmonary artery stenosis* have an abnormally higher pulmonary blood flow to the left lung. The jet flow formed by the stenotic valve is directed preferentially to the left pulmonary artery.[48,49] In these patients, the left lung also has relatively greater perfusion of the upper zone. Infants with pulmonic stenosis and left-to-right shunts have perfusion abnormalities in both lungs. There is increased flow to both upper zones and overperfusion of the left lung.

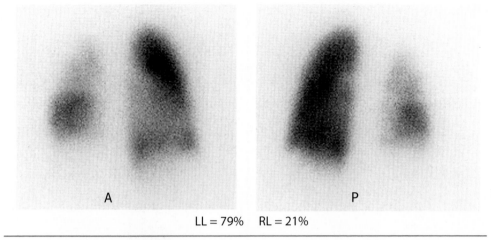

LL = 79%   RL = 21%

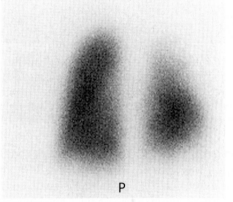

LL = 61%   RL = 39%

FIGURE 5.15. Right pulmonary artery angioplasty. Technetium-99m-MAA scintigraphy before (top) and after (bottom) right pulmonary artery angio-plasty demonstrated improvement of blood flow to the right lung (RL). LL, left lung.

Septal Defects

Patients with *ventricular septal defect* may have decreased perfusion in the left lung because of enlargement of the left side of the heart compressing the left lung.[50] In patients who have had a *pulmonary artery band*, distal migration of the band may impinge on either the right or left pulmonary arteries, resulting in abnormal ventilation and perfusion balance. This imbalance in the distribution of pulmonary blood flow does not reverse in most patients after surgical removal of the band and repair of the ventricular septal defect.[51] Normal children, even infants held in the erect position, have rela-

tively more pulmonary perfusion in the lower lung fields than in the upper lung fields. The normal upper/lower lung pulmonary perfusion ratio is 0.5 to 0.6. Children with intracardiac left-to-right shunts have an abnormally higher fraction of pulmonary blood flow going to their upper lung fields with equal distribution between the right and left lungs. In older children with atrial septal defect, a greater than normal proportion of blood flows to the right lung. Enlargement of the heart into the left hemithorax has been called a causative factor for this increased flow.[52] With *partially anomalous pulmonary venous return* (PAPVR), one or more of the pulmonary veins enter the right

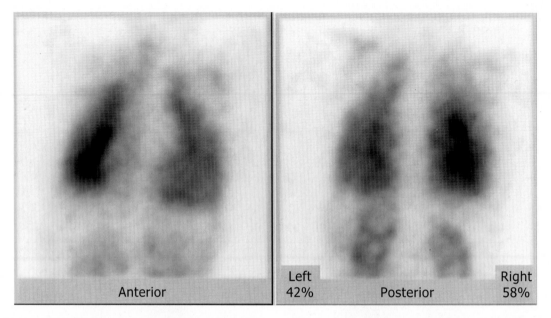

| Left | | Right |
| 42% | Posterior | 58% |

Anterior

FIGURE 5.16. Right-to-left shunt. Technetium-99m-MAA pulmonary scintigraphy from a child with tetralogy of Fallot being evaluated prior to pulmonary artery angioplasty to determine left-right pulmonary perfusion distribution. A significant portion of the ^{99m}Tc-MAA has reached the systemic circulation through a large right-to-left shunt. Fewer than 10,000 particles of MAA were used.

atrium instead of the left. In one series, this condition was found in approximately 0.7% of routine autopsies.[53] The right lung is involved in some form of anomalous venous return almost twice as often as the left. The most frequent association of anomalous draining right pulmonary veins is an atrial septal defect of the sinus venosus type. Also, the anomalous draining vein(s) can enter the superior vena cava or inferior vena cava (scimitar syndrome); only rarely do they enter the right atrium directly. With PAPVR from the left lung, the return is typically to a persistent left-sided superior vena cava; rarely is there subdiaphragmatic return of the lower pulmonary vein. The clinical and physiologic features of PAPVR are similar to those of atrial septal defect with left-to-right shunting. The left-to-right shunt of PAPVR can be detected and quantified with first-pass radionuclide angiography.

Pulmonary Arteriovenous Malformations

Pulmonary arteriovenous malformations (AVMs) are congenital or acquired anomalies with direct connections between the pulmonary artery and vein. Acquired AVMs are typically associated with hepatic disease or systemic venous-to-pulmonary shunts (Glenn or Fontan procedures). The abnormalities are usually cavernomatous and cause physiologic right-to-left shunting and arterial desaturation. These lesions can be solitary, multiple, diffuse (telangiectatic), or mixed. More than 60% are solitary, and most occur on the lower lobes. In approximately half these patients there is associated familial telangiectasis and hemangiomas of the skin and mucous membranes. Clinical symptoms are secondary to abnormal oxygenation related to the right-to-left shunt (cyanosis, dyspnea, hemoptysis, epistaxis, exercise intolerance) and secondary embolic pneumonia. Physical examination of patients with pulmonary AVMs may reveal conjunctival hemorrhages, digital clubbing, or murmur. Polycythemia or cerebrovascular accidents may occur. Radiographs of the chest show single or multiple lesions with linear, vascular shadows. Pulmonary angiography is diagnostic. Detection with radionuclide angiography depends on the size and location of the lesion. The appearance on radionuclide angiography is that of a distinct, localized blush of activity within a lung field immediately after the appearance of the right side of the heart.[54–56] The right-to-left shunt can be measured with ^{99m}Tc-MAA.

Surgery and Changes in Regional Pulmonary Blood Flow

A number of recent surgical modifications have been introduced in patients with single ventricle to directly connect the systemic venous return into the pulmonary arteries and provide more effective pulmonary blood flow. In the classic Glenn shunt, the superior vena cava is directly connected to the right pulmonary artery, with ligation of the connection between the cardiac end of the superior vena cava and the right atrium and division of the connection between the right pulmonary artery and the main pulmonary artery. This operation results in all the systemic venous return from the head, neck, and arms entering the right lung. However, the "bidirectional" Glenn shunt does not result in pulmonary vascular discontinuity; injection of tracer into the upper extremity veins in these patients more accurately reflects the distribution of pulmonary blood flow. In patients who have had a classic Glenn shunt, injection of ^{99m}Tc-MAA into a vein of the upper body will concentrate almost entirely in the right lung, thereby making calculations of asymmetric pulmonary blood flow difficult or impossible. If the injection is made in the lower extremity, most of the tracer ends up entering the left lung, and a larger right-to-left shunt will be detected. It is therefore critical that the precise surgical anatomy of these patients be determined so that proper interpretation of the results can be made.

Pulmonary Embolism

With pulmonary emboli there is partial or total occlusion of pulmonary arteries that may or may not be accompanied by pulmonary infarction. Arterial thrombi occur most frequently in association with a damaged vessel wall. Venous thrombi occur in association with reduced blood flow in the absence of a vascular lesion. Platelets are an important factor in arterial thrombosis, whereas components of the intrinsic plasma clotting mechanism are involved in venous thrombosis.[57]

Pulmonary embolism remains one of the most common and difficult problems in medicine. It is more common in adults, with only approximately 10% of all emboli occurring in the pediatric population.[58] Necropsy studies reveal that approximately 50% of patients who die of pulmonary embolism are not diagnosed before death.[59] The incidence of symptomatic pulmonary embolism in the United States is approximately 650,000 cases per year. The mortality of patients with pulmonary embolism is far greater in those patients in whom the diagnosis is not made.[60] Emery[61] reported an incidence of pulmonary embolism in infants and toddlers of 1.25%. Jones and Sabiston[62] reported a 0.70% incidence of pulmonary embolism at autopsy in children less than 16 years of age. In a review of autopsies in children, Buck and coworkers[63] found an incidence of pulmonary embolism of approximately 4.0% in patients from 0 to 19 years of age; patients with known tumor emboli, fat emboli, or foreign material and those thought to have pulmonary thrombosis were not included.

Venous thromboses have been found in approximately 40% of patients with pulmonary emboli and were located, in order of frequency, in the heart, superior vena cava, mesenteric veins, brain, iliofemoral veins, inferior vena cava, and lower and upper extremities. In approximately 30% of these patients, pulmonary embolism was thought to contribute to their death. In the remaining 70%, pulmonary embolism did not have a demonstrable effect on the clinical course or was thought to be an incidental finding at autopsy. Buck et al.[63] stated that pulmonary embolism in children is underdiagnosed, and an increased use of perfusion scintigraphy should be encouraged. Almost half (17 of 36) of their patients in whom pulmonary embolism was thought at autopsy to have had clinical importance had signs and symptoms usually attributable to pulmonary embolism. Pulmonary embolism was suspected clinically in only five of the 17 patients, and only two were on anticoagulant therapy at the time of death. There was no apparent age effect in the incidence of pulmonary embolism, although infants made up 25% of the patients in this series.

The risk of developing pulmonary embolism in children after surgery was more than twice as great as in nonsurgical patients.[63] Pulmonary embolism has also been found as a complication of legally induced abortions.[64] Other causes include oral contraceptives, infected arteriovenous (AV) shunts, fat, and air.[65] Fat emboli may occur after bone fractures or orthopedic procedures involving bone.[66–68] Central venous catheters used for hyperalimentation carry a risk for developing pulmonary emboli associated with the chronic venous trauma and the thrombotic effect of the catheter.[69–71] Pulmonary embolism during cardiac catheterization may be caused by detachment of synthetic fibers from nondisposable catheters.[72] Pulmonary emboli caused during catheterization remain undetected in many instances. Heart disease is a major factor associated with pulmonary emboli in children and adults.[73,74]

Victims of accidental trauma, especially those with fractures of the hip or pelvis, have a 15% incidence of pulmonary embolism.[75] Septic emboli may originate from any infectious focus. Young drug addicts may present with septic pulmonary emboli. With sickle cell disease, microthrombosis frequently results in infarction of the lung, spleen, kidney, and bone, but medically important pulmonary embolism in these patients is rare. With polycythemia, increased blood viscosity and vascular stasis lead to thrombosis.[76] Pulmonary embolism may result from birth injury that dislodges cerebral or cerebellar tissue.[77–79] Homocystinuria, an inborn error of metabolism, is characterized by the absence of cystathionine synthetase in several body tissues. In patients affected with this disorder, platelet abnormalities are believed to cause thrombosis. Also, homocystine may induce vascular endothelial damage that facilitates platelet plug formation and thrombosis.[80]

Pulmonary embolism may present acutely as an overwhelming catastrophic disease or insidiously as a chronic cardiopulmonary problem or fever of unknown origin. It may occur in previously healthy individuals or those with a chronic or acute illness. The clinical presentation of pulmonary embolism varies. Commonly it suggests congestive heart failure or pneumonia, or, less frequently, myocardial infarction, chronic obstructive lung disease, or pleurisy. Hemoptysis and fever may be present in subacute cases. Tachypnea or dyspnea and elevation of venous pressure are present frequently.[73,81,82] Other signs and symptoms found with pulmonary embolism include cough, wheezing, rales, sweats, palpitations, nausea, vomiting, chills, syncope, tachycardia, phlebitis, edema, murmur, and cyanosis. A pleural friction rub is common. Hepatomegaly and occasionally splenomegaly may be present. None of these signs and symptoms is specific for or establishes the diagnosis of pulmonary embolism.

Arterial blood oxygen is frequently but not always reduced in pulmonary embolism. Therefore, the presence of normal blood gases does not exclude the diagnosis of pulmonary embolism. Serum enzyme determinations [lactic dehydrogenase (LDH) and aspartate aminotransferase (serum glutamic-oxaloacetic transaminase, SGOT)] are of limited or minimal value, and blood coagulation tests are not useful. The erythrocyte sedimentation rate (ESR) is elevated in approximately 40% of the patients. The electrocardiogram (ECG) may demonstrate right ventricular strain, but the test has no specific value. The ECG is abnormal in most patients with massive or submassive pulmonary embolism.

The signs of pulmonary embolism on radiographs of the chest are variable and nonspecific (elevated hemidiaphragm, pleural effusion, infiltrate or consolidation, atelectasis, changes in pulmonary vessels). Radiographs of the chest may show increased density in the area involved, and pleural effusion is found in most patients with pulmonary embolism. Many patients with proven pulmonary embolism have normal radiographs of the chest.[83] Computed tomography (CT) angiography is a very good method to diagnose pulmonary embolism.

Pulmonary function tests may be normal or abnormal and have limited value in the diagnosis of pulmonary embolism. Pulmonary emboli result in vasoconstriction and bronchoconstriction, and these changes lead to ventilation-perfusion abnormalities. Hemodynamic studies reveal a reduction in systemic pressure with an increase in pulmonary artery pressure, but such studies are usually done at the time of pulmonary angiography.

Pulmonary scintigraphy using ^{99m}Tc-MAA provides a simple, safe, sensitive, and precise method to evaluate pulmonary artery perfusion. Any disorder that affects pulmonary blood flow, including pulmonary embolism, can cause abnormal perfusion scintigraphy.[84] With pulmonary embolism, perfusion defects may be single or multiple and follow a segmental or subsegmental distribution. An entire lobe of lung may be affected (Fig. 5.17). In a patient

suspected of having an acute pulmonary embolism with a perfusion defect on scintigraphy and a normal radiograph of the chest, the likelihood of pulmonary embolism is high.

In some cases the addition of ventilation studies using radioactive gases further assists in the diagnosis of pulmonary embolism. In many patients with pulmonary embolism, ventilation is preserved in the area of the affected lung. It is important to remember, however, that processes affecting the ventilatory areas first may affect the vascular network and produce a reduction in blood flow. Conversely, lesions that affect the pulmonary vasculature first can

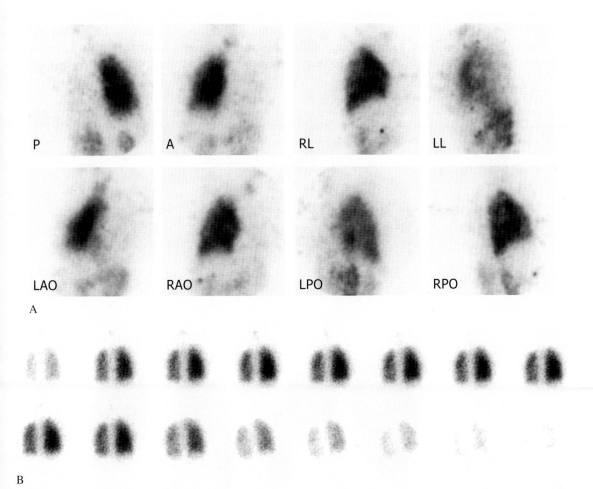

FIGURE 5.17. Massive pulmonary embolism. A: Scintigraphy using ^{99m}Tc-MAA demonstrates no pulmonary blood flow to the entire left lung. In addition, there is a large right-to-left shunt. The patient was a 21-year-old man with a ventricular septal defect and left pulmonary artery hypoplasia who presented with acute chest pain and dyspnea. B: This ^{133}Xe ventilation study reveals significant ventilation (40%) of the left lung.

compromise regional ventilation. Atelectasis causes a defect in perfusion and ventilation. Emphysema, chronic obstructive lung disease, or bronchitis may compromise the vascular network of the lung and disrupt blood flow. Infectious diseases of the lung invade both ventilatory and vascular spaces. Although it is believed that pulmonary embolism is characterized by ventilation-perfusion mismatch, it can also cause ventilation-perfusion match.[85–89]

Resolution of pulmonary embolism occurs principally by fibrinolysis. This mechanism can result in resolution as quickly as 24 hours. More commonly, restoration of pulmonary blood flow after pulmonary embolism takes a few days or even a few weeks. Resolution of pulmonary embolism is more rapid in young patients than in older patients.[90]

Pulmonary angiography is a specific and precise test for the diagnosis of pulmonary embolism. With this method the hemodynamics and cardiac function can be measured simultaneously. Unfortunately, the procedure is invasive and carries a definite risk. The decision to perform arteriography is arrived at only after careful analysis of the clinical situation, physical examination, radiography of the chest, pulmonary scintigraphy, and therapeutic considerations. Computed tomography angiography has gained wide acceptance in the diagnosis of pulmonary embolism and has significantly reduced the use of pulmonary angiography.

Airway Obstruction

Diffuse airway obstruction in children occurs in asthma, infection, CF, and α_1-antitrypsin deficiency. Local airway obstruction can be caused by mucous plugs (Fig. 5.18), foreign bodies

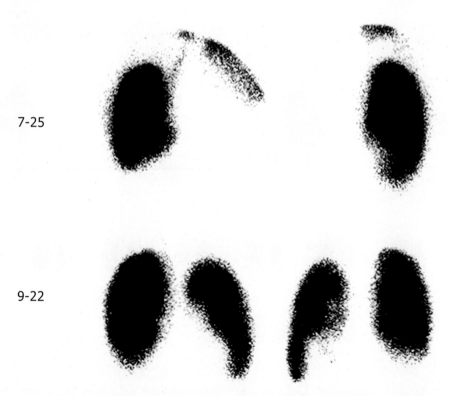

7-25

9-22

FIGURE 5.18. Complete airway obstruction, left lung. Krypton-81m images show no ventilation to the entire left lung (top), thought to be due to a mucous plug. A follow-up study 2 months later (bottom) reveals restoration of ventilation to the left lung.

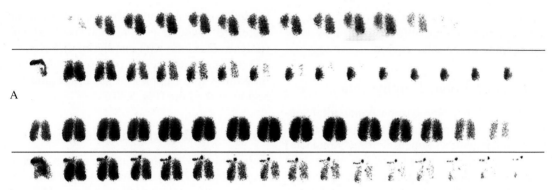

FIGURE 5.19. Airway obstruction due to a foreign body: ^{133}Xe ventilation and perfusion studies. A: Series of images during inhalation (top) reveal absence of ventilation to the left lower lung field. Xenon-133 perfusion images (bottom) reveal normal perfusion to the lungs including the left lower lung field. There is significant air trapping in the left lower lung, which is strongly suggestive of airway obstruction. B: Follow-up study on the same patient 20 days after removal of a peanut in the left lower lung bronchus reveals restoration of ventilation to the left lung field (top) and some residual air trapping following intravenous ^{133}Xe.

(Fig. 5.19), pneumonia, CF, or congenital lobar emphysema. Xenon-133 studies characteristically show delayed washout of the tracer within the involved region of the lung. With airway obstruction, equilibrium of ^{133}Xe within the lungs cannot be achieved. The pulmonary distribution of radioxenon depends on the degree and distribution of airway obstruction and on the length of the rebreathing period. Depending on penetration of the gas in the obstructed lung regions, the images may or may not reflect air trapping. Images after short periods of rebreathing ^{133}Xe may show one or several areas of reduced to no accumulation of the tracer corresponding to lung regions supplied by obstructed airways. Longer periods of rebreathing result in greater penetration and even accumulation of the tracer in the obstructed lung tissue. Increased accumulation of gas in these obstructed lung regions represents decreased ventilation. Images obtained during the washout phase reveal the delayed clearance of radiotracer (trapping) in areas of airway obstruction. When ^{133}Xe in saline is administered by intravenous injection, it usually attains a more uniform distribution in the lung than that obtained with short rebreathing periods. Regions of airway obstruction may

show perfusion with delayed washout. This pattern of delayed wash-in during inhalation and delayed washout after intravenous ^{133}Xe is characteristic of airway obstruction. With severe acute airway obstruction, trapping may be detected only after intravenous injection of ^{133}Xe because the inhaled gas may not reach the obstructed lung at all. Acute bronchial obstruction may be accompanied by pulmonary hypoperfusion, which is reversible. We have seen patients, however, in whom perfusion to the obstructed area is not affected (Fig. 5.19). A mucous plug occluding a main stem bronchus results in severe reduction of airflow to the involved lung (Fig. 5.18). After removal of the plug, ventilation usually returns to normal.[91-93] In addition, obstruction by a mucous plug results in secondary mild to severe reduction in regional blood flow. The mechanism by which abnormal ventilation causes diminished perfusion may be related to reduced oxygen in the alveoli rather than changes in airflow.[94] Xenon-133 studies in patients with mucous plugs are similar to those found after aspiration of foreign objects. The involved region of lung typically shows reduced or absent ventilation during inhalation of ^{133}Xe. After administration of intravenous ^{133}Xe in saline, the affected region of lung may reveal normal, reduced, or even absent pulmonary blood flow followed by air trapping in the same region.

Congenital Lobar Emphysema

Congenital lobar emphysema (congenital segmental lobar emphysema, emphysema of infancy, or congenital segmental bronchomalacia) exists in several forms and probably has several etiologies, although the precise cause or causes are unknown. Patients with congenital lobar emphysema present with early onset of respiratory distress. Approximately 80% have symptoms within the first 6 months of life, but the disorder has been discovered as late as 8 years of age.[95] Sometimes the abnormality is recognized incidentally on roentgenograms of the chest obtained for other reasons. Approximately 10% to 30% of the patients are found to have associated cardiovascular abnormalities, such as ventricular septal defect or patent ductus arteriosus. The male/female ratio is 2:1. Radiographically, overaeration of the lobe can be seen to cause compression of the adjacent lung, spreading of the ribs, and mediastinal shift. The hyperlucent overdistended lobe may herniate across the midline. In the newborn the overdistended lobe may be filled with fluid. Most commonly, a single lobe is involved (50% left upper lobe, 25% right middle lobe, 20% right upper lobe, other lobes less frequently). Histologically, there are distended alveoli with

minimal or no interstitial involvement and an increased number of normal-sized alveoli (polyalveolar lobe with emphysema).[96] Xenon-133 studies show reduced or absent pulmonary blood flow and trapping of gas in the affected region of the lung (Fig. 5.20).

Unilateral Hyperlucent Lung

Repeated airway infection in children causing bronchiolitis obliterans may result in a unilateral hyperlucent lung (Swyer-James-McLeod syndrome). This disorder most frequently follows pulmonary infection by adenovirus. Measles, pertussis, and tuberculosis have also been implicated. The affected lung usually has a normal main bronchus with marked bronchiectatic changes in the more peripheral bronchi. Radiographs of the chest demonstrate diminished or normal lung volume and marked decrease in bronchovascular markings. Radionuclide studies using ^{133}Xe usually reveal markedly reduced perfusion and ventilation as well as air trapping in the affected lung. Pulmonary angiography shows a small ipsilateral pulmonary artery with thin branches and greatly reduced peripheral vascularity.[13,97–99]

Asthma

In patients with bronchial asthma in remission, ^{99m}Tc-MAA scintigraphy may show normal or markedly improved perfusion.[100] Macroag-

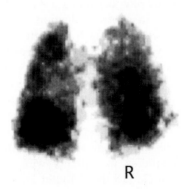

R

FIGURE 5.20. Congenital lobar emphysema. Perfusion image (left) after intravenous ^{133}Xe in saline shows apparent symmetric distribution of pulmonary blood flow. Thirty seconds after the arrival of ^{133}Xe in the lungs, a large region of significant trapping is evident. It corresponded to a hyperlucent right middle lobe on the chest radiograph.

gregated pulmonary scintigraphy during acute asthmatic attacks reveals focal perfusion abnormalities. Regional ventilation becomes increasingly abnormal as symptoms increase but is reversible with treatment. Perfusion usually decreases in the area of decreased ventilation, but the degree of change is not as great.[101,102] Xenon-133 distribution indices for ventilation and perfusion in asthmatic patients in remission generally agree with findings in normal subjects. In some asthmatic patients in remission, however, there are slight residual regional irregularities on the ventilation studies. Such ventilatory abnormalities do not seem to be accompanied by a significant alteration in perfusion.[103] The use of bronchodilators is helpful for assessing of regional lung function in patients with asthma (Fig. 5.21).

Pulmonary Air Cysts

All thin-walled, air-containing intrapulmonary spaces that are radiographically visible regardless of their pathogenesis are called pulmonary air cysts. Their clinical significance varies widely.[104] It is important to determine whether a cyst is solitary or part of generalized pulmonary disease. Air cysts (bullae or blebs) range from 1 cm in diameter to the volume of an entire hemithorax and possess a smooth wall of minimal thickness. These lesions may be congenital or acquired. Congenital types include bronchogenic cysts, whose fluid content has been expelled, and congenital cystic disease of the lung. Air cysts may also be part of congenital intrapulmonary sequestration. Acquired cysts may arise de novo or occur as part of other disorders, usually infectious; they are frequently associated with parenchymal damage. Acquired cysts include blebs and bullae. Blebs are usually less than 1 to 2 cm in diameter and immediately subpleural. They have been implicated as a cause of spontaneous pneumothorax. Bullae, which are intrapulmonary, are usually attributable to excessive rupture of alveolar walls. Their walls are composed of compressed parenchymal tissue. The exact cause of this problem is not clear; obstruction, postinfection lung abscess (tuberculosis, staphylococcus), resolution of acute pneumonia, and trauma have

been suggested.[105] Most bronchogenic cysts are located near the trachea, stem bronchi, or carina, although intrapulmonary and cervical locations have been found. The cysts are usually unilocular structures containing clear fluid; but mucoid, hemorrhagic, or purulent material may be present. The walls may contain bronchial elements (cartilage, fibrovascular connective tissue, pseudostratified columnar epithelium). Patients may be asymptomatic or present with respiratory distress, cough, or recurrent respiratory infections. Radiographs of the chest usually reveal a rounded mass in proximity to the stem bronchi and carina. Cysts may compress a major bronchus leading to air trapping and collapse. At fluoroscopy, during expiration the cysts appear to inflate while the rest of the lung deflates. Computed tomography can help differentiate cyst from tumor, lymph nodes, or other structures. Xenon-133 studies may demonstrate lack of ventilation and perfusion within the cyst, provided it is large enough to be detected. Alternatively, a cyst may cause air trapping.

Pneumonia

With acute pneumonia, regional ventilation and perfusion may be affected. Ventilation is usually reduced to a greater degree than perfusion, resulting in a low ventilation/perfusion ratio. During recovery, residual trapping of ^{133}Xe is common in the areas previously affected even in the presence of a normal roentgenogram of the chest (Fig. 5.22).[2] With time, and providing there are no complications, normal regional lung function is eventually restored. Xenon-133 studies are sensitive to alterations in regional lung function caused by infection.

Bronchopulmonary Dysplasia

Bronchopulmonary dysplasia is a form of chronic lung disease that occurs in infants treated for prolonged periods of time with mechanical ventilation and oxygen. It occurs most commonly in premature infants who require mechanical ventilation for hyaline membrane disease and is rare in infants of

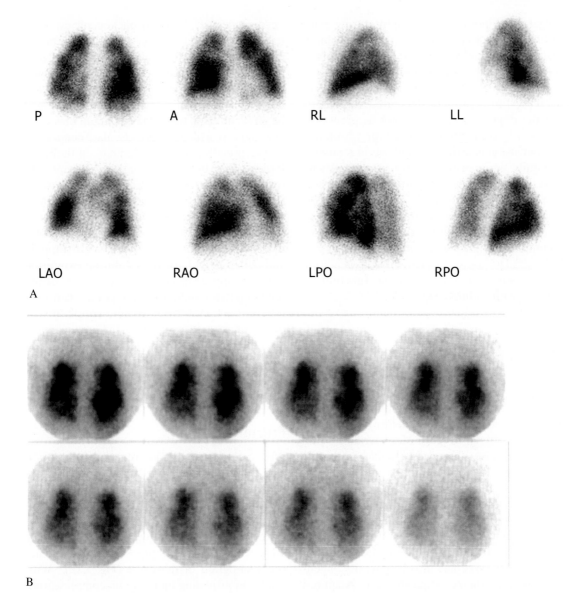

P   A   RL   LL

LAO   RAO   LPO   RPO

A

B

FIGURE 5.21. Asthma: effect of bronchodilators. This 17-year-old boy, suffering from asthma and acute chest pain, underwent pulmonary scintigraphy to rule out pulmonary embolism. A,B: Initial study reveals multiple nonsegmental perfusion defects (^{99m}Tc-MAA) and an irregular ventilation pattern (^{133}Xe). C,D: Perfusion and ventilation studies done immediately after nebulized bronchodilation reveals more uniform distribution of lung function, except for an area of decreased ventilation in the left lower lung that subsequently was shown radiographically to correspond to left lower lobe atelectasis.

advanced gestational age. Oxygen concentrations of more than 40% are frequently used for more than 4 to 6 days.

Although the precise etiology of bronchopulmonary dysplasia is not known, it is likely that disease results from pulmonary immaturity combined with one or more of the following factors: oxygen, mechanical ventilation, patent ductus arteriosus, and fluid overload. At an early stage, the patient exhibits tachypnea, interstitial retraction, and rales. Congestive heart failure with hepatomegaly

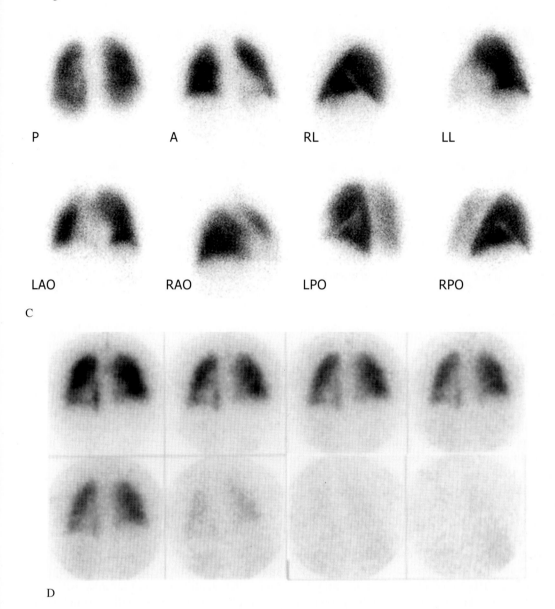

P   A   RL   LL

LAO   RAO   LPO   RPO

C

D

FIGURE 5.21. *Continued*

and cyanosis are present. Radiographs of the chest reveal various degrees of abnormality. Initially there is interstitial emphysema that appears as small radiolucent bubbles or streaks in an interstitial pattern. Later the radiologic appearance is one of white-out lung with diffuse bilateral opacification. As the condition progresses, there is extensive disruption of pulmonary parenchyma with hyperinflation, bilateral cystic appearance, and coarse interstitial markings. Left-to-right shunting and congestive heart failure result in cardiomegaly and hepatomegaly. The ECG reveals right ventricular strain.

Echocardiography helps when evaluating cardiac anomalies often associated with bronchopulmonary dysplasia or demonstrating right and left ventricular hypertrophy. Radionuclide

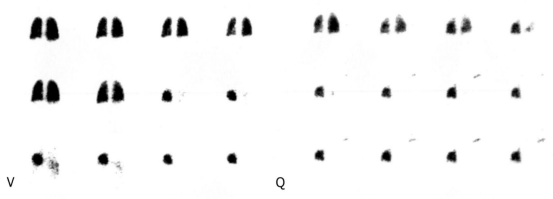

V   Q

FIGURE 5.22. Pneumonia. Residual air trapping after pneumonia in a 5-year-old girl with a history of recurrent respiratory infections. At the time of this ^{133}Xe study, the chest radiograph was normal. The ventilatory phase (left) reveals reduced wash-in and washout of ^{133}Xe from the left lower lung field. The perfusion phase, following intravenous ^{133}Xe in saline, reveals reduced blood flow and air trapping in the left lower lung field.

angiocardiography may assist in assessing the magnitude of left-to-right shunting through a patent ductus arteriosus.[106] Studies using ^{133}Xe or ^{81m}Kr in infants with bronchopulmonary dysplasia reveal diffuse or multifocal abnormal distribution of ventilation and perfusion. Evidence of air trapping is common.

Long-term studies of patients with bronchopulmonary dysplasia between ages 1 and 5 years show persistent alterations of global or regional lung function.[107] With Wilson-Mikity lung, there is fine collagenation and elastosis of structured portions of the lobule. The areas of hyperaeration and atelectasis follow lobular or subsegmental patterns. These infants generally do not develop cor pulmonale, although some minor hypertrophy of fetal arterioles may be present. This condition is not usually preceded by respiratory distress syndrome, and it appears after a longer interval than bronchopulmonary dysplasia (4 to 6 weeks of age).[108–110]

Neonatal Interstitial Emphysema

Intensive ventilatory treatment for premature infants with respiratory failure may become complicated by persistent interstitial emphysema involving one lobe or an entire lung. A suggested mechanism is alveolar rupture followed by dissection and entrapment of air in the pulmonary interstitium.[56,111–114] It is generally assumed that the overexpanded lobe has no functional value and compromises adjacent lung tissue, causing alteration of respiratory function. Leonidas et al.[113,115] found ventilation-perfusion scintigraphy useful for assessing neonatal emphysema. The scintigraphic findings on ^{133}Xe studies are those of airway obstruction: reduced perfusion accompanied by reduced ventilation and air trapping of gas in the affected lung region.

Bronchiectasis

Vandevivere et al.[116] compared chest radiographs, ^{99m}Tc-MAA perfusion scintigraphy, and ^{81m}Kr ventilation scintigraphy with bronchography in patients with bronchiectasis. They found 73% sensitivity and 76% specificity for radiographs of the chest. For lung scintigraphy, the sensitivity was 92% and the specificity 60%. In this study, approximately 40% of the bronchograms performed might have been avoided on the basis of a normal chest radiograph and pulmonary scintigraphy. The combination of pulmonary scintigraphy and chest radiography thus provides excellent screening when a decision on the advisability of bronchography is being made in children (Fig. 5.23).

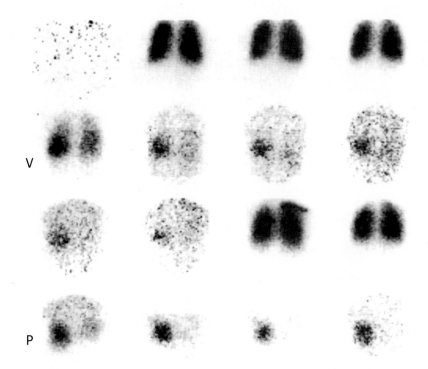

FIGURE 5.23. Bronchiectasis. Xenon-133 study shows trapping of gas in the left lower lung field after both inhalation (V) and perfusion (P) of the tracer. This patient had repeated respiratory infections; on the chest radiograph it was not clear if there were bronchiectasis.

Congenital Diaphragmatic Hernia

Herniation of intraabdominal organs through the diaphragm is much more common in the left hemidiaphragm (Bochdalek's hernia). Diaphragmatic hernia results in hypoplasia of the ipsilateral lung with a reduction in the lung volume and the number of airways and pulmonary arteries. Wohl et al.,[117] in our institution, studied 19 patients after repair of congenital diaphragmatic hernia. Their total lung capacity and vital capacity averaged 99% of predicted value. Forced expiratory volume in 1 second (FEV$_1$) averaged 89% of predicted value. Maximum expiratory flow volumes were normal. Lung volume was equally distributed in both lungs. Ventilation to the ipsilateral lung was reduced in two of nine patients. Blood flow to the affected lung was reduced in all patients studied. These findings are consistent with persistence of a reduced number of branches or generations of pulmonary arteries and bronchi on the side of the hernia. Because a substantial part of the vascular resistance resides in the peripheral vessels, this developmental abnormality influences the distribution of pulmonary blood flow even though it has little effect on tests reflecting airway resistance or the distribution of ventilation (Figs. 5.24 and 5.25).

Pectus Excavatum

Patients with pectus excavatum frequently exhibit left-right ventilation and perfusion imbalance. Most commonly, the left lung shows a reduction in ventilation and an even greater reduction in perfusion. Commonly, ventilation/perfusion (V/Q) ratios in each lung are either high or low before surgery. Postoperative evaluation of these patients reveals a tendency

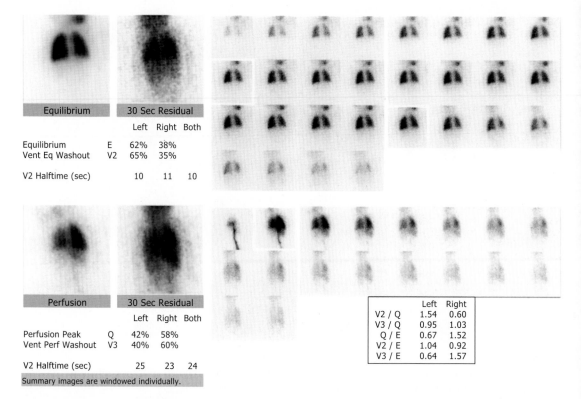

		Left	Right	Both
Equilibrium	E	62%	38%	
Vent Eq Washout	V2	65%	35%	
V2 Halftime (sec)		10	11	10

		Left	Right	Both
Perfusion Peak	Q	42%	58%	
Vent Perf Washout	V3	40%	60%	
V2 Halftime (sec)		25	23	24

	Left	Right
V2 / Q	1.54	0.60
V3 / Q	0.95	1.03
Q / E	0.67	1.52
V2 / E	1.04	0.92
V3 / E	0.64	1.57

Summary images are windowed individually.

FIGURE 5.24. Congenital diaphragmatic hernia of the left lung after surgical repair. This study is from a 10-month-old girl after surgical repair of a left congenital diaphragmatic hernia. Xenon-133 ventilation study (top) reveals a larger air volume in the left lung. The perfusion study with intravenous ^{133}Xe in saline reveals poor perfusion of the left lung.

toward a more even distribution of lung function (Figs. 5.26 and 5.27).

Bronchopulmonary Sequestration

Bronchopulmonary sequestration is part of a wide spectrum of bronchopulmonary developmental abnormalities resulting from abnormal bronchial vascular supply and drainage of normal, hypoplastic, or dysplastic segments of the lung. This uncommon disorder enters in the differential diagnosis of certain intrathoracic masses. It is usually asymptomatic and often discovered by chance when a chest radiograph

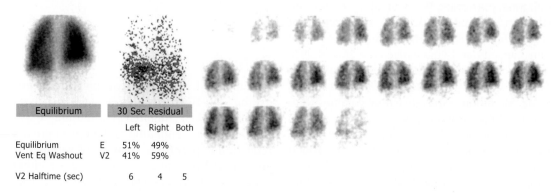

		Left	Right	Both
Equilibrium	E	51%	49%	
Vent Eq Washout	V2	41%	59%	
V2 Halftime (sec)		6	4	5

FIGURE 5.25. Surgical repair of a left congenital diaphragmatic hernia. Xenon-133 ventilation and perfusion images reveal rather symmetric distribution of ventilation. Pulmonary blood flow to the left lung is reduced.

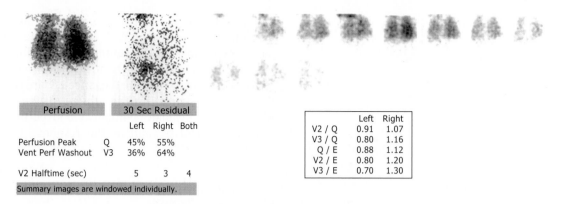

Perfusion	30 Sec Residual		
	Left	Right	Both
Perfusion Peak	Q	45%	55%
Vent Perf Washout	V3	36%	64%
V2 Halftime (sec)		5	3	4

Summary images are windowed individually.

	Left	Right
V2 / Q	0.91	1.07
V3 / Q	0.80	1.16
Q / E	0.88	1.12
V2 / E	0.80	1.20
V3 / E	0.70	1.30

FIGURE 5.25. *Continued*

is obtained for other reasons. When sequestration is symptomatic, it manifests by repeated episodes of pneumonia or atelectasis. Approximately two thirds of the reported cases involve the left lower lobe. Systemic blood supply may arise from the descending thoracic aorta or the abdominal aorta in patients with bronchopulmonary sequestration.[118] In one report of the radionuclide angiographic findings in five patients with bronchopulmonary sequestration, the sequestered lobe did not perfuse during the pulmonary phase; it was supplied by the systemic circulation in all patients.[119] Bronchopulmonary sequestration may be classified as

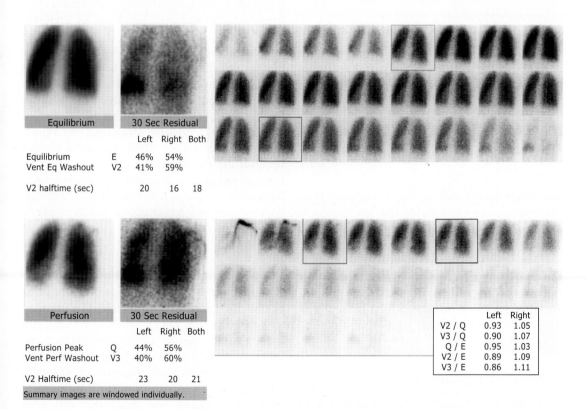

Equilibrium	30 Sec Residual		
	Left	Right	Both
Equilibrium	E	46%	54%
Vent Eq Washout	V2	41%	59%
V2 halftime (sec)		20	16	18

Perfusion	30 Sec Residual		
	Left	Right	Both
Perfusion Peak	Q	44%	56%
Vent Perf Washout	V3	40%	60%
V2 Halftime (sec)		23	20	21

Summary images are windowed individually.

	Left	Right
V2 / Q	0.93	1.05
V3 / Q	0.90	1.07
Q / E	0.95	1.03
V2 / E	0.89	1.09
V3 / E	0.86	1.11

FIGURE 5.26. Pectus excavatum. Xenon-133 ventilation and perfusion studies from an 11-year-old girl with pectus excavatum. The study reveals a slight reduction in ventilation (41% of the total) in the left lung with air trapping in the left lower lung field. Perfusion is slightly reduced in the left lung.

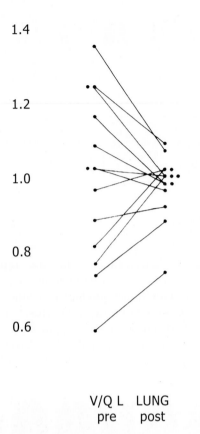

1.4

1.2

1.0

0.8

0.6

V/Q L LUNG
pre   post

FIGURE 5.27. Improvement of V/Q in pectus excavatum after surgery. Ventilation-perfusion ratios from the left lung in 12 patients with pectus excavatum before and after surgical repair, showing an improvement of the ventilation-perfusion balance.

intralobar or extralobar. The extralobar type involves an ectopic lobe of the lung situated above or below the diaphragm and enclosed in its own visceral pleura. The intralobar type involves malformation of a perfused, but often unventilated, lung segment sequestered within the normal lung without its own visceral pleura. In addition, the sequestered lobe or segment may not communicate with the tracheo-bronchial tree.

Pulmonary Papillomatosis

Espinola et al.[120] studied three children with pulmonary papillomatosis using ^{133}Xe and ^{99m}Tc microspheres. They observed different imaging patterns depending on the size, number, and distribution of the lesions. With early parenchymal involvement, a ventilation-perfusion imbalance was seen with relatively less perfusion than ventilation in the affected areas. Pulmonary scintigraphy in these patients was useful to evaluate ventilatory and perfusion impairment as well as the response to treatment.

Abnormalities of Airway Connective Tissues

When unexplained maldistribution of inhaled air in the lungs is present, one should consider disorders of the airways. Several disorders of the airways may cause air turbulence and secondary maldistribution of radioactive gases within the lungs during tidal breathing and particularly during deep breathing. Tracheomalacia is caused by a weak or flaccid tracheal wall that allows excessive tracheal collapse during respiration. Tracheomalacia may be found after tracheostomy and prolonged use of endotracheal tubes, especially those with cuffed attachments. Other causes include mediastinal masses, vascular anomalies, tracheoesophageal fistula, and cutis laxa. Stridor is present in some of these patients. Children with laryngomalacia (infantile supraglottic hypermotility) often present with loud and stridorous breathing. During inspiration, the larynx collapses because the cartilages are not stiff enough to support the airway. Tracheal stenosis is a fixed narrowing of the trachea caused by external compression or intrinsic congenital or acquired lesions.

Pulmonary Alveolar Proteinosis

Pulmonary alveolar proteinosis is a syndrome of unknown etiology characterized by progressive dyspnea and cough. Most cases occur at older ages; the number of affected children and infants is small. The most striking histologic features are intraalveolar deposits of granular, eosinophilic, or proteinaceous material. On gross examination, one finds multiple, firm, gray or yellow nodules of various sizes often located subpleurally throughout the lung. The bronchial tree appears normal, but there is evidence of alveolar wall damage. In children, productive cough with yellow sputum may be present. Cyanosis, fatigue, weight loss, and occasionally hemoptysis may be encountered. Chest radiographs show a fine, diffuse perihilar increase in lung density following a pattern similar to that of pulmonary edema without cardiac enlargement. The radiographic changes are due to the alveolar fluid. Occasionally, the pattern may be nodular in appearance. The prognosis of pulmonary alveolar proteinosis is not favorable because the alveoli progressively fill and complicating infections are common. Variable changes in the distribution of ventilation and perfusion can be identified by ^{133}Xe pulmonary scintigraphy.[121–124]

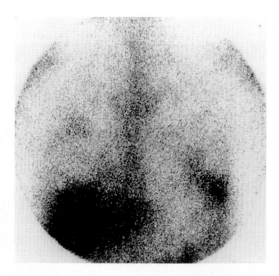

FIGURE 5.29. Cystic fibrosis and infection. Anterior image from a teenage girl with cystic fibrosis. Bilateral focal accumulation of ^{67}Ga indicating active infection in both lungs, though worse in the left.

Inflammatory and Other Lesions Causing Uptake of ^{67}Ga in the Lungs

Cystic fibrosis (Figs. 5.28 and 5.29), granulomatous lesions seen with immunodeficiency, sarcoidosis (Fig. 5.30), pneumonitis (Fig. 5.31), and chemotoxicity cause ^{67}Ga uptake in the lungs. *Sarcoidosis* is a granulomatous disease of unknown origin that affects several systems in the body but most frequently the lungs, lymph nodes, eyes, skin, liver, and spleen. In patients with sarcoidosis, decreased and delayed hypersensitivity suggests impaired cell immunity as well as elevated or abnormal immunoglobulins. Histologically, there are widespread noncaseating epithelioid granulomas in more than one organ. Dry cough, wheezing, pleuritic pain, and mild to moderate dyspnea are the symptoms of pulmonary sarcoidosis.

Most cases of sarcoidosis are found in adults between ages 20 and 40 years. The disease is occasionally seen in children, especially those between ages 9 and 15, and it has been described in infants as young as 2 months.

Thoracic adenopathy is observed in most pediatric patients. Usually radiography of the chest reveals a mix of small irregular nodular shadows and fine linear densities diffusely scattered in the lungs. Rarely, sarcoidosis exists with normal chest radiography. Approximately one third of patients have discrete, painless lymphadenopathy. Uveitis, iritis, conjunctivitis, keratosis, retinitis, glaucoma, and involvement of the eyelids and lacrimal glands can be seen with this disease. Swelling of the parotid gland and induration can also be seen.[125–127]

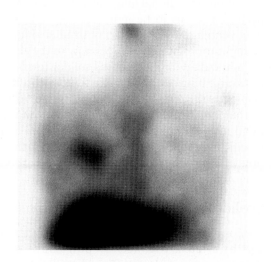

FIGURE 5.28. Lung infection in cystic fibrosis patient. Anterior ^{67}Ga scintiscan of the chest from a 17-year-old girl with cystic fibrosis. The intense uptake of the tracer in the right hemithorax is indicative of an active infection.

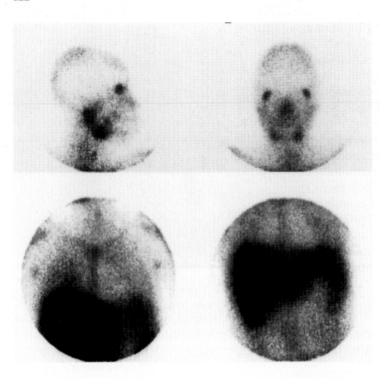

FIGURE 5.30. Sarcoidosis. Gallium-67 scintigraphy showing increased tracer uptake in both lung fields. Other areas of increased uptake include the axillary lymph nodes and the salivary and lacrimal glands.

Gallium-67 citrate scintigraphy demonstrates areas of active sarcoidosis in the body and may be useful for assessing the extent and activity of the intrathoracic lesions. Serum lysozyme and angiotensin-converting enzyme measurements are usually helpful, although normal values do not exclude activity and progression of pulmonary sarcoidosis.[128]

Klech et al.[129] examined the value of several factors to assess activity in sarcoidosis. Gallium-67 scintigraphy proved the most sensitive method (94%) followed by serum angiotensin-converting enzyme levels, chest radiography, and lymphocyte assays. Despite poor specificity, negative ^{67}Ga scintigraphy together with normal angiotensin-converting enzyme is of value for excluding a diagnosis of active sarcoidosis. Klech et al. also found that in patients with peripheral pulmonary lesions chest radiographs have doubtful value for staging involvement and assessment of activity. Gallium-67 also may concentrate in sarcoid lesions of the heart. Normal ^{67}Ga scintigraphy can be used to support clinical identification of inactive sarcoidosis.[130]

Radiation Therapy

After radiation therapy to the mediastinum or pulmonary parenchyma, there are marked alterations in regional lung function. Generally, perfusion seems to be more severely affected than ventilation in the areas of irradiated lung. Complications of radiation therapy to the chest include radiation pneumonitis, milder forms of restrictive lung disease, constrictive pericarditis, and growth retardation of the spine, ribs, sternum, and clavicle. Irradiation given during rapid lung growth affects the parenchyma and results in smaller lungs and chest wall than predicted. Reduced lung volume and carbon monoxide-diffusing capacity also occur.

Scoliosis

Scoliosis may cause alveolar hypoventilation and hypoxemia followed by progressive cardiopulmonary failure. The distribution of perfusion and ventilation improves in the supine position when the spinal curvature is diminished. Abnormal ventilation occurs primarily on the concave side of the spine.[131]

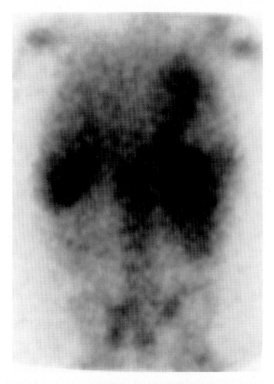

FIGURE 5.31. Pneumonitis. Gallium-67 scintiscan from a 3-year-old girl with persistent fever. Posterior image shows intense radiotracer uptake in the right lung and less in the left lung, indicating an active inflammatory process.

Acknowledgment. Some concepts and part of the wording in this chapter were contributed by C.B.G. Harris, M.D., formerly at Children's Hospital Boston, who was a coauthor of this chapter in the first edition of *Pediatric Nuclear Medicine.*

References

1. Lassen NA. Assessment of tissue radiation dose in clinical use of radioactive inert gases with examples of absorbed dose from 3H, 85Kr, and 133Xe. Radioakt Isot Klin Fortschr 1965;6:37–47.
2. Kjellman B. Regional lung function studied with Xe133 in children with pneumonia. Acta Paediatr Scand 1967;56(5):467–76.
3. Treves S, Ahnberg DS, Laguarda R, Strieder DJ. Radionuclide evaluation of regional lung function in children. J Nucl Med 1974;15(7): 582–7.
4. Treves S, Strieder DJ, Adelstein SJ. Scintillation camera radiospirometry. Prog Nucl Med 1973;3: 149–65.
5. Miorner G. 133 Xe-radiospirometry. A clinical method for studying regional lung function. Scand J Respir Dis Suppl 1968;64:1–84.
6. Wartak J, Overton TR, Friedenberg LW, Sproule BJ. Computer-aided evaluation of regional pulmonary function. Comput Biomed Res 1972;5(4):429–39.
7. Fazio F, Jones T. Assessment of regional ventilation by continuous inhalation of radioactive krypton-81m. Br Med J 1975;3(5985): 673–6.
8. Li DK, Treves S, Heyman S, et al. Krypton-81m: a better radiopharmaceutical for assessment of regional lung function in children. Radiology 1979;130(3):741–7.
9. Schor RA, Shames DM, Weber PM, Dos Remedios LV. Regional ventilation studies with Kr-81m and Xe-133: a comparative analysis. J Nucl Med 1978;19(4):348–53.
10. Coates G, O'Brodovich H. Extrapulmonary radioactivity in lung permeability measurements. J Nucl Med 1987;28(5):903–6.
11. Meignan M, Rosso J, Leveau J, et al. Exercise increases the lung clearance of inhaled technetium-99m DTPA. J Nucl Med 1986;27(2): 274–80.
12. Jefferies AL, Coates G, O'Brodovich H. Pulmonary epithelial permeability in hyaline-membrane disease. N Engl J Med 1984;311(17): 1075–80.
13. O'Dell CW, Taylor A, Higgins CB, Ashburn WL, Schillaci RF, Alazraki NP. Ventilation-perfusion lung images in the Swyer-James syndrome. Radiology 1976;121(2):423–6.
14. Rosso J, Guillon JM, Parrot A, et al. Technetium-99m-DTPA aerosol and gallium-67 scanning in pulmonary complications of human immunodeficiency virus infection. J Nucl Med 1992;33(1):81–7.
15. Schiff RG, Kabat L, Kamani N. Gallium scanning in lymphoid interstitial pneumonitis of children with AIDS. J Nucl Med 1987;28(12): 1915–9.
16. Dusser DJ, Collignon MA, Stanislas-Leguern G, Barritault LG, Chretien J, Huchon GJ. Respiratory clearance of 99mTc-DTPA and pulmonary involvement in sarcoidosis. Am Rev Respir Dis 1986;134(3):493–7.
17. Jackson P, Mackey D, Van der Wall H. Physical and chemical nature of technegas. J Nucl Med 1998;39(9):1646–9.

18. Senden TJ, Moock KH, Gerald JF, Burch WM, Browwitt RJ, Ling CD, Heath GA. The physical and chemical nature of technegas. J Nucl Med 1997;38(8):1327–33.
19. Lloyd JJ, Shields RA, Taylor CJ, Lawson RS, James JM, Testra HJ. Technegas and pertechnegas particle size distribution. Eur J Nucl Med 1995;22(5):473–6.
20. Burch WM, Boyd MM, Crellin DE. Technegas: particle size and distribution. Eur J Nucl Med 1994;21(4):365–7.
21. Kropp J, Buhr W, Biersack HJ. Lung inhalation scintigraphy in newborns: a study with the new tracer Technegas. J Nucl Med 1989;30:1989.
22. Amis TC, Crawford AB, Davison A, Engel LA. Distribution of inhaled 99m-technetium labelled ultrafine carbon particle aerosol (Technegas) in human lungs. Eur Respir J 1990;3(6):679–85.
23. Cook G, Clarke SE. An evaluation of Technegas as a ventilation agent compared with krypton-81m in the scintigraphic diagnosis of pulmonary embolism. Eur J Nucl Med 1992;19(9):770–4.
24. Peltier P, De Faucal P, Chetanneau A, Chatal JF. Comparison of technetium-99m aerosol and krypton-81m in ventilation studies for the diagnosis of pulmonary embolism. Nucl Med Commun 1990;11(9):631–8.
25. Sullivan PJ, Burke WM, Burch WM, Lomas FE. A clinical comparison of Technegas and xenon-133 in 50 patients with suspected pulmonary embolus. Chest 1988;94(2):300–4.
26. James JM, Lloyd JJ, Leahy BC, Shields RA, Prescott MC, Testa HJ. The incidence and severity of hypoxia associated with 99Tcm Technegas ventilation scintigraphy and 99Tcm MAA perfusion scintigraphy. Br J Radiol 1992;65(773):403–8.
27. Monaghan P, Provan I, Murray C, et al. An improved radionuclide technique for the detection of altered pulmonary permeability. J Nucl Med 1991;32(10):1945–9.
28. Scalzetti EM, Grossman ZD, Gagne GM. Experimentally produced pulmonary arterial occlusion in the dog: identification with pertechnegas inhalation. Radiology 1993;186(2):423–6.
29. Alavi A. Scintigraphic demonstration of acute gastrointestinal bleeding. Gastrointest Radiol 1980;5(3):205–8.
30. Davies G, Reid L. Growth of the alveoli and pulmonary arteries in childhood. Thorax 1970;25(6):669–81.
31. Thurlbeck WM. Postnatal growth and development of the lung. In: Murray JF, ed. Lung Disease State of the Art (1974–1975). New York: American Lung Association, 1976.
32. Emery JL, Mithal A. The number of alveoli in the terminal respiratory unit of man during late intrauterine life and childhood. Arch Dis Child 1960;35:54–7.
33. Heyman S. Toxicity and safety factors associated with lung perfusion studies with radiolabeled particles. J Nucl Med 1979;20(10):1098–9.
34. Di Sant'Agnese PA, Davis PB. Research in cystic fibrosis (first of three parts). N Engl J Med 1976;295(9):481–5.
35. Shwachman H, Kulczycki LL, Khaw KT. A report on sixty-five patients over 17 years of age. Pediatrics 1965;36(5):689–99.
36. Wood RE, Boat TF, Doershuk CF. Cystic fibrosis. Am Rev Respir Dis 1976;113(6):833–78.
37. Piepsz A, Decostre P, Baran D. Scintigraphic study of pulmonary blood flow distribution in cystic fibrosis. J Nucl Med 1973;14(6):326–30.
38. Alderson PO, Secker-Walker RH, Strominger DB, McAlister WH, Hill RL, Markham J. Quantitative assessment of regional ventilation and perfusion in children with cystic fibrosis. Radiology 1974;111(1):151–5.
39. Gyepes MT, Bennett LR, Hassakis PC. Regional pulmonary blood flow in cystic fibrosis. AJR Radium Ther Nucl Med 1969;106(3):567–75.
40. Bateman JR, Newman SP, Daunt KM, Pavia D, Clarke SW. Regional lung clearance of excessive bronchial secretions during chest physiotherapy in patients with stable chronic airways obstruction. Lancet 1979;1(8111):294–7.
41. DeCesare JA, Babchyck BM, Colten HR, Treves S. Radionuclide assessment of the effects of chest physical therapy on ventilation in cystic fibrosis. Phys Ther 1982;62(6):820–7.
42. Coel MN, Druger G. Radionuclide detection of the site of hemoptysis. Chest 1982;81(2):242–3.
43. Winzelberg GG, Wholey MH, Sachs M. Scintigraphic localization of pulmonary bleeding using technetium Tc 99m sulfur colloid: a preliminary report. Radiology 1982;143(3):757–62.
44. Alavi A, Dann RW, Baum S, Biery DN. Scintigraphic detection of acute gastrointestinal bleeding. Radiology 1977;124(3):753–6.
45. Barry J, Alazraki NP, Heaphy JH. Scintigraphic detection of intrapulmonary bleeding using

technetium-99m sulfur colloid: concise communication. J Nucl Med 1981;22(9):777–80.

46. Miller T, Tanaka T. Nuclear scan of pulmonary hemorrhage in idiopathic pulmonary hemosiderosis. AJR 1979;132(1):120–1.

47. Mishkin F, Knote J. Radioisotope scanning of the lungs in patients with systemic-pulmonary anastomoses. AJR Radium Ther Nucl Med 1968;102(2):267–73.

48. Chen JT, Robinson AE, Goodrich JK, Lester RG. Uneven distribution of pulmonary blood flow between left and right lungs in isolated valvular pulmonary stenosis. AJR Radium Ther Nucl Med 1969;107(2):343–50.

49. Dunne EF. Cardiac Radiology. Philadelphia: Lea & Febiger, 1967.

50. Wagner HN Jr, Sabiston DC Jr, Iio M, McAfee JG, Meyer JK, Langan JK. Regional pulmonary blood flow in man by radioisotope scanning. JAMA 1964;187:601–3.

51. Sade RM, Williams RG, Castaneda AR, Treves S. Abnormalities of regional lung function associated with ventricular septal defect and pulmonary artery band. J Thorac Cardiovasc Surg 1976;71(4):572–80.

52. Fleming HA. Differential lung function in atrial septal defect. Circulation 1959;19(6):856–62.

53. Hughes JM, Glazier JB, Maloney JE, West JB. Effect of interstitial pressure on pulmonary blood-flow. Lancet 1967;1(7483):192–3.

54. Higgins CB, Wexler L. Clinical and angiographic features of pulmonary arteriovenous fistulas in children. Radiology 1976;119(1):171–5.

55. Moyer JH, Glantz G, Brest AN. Pulmonary arteriovenous fistulas; physiologic and clinical considerations. Am J Med 1962;32:417–35.

56. Utzon F, Brandrup F. Pulmonary arteriovenous fistulas in children. A review with special reference to the disperse telangiectatic type, illustrated by report of a case. Acta Paediatr Scand 1973;62(4):422–32.

57. Chandler AB. The anatomy of a thrombus. In: Sherry SBK, Genton E, Stengle JM, eds. Thrombus. Washington, DC: National Academy of Science, 1969.

58. Jones DR, Macintyre IM. Venous thromboembolism in infancy and childhood. Arch Dis Child 1975;50(2):153–5.

59. Freiman DG, Suyemoto J, Wessler S. Frequency of pulmonary thromboembolism in man. N Engl J Med 1965;272:1278–80.

60. Bell WR, Simon TL. Current status of pulmonary thromboembolic disease: pathophysiology, diagnosis, prevention, and treatment. Am Heart J 1982;103(2):239–62.

61. Emery JL. Pulmonary embolism in children. Arch Dis Child 1962;37:591–5.

62. Jones RH, Sabiston DC Jr. Pulmonary embolism in childhood. Monogr Surg Sci 1966;3(1):35–51.

63. Buck JR, Connors RH, Coon WW, Weintraub WH, Wesley JR, Coran AG. Pulmonary embolism in children. J Pediatr Surg 1981;16(3):385–91.

64. Kimball AM, Hallum AV, Cates W Jr. Deaths caused by pulmonary thromboembolism after legally induced abortion. Am J Obstet Gynecol 1978;132(2):169–74.

65. Gandilo SB, Tanswell AK, Mackie KW. Pulmonary vascular air embolism in hyaline membrane disease. J Can Assoc Radiol 1977;28(4):294–6.

66. Buchanan D, Mason JK. Occurrence of pulmonary fat and bone marrow embolism. Am J Forensic Med Pathol 1982;3(1):73–8.

67. Gittman JE, Buchanan TA, Fisher BJ, Bergeson PS, Palmer PE. Fatal fat embolism after spinal fusion for scoliosis. JAMA 1983;249(6):779–81.

68. Moore P, James O, Saltos N. Fat embolism syndrome: incidence, significance and early features. Aust N Z J Surg 1981;51(6):546–51.

69. Firor HV. Pulmonary embolization complicating total intravenous alimentation. J Pediatr Surg 1972;7(1):81.

70. Nichols MM, Tyson KR. Saddle embolus occluding pulmonary arteries. Am J Dis Child 1978;132(9):926.

71. Wesley JR, Keens TG, Miller SW, Platzker AC. Pulmonary embolism in the neonate: occurrence during the course of total parenteral nutrition. J Pediatr 1978;93(1):113–5.

72. Tang TT, Chambers CH, Gallen WJ, McCreadie SR. Pulmonary fiber embolism and granuloma. JAMA 1978;239(10):948–50.

73. Bell WR, Simon TL, DeMets DL. The clinical features of submassive and massive pulmonary emboli. Am J Med 1977;62(3):355–60.

74. Coon WW. Risk factors in pulmonary embolism. Surg Gynecol Obstet 1976;143(3):385–90.

75. Salzman EW, Harris WH, DeSanctis RW. Anticoagulation for prevention of thromboembolism following fractures of the hip. N Engl J Med 1966;275(3):122–30.

76. Walker BK, Ballas SK, Burka ER. The diagnosis of pulmonary thromboembolism in sickle cell disease. Am J Hematol 1979;7(3):219–32.

77. Bohm N, Keller KM, Kloke WD. Pulmonary and systemic cerebellar tissue embolism due to birth injury. Virchows Arch A Pathol Anat Histopathol 1982;398(2):229–35.

78. Pillay SV. Pulmonary embolism of cerebral tissue in a neonate. A case report. S Afr Med J 1980;58(12):498.

79. Tan KL, Hwang WS. Neonatal brain tissue embolism in the lung. Aust N Z J Med 1976;6(2):146–9.

80. Harker LA, Slichter SJ, Scott CR, Ross R. Homocystinemia. Vascular injury and arterial thrombosis. N Engl J Med 1974;291(11):537–43.

81. Esposito AL, Gleckman RA. A diagnostic approach to the adult with fever of unknown origin. Arch Intern Med 1979;139(5):575–9.

82. Sasahara AA, Cannilla JE, Morse RL, Sidd JJ, Tremblay GM. Clinical and physiologic studies in pulmonary thromboembolism. Am J Cardiol 1967;20(1):10–20.

83. Moses DC, Silver TM, Bookstein JJ. The complementary roles of chest radiography, lung scanning, and selective pulmonary angiography in the diagnosis of pulmonary embolism. Circulation 1974;49(1):179–88.

84. Kelley MJ, Elliott LP. The radiologic evaluation of the patient with suspected pulmonary thromboembolic disease. Med Clin North Am 1975;59(1):3–36.

85. Epstein J, Taylor A, Alazraki N, Coel M. Acute pulmonary embolus associated with transient ventilatory defect: case report. J Nucl Med 1975;16(11):1017–20.

86. Kessler RM, McNeil BJ. Impaired ventilation in a patient with angiographically demonstrated pulmonary emboli. Radiology 1975;114(1):111–2.

87. Kim EE, DeLand FH. V/Q mismatch without pulmonary emboli in children with histoplasmosis. Clin Nucl Med 1978;3(8):328–30.

88. Li DK, Seltzer SE, McNeil BJ. V/Q mismatches unassociated with pulmonary embolism: case report and review of the literature. J Nucl Med 1978;19(12):1331–3.

89. Medina JR, L'Heureux P, Lillehei JP, Liken MK. Regional ventilation in the differential diagnosis of pulmonary embolism. Circulation 1969;39(6):831–5.

90. McGoldrick PJ, Rudd TG, Figley MM, Wilhelm JP. What becomes of pulmonary infarcts? AJR 1979;133(6):1039–45.

91. Makler PT, Malmud LS, Charkes ND. Diminished perfusion to an entire lung due to mucous plug. Clin Nucl Med 1977;2:160–2.

92. Stinnett RG, Hietala S, Fratkin MJ. Reversible unilateral pulmonary hypoperfusion secondary to mucous plugs. Clin Nucl Med 1977;2:157–9.

93. Treves ST, Harris CBC. Lung. In: Treves ST, ed. Pediatric Nuclear Medicine. New York: Springer-Verlag, 1985:289–330.

94. Arborelius M Jr. Influence of moderate hypoxia in one lung on the distribution of the pulmonary circulation and ventilation. Scand J Clin Lab Invest 1965;17:257–9.

95. Stocker JT, Drake RM, Madewell JE. Cystic and congenital lung disease in the newborn. Perspect Pediatr Pathol 1978;4:93–154.

96. Hislop A, Reid L. New pathological findings in emphysema of childhood. 1. Polyalveolar lobe with emphysema. Thorax 1970;25(6):682–90.

97. Cumming GR, Macpherson RI, Chernick V. Unilateral hyperlucent lung syndrome in children. J Pediatr 1971;78(2):250–60.

98. Lee HK, Granada M. Swyer-James syndrome: diagnostic application of combined radionuclide ventilation and perfusion scanning. Clin Nucl Med 1977;2:100–2.

99. Zeiger LS, Moss EG. Ventilation and perfusion imaging in the Swyer-James syndrome. Clin Nucl Med 1977;2:103–5.

100. Mishkin F, Wagner HN Jr. Regional abnormalities in pulmonary arterial blood flow during acute asthmatic attacks. Radiology 1967;88(1):142–4.

101. Rao M, Steiner P, Victoria MS, et al. Regional lung functions in children with asthma. J Asthma Res 1977;14(3):107–10.

102. Wilson AF, Surprenant EL, Beall GN, Siegel SC, Simmons DH, Bennett LR. The significance of regional pulmonary function changes in bronchial asthma. Am J Med 1970;48(4):416–23.

103. Bentivoglio LG, Beerel F, Bryan AC, Stewart PB, Rose B, Bates DV. Regional pulmonary function studied with xenon in patients with bronchial asthma. J Clin Invest 1963;42:1193–200.

104. Bates DV, Macklem PT, Christie RV. Respiratory Function in Disease: An Introduction to the Integrated Study of the Lung, 2d ed. Philadelphia: Saunders, 1971.

105. Fraser RG, Parâe JAP. Diagnosis of Diseases of the Chest, 2d ed. Philadelphia: Saunders, 1977.

106. Treves S, Fogle R, Lang P. Radionuclide angiography in congenital heart disease. Am J Cardiol 1980;46(7):1247–55.

107. Harrod JR, L'Heureux P, Wangensteen OD, Hunt CE. Long-term follow-up of severe respi-

ratory distress syndrome treated with IPPB. J Pediatr 1974;84(2):277–85.

108. Baghdassarian OM, Avery ME, Neuhauser EB. A form of pulmonary insufficiency in premature infants. Pulmonary dysmaturity? AJR Radium Ther Nucl Med 1963;89:1020–31.

109. Grossman H, Berdon WE, Mizrahi A, Baker DH. Neonatal focal hyperaeration of the lungs (Wilson-Mikity syndrome). Radiology 1965; 85(3):409–17.

110. Wilson MG, Mikity VG. A new form of respiratory disease in premature infants. Am J Dis Child 1960;99:489–99.

111. Fletcher BD, Outerbridge EW, Youssef S, Bolande RP. Pulmonary interstitial emphysema in a newborn infant treated by lobectomy. Pediatrics 1974;54(6):808–11.

112. Hall RT, Rhodes PG. Pneumothorax and pneumomediastinum in infants with idiopathic respiratory distress syndrome receiving continuous positive airway pressure. Pediatrics 1975;55(4):493–6.

113. Leonidas JC, Moylan FM, Kahn PC, Ramenofsky ML. Ventilation-perfusion scans in neonatal regional pulmonary emphysema complicating ventilatory assistance. AJR 1978; 131(2):243–6.

114. Macklin MT, Macklin CC. Malignant interstitial emphysema of the lungs and mediastinum as an important occult complication in many respiratory disease and other conditions: an interpretation of the clinical literature in the light of laboratory experiment. Medicine (Baltimore) 1944;23:281–358.

115. Leonidas JC, Hall RT, Rhodes PG. Conservative management of unilateral pulmonary interstitial emphysema under tension. J Pediatr 1975;87(5):776–8.

116. Vandevivere J, Spehl M, Dab I, Baran D, Piepsz A. Bronchiectasis in childhood. Comparison of chest roentgenograms, bronchography and lung scintigraphy. Pediatr Radiol 1980;9(4):193–8.

117. Wohl ME, Griscom NT, Strieder DJ, Schuster SR, Treves S, Zwerdling RG. The lung following repair of congenital diaphragmatic hernia. J Pediatr 1977;90(3):405–14.

118. Felson B. Chest Roentgenology. Philadelphia: WB Saunders, 1973.

119. Gooneratne N, Conway JJ. Radionuclide angiographic diagnosis of bronchopulmonary sequestration. J Nucl Med 1976;17(12):1035–7.

120. Espinola D, Rupani H, Camargo EE, Wagner HN, Jr. Ventilation-perfusion imaging in pulmonary papillomatosis. J Nucl Med 1981; 22(11):975–7.

121. Liebow AA, Steer A, Billingsley JG. Desquamative Interstitial Pneumonia. Am J Med 1965;39:369–404.

122. Plenk HP, Swift SA, Chambers WL, Peltzer WE. Pulmonary alveolar proteinosis—a new disease? Radiology 1960;74:928–38.

123. Rosen SH, Castleman B, Liebow AA. Pulmonary alveolar proteinosis. N Engl J Med 1958;258(23):1123–42.

124. Wilkinson RH, Blanc WA, Hagstrom JW. Pulmonary alveolar proteinosis in three infants. Pediatrics 1968;41(2):510–5.

125. Cone RB. A review of Boeck's sarcoid with analysis of twelve cases occurring in children. J Pediatr 1948;32:629–40.

126. James DG, Turiaf J, Hosoda Y, et al. Description of sarcoidosis: report of the Subcommittee on Classification and Definition. Ann N Y Acad Sci 1976;278:742.

127. Merten DF, Kirks DR, Grossman H. Pulmonary sarcoidosis in childhood. AJR 1980;135(4): 673–9.

128. Alberts C, van der Schoot JB, van Daatselaar JJ, Braat MC, Roos CM. 67Ga scintigraphy, serum lysozyme and angiotensin-converting enzyme in pulmonary sarcoidosis. Eur J Respir Dis 1983;64(1):38–46.

129. Klech H, Kohn H, Kummer F, Mostbeck A. Assessment of activity in sarcoidosis. Sensitivity and specificity of 67 gallium scintigraphy, serum ACE levels, chest roentgenography, and blood lymphocyte subpopulations. Chest 1982;82(6):732–8.

130. Gupta RG, Bekerman C, Sicilian L, Oparil S, Pinsky SM, Szidon JP. Gallium 67 citrate scanning and serum angiotensin converting enzyme levels in sarcoidosis. Radiology 1982;144(4): 895–9.

131. Shannon DC, Riseborough EJ, Valenca LM, Kazemi H. The distribution of abnormal lung function in kyphoscoliosis. J Bone Joint Surg Am 1970;52(1):131–44.

6
Cardiovascular System

S.T. Treves, Elizabeth D. Blume, Laurie Armsby, Jane W. Newburger, and Alvin Kuruc

The application of radionuclides to study the cardiovascular system was first investigated by Blumgart and Yens[1] and Blumgart and Weiss[2] in 1927. These investigators used radium C and a primitive radiation detector to study blood-flow velocity. In 1948 and 1949, Prinzmetal et al.[3,4] described radiocardiograms of three patients with congenital heart disease using iodine-131 (^{131}I), sodium iodine, and a Geiger-Mueller counter.

Congenital heart disease affects 0.8 per 100 live births. Approximately one third of these children require treatment by interventional catheterization or surgery during the first year of life.[5] Significant advances in interventional catheterization, cardiac surgery, and cardiac intensive care during the past three decades have enabled corrective and palliative interventions to be performed in even the smallest neonates.[6,7]

In the past three decades, tremendous advances in imaging techniques such as echocardiography, computed tomography (CT), magnetic resonance imaging (MRI), and angiography have helped in the evaluation of anatomy and the understanding of physiology in children with heart disease in ways not possible before. Furthermore, with dramatic improvements in technology (radiopharmaceuticals and imaging instrumentation), nuclear medicine offers several methods applicable to the diagnosis and assessment of pediatric cardiovascular disorders. These include single photon emission computed tomography (SPECT), positron emission tomography (PET), first-pass radionuclide angiocardiography, radionuclide ventriculography (gated blood pool scan), and venography. Nuclear medicine techniques play an important role in the diagnostic and functional armamentarium of the pediatric cardiologist.

Myocardial Imaging

Radionuclide imaging of the myocardium can be carried out with SPECT or PET, which can image myocardial perfusion, metabolism, neuronal innervation, and inflammation/infection. This chapter focuses primarily on myocardial perfusion using SPECT, as the other methods are not utilized as frequently in pediatric practice and are not widely available now. Myocardial perfusion SPECT is useful in the assessment of disorders of coronary perfusion, such as Kawasaki disease, transposition of the great arteries following arterial switch operation, cardiac transplantation, cardiomyopathy, chest pain, chest trauma, and anomalous left coronary artery arising from the pulmonary artery. Other less frequent indications include hyperlipidemia, supravalvular aortic stenosis, syncope, coarctation of the aorta, and pulmonary atresia with intact ventricular septum.

Clinical Applications

Kawasaki Disease

Kawasaki disease, also known as mucocutaneous lymph node syndrome, was first described in 1967 by Tomisaku Kawasaki.[8] Kawasaki disease is an acute, self-limited vasculitis of unknown etiology that occurs predominantly in infants and young children of all races. The disease is characterized by fever, bilateral nonexudative conjunctivitis, erythema of the lips and oral mucosa, changes in the extremities, rash, and cervical lymphadenopathy. Coronary artery aneurysms or ectasia develop in 15% to 25% of untreated children with the disease and may lead to ischemic heart disease, myocardial infarction, or even sudden death.[9,10] In the United States, Kawasaki disease has surpassed acute rheumatic fever as the leading cause of acquired heart disease in children. The cause of Kawasaki disease is unknown, although an infectious agent seems likely, as there is a seasonal incidence with peaks during the winter and spring, and cases are usually clustered geographically. The peak incidence of Kawasaki disease is in the toddler and preschool age group (75% of cases in children under 5 years in the U.S.)[11]; it is rare in adults. The case fatality ratio of Kawasaki disease is approximately 0.08%, with virtually all deaths caused by the cardiac complications of this disease.[12]

Upon histopathologic examination, initial findings at 0 to 9 days are characterized by acute perivasculitis and vasculitis of the microvessels and small arteries throughout the body.[13] At 12 to 25 days there is panvasculitis of the coronary arteries with aneurysm and thrombosis. Aneurysms with internal diameters greater than 8mm are labeled "giant aneurysms" and carry a disproportionately high risk of myocardial infarction. Myocarditis, pericarditis, and endocarditis may be present during this phase as well. Disappearance of inflammation in the microvessels, marked intimal thickening, and granulation of the coronary arteries is seen at between 28 and 31 days. Subsequently, coronary artery aneurysms may either regress by myointimal proliferation to normal lumen diameter, or stenosis may develop, often at either end of an aneurysm. Among patients with persistent coronary artery aneurysms, the prevalence and severity of stenoses increases steadily over many years and is most highly predicted by the original size of the aneurysm.[14]

The risk of coronary artery thrombosis is greatest after the acute phase subsides (beyond 12 days), when coronary vasculitis occurs concomitantly with marked elevation of the platelet count and a hypercoagulable state. Standard treatment currently involves intravenous immunoglobulin (IVIG), other anti-inflammatory agents, and oral anticoagulant therapy. Intravenous anticoagulant therapy or thrombolytic therapy may be necessary, and in rare cases coronary artery bypass grafting is required.[15]

Echocardiography is helpful for delineating aneurysms and assessing ventricular function. Myocardial perfusion SPECT has been widely used in the assessment of these patients. The presence of aneurysm may or may not be correlated with abnormalities in regional myocardial perfusion. Perfusion SPECT, with exercise or pharmacologic stress, may demonstrate regional myocardial perfusion impairment or improvement in perfusion after medical therapy.[16] Examples of myocardial perfusion SPECT in Kawasaki disease are illustrated in Figures 6.1 to 6.3.

Transposition of the Great Arteries: Arterial Switch Operation

In dextro-transposition of the great arteries (d-TGA), the aorta arises anterior from the anatomic right ventricle and the pulmonary artery arises from the anatomic left ventricle. This defect accounts for 5% to 7% of all congenital cardiac malformations.[17] Without treatment, approximately 30% of these infants die in the first week of life, 50% within the first month, and more than 90% within the first year.[18] Current medical and surgical treatment, which includes the arterial switch operation (ASO), provide greater than 95% early and midterm survival. The most technically challenging portion of the ASO surgery involves the transfer of the coronary arteries from the

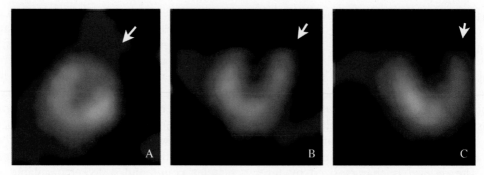

FIGURE 6.1. A 6-year-old boy with Kawasaki disease and severe aneurysms in the left anterior descending and the right coronary arteries. Short axis (A), hori- zontal long axis (B), and vertical long axis (C) slices reveal a perfusion defect in the anterior wall of the left ventricle (arrows).

anterior semilunar root to the reconstructed neoaorta. The short- and long-term success of this operative approach depends principally on the continued patency and adequate function-

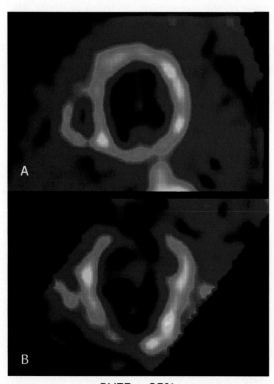

RVEF = 35%
LVEF = 25%

FIGURE 6.2. Kawasaki disease. Dilated cardio-myopathy with focal myocardial defects and poor function. A: short axis. B: transverse long axis.

ing of the coronary arteries.[19–23] Vogel et al.[24,25] have previously reported areas of myocardial hypoperfusion after the ASO. Using thallium-201 (^{201}Tl) perfusion scintigraphy with isopro-terenol stress, we investigated the prevalence of myocardial perfusion abnormalities in chil-dren after the arterial switch operation at rest and with the physiologic stress of exercise using technetium-99m hexakis (2-methoxy-isobutylisonitrile) sestamibi (^{99m}Tc-MIBI) myocardial perfusion SPECT. Abnormalities of myocardial perfusion present in nearly all patients. These perfusion abnormalities did not correlate with echocardiographic indices of wall motion abnormalities and most likely were related to small areas of hyperperfusion resulting from aortic cross-clamping at surgery (Fig. 6.4).

Cardiac Transplantation

Pediatric cardiac transplantation has evolved into a viable treatment option for neonates, infants, and children with end-stage cardio-myopathy or congenital heart disease not amenable to conventional surgical repair or palliation. Although early mortality generally results from acute rejection or infectious com-plications, accelerated coronary vasculopathy has become the major cause of late morbidity and mortality following transplantation.[26,27] The specific pathogenesis of transplant coronary disease is unknown, but it is presumed to involve some form of vascular immunologic

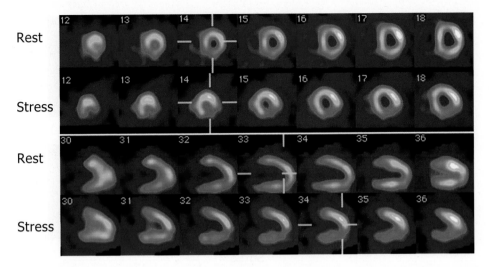

FIGURE 6.3. Patient with Kawasaki disease with severe ischemia of the inferior wall of the left ventricle, most pronounced during stress.

injury. In severe cases, coronary arteriography shows progressive distal obliterative disease in the absence of collateral vessel development.[28] Myocardial perfusion SPECT has been used to evaluate these patients on a regular basis. Along with coronary angiography, it helps in the diagnosis of coronary artery disease and myocardial viability. In cases showing perfusion defects, fluorine-18 fluorodeoxyglucose (^{18}F-

FDG)-PET can determine myocardial viability. Examples of ^{99m}Tc-MIBI SPECT in patients following heart transplant can be seen on Figures 6.5 to 6.8).

Anomalous Left Coronary Artery

Anomalous origin of the left coronary artery from the pulmonary artery (ALCAPA) results

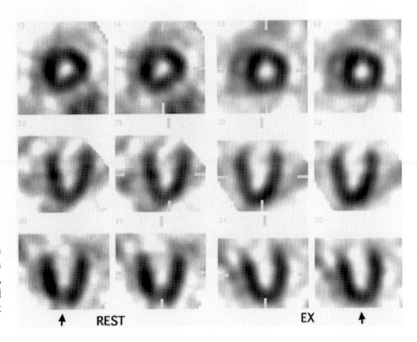

FIGURE 6.4. Arterial switch operation for transposition of the great arteries. At rest, there is an apparent apical defect that is not present at exercise (arrows).

REST   EX

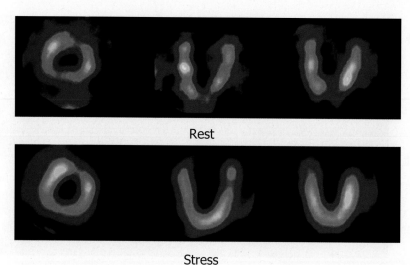

Rest

Stress

FIGURE 6.5. Cardiac transplant. Images at rest reveal irregular distribution of myocardial perfusion. This pattern changes during stress. The defect in the ante- rior wall remains, while the apical defect improves with stress. A coronary angiogram revealed col- lateral circulation feeding the apex.

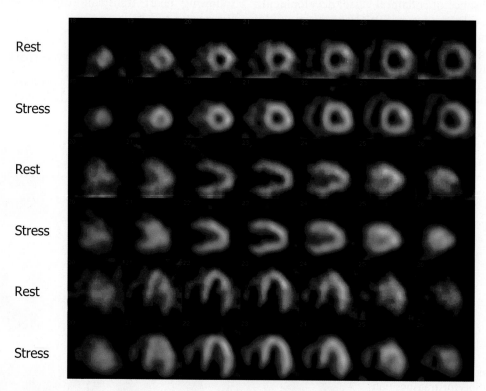

Rest

Stress

Rest

Stress

Rest

Stress

FIGURE 6.6. Cardiac transplant. Images at rest reveal irregular distribution of myocardial perfusion with defects in the mid-anterior, mid-septal, and mid-infe- rior wall of the left ventricle. The images at stress show a more normal distribution of myocardial blood flow. There were collaterals that were recruited during the stress.

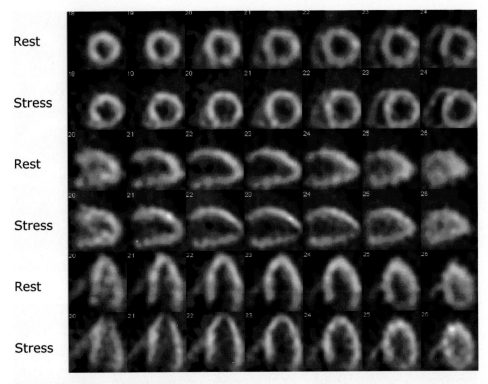

Figure 6.7. Cardiac transplant. ^{99m}Tc-MIBI single photon emission computed tomography (SPECT) demonstrates an apical perfusion defect that is seen at stress.

in severe myocardial dysfunction and ischemia during early infancy.[29,30] Following birth, the left ventricle becomes perfused with desaturated blood at pressures that rapidly fall below systemic pressures. Classic findings include infarction of the anterolateral left ventricular free wall followed by mitral valve incompetence secondary to an infarcted anterior papillary muscle. This leads to symptomatic congestive heart failure in the first year of life. A number of surgical techniques have been utilized to transfer the anomalous coronary back to the aortic cusp.[31-33] The diagnosis can usually be made by history, physical examination, electrocardiogram, and echocardiogram with color Doppler. Myocardial perfusion scintigraphy may be helpful for assessing the severity of hypoperfusion and for the serial evaluation during recovery of function following repair[34] (Figs. 6.9 and 6.10).

Cardiomyopathy

Primary cardiomyopathies (CMs) include a diverse group of diseases affecting the heart muscle itself. There are three types of CM based on anatomic and functional features: hypertrophic (HCM), dilated (DCM), and restrictive (RCM). Each type of CM is distinct in its set of etiologies, functional characteristics, clinical features, and therapeutic approach. Based on the form of cardiomyopathy, the ventricle may become hypertrophied or dilated with increasingly diminished diastolic or systolic function, ultimately leading to heart failure, arrhythmia, or sudden death. Depending on the type and severity of the disease, myocardial perfusion SPECT can diagnose myocardial dilatation, myocardial thinning, focal ischemia, or infarction as well as myocardial contractility and wall motion abnormalities.

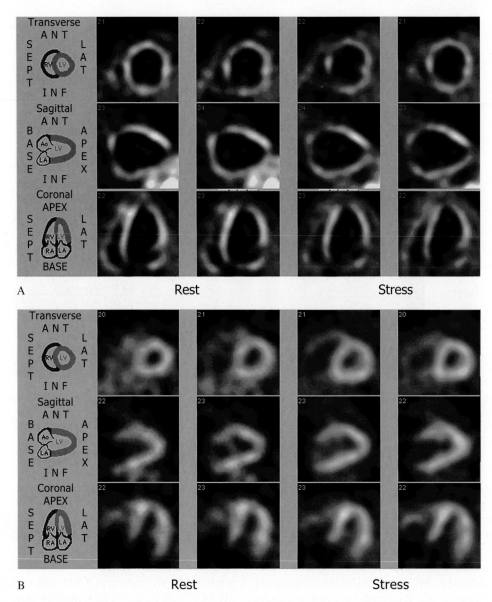

FIGURE 6.8. A: Patient with severe dilated cardiomyopathy. B: Same patient following successful cardiac transplantation.

Chest Pain and Trauma

Chest pain is a common complaint in children, often idiopathic, commonly chronic, and most often benign. Cardiac causes of chest pain account for a small minority of potential etiologies including idiopathic (12% to 85%), musculoskeletal (15% to 31%), pulmonary (12% to 21%), psychiatric (5% to 17%), gastrointestinal (4% to 7%), other (4% to 21%), and cardiac (4% to 6%).[35] Cardiac-related causes of chest pain include anatomic lesions (such as aortic stenosis, anomalous coronary artery from the pulmonary artery, and coarctation), acquired lesions (cardiomyopathies, Kawasaki disease, dissecting aortic aneurysm,

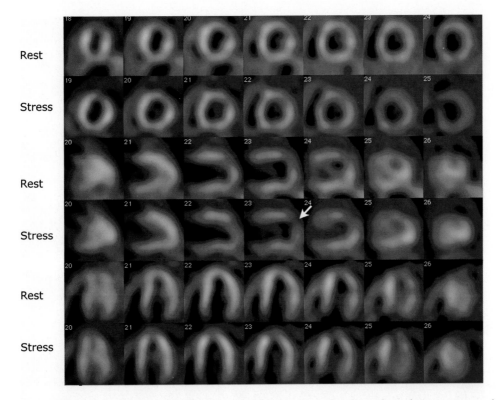

FIGURE 6.9. A 5-year-old boy with anomalous coronary artery departing from the pulmonary artery. A perfusion defect gets worse with stress (arrow).

and pericarditis), and tachyarrhythmias. Chest pain is not a frequent referral diagnosis for myocardial perfusion SPECT. However, in our practice we have observed that this method has been utilized to help rule out cardiac ischemia as a cause of chest pain.

Right Ventricular Hypertrophy and Hypertension

In normal individuals, the right-ventricular myocardium has lower tracer uptake compared to the left ventricle, and therefore may not be clearly visible on myocardial perfusion SPECT. The right-ventricular wall can be seen in the normal individual if the injection is made during or just after exercise. Increased ^{99m}Tc-MIBI and ^{201}Tl uptake in the right ventricular myocardium at rest is seen in patients with right ventricular hypertrophy[36–39] (Figs. 6.11 to 6.13).

Visualization of the right ventricle on myocardial perfusion scintigraphy occurs in patients with congenital heart disease, such as tetralogy of Fallot (pre- and postoperatively), transposition of the great arteries (following Senning or Mustard's repair when the right ventricle is at systemic pressure) (Table 6.1), or after an ASO (with residual supravalvular pulmonary stenosis and secondary right-ventricular hypertrophy).

We have studied the effect of right-ventricular hypertrophy on the myocardial distribution of ^{201}Tl in a small group of rats maintained in a hypobaric chamber (air at 380 mm Hg) for 2 weeks to cause pulmonary arterial hypertension.[40] The hypoxic rats showed significant right ventricular hypertrophy, and the ratio between left-ventricle (LV) mass and right-ventricle (RV) mass decreased from 4.2 ± 0.2 (SD) in controls to 2.4 ± 0.1 in

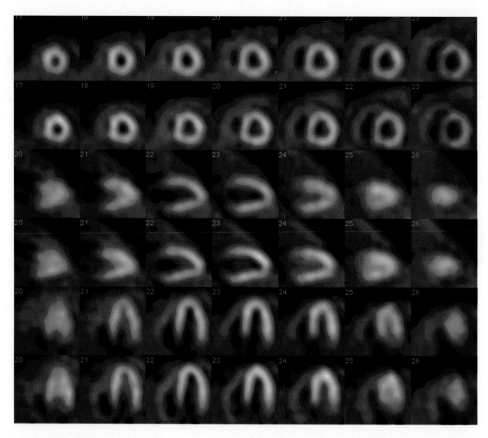

FIGURE 6.10. Anomalous origin of the left anterior descending coronary artery from the right coronary artery. Successful repair.

hypoxic animals. The LV/RV activity ratios in both the hypoxic and control rats were nearly identical to the respective mass ratios ($r = -0.97$). Radiographic and microscopic studies confirmed the changes of pulmonary arterial hypertension in the lungs of hypoxic rats. The right ventricle hypertrophied in response to this increased pressure load, whereas the left ventricle remained the same in weight-adjusted comparisons of the two groups.[41] In another study, ^{201}Tl myocardial scintigraphy was performed in patients with congenital heart defects to determine if quantitative right-ventricular uptake correlated with the degree of right-ventricular hypertrophy and therefore the degrees of right-ventricular pressure.[42] A total of 24 patients ranging from 7 months to 30 years were studied; 18 were studied before corrective surgery and six postoperatively. All but three had congenital heart defects that had resulted in pressure or volume overload (or both) of the right ventricle. During routine cardiac catheterization, ^{201}Tl was injected through the venous catheter and myocardial images were recorded in anterior and left anterior oblique projections.

Insignificant right-ventricular ^{201}Tl counts were present in six patients, all with a right-ventricular peak-systolic pressure of less than 30 mm Hg. In the remaining 18 patients, there was a good correlation between the right-ventricular/left-ventricular peak-systolic pressure ratio and the right-ventricular/left-ventricular ^{201}Tl counts ratio. All patients with right-ventricular/left-ventricular peak systolic pressure of less than 0.5 mm Hg had a right-ventricular/left-ventricular ^{201}Tl count ratio of less than 0.4. Qualitative evaluation of right-ventricular uptake was able to distinguish patients with right-ventricular pressure at or above systemic levels.

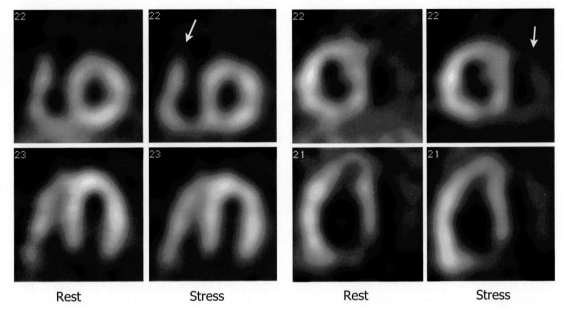

Rest   Stress   Rest   Stress

FIGURE 6.11. An 11-year-old girl with truncus arteriosus. The ^{99m}Tc-MIBI SPECT reveals increased right ventricular tracer uptake due to hypertrophy (arrow). Post-repair magnetic resonance imaging (MRI) shows mild narrowing of the distal conduit, a left pulmonary artery of small caliber, and regurgitant fraction of 43%. Pulmonary hypertension and mild-to-moderate right ventricular dilatation are present.

FIGURE 6.12. A 28-year-old man who had a Mustard operation for transposition of the great arteries. The patient had a dilated and hypertrophic right (systemic) ventricle with depressed function, mild to moderate TR, chest pain with exertion, and systemic hypertension. The left ventricle (pulmonary) is small and takes relatively much lower amount of tracer.

Similarly, myocardial perfusion SPECT with ^{99m}Tc-MIBI can be used to estimate right-ventricular pressure and right-ventricular overload in children with congenital heart disease.[43]

External quantitation of ^{201}Tl myocardial uptake could be used as an index of right-ventricular mass and may correlate with increased pressure in the right ventricle,[42,44,45] especially in patients with echocardiographic parameters inadequate for estimating right-ventricular pressure. Such information may be useful for right-sided obstructive lesions, septal defects altering the pulmonary vasculature, and primary pulmonary disorders such as cystic fibrosis.

patients with a spectrum of disease ranging from a nearly normal-sized RV and tricuspid valve to an extremely hypoplastic RV and tricuspid valve with coronary sinusoids.[46–49] In many of these patients the combination of RV-to-coronary sinusoids and proximal coronary-

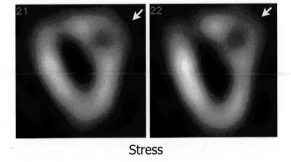

Stress

FIGURE 6.13. A 13-year-old boy with double outlet right ventricle, hypoplastic left heart syndrome, multiple septal defects, mitral atresia, and moderate RV dysfunction. Ventricular ejection fraction was 36%.

Pulmonary Atresia with Intact Ventricular Septum

Pulmonary atresia with intact ventricular septum represents a heterogeneous group of

TABLE 6.1. Uses of radionuclide angiography for quantitative assessment of ventricular function

Ventricle morphology	Physiology	Location	Clinical examples
Right	Pulmonary ventricle	Anterior/rightward	Tetralogy of Fallot Truncus arteriosus Valvar pulmonary stenosis Cystic fibrosis
Right	Systemic ventricle	Anterior/rightward Posterior/leftward	D-TGA L-TGA
Left	Systemic ventricle	Posterior/leftward	Kawasaki disease s/p chemotherapy s/p transplantation s/p corrective cardiac surgery
Left	Pulmonary ventricle	Anterior/rightward	L-TGA
Variable	Systemic ventricle	Variable	s/p Fontan surgery

s/p, status post; TGA, transposition of the great arteries.

artery stenoses create an RV-dependent coronary circulation in which a significant portion of coronary blood supply arises from the hypertensive RV. Decompression of the right ventricle at surgical repair may thus result in significant areas of myocardial ischemia. Myocardial perfusion imaging is helpful for evaluating infarcted areas.

Radiopharmaceuticals for Myocardial Perfusion Single Photon Emission Computed Tomography

Myocardial SPECT in children can be carried out using one of the following agents: ^{99m}Tc-MIBI (Cardiolite, Bristol-Meyers-Squibb Co.), ^{99m}Tc-tetrofosmin (Myoview, GE Healthcare, Boston, MA), or thallium-201 (^{201}Tl). In our laboratory, the radiopharmaceutical of choice for myocardial perfusion SPECT is ^{99m}Tc-MIBI.

Technetium-99m-MIBI

Technetium-99m-MIBI is a cationic complex that accumulates in the myocardium according to regional myocardial perfusion. After intravenous administration, this agent is distributed throughout the body and concentrates in several organs including the thyroid, myocardium, kidneys, and striated muscle. The agent clears rapidly from the blood with a fast initial component with a half-time of 4.3 minutes. There is less, approximately 8%, of the administered tracer activity in blood by 5 minutes, and less than 1% of the tracer is protein-bound in the plasma. The major route of elimination of ^{99m}Tc-MIBI is the hepatobiliary system. Tracer activity appears within the intestine within the first hour after injection. The cumulative excretion of this agent in 48 hours is 27% of the amount administered in urine and 33% in the feces. The biologic half-lives of ^{99m}Tc-MIBI in myocardium and liver are 6 hours and 30 minutes, respectively. The effective half-lives are 3 hours and 28 minutes, respectively. At rest, approximately 1.5% of the injected dose is taken up in the myocardium. Once ^{99m}Tc-MIBI is taken up by the myocardium, it remains fixed there and it shows no redistribution over time.

With ^{99m}Tc-MIBI, both resting and exercise stress evaluations can be performed; physiologic stress evaluations may be performed in patients old enough to cooperate with exercise testing (usually 7 years or older), and the pharmacologic stress can be used in all age groups.

Technetium-99m-Tetrofosmin

This agent is taken up in the myocardium to a maximum of 1.2% of the injected dose at 5

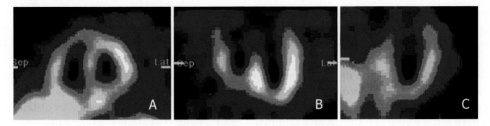

FIGURE 6.14. ^{123}I-MIBG SPECT in a 10-year-old boy who was followed for neuroblastoma. (A) short axis, (B) transverse long axis, (C) vertical long axis.

minutes and 1% at 2 hours, respectively. Activity in the blood, liver, and lung is less than 5% of the administered activity at 10 minutes and less than 2% at 30 minutes. Tracer activity is eliminated in the urine (approximately 40%) and in the feces (26%) within 48 hours.

Thallium-201

Thallium-201 is cyclotron produced; it has a physical half-life of 73 hours and decays by electron capture. During its decay, it produces mercury K x-rays of 69 to 83 keV (98% abundance) and gamma rays of 135 and 167 keV (10% abundance).[50] A minimum dose of 0.150 mCi (5.55 MBq) and a maximum dose of 2.0 mCi (74 MBq) are suggested dose guidelines. See Chapter 20 for absorbed dose estimates.

Thallium-201 is considered a potassium analogue.[50,51] Clearance of potassium from the myocardium is faster than that of thallium, however.[52,53] After intravenous injection, the blood disappearance half-time of ^{201}Tl is less than 1 minute. The peak myocardial uptake, about 3% to 4% of the injected dose, occurs at approximately 10 minutes. At this time, the distribution of radiothallium in the heart appears to correlate with myocardial perfusion.[53] Thallium-201 is not fixed to the myocardium; it redistributes with time, exercise, drugs, and ischemia.

Neuronal Single Photon Emission Computed Tomography Tracer (^{123}I-MIBG)

Iodine-123-metaiodobenzylguanidine (^{123}I-MIBG) is a norepinephrine analogue. (Iodine-

123 has a physical half-life of 13.3 hours and decays with the emission of a 159-keV photon in 85% abundance.) As such, this agent allows noninvasive assessment of cardiac adrenergic function. Metaiodobenzylguanidine shares the same uptake and storage mechanisms as norepinephrine. It is actively transported into the presynaptic nerve terminals by the uptake 1 system and it is stored within vesicles.[54-61] Single photon emission computed tomography can be obtained at 2 to 4 hours (or even later) following the intravenous administration of the agent. The images reflect neuronal uptake. There are a number of drugs that interfere with MIBG uptake. MIBG imaging has been used to evaluate patients with cardiomyopathy, chronic heart failure, heart transplantation, and ventricular arrhythmias (Fig. 6.14).

Positron Emission Tomography Perfusion Tracers

Rubidium-82 (^{82}Rb), nitrogen-13 (^{13}N), ammonia, and oxygen-15 (^{15}O) water can be used to assess myocardial perfusion with PET. Rubidium-82 is a generator-produced radionuclide with a half-life of 75 seconds. The parent radioisotope is strontium-82 with a physical half-life of 25.5 days. The generator eluant is injected intravenously into the patient as a continuous infusion. It is extracted rapidly in the myocardium depending on the flow. The short half-life of ^{82}Rb permits studies to be performed in rapid succession. The ^{82}Rb generator can be used for approximately a month. Nitrogen-13 and ^{15}O require a medical cyclotron in proximity to a PET scanner. Nitrogen-13 has a physical half-life of 10 minutes; in the form of ammonia it is rapidly extracted by the myocardium (70% extraction fraction). It is trapped there by the glutamic-acid glutamate reaction. The amount of tracer in the myocardium also depends on the metabolic state of the cardiac muscle. Therefore, accurate measurement of myocardial blood flow is difficult. Oxygen-15 has a physical half-life of 2 minutes, and as oxygen-water it is taken up by the myocardium with an extraction fraction of almost 100%. However, intravenously injected ^{15}O-H$_2$O also resides within the blood pool, and special processing techniques are needed to outline the myocardial image separate from the blood pool.

Positron Emission Tomography Metabolic Tracers

Fluorine-18-fluoro-2-deoxyglucose (^{18}F-FDG) is a glucose analogue. Fluorine-18 has a physical half-life of 111 minutes. Fluoro-2-deoxyglucose PET images regional myocardial glucose metabolism. Blood disappearance of ^{18}F-FDG is rapid. Most of the activity leaves within 1 minute after intravenous injection, most of the remainder leaves within 10 minutes, and a small fraction of the tracer remains in the blood pool in 90 minutes. Imaging can begin within a few minutes following tracer injection. Fluoro-2-deoxyglucose is phosphorylated in the myocardial cell and no further metabolism occurs, and the radiotracer is trapped within the cell. There is no significant tissue clearance over 4 hours.

Technique for Myocardial Perfusion Single Photon Emission Computed Tomography

Usual Administered Doses of ^{99m}Tc-MIBI

The patient should fast for 2 hours prior to administration of the tracer. An intravenous needle or a short catheter is placed and secured to the skin with tape, and the line is kept open with normal saline. The intravenous line is kept in place so it can be used to inject the tracer during exercise studies. Because ^{99m}Tc-MIBI has no significant redistribution over a 4- to 6-hour period,[62] two injections of the radiopharmaceutical are necessary to obtain resting and peak exercise myocardial perfusion imaging.[63]

Single ^{99m}Tc-MIBI SPECT

For a single study (rest or exercise) done alone, a dose of 0.25 mCi (9.25 MBq)/kg is used with a minimum total dose of 2 mCi (74 MBq) and a maximum dose of 10 mCi (370 MBq). If rest and exercise studies are done on separate days, the same dose of ^{99m}Tc-MIBI can be used.

Rest and Exercise ^{99m}Tc-MIBI SPECT Studies (Same Day)

For rest and exercise studies performed on the same day, the following dose schedule is suggested:

Rest ^{99m}Tc-MIBI SPECT study: 0.15 mCi (5.55 MBq)/kg, with a minimum dose 2.0 mCi (74 MBq) and a maximum dose of 10 mCi (370 MBq).

Exercise ^{99m}Tc-MIBI SPECT study: at 2 to 4 hours after the rest study, the exercise study is performed using a dose of 0.35 mCi (12.95 MBq)/kg, with a minimum dose of 4 mCi (148 MBq) and a maximum dose of 20 mCi (740 MBq), given at peak exercise. After this injection, the child is encouraged to run for an additional 30 to 60 seconds.

Imaging

Imaging is performed 0.5 to 1.0 hour after tracer administration. The patient lies supine on the imaging table. Acquisition protocols should be adapted to individual SPECT systems. Single photon emission computed tomography is acquired using the following parameters: 120 total projections (i.e., 120 stops with a single detector and 60 stops with a dual detector system) with a 128×128 matrix for a total acquisition of 30 minutes. Appropriate magnifi-

FIGURE 6.15. Gated myocardial perfusion SPECT. Selected end-diastole and end-systole slices in the short axis and horizontal and vertical long axes are shown. Ventricular time-activity curve of a cardiac cycle is represented in the right upper quadrant.

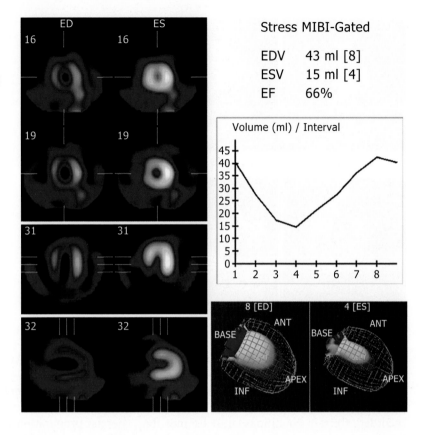

cation is used depending on the patient's heart size. After acquisition and reconstruction, the study is reoriented along the long axis of the left ventricle. Gated myocardial perfusion SPECT provides additional information regarding myocardial contractility, wall motion, end-diastolic and end-systolic ventricular volumes, ejection fraction, regurgitant fraction, and cardiac output (Fig. 6.15).

Assessment of Ventricular Function

Clinical Applications

Several nuclear medicine methods for the assessment of ventricular function in children are available. These include electrocardiogram (ECG)-gated myocardial-perfusion SPECT, gated metabolic PET (^{18}F-FDG), gated blood-pool scintigraphy, and first-pass radionuclide angiography. Radionuclide assessments of ventricular function include right and left ejection fractions, detection of wall-motion abnormalities, ventricular volume, cardiac output, and regurgitant fraction. Clinical applications of radionuclide studies to assess ventricular function have been applied to Kawasaki disease, anomalous origin of the coronary artery, cardiomyopathies, cardiac transplants, atrial and ventricular septal defects, cystic fibrosis, cardiac tumors, and certain congenital heart diseases, before and after catheter intervention or corrective surgery.

Gated Studies (Blood Pool or Myocardial Perfusion Imaging)

Gated studies are frequently done in adult patients. The method can also be employed in children.

Gated blood-pool scintigraphy is a means of imaging the cardiac blood pool by synchroniz-

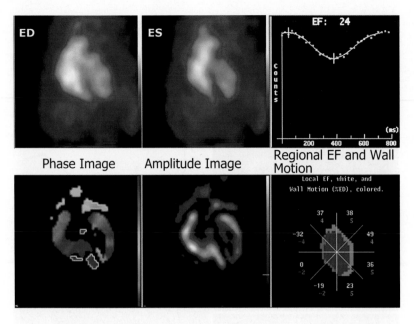

ED   ES   EF: 24

Phase Image   Amplitude Image   Regional EF and Wall Motion
Local EF, white, and Wall Motion (%ED), colored.

FIGURE 6.16. Gated blood pool scan showing end-diastolic (ED) and end-systolic (ES) frames and a ventricular time-activity curve of an average cardiac cycle. The ejection fraction is 24%. On the bottom of the image a phase image, an amplitude image, and an image of regional ejection fraction are shown.

ing the recording of scintillation data with the ECG.[64,65] This technique permits repetitive sampling of the cardiac cycle from many cycles until an image of appropriate count density is recorded. Certain conditions must be met for the gated scan to be performed adequately: regular heart rate and rhythm, limited beat-to-beat variability during the study, no patient motion, minimal diaphragmatic motion, largely intravascular location of the tracer, and sufficient count density.

Gated cardiac studies permit an evaluation of both global and regional ventricular function. Generally, no patient preparation is needed for this study, but patients under 3 years of age may require sedation in order to keep them still for the 20 to 30 minutes required for the recording (Fig. 6.16).

Radiopharmaceuticals

The myocardial-perfusion radiopharmaceuticals and their suggested administered doses have been described under the section on myocardial imaging. A good blood-pool label is critical for an adequate study.

In Vitro Labeling of Red Blood Cells

A 1- to 3-mL specimen of the patient's blood is obtained and treated with heparin or acid-citrate-dextrose (ACD). Ethylenediaminetetraacetic acid (EDTA) or oxalate should not be used as an anticoagulant. The red blood cells (RBCs) are labeled with ^{99m}Tc using a commercial preparation (Ultratag RBC, Mallinckrodt, St. Louis, MO). The labeled RBCs are reinjected slowly into the patient. *Caution: The labeled blood cells must be reinjected only into the patient from whom the blood was drawn.* Technetium-99m-labeled RBCs (^{99m}Tc-RBCs) are used in a dose of 0.2 mCi (7.4 MBq)/kg, with a minimum dose of 2.0 mCi (74 MBq) and a maximum of 20 mCi (740 MBq).

Imaging Technique

The patient is usually studied in the supine position. Sitting or upright positions are also possible. An intravenous needle (butterfly type, 23 or 25 gauge) or a short IV catheter is inserted and used to obtain blood for radiopharmaceutical labeling and injection. Once one is certain the needle/catheter is properly placed and that there is no possibility of extravasation, it should be secured with tape to the patient's skin. The patient's arm should be free of any object that could interfere with venous return. Venous access is kept patent with normal saline while the patient is being readied for the angiogram. Electrocardiographic electrodes are placed on both shoulders and on the patient's right costal margin. After intravenous injection of the ^{99m}Tc-RBCs, recording proceeds almost immediately. The gamma camera is usually equipped with a high-resolution parallel-hole collimator in the left anterior oblique projection in order to obtain maximal separation between the right and the left sides of the heart and tilted caudally so there is a separation between the aria and the ventricles. If available, a 30-degree slanted parallel-hole collimator positioned on contact with the patient's chest on a left anterior oblique projection and tilted caudally is preferred. Adjustments for abnormal cardiac positions may be necessary. Typically, recording consists of 32 frames per heartbeat on a 128 × 128 matrix for an appropriate amount of counts.

Data Recording

Data recording programs allow tailoring studies to each individual patient. The recording rate should be adjusted depending on the patient's heart rate.

If aberrant beats occur frequently (more than 10% of the beats) or if other arrhythmias are present (e.g., atrial fibrillation), this method of recording may not be effective. Alternatively, it is possible to record all scintigraphic events and the electrocardiogram in list mode and then evaluate various R-R intervals after the study is recorded. The end of the study can be determined by a preset number of cardiac cycles or a preset amount of time.

Analysis

Before analyzing the gated study, it is important to assess the technical adequacy of the study. The following items should be evaluated: adequate tracer labeling, patient motion, positioning, sharpness of the image, and adequate gating.

The study is viewed to assess global cardiac function, chamber sizes, and to detect abnormal wall motion. Analysis of the study can be performed manually or by several available automated methods. Time-activity curves of ventricular activity are calculated. Maps of regional ejection fraction and stroke volume are also displayed for analysis.

There are two parts to the analysis of gated scans: visual evaluation of the study on a series of images or on a movie mode display of the heart cycle, and measurement of ventricular function and volumes. Ventricular volume changes can be quantitated by analyzing time-activity curves from regions of interest (ROIs) over the ventricles. Global ventricular ejection fraction, ejection rate, filling rates, and ventricular volumes can be estimated.

Valvar Regurgitation

This technique is useful for quantitating mitral-valve or aortic-valve regurgitation, both prospectively following the natural history as well as assessing the results of surgical or catheter intervention. In gated blood-pool studies, a ratio of the change in count rates in the left ventricle between end-diastole and end-systole divided by the change in count rates in the right ventricle between end-systole and end-diastole (regurgitant volume index, stroke-volume ratio) provides a unique way to quantitate left-sided valvular regurgitation.[66-71] Rigo et al.[69] developed the method based on cardiac blood pool scintigraphy. In the left anterior oblique projection, this study permits simultaneous assessment of the left and right ventricles. The mean left ventricular/right ventricular stroke ratio (LV/RV) in normal patients is 1.19. In patients with aortic or mitral regurgitation, this ratio is elevated. These authors found good agreement between the LV/RV stroke volume ratio and angiographic grading of valvular regurgitation. The technique is simple and does not require elaborate data processing. Hurwitz et al.,[72] in our laboratory, evaluated this method to quantitate aortic or mitral regurgitation in children and young adults at rest and during isometric exercise. There was good correlation with cineangiographic results in 47 of 48 patients. The stroke-volume ratio was used to classify severity. The group with equivocal regurgitation differed from the group with mild regurgitation ($p < .02$); patients with mild regurgitation differed from those with moderate regurgitation ($p < .001$); and those with

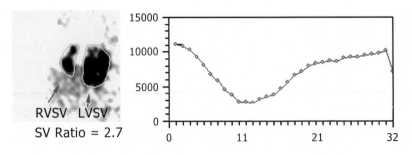

FIGURE 6.17. Regurgitant fraction estimated by gated blood pool scanning. The stroke volume ratio (SV ratio) is 2.7.

moderate regurgitation differed from those with severe regurgitation ($p < .01$). The stroke-volume ratio was responsive to isometric exercise, remaining constant or increasing in 16 of 18 patients. After corrective surgery in seven patients, the stroke-volume ratio significantly decreased from preoperative measurements in all patients. As in adult patients, the stroke-volume ratio in normals varied between 1.0 and 1.3. This study suggested that a stroke-volume ratio of more than 2.0 is compatible with moderate to severe regurgitation, and that a ratio greater than 3.0 indicates severe regurgitation (Fig. 6.17).

Diagnosis and Quantitation of Left-to-Right Shunts and Ventricular Function with First-Pass Radionuclide Angiocardiography

Clinical Applications

First-pass radionuclide angiocardiography (Fig. 6.18) is a rapid, accurate, and noninvasive method that is useful in the diagnosis and measurement of left-to-right shunts in certain congenital lesions, including the following:

Atrial septal defect
Ventricular septal defect

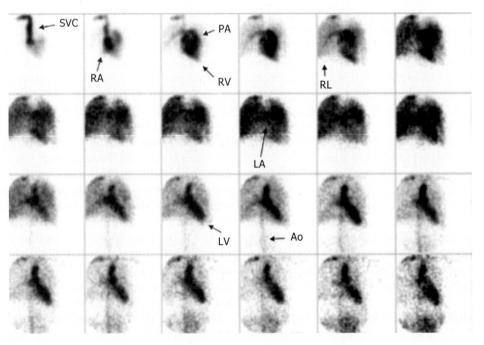

FIGURE 6.18. Normal radionuclide angiocardiogram. Tracer circulates in the superior vena cava (SVC), right atrium (RA), right ventricle (RV), pulmonary artery (PA), right lung (RL), left atrium (LA), left ventricle (LV), and aorta (Ao).

Truncus arteriosus
Patent ductus arteriosus
Complete atrioventricular canal
Aortopulmonary collaterals

This method is useful for assessing the magnitude of the shunt in patients before and after repair.

Determination of ventricular function with first-pass radionuclide angiocardiography is also possible in patients with most of the indications described earlier (see Assessment of Ventricular Function).

The method for determination and measuring left-to-right shunts is described below. The following section discusses the use of radionuclide angiocardiography for the determination of right and left ventricular ejection fraction.

Left-to-Right Shunts

Radiopharmaceuticals

Technetium-99m as pertechnetate is the most commonly used radiopharmaceutical for first-pass radionuclide angiocardiography. Other radiopharmaceuticals labeled with ^{99m}Tc can be used so long as they remain largely within the blood during the time required for the angiocardiogram [e.g., ^{99m}Tc-methylene diphosphonate (^{99m}Tc-MDP), ^{99m}Tc–diethylenetriamine pentaacetic acid (^{99m}Tc-DTPA), technetium-99m-disodium [N-[N-N-(mercaptoacetyl) glycyl]-glycinato(2-)-N,N′,N″,S]oxotechnetate (2-) (^{99m}Tc-MAG$_3$)]. Clearly agents such as ^{99m}Tc–macroaggregated albumin (^{99m}Tc–MAA) are not adequate for this purpose. Radiopharmaceuticals with rapid blood disappearance rate (^{99m}Tc-MAG$_3$ or ^{99m}Tc-DTPA) enable repeated angiocardiograms with lower residual background than pertechnetate.

When using ^{99m}Tc-pertechnetate, the patient should be premedicated with sodium (intravenous) or potassium (oral) perchlorate to reduce thyroid uptake of the tracer. When other ^{99m}Tc-labeled radiopharmaceuticals are used, perchlorate premedication is not necessary. Recommended administered doses of ^{99m}Tc are 0.2 mCi (7.4 MBq)/kg, with a minimum total dose of 2 to 3 mCi (74–111 MBq) and a maximum of 20 mCi (740 MBq). The total volume of radiopharmaceutical should be 0.2 mL so that a small rapid bolus can be administered.

Imaging Technique

The majority of patients do not need sedation for this short procedure. If sedation is needed, it should be prescribed for each patient individually. Prior to positioning the patient under the gamma camera for the angiocardiogram, an intravenous needle (butterfly type, 23 to 25 gauge) or a short IV catheter is inserted. Once one is assured that the needle/catheter is properly placed and that there is no possibility of extravasation, it should be secured with tape to the patient's skin. If possible, an antecubital vein is selected for the injection. In instances when the bolus of tracer is fragmented, the application of deconvolution analysis ensures a high percentage of successful studies.

The patient is placed supine on the imaging table. The gamma camera, equipped with a parallel-hole, high-sensitivity collimator is positioned anteriorly over the patient's chest. The field of view should extend from the suprasternal notch to just below the xiphoid and should cover both pulmonary fields.

Data Recording

Radionuclide angiocardiography for the assessment of left-to-right shunting is recorded at two or four frames per second for 25 seconds on a 128×128 matrix. Alternatively, a list mode acquisition can be used. For determination of right and left ventricular ejection fraction, radionuclide angiocardiography should be recorded at a minimum recording rate of 25 frames per second. The study is recorded for 25 seconds on a 128×128 matrix. Alternatively, the study can be recorded on a list mode.

Injection Technique

For the evaluation of left-to-right shunts, the technique of injection is of utmost importance in order to obtain a good-quality angiogram with high temporal resolution. Qualitative and quantitative analyses of radionuclide angiocardiography are best done when the radiotracer is delivered as a single, small, rapid intravenous bolus injection, a point that cannot be overemphasized. We prefer a disposable injector (bolus injector unit, International Medical Industries, Pompano Beach, FL) to deliver the tracer and saline flush. The volume of saline flush varies from approximately 0.5 mL in infants to 15.0 mL in adults. Before the tracer is injected, a trial flush with saline alone should be made to ensure against the possibility of accidental tracer extravasation. If there is no free flow into the vein or there are any doubts about the adequacy of venous access, the tracer must not be injected and another site for the injection should be selected. The tracer should not be injected while the patient is crying or producing Valsalva maneuvers. Increased or widely variable changes of intrathoracic changes will most likely cause bolus fragmentation and render the study inadequate. Injecting the tracer with the saline simultaneously through the injector allows rapid, uniform delivery of the tracer with uninterrupted saline flushing. The injection should be given in one continuous motion, and recording should begin simultaneously with tracer injection.

Initial Quality Control

Without moving the patient, the angiocardiogram is reviewed on a cine display. Then a small ROI is placed over the superior vena cava, and a time-activity curve is generated. This curve serves to determine the adequacy of the bolus. Acceptable bolus injections reveal a single peak with a FWHM (full width at half maximum) of less than 3 seconds. As mentioned, some fragmented boluses can be corrected by deconvolution analysis. If the study still appears inadequate for analysis, a second study may be performed using approximately twice the amount of the initial dose. Recording for the second angiogram is begun 3 to 5 seconds after the injection to allow background correction. If both injections fail, the study should be rescheduled for another day.

Analysis

The ROIs are marked over the lung fields. These regions should be placed carefully so they do not overlap the heart and great vessels. A series of images at 0.5 to 1.0 frames per second should be displayed. Superior vena cava time-activity curves are used to evaluate the quality of the bolus and to select the input for deconvolution analysis. Pulmonary time-activity curves are used for left-to-right detection and quantitation.

In a normal radionuclide angiocardiogram, tracer is seen as it circulates sequentially through the superior vena cava, right atrium, right ventricle, pulmonary artery, lungs, left atrium, left ventricle, and aorta. The left ventricle and the aorta are clearly visualized with only minimal pulmonary activity. The relative sizes of the heart chambers can be appreciated on the angiocardiogram (Fig. 6.18). A normal pulmonary time-activity curve is characteristic. Following an initial almost flat segment, the curve rapidly rises to a single peak and descends less rapidly to a "valley," almost reaching the baseline. This first peak represents the initial passage of the bolus through the pulmonary circulation and is followed by a second peak of less amplitude and broader than the first one. The second peak represents the portion of the initial bolus returning to the lungs after it circulates through the systemic circuit (Fig. 6.19).

With left-to-right shunting, the radionuclide angiocardiogram reveals a persistence of tracer activity in the lungs caused by premature pulmonary recirculation of the tracer through the intracardiac shunt (Figs. 6.20 and 6.21). The amount of persistent tracer activity in the lungs is directly related to the magnitude of shunt flow. In addition, in moderate to severe left-to-right shunting, the left side of the heart and the aorta are not well visualized on the angiogram. These two radionuclide angiocardiographic features—persistent pulmonary tracer activity and poor visualization of the left side of the heart and aorta—are diagnostic for left-to-right shunting. The pulmonary time-activity curve in left-to-right shunting characteristically reveals an early secondary peak that interrupts the initial down-slope of the curve. This premature secondary peak is due to premature reentry of tracer into the pulmonary circulation through the left-to-right shunt and is diagnostic. The pulmonary time-activity curve can be used to

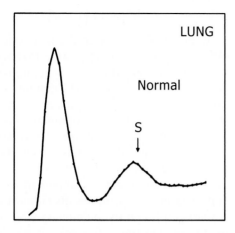
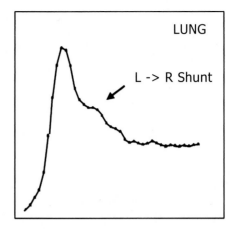

FIGURE 6.19. Pulmonary time-activity curves. Left: Normal. S, systemic peak. Right: Left-to-right shunt.

calculate the pulmonary-to-systemic flow ratio (Q_p/Q_s) (Figs. 6.22 and 6.23).

Quantitation of Left-to-Right Shunts

Analytic Model

The pulmonary time-activity curve recorded from a normal subject is composed of several sequential components. The first component, appearing at time t_p, is due to detection of radiotracer passing through the pulmonary vascular bed for the first time. We term this component $P(t)$. The second component, appearing at time tr_l, is due to detection of radiotracer passing through the pulmonary vascular bed for the second time, after one circuit through the systemic vascular bed. We term this component $R1(t)$. The third and later components are due

to detection of radiotracer passing through the pulmonary vascular bed for the third or later time, after two or more circuits of the systemic vascular bed. The observed normal pulmonary curve, $O(t)$, may therefore be decomposed according to the following formula:

$$O(t) = P(t) + R1(t) + \ldots .$$

In the case of a subject with a *left-to-right shunt*, a fraction (K) of radiotracer leaving the pulmonary vascular bed bypasses the systemic vascular bed by traveling through the shunt. The remaining fraction ($1 - K$) of radiotracer passes through the systemic vascular bed. Assuming the radiotracer is well mixed with the blood in the pulmonary vascular bed, these fractions are equal to the relative blood flows through the shunt and systemic vascular beds. It follows that

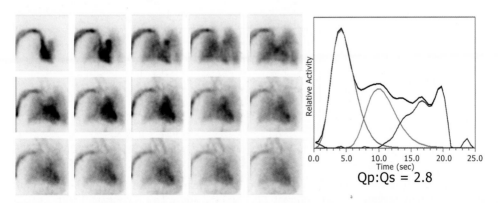

FIGURE 6.20. Left-to-right shunt. Radionuclide angiocardiogram from a patient with a moderate left-to-right shunt ($Q_p:Q_s = 2.8$). The angiocardiogram reveals premature pulmonary recirculation.

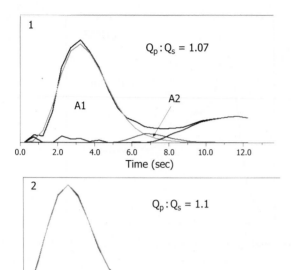

$$Q_p/Q_s = 1/(1 - K)$$

As in a normal subject, the first component of the observed pulmonary curve, $P(t)$, is due to radiotracer passing through the pulmonary vascular bed for the first time. The minimum transit time for the radiotracer passing through the shunt and back to the pulmonary system is generally less than that for the radiotracer passing through the systemic vascular bed before returning to the pulmonary system. Therefore, the second component of $O(t)$, appearing at time t_{s1}, represents radiotracer that is passing through the pulmonary vascular bed for the second time, after one circuit through the shunt. We term this component $S1(t)$. The area under $S1(t)$ is equal to K times the area under $P(t)$. The next two components of $O(t)$, appearing at times t_{r1} and t_{s2}, are due to detection of radiotracer passing through the pulmonary vascular bed after one circuit of the systemic vascular bed and two circuits of the shunt, respectively. We term these components $R1(t)$ and $S2(t)$. The remaining components of

FIGURE 6.21. Pulmonary time-activity curves for two patients without intracardiac shunting.

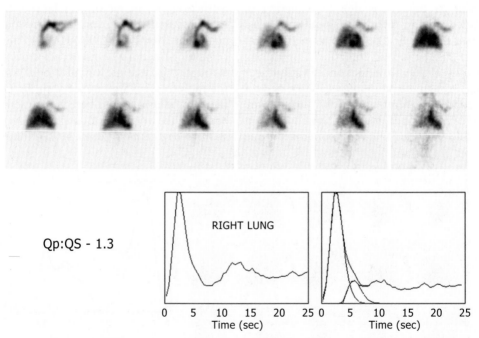

FIGURE 6.22. Small left-to-right shunt. The radionuclide angiocardiogram reveals a small amount of early pulmonary recirculation accompanied by a rather clear visualization of the left side of the heart and the aorta. This is consistent with a small left-to-right shunt ($Q_p : Q_s = 1.3$).

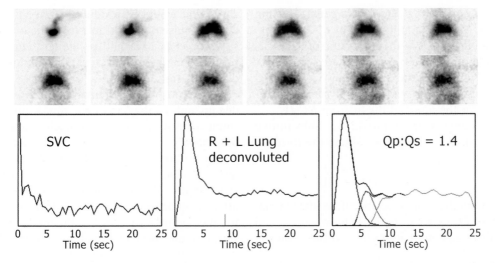

FIGURE 6.23. Radionuclide angiocardiogram from a 4–month-old girl after repair of tetralogy of Fallot 8 weeks prior to this examination. SVC, superior vena cava.

$O(t)$ are due to radiotracer passing through the pulmonary vascular bed following multiple circuits of the shunt or systemic vascular bed (or both). The observed pulmonary curve may therefore be decomposed as

$$O(t) = P(t) + S1(t) + R1(t) + S2(t) + \ldots$$

Shunt quantification is the problem of determining K. From the above,

$$K = \text{area under } S1(t)/\text{area under } P(t)$$

Thus, we can compute K by recovering $P(t)$ and $S1(t)$ from $O(t)$.

Gamma Variate Analysis

We now describe the gamma-variate method for recovering $P(t)$ and $S1(t)$ from the observed pulmonary curve, $O(t)$. Consider the $O(t)$ obtained from a normal subject. The portion of $O(t)$ for t between t_p and t_{r1} is due solely to the component $P(t)$. At time t_{r1}, the component $R1(t)$ appears. In most cases, almost the entire area of $P(t)$ is to the left of t_{r1}. It is therefore possible to recover $P(t)$ almost perfectly.

It has been found empirically that the $P(t)$ obtained after a compact bolus injection of radiotracer can be closely approximated by a gamma-variate function of the form

$$P(t) = C(t - t_p)^A e_p^{-(t-t)/B}$$

where t_p is the time at which activity first appears and C, A, and B are variable parameters. The gamma-variate function can be fitted to a portion of an observed data curve by a weighted least-squares technique.[73] Thus, it is possible to estimate $P(t)$ by fitting the gamma variate function to $O(t)$ for t between t_p and t_{r1} and extrapolating.

Consider the $O(t)$ obtained from a subject with a left-to-right shunt. The initial portion of the curve is again solely due to the component $P(t)$. At time t_{s1}, the component $S1(t)$ begins to appear. Because t_{s1} is smaller than t_{r1}, a substantial portion of the area under $P(t)$ may be to the right of t_{s1}. However, it is usually still possible to recover $P(t)$ approximately by fitting a gamma variate to $O(t)$ for t between t_p and t_{s1} and extrapolating. We denote the area under $P(t)$ by $A1$. Note that, in practice, it is necessary to infer the limits of the gamma-variate fit from $O(t)$. It can be done by visually interpreting the curve and manually choosing the points or by using a computer algorithm that automatically chooses the points.[74]

We now need to recover the component $S1(t)$. Subtracting the gamma variate fit for $P(t)$ from $O(t)$ yields the recirculation curve

$$RC(t) = S1(t) + R1(t) + S2(t) + \ldots$$

which is equal to $S1(t)$ for t between t_{s1} and min (t_{s2}, t_{r1}). We denote min (t_{s2}, t_{r1}) by t_{rc}. A gamma-variate function is fit to this portion of the recirculation curve and extrapolated to recover $S1(t)$. We denote the area under $S1(t)$ by $A2$. Again it is necessary to manually or automatically infer the limits of the fit from $RC(t)$.

K is equal to the ratio $A2/A1$. Substituting $A2/A1$ for K in Eq. (1), we obtain the formula

$$Q_p/Q_s = 1/(1 - A2/A1)$$
$$= A1/(A1 - A2).$$

This method provides accurate determinations of Q_p/Q_s when Q_p/Q_s is between 1.0 and 3.0, the range most important to the clinician. Q_p/Q_s values of greater than 3.0 are difficult to quantify precisely. However, large shunts (Q_p/Q_s <3.0) are usually clinically apparent, and more precise quantitation is unimportant.[72] Q_p/Q_s values between 1.0 and 1.2 may be obtained in patients with no shunt.[75–80] When the flow ratio is Q_p/Q_s <1.5, the shunt may not be recognized by visual inspection of the angiogram alone.

A number of alternative methods to estimate Q_p/Q_s from pulmonary time-activity curves have been suggested. We refer the interested reader to the available literature.[81–86]

Correction for Radiotracer Delivery

Shunt quantification by the gamma-variate method assumes that $P(t)$ and $S1(t)$ can be described by gamma-variate functions. In addition, the method assumes that sufficiently large portions of $P(t)$ and $S1(t)$ occur before t_{s1} and t_{rc}, respectively, to allow accurate extrapolation. The validity of both of these assumptions depends on the time course of delivery of the radiotracer to the cardiopulmonary system. This delivery can be monitored using an ROI over the superior vena cava.

Ideally, one would like to deliver the radiotracer to the cardiopulmonary system as an instantaneous pulse because it would maximize the separation of the components of the pulmonary curve and thus facilitate shunt quantitation. In practice, it is impossible to attain this goal by peripheral intravenous injection. It is possible, however, to estimate the pulmonary

curve that would be produced from an instantaneous pulse of radiotracer from the observed superior vena cava and pulmonary curves by using a mathematical technique known as deconvolution.[40,87,88]

Studies on dogs and humans have shown that deconvolution may improve the accuracy of shunt quantification by radionuclide angiocardiography.[66,89,90] Figure 6.22 shows the effect of deconvolution on [191m]Ir radionuclide angiocardiography performed on a dog with a left-to-right shunt. The pulmonary curve obtained after a fragmented injection is distorted relative to the pulmonary curve obtained after a compact injection in the same animal. After deconvolution, both lung curves are nearly identical.

Analysis of Ventricular Ejection Fraction

For assessment of ventricular ejection fraction, the radionuclide angiocardiogram should be first evaluated on a cinematic mode. This provides an overall view of the study and allows quality control. Regions of interest are drawn over the left and right ventricles, and time-activity curves are calculated (see below). These curves are used to identify the frames in the study corresponding to end-diastole and end-systole. An adaptive low-pass filter is applied to eliminate high-frequency noise. Consecutive end-diastolic and end-systolic frames are selected over several cardiac cycles during the first pass of radionuclide through the right and left ventricles. Composite images of each ventricle at end-diastole and end-systole are formed by adding the selected frames. Subtracting the end-systolic image from the end-diastolic image results in a "stroke volume" image, which is useful for identifying the atrioventricular plane. Regions of interest are then marked over the summed right and left diastolic and systolic frames. Ejection fractions are calculated by the formula

$$EF = \frac{EDC - ESC}{EDC}$$

where EF is the right (RV) or left (LV) ventricular ejection fraction, EDC is the end-diastolic counts, and ESC is the end-systolic

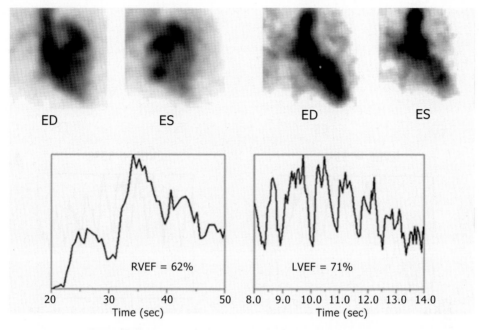

FIGURE 6.24. Determination of right and left ventricular ejection fractions (RVEF, LVEF) by first-pass radionuclide angiocardiography. Upper left: Right ventricle. ED, end diastolic image; ES, end systolic image. Upper right: Left ventricle. Lower quadrants: right and left ventricular time-activity curves.

counts. This method is accurate and ideally suited for children because it can be performed in just a few seconds, with no need for prolonged immobilization or sedation. First-pass radionuclide angiocardiography (FPRA) has been compared in our laboratory with biplane angiocardiography, and a good correlation was found (Figs. 6.24 and 6.25).[91]

To determine normal pediatric values of EF, we measured right and left ventricular ejection fractions in 74 children with normal cardiovascular function who were referred for skeletal scintigraphy.[92] These normal values are listed in Table 6.2. First-pass radionuclide angiocardiography requires meticulous attention to detail in the delineation of the edges of the ventricular margins and careful injection technique.

Right-to-Left Shunts

With right-to-left shunting, the first-pass radionuclide angiogram reveals passage of the radiotracer within the superior (or inferior) vena cava, the right atrium, and the right ventricle. There is, depending on the level of the shunt, rapid appearance of the tracer within the left atrium or the left ventricle and the aorta (or both), which on the angiogram appears to occur at the same time or before the tracer reaches the lungs. For example, with tricuspid atresia, the tracer is seen to circulate from the right atrium into the left ventricle via the left atrium, presenting a rather unique angiographic pattern. Some examples of congenital lesions where radionuclide angiocardiography may be used to detect and quantify right-to-left shunts are as follows:

Tetralogy of Fallot
Tricuspid atresia
Pulmonary atresia/intact ventricular septum
Tetralogy of Fallot with pulmonary atresia

Two approaches to the detection and quantitation of right-to-left shunts have been taken. The angiocardiographic technique is the same as that described for left-to-right shunting

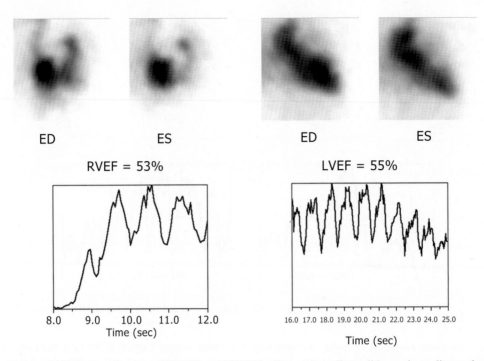

FIGURE 6.25. Determination of RVEF and LVEF by first-pass radionuclide angiocardiography.

except that the patient (with levocardia) should be imaged in the left anterior oblique projection to obtain maximum separation between the right and left ventricles. The ROIs are marked over the superior vena cava, right ventricle, left ventricle, and lungs. The time-activity curve from a small ROI over the left ventricle is analyzed. Care must be taken to avoid contamination of counts from the right side of the heart in the ROI selected. A first peak of activity, due to blood shunted from the right to the left side of the heart, is followed by a second peak of activity due to the radioactive blood that has circulated through the lungs.

Using an exponential extrapolation of the down-slope following these peaks, shunt flow can be estimated as the ratio of the area under the first peak to the whole area under both peaks.[93–96]

Another technique uses large-molecular-weight radioactive particles (^{99m}Tc-MAA) (Fig. 6.26). The major assumption in this method is that the particles are completely extracted from the circulation in one pass through either the pulmonary or the systemic capillary beds. This condition is largely met for particles larger than 10 μm in diameter. It is also assumed that the particles are mixed uniformly in the blood, that

TABLE 6.2. Right and left ventricular ejection fractions in children

	Right ventricle		Left ventricle	
Age (years)	No. of patients	RVEF	No. of patients	LVEF
<1	5	0.54 ± 0.09	5	0.68 ± 0.13
1–5	12	0.53 ± 0.07	11	0.62 ± 0.09
6–10	16	0.52 ± 0.05	15	0.69 ± 0.08
11–15	19	0.54 ± 0.03	18	0.65 ± 0.09
16–20	22	0.53 ± 0.06	23	0.70 ± 0.08
Totals/mean	74	0.53 ± 0.06	72	0.68 ± 0.09

RVEF, right ventricular ejection fraction; LVEF, left ventricular ejection fraction.

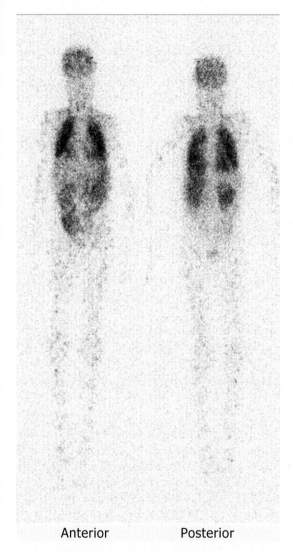

Anterior   Posterior

FIGURE 6.26. Right-to-left shunt. The patient received ⁹⁹ᵐTc-macroaggragated albumin intravenously. The whole-body scan reveals systemic penetration of the particles. This extrapulmonary activity is noted in the brain, thyroid, myocardium, spleen, kidneys, intestine, and muscles.

the particles themselves do not affect the blood flow, and that the particles traverse the system in the same manner as the blood. After intravenous administration of radioactive particles to a patient with a right-to-left shunt, the ratio of particles that enter the pulmonary and systemic circulations equals the pulmonary blood flow/systemic blood flow ratio.

The activity in the whole body is measured and compared with that in the lungs. Gates et al.,[97] using posterior scintiphotographs, and Lin,[98] using a whole-body profile device, employed this method. The theoretic difficulty is that the pulmonary and systemic circulations may be detected with different sensitivities owing to counting geometry and self-absorption. Complete separation of pulmonary and systemic activities may pose a minor difficulty, but good clinical results have been reported with this method. Although no adverse reactions have been reported from the intravenous administration of particles in patients with right-to-left shunting, one should be reminded that these particles produce microembolization in the systemic vascular bed, including the brain and kidneys. When necessary in patients with right-to-left shunts, we empirically employ a small number of particles (<10,000) in order to reduce systemic embolization.

Assessment of right-to-left shunting with ⁹⁹ᵐTc-MAA may be particularly useful in cyanotic patients with congenital heart disease to differentiate intrapulmonary versus intracardiac or extracardiac shunting. For example, in patients who have had either a Glenn or Fontan operation for a single ventricle, a number of "decompressing" or "short-cut" venous collaterals may develop, diverting blood from the high-pressure venous circuit in the superior vena cava to the lower pressure left atrium. Injections in the upper extremities with visualization of the particles in territories such as the brain and the kidneys suggest an extracardiac connection between the upper venous system and the left atrium.

Right-to-left shunting can also be detected by angiocardiography with an inert gas. An inert gas is almost completely removed from the blood in one transit through the lungs. The appearance of systemic activity after intravenous injection of an inert gas (dissolved in saline) indicates a right-to-left shunt. Prior to high-resolution echocardiography and cine-MRI, some investigators used both an inert gas and a nondiffusable indicator to define the nature of the cardiac defect, especially in complicated cases.[99–103]

Venography and Evaluation of Central Venous Lines

Radionuclide venography can be used to evaluate venous drainage in patients who have had multiple venous lines to determine venous patency and to help decide a site for placement of a new line. Also, this technique is indicated to evaluate venous drainage in patients with suspected superior vena cava syndrome. Another indication is the assessment of patency of central venous lines. Finally, the presence of a left superior vena cava is common in certain complex congenital heart diseases and may not be visible on the transthoracic echocardiogram. In these cases, a left-hand injection is helpful for determining the venous route to the heart. Radionuclide venography employs small volumes of material and can be done using simple intravenous needles. Radionuclide venography is a sensitive technique, as well as being safe and effective.

Radionuclide Venography

Radiopharmaceuticals

Technetium-99m (^{99m}Tc) pertechnetate is commonly used, although other radiopharmaceuticals, including ^{99m}Tc-DTPA and ^{99m}Tc-MAG$_3$, may be used as well.

Imaging Technique

When evaluating venous drainage from a single extremity, the imaging method is simple. Once venous access has been gained as described above, the gamma camera equipped with a high-resolution collimator is positioned anteriorly over the patient, covering an area including the injection site, the extremity, and the heart. The tracer is injected as a bolus, as described above. The venogram is recorded beginning at the time of injection at a rate of two frames per second for 60 seconds on a 64 × 64 or 128 × 128 matrix. Recommended administered dose for a single study is 0.03 mCi (11.1 MBq)/kg, with a minimum of 1 mCi (37 MBq) and a maximum of 2 mCi (74 MBq) (Fig. 6.27).

Patients with central venous lines are best evaluated using three injections: one in the right arm, one in the left arm, and one in the central line itself.

Three injections may be necessary, as clotting and other complications may occur in the proximal veins and not the central venous line itself. The venography technique is essentially the same as above, except it is modified by using three consecutive injections of graded amounts of radiotracer. The three sites for injection are prepared, and butterfly-type needles are placed in veins of both arms and secured with tape to the skin. The entry port of the central venous line is identified. Three syringes containing the radiopharmaceutical are prepared. The recommended administered doses for three sequential doses are as follows:

First injection: 0.03 mCi (1.11 MBq)/kg; minimum 1 mCi (37 MBq), maximum 2 mCi (74 MBq)
Second injection: 0.06 mCi (2.22 MBq)/kg; minimum 2 mCi (74 MBq), maximum 4 mCi (148 MBq)
Third injection: 0.12 mCi (4.44 MBq)/kg; minimum 4 mCi (148 MBq), maximum 8 mCi (296 MBq)

The computer is set to record at a rate of two frames per second for 5 minutes, and the recording is interrupted as soon as the last venography phase is completed. Alternatively, three sequential recording phases are preset, each at a rate of two frames per second for 60 seconds. First the arms are injected in sequence (the right and then the left, or vice versa), and the central line is injected last. Once the venogram is completed, it is evaluated by viewing it on cinematic mode on the computer monitor.

Assessment of Pulmonary Blood Flow

Abnormalities of pulmonary artery blood flow and distribution are common with complex congenital heart disease. A number of complex lesions require the combined surgical catheter and intervention approaches.[104–112] Quantitative pulmonary-perfusion scintigraphy has assumed an important role in the assessment of these repairs.

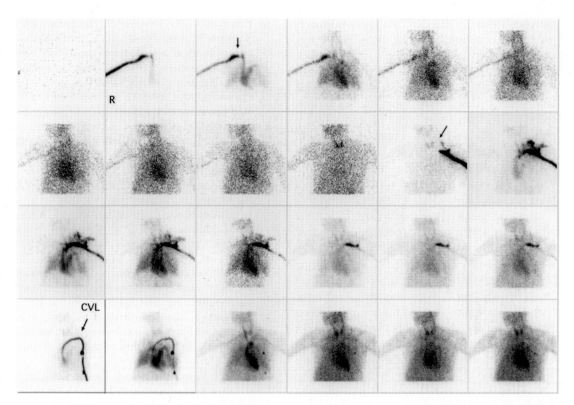

FIGURE 6.27. Radionuclide venography. This patient had had several central venous lines (CVLs) in the past and now has a left one. Technetium-99m pertechnetate was injected first into a right antecubital vein, which shows some impediment of flow at the junction of the innominate vein and the superior vena cava (arrow in top row). The second injection was in a left antecubital vein, which shows obstruction (arrow in second row) with collaterals. The third injection in the CVL demonstrates its patency.

Appendix: Ultrashort-Lived Radionuclides

Although commonly used, ^{99m}Tc has limitations as a tracer for first-pass radionuclide angiography: (1) Radiation-dose constraints limit the injected dose, which, in turn, limits the number of counts present in the study and thus the statistical accuracy. (2) It is difficult to perform repeated studies within a short time (as would be required to assess the effects of an intervention such as a pharmacologic intervention or exercise) because of background interference from the previous study. (3) In small children the temporal and spatial resolution of the study may be limited because of absorbed dose con-

siderations. These limitations are primarily a consequence of the 6-hour half-life of ^{99m}Tc compared to the short time required to perform the study (<30 seconds).

The most obvious way to eliminate these problems is to use a tracer with a shorter half-life.[113] This group of tracers is collectively known as ultrashort-lived radionuclides and includes gold-195m (^{195M}Au, $t_{1/2} = 30.5$ seconds), iridium-191m (^{191m}Ir, $t_{1/2} = 5$ seconds), and tantalum-178 (^{178}Ta, $t_{1/2} = 9.3$ minutes).[114] Because of their short half-lives, these tracers are produced at the bedside using radionuclide generators analogous to the molybdenum (^{99}Mo → ^{99m}Tc) generator.

Gold-195m was the subject of several clinical studies[115–120] during the 1980s when the mercury-195m (^{195m}Hg → ^{195m}Au) generator was produced commercially, but it is no longer available.

We[121–125] and others[126,127] have found that ^{191m}Ir is well suited for first-pass radionuclide angiography despite its short half-life (4.96 seconds). Iridium-191m emits 65 and 129 keV photons (65% and 26% abundance, respectively),[123] both of which can be imaged with modern scintillation cameras. In addition, the 65-keV x-rays can be imaged with the multiwire proportional camera.[128] The short half-life of ^{191m}Ir allows much larger amounts of ^{191m}Ir to be administered with an absorbed radiation dose to the patient lower than would be experienced with the normal dose of ^{99m}Tc. The resulting high photon flux permits images with high count density and thus greater statistical accuracy. The short half-life and low-radiation dose allow multiple studies to be performed within a short time to assess the cardiovascular changes that result from exercise, drugs, or catheter interventions.

Iridium-191m is the product of beta decay of osmium-191m (^{191m}Os), which has a physical half-life of 15.4 days. An ^{191}Os-^{191m}Ir generator system, which can deliver multiple doses of ^{191m}Ir for rapid intravenous injection, has been developed in our laboratory and used in humans.[123] If ^{191m}Ir is used, the time-activity curve from the angiogram is corrected for radioactive decay and count losses due to gamma-camera dead time before analysis.

Tantalum-178 has a somewhat longer half-life than ^{195m}Au or ^{191m}Ir but is still a significant improvement over ^{99m}Tc for first-pass radionuclide angiocardiography (FPRA). Lacy et al.[129–132] have described an automated generator that facilitates clinical use of ^{178}Ta.

References

1. Blumgart HL, Yens OC. Studies on the velocity of blood flow. I. The method utilized. J Clin Invest 1927;4:1–13.
2. Blumgart HL, Weiss S. Studies on the velocity of blood flow. VII. The pulmonary circulation time in normal resting individuals. J Clin Invest 1927;4:399–425.
3. Prinzmetal M, Corday E, Bergman HC, Schwartz L, Spritzler RJ. Radiocardiography: a new method for studying the blood flow through the chambers of the heart in human beings. Science 1948;108:340–1.
4. Prinzmetal M, Corday E, Spritzler RJ, Flieg W. Radiocardiography and its clinical applications. JAMA 1949;149:617–22.
5. Fyler DC. Report of the New England Regional Infant Cardiac Program. J Pediatr 1980; 65(supp):377.
6. Castaneda AR, Mayer JE Jr, Jonas RA, Lock JE, Wessel DL, Hickey PR. The neonate with critical congenital heart disease: repair—a surgical challenge. J Thorac Cardiovasc Surg 1989;98(5 pt 2):869–75.
7. Chang AC, Hanley FL, Lock JE, Castaneda AR, Wessel DL. Management and outcome of low birth weight neonates with congenital heart disease. J Pediatr 1994;124(3):461–6.
8. Kawasaki T. Acute febrile mucocutaneous syndrome with lymphoid involvement with specific desquamation of the fingers and toes in children. Arerugi 1967;16(3):178–222.
9. Kato H, Sugimura T, Akagi T, et al. Long-term consequences of Kawasaki disease. A 10- to 21-year follow-up study of 594 patients. Circulation 1996;94(6):1379–85.
10. Dajani AS, Taubert KA, Gerber MA, et al. Diagnosis and therapy of Kawasaki disease in children. Circulation 1993;87(5):1776–80.
11. Holman RC, Curns AT, Belay ED, Steiner CA, Schonberger LB. Kawasaki syndrome hospitalizations in the United States, 1997 and 2000. Pediatrics 2003;112(3 pt 1):495–501.
12. Yanagawa H, Nakamura Y, Yashiro M, et al. Results of the nationwide epidemiologic survey of Kawasaki disease in 1995 and 1996 in Japan. Pediatrics 1998;102(6):E65.
13. Fujiwara H, Hamashima Y. Pathology of the heart in Kawasaki disease. Pediatrics 1978; 61(1):100–7.
14. Tsuda E, Kamiya T, Ono Y, Kimura K, Kurosaki K, Echigo S. Incidence of stenotic lesions predicted by acute phase changes in coronary arterial diameter during Kawasaki disease. Pediatr Cardiol 2005;26(1):73–9.
15. Suzuki A, Kamiya T, Ono Y, Okuno M, Yagihara T. Aortocoronary bypass surgery for coronary arterial lesions resulting from Kawasaki disease. J Pediatr 1990;116(4):567–73.
16. Nienaber CA, Spielmann RP, Hausdorf G. Dipyridamole-thallium-201 tomography docu-

menting improved myocardial perfusion with therapy in Kawasaki disease. Am Heart J 1988;116(6 pt 1):1575–9.

17. Fyler DC. Report of the New England Regional Infant Cardiac Program. Pediatrics 1980;65(2 pt 2):377.

18. Liebman J, Cullum L, Belloc NB. Natural history of transposition of the great arteries. Anatomy and birth and death characteristics. Circulation 1969;40(2):237–62.

19. Arensman FW, Sievers HH, Lange P, et al. Assessment of coronary and aortic anastomoses after anatomic correction of transposition of the great arteries. J Thorac Cardiovasc Surg 1985;90(4):597–604.

20. Day RW, Laks H, Drinkwater DC. The influence of coronary anatomy on the arterial switch operation in neonates. J Thorac Cardiovasc Surg 1992;104(3):706–12.

21. Goor DA, Shem-Tov A, Neufeld HN. Impeded coronary flow in anatomic correction of transposition of the great arteries: prevention, detection, and management. J Thorac Cardiovasc Surg 1982;83(5):747–54.

22. Mayer JE Jr, Jonas RA, Castaneda AR. Arterial switch operation for transposition of the great arteries with intact ventricular septum. J Cardiovasc Surg 1986;1(2):97–104.

23. Tsuda E, Imakita M, Yagihara T, et al. Late death after arterial switch operation for transposition of the great arteries. Am Heart J 1992;124(6):1551–7.

24. Vogel M, Smallhorn JF, Gilday D, et al. Assessment of myocardial perfusion in patients after the arterial switch operation. J Nucl Med 1991;32(2):237–41.

25. Vogel M, Smallhorn JF, Trusler GA, Freedom RM. Echocardiographic analysis of regional left ventricular wall motion in children after the arterial switch operation for complete transposition of the great arteries. J Am Coll Cardiol 1990;15(6):1417–23.

26. Hunt SA. Complications of heart transplantation. J Heart Transplant 1983;3:70–4.

27. Pahl E, Naftel DC, Kuhn M, et al. The incidence and impact of transplant coronary artery disease in pediatric recipients: a 9 year multi-institutional study abstract. Circulation 2002; 106:II-396.

28. Gao SZ, Alderman EL, Schroeder JS, Silverman JF, Hunt SA. Accelerated coronary vascular disease in the heart transplant patient: coronary arteriographic findings. J Am Coll Cardiol 1988;12(2):334–40.

29. Rein AJ, Colan SD, Parness IA, Sanders SP. Regional and global left ventricular function in infants with anomalous origin of the left coronary artery from the pulmonary trunk: preoperative and postoperative assessment. Circulation 1987;75(1):115–23.

30. Sauer U, Stern H, Meisner H, Buhlmeyer K, Sebening F. Risk factors for perioperative mortality in children with anomalous origin of the left coronary artery from the pulmonary artery. J Thorac Cardiovasc Surg 1992;104(3):696–705.

31. Bunton R, Jonas RA, Lang P, Rein AJ, Castaneda AR. Anomalous origin of left coronary artery from pulmonary artery. Ligation versus establishment of a two coronary artery system. J Thorac Cardiovasc Surg 1987;93(1):103–8.

32. Montigny M, Stanley P, Chartrand C, Selman E, Fournier A, Davignon A. Postoperative evaluation after end-to-end subclavian-left coronary artery anastomosis in anomalous left coronary artery. J Thorac Cardiovasc Surg 1990;100(2):270–3.

33. Vouhe PR, Tamisier D, Sidi D, et al. Anomalous left coronary artery from the pulmonary artery: results of isolated aortic reimplantation. Ann Thorac Surg 1992;54(4):621–6; discussion 7.

34. Hurwitz RA, Caldwell RL, Girod DA, Brown J, King H. Clinical and hemodynamic course of infants and children with anomalous left coronary artery. Am Heart J 1989;118(6):1176–81.

35. Kocis KC. Chest pain in pediatrics. Pediatr Clin North Am 1999;46(2):189–203.

36. Khaja F, Alam M, Goldstein S, Anbe DT, Marks DS. Diagnostic value of visualization of the right ventricle using thallium-201 myocardial imaging. Circulation 1979;59(1):182–8.

37. Kondo M. Thallium-201 myocardial imaging in patients with various heart diseases (author's transl). Nippon Igaku Hoshasen Gakkai Zasshi 1979;39(9):942–54.

38. Kondo M, Kubo A, Yamazaki H, et al. Thallium-201 myocardial imaging for evaluation of right ventricular overloading. J Nucl Med 1978;19:1197–203.

39. Stevens RM, Baird MG, Fuhrmann CF, et al. Detection of right ventricular hypertrophy by thallium-201 myocardial perfusion imaging abstract. Circulation 1975;51/52(suppl II):243.

40. Bassingthwaighte JB. Circulatory transport and the convolution integral. Mayo Clin Proc 1967;42(3):137–54.

41. Rabinovitch M, Fisher K, Gamble W, Reid L, Treves S. Thallium-201: quantitation of right ventricular hypertrophy in chronically hypoxic rats. Radiology 1979;130(1):223–5.

42. Rabinovitch M, Fischer KC, Treves S. Quantitative thallium-201 myocardial imaging in assessing right ventricular pressure in patients with congenital heart defects. Br Heart J 1981;45(2):198–205.

43. Nakajima K, Taki J, Taniguchi M, Tonami N, Hisida K. Comparison of 99Tcm-sestamibi and 201Tl-chloride to estimate right ventricular overload in children. Nucl Med Commun 1995;16(11):936–41.

44. Cohen HA, Baird MG, Rouleau JR, et al. Thallium 201 myocardial imaging in patients with pulmonary hypertension. Circulation 1976; 54(5):790–5.

45. Strauer BE, Burger S, Bull U. Multifactorial determination of 201thallium uptake of the heart: an experimental study concerning the influence of ventricular mass, perfusion and oxygen consumption. Basic Res Cardiol 1978;73(3):298–306.

46. Bull C, de Leval MR, Mercanti C, Macartney FJ, Anderson RH. Pulmonary atresia and intact ventricular septum: a revised classification. Circulation 1982;66(2):266–72.

47. Gentles TL, Colan SD, Giglia TM, Mandell VS, Mayer JE Jr, Sanders SP. Right ventricular decompression and left ventricular function in pulmonary atresia with intact ventricular septum. The influence of less extensive coronary anomalies. Circulation 1993;88(5 pt 2): II183–8.

48. Giglia TM, Mandell VS, Connor AR, Mayer JE Jr, Lock JE. Diagnosis and management of right ventricle-dependent coronary circulation in pulmonary atresia with intact ventricular septum. Circulation 1992;86(5):1516–28.

49. Hanley FL, Sade RM, Blackstone EH, Kirklin JW, Freedom RM, Nanda NC. Outcomes in neonatal pulmonary atresia with intact ventricular septum. A multiinstitutional study. J Thorac Cardiovasc Surg 1993;105(3):406–23, 24–7; discussion 23–4.

50. Lebowitz E, Greene MW, Fairchild R, et al. Thallium-201 for medical use. I. J Nucl Med 1975;16(2):151–5.

51. Kawana N, Krizeh H, Porter J, et al. Use of Tl-201 as a potassium analog in scanning abstract. J Nucl Med 1970;11:333.

52. Gehring PJ, Hammond PB. The interrelationship between thallium and potassium in animals. J Pharmacol Exp Ther 1967;155(1): 187–201.

53. Strauss HW, Harrison K, Langan JK, Lebowitz E, Pitt B. Thallium-201 for myocardial imaging. Relation of thallium-201 to regional myocardial perfusion. Circulation 1975;51(4): 641–5.

54. Karasawa K, Ayusawa M, Noto N, Sumitomo N, Okada T, Harada K. Assessment of cardiac sympathetic nerve activity in children with chronic heart failure using quantitative iodine-123 metaiodobenzylguanidine imaging. J Cardiol 2000;36(6):387–95.

55. Acar P, Merlet P, Iserin L, et al. Impaired cardiac adrenergic innervation assessed by MIBG imaging as a predictor of treatment response in childhood dilated cardiomyopathy. Heart 2001;85(6):692–6.

56. Sakurai H, Maeda M, Miyahara K, et al. Evaluation of cardiac autonomic nerves by iodine-123 metaiodobenzylguanidine scintigraphy and ambulatory electrocardiography in patients after arterial switch operations. J Cardiol 2000;35(5):353–62.

57. Maunoury C, Agostini D, Acar P, et al. Impairment of cardiac neuronal function in childhood dilated cardiomyopathy: an 123I-MIBG scintigraphic study. J Nucl Med 2000; 41(3):400–4.

58. Momose M, Kobayashi H, Kasanuki H, et al. Evaluation of regional cardiac sympathetic innervation in congenital long QT syndrome using 123I-MIBG scintigraphy. Nucl Med Commun 1998;19(10):943–51.

59. Acar P, Merlet P, Iserin L, et al. Cardiac MIBG imaging: a new marker for myocardial function in children?. Arch Mal Coeur Vaiss 1996;89(5): 599–604.

60. Olgunturk R, Turan L, Tunaoglu FS, et al. Abnormality of the left ventricular sympathetic nervous function assessed by I-123 metaiodobenzylguanidine imaging in pediatric patients with neurocardiogenic syncope. Pacing Clin Electrophysiol 2003;26(10):1926–30.

61. Muller KD, Jakob H, Neuzner J, Grebe SF, Schlepper M, Pitschner HF. 123I-metaiodobenzylguanidine scintigraphy in the detection of irregular regional sympathetic innervation in long QT syndrome. Eur Heart J 1993;14(3): 316–25.

62. Stirner H, Buell U, Kleinhans E, Bares R, Grosse W. Myocardial kinetics of 99Tcm hexakis-(2-methoxy-isobutyl-isonitrile) (HMIBI) in patients with coronary heart

disease: a comparative study versus 201Tl with SPECT. Nucl Med Commun 1988;9(1):15–23.

63. Magrina J, Bosch X, Garcia A, et al. Diagnostic value of technetium-99m-MIBI as a myocardial perfusion imaging agent: comparison of long and short intervals between rest and stress injections. Clin Cardiol 1992;15(7):497–503.

64. Berman DS, Salel AF, DeNardo GL, Bogren HG, Mason DT. Clinical assessment of left ventricular regional contraction patterns and ejection fraction by high-resolution gated scintigraphy. J Nucl Med 1975;16(10):865–74.

65. Strauss HW, Zaret BL, Hurley PJ, Natarajan TK, Pitt B. A scintiphotographic method for measuring left ventricular ejection fraction in man without cardiac catheterization. Am J Cardiol 1971;28(5):575–80.

66. Alderson PO, Douglass KH, Mendenhall KG, et al. Deconvolution analysis in radionuclide quantitation of left-to-right cardiac shunts. J Nucl Med 1979;20(6):502–6.

67. Bough EW, Gandsman EJ, North DL, Shulman RS. Gated radionuclide angiographic evaluation of valve regurgitation. Am J Cardiol 1980;46(3):423–8.

68. Lam W, Pavel D, Byrom E, Sheikh A, Best D, Rosen K. Radionuclide regurgitant index: value and limitations. Am J Cardiol 1981;47(2):292–8.

69. Rigo P, Alderson PO, Robertson RM, Becker LC, Wagner HN Jr. Measurement of aortic and mitral regurgitation by gated cardiac blood pool scans. Circulation 1979;60(2):306–12.

70. Sorensen SG, O'Rourke RA, Chaudhuri TK. Noninvasive quantitation of valvular regurgitation by gated equilibrium radionuclide angiography. Circulation 1980;62(5):1089–98.

71. Urquhart J, Patterson RE, Packer M, et al. Quantification of valve regurgitation by radionuclide angiography before and after valve replacement surgery. Am J Cardiol 1981;47(2):287–91.

72. Hurwitz RA, Treves S, Keane JF, Girod DA, Caldwell RL. Current value of radionuclide angiocardiography for shunt quantification and management in patients with secundum atrial septal defect. Am Heart J 1982;103(3):421–5.

73. Starmer CF, Clark DO. Computer computations of cardiac output using the gamma function. J Appl Physiol 1970;28(2):219–20.

74. Kuruc A, Treves S, Smith W, Fujii A. An automated algorithm for radionuclide angiocardiographic quantitation of circulatory shunting. Comput Biomed Res 1984;17(5):481–93.

75. Alderson PO, Gaudiani VA, Watson DC, Mendenhall KG, Donovan RC. Quantitative radionuclide angiocardiography in animals with experimental atrial septal defects. J Nucl Med 1978;19(4):364–9.

76. Alderson PO, Jost RG, Strauss AW, Boonvisut S, Markham J. Detection and quantitation of left-to-right cardiac shunts in children: a clinical comparison of count ratio and area ratio techniques. J Nucl Med 1975;16:511.

77. Askenazi J, Ahnberg DS, Korngold E, LaFarge CG, Maltz DL, Treves S. Quantitative radionuclide angiocardiography: detection and quantitation of left to right shunts. Am J Cardiol 1976;37(3):382–7.

78. Maltz DL, Treves S. Quantitative radionuclide angiocardiography: determination of Qp: Qs in children. Circulation 1973;47(5):1049–56.

79. Treves S, Maltz DL. Radionuclide angiocardiography. Postgrad Med 1974;56(1):99–107.

80. Treves S, Maltz DL, Adelstein SJ. Intracardiac shunts. In: James AE, Wagner HN Jr, Cooke RE, eds. Pediatric Nuclear Medicine. Philadelphia: Saunders, 1974.

81. Bourguignon MH, Links JM, Douglass KH, Alderson PO, Roland JM, Wagner HN Jr. Quantification of left to right cardiac shunts by multiple deconvolution analysis. Am J Cardiol 1981;48(6):1086–90.

82. Kveder M, Bajzer Z, Nosil J. A mathematical model for the quantitative study of left to right cardiac shunt. Phys Med Biol 1985;30(3):207–15.

83. Kveder M, Bajzer Z, Zadro M. Theoretical aspects of multiple deconvolution analysis for quantification of left to right cardiac shunts. Phys Med Biol 1987;32(10):1237–43.

84. Madsen MT, Argenyi E, Preslar J, Grover-McKay M, Kirchner PT. An improved method for the quantification of left-to-right cardiac shunts. J Nucl Med 1991;32(9):1808–12.

85. Nakamura M, Suzuki Y, Nagasawa T, Sugihara M, Takahashi T. Detection and quantitation of left-to-right shunts from radionuclide angiocardiography using the homomorphic deconvolution technique. IEEE Trans Biomed Eng 1982;29(3):192–201.

86. Parker JA, Treves S. Radionuclide detection, localization, and quantitation of intracardiac shunts and shunts between the great arteries. Prog Cardiovasc Dis 1977;20(2):121–50.

87. Gamel J, Rousseau WF, Katholi CR, Mesel E. Pitfalls in digital computation of the impulse response of vascular beds from indicator-

dilution curves. Circ Res 1973;32(4):516–23.

88. Kuruc A, Treves S, Parker JA. Accuracy of deconvolution algorithms assessed by simulation studies: concise communication. J Nucl Med 1983;24(3):258–63.

89. Ham HR, Dobbeleir A, Virat P, Piepsz A, Lenaers A. Radionuclide quantitation of left-to right cardiac shunts using deconvolution analysis: concise communication. J Nucl Med 1981; 22(8):688–92.

90. Kuruc A, Treves S, Parker JA, Cheng C, Sawan A. Radionuclide angiocardiography: an improved deconvolution technique for improvement after suboptimal bolus injection. Radiology 1983;148(1):233–8.

91. Kurtz D, Ahnberg DS, Freed M, LaFarge CG, Treves S. Quantitative radionuclide angiocardiography. Determination of left ventricular ejection fraction in children. Br Heart J 1976;38(9):966–73.

92. Hurwitz RA, Treves S, Kuruc A. Right ventricular and left ventricular ejection fraction in pediatric patients with normal hearts: first-pass radionuclide angiocardiography. Am Heart J 1984;107(4):726–32.

93. Hurley PJ, Poulose KP, Wagner HN Jr. Radionuclide angiocardiography for detecting right-to-left intracardiac shunts abstract. J Nucl Med 1969;10:344.

94. Riihimaki E, Heiskanen A, Tahti E. Theory of quantitative determination of intracardiac shunts by external detection. Ann Clin Res 1974;6(1):45–9.

95. Treves S. Detection and quantitation of cardiovascular shunts with commonly available radionuclides. Semin Nucl Med 1980;10(1):16–26.

96. Weber PM, Dos Remedios LV, Jasko IA. Quantitative radioisotopic angiocardiography. J Nucl Med 1972;13(11):815–22.

97. Gates GF, Orme HW, Dore EK. Measurement of cardiac shunting with technetium-labeled albumin aggregates. J Nucl Med 1971;12(11):746–9.

98. Lin CY. Lung scan in cardiopulmonary disease. I. Tetralogy of Fallot. J Thorac Cardiovasc Surg 1971;61(3):370–9.

99. Bosnjakovic VB, Bennett LR. Dynamic isotope studies in cardiology. AEC Symp Series 1972;27:562.

100. Braunwald E, Long RTL, Morrow AG. Injections of radioactive krypton (KR[85]) solutions in the detection of cardiac shunts. J Clin Invest 1959;38:990.

101. Long RT, Braunwald E, Morrow AG. Intracardiac injection of radioactive krypton. Clinical applications of new methods for characterization of circulatory shunts. Circulation 1960;21:1126–33.

102. Long RT, Waldhausen JA, Cornell WP, Sanders RJ. Detection of right-to-left circulatory shunts: a new method utilizing injections of krypton. Proc Soc Exp Biol Med 1959;102:456–8.

103. Parker JA, Secker-Walker R, Hill R, Siegel BA, Potchen EJ. A new technique for the calculation of left ventricular ejection fraction. J Nucl Med 1972;13(8):649–51.

104. Driscoll DJ, Hesslein PS, Mullins CE. Congenital stenosis of individual pulmonary veins: clinical spectrum and unsuccessful treatment by transvenous balloon dilation. Am J Cardiol 1982;49(7):1767–72.

105. Gentles TL, Lock JE, Perry SB. High pressure balloon angioplasty for branch pulmonary artery stenosis: early experience. J Am Coll Cardiol 1993;22(3):867–72.

106. O'Laughlin MP, Perry SB, Lock JE, Mullins CE. Use of endovascular stents in congenital heart disease. Circulation 1991;83(6):1923–39.

107. O'Laughlin MP, Slack MC, Grifka RG, Perry SB, Lock JE, Mullins CE. Implantation and intermediate-term follow-up of stents in congenital heart disease. Circulation 1993;88(2):605–14.

108. Rothman A, Perry SB, Keane JF, Lock JE. Balloon dilation of branch pulmonary artery stenosis. Semin Thorac Cardiovasc Surg 1990;2(1):46–54.

109. Rothman A, Perry SB, Keane JF, Lock JE. Early results and follow-up of balloon angioplasty for branch pulmonary artery stenoses. J Am Coll Cardiol 1990;15(5):1109–17.

110. Stewart JA, Silimperi D, Harris P, Wise NK, Fraker TD Jr, Kisslo JA. Echocardiographic documentation of vegetative lesions in infective endocarditis: clinical implications. Circulation 1980;61(2):374–80.

111. Tamir A, Melloul M, Berant M, et al. Lung perfusion scans in patients with congenital heart defects. J Am Coll Cardiol 1992;19(2):383–8.

112. Vogel M, Ash J, Rowe RD, Trusler GA, Rabinovitch M. Congenital unilateral pulmonary vein stenosis complicating

transposition of the great arteries. Am J Cardiol 1984;54(1):166–71.

113. Yano Y, Anger HO. Ultrashort-lived radioisotopes for visualizing blood vessels and organs. J Nucl Med 1968;9(1):2–6.

114. Paras T, Thiessen JW. Single-photon ultrashort-lived radionuclides. In: U.S. Department of Energy Symposium Series. Washington, DC: DOE, 1985:57.

115. Caplin JL, Dymond DS, O'Keefe JC, et al. Relation between exercise: a study using first-pass radionuclide angiography with gold-195m. Br Heart J 1986;55:120–8.

116. Kipper SL, Ashburn WL, Norris SL, Rimkus DS, Dillon WA. Gold-195m first-pass radionuclide ventriculography, thallium-201 single-photon emission CT, and 12–lead ECG stress testing as a combined procedure. Radiology 1985;156(3):817–21.

117. Lahiri A, Zanelli GD, O'Hara MJ, et al. Simultaneous measurement of left ventricular function and myocardial perfusion during a single exercise test: dual isotope imaging with gold-195 m and thallium-201. Eur Heart J 1986;7(6):493–500.

118. Miller DD, Gill JB, Fischman AJ, et al. New radionuclides for cardiac imaging. Prog Cardiovasc Dis 1986;28(6):419–34.

119. Stone DL, Barber RW, Ormerod OJ, Petch MC, Wraight EP. Quantification of intracardiac shunts by gold-195m, a new radionuclide with a short half life. Br Heart J 1985;54(5):495–500.

120. Van der Wall EE, van Lingen A, den Hollander W, et al. Short-lived 195mAu for evaluation of left ventricular function by first-pass radionuclide angiography. Nuklearmedizin 1985;24(4):191–2.

121. Heller GV, Treves ST, Parker JA, et al. Comparison of ultrashort-lived iridium-191m with technetium-99m for first pass radionuclide angiocardiographic evaluation of right and left ventricular function in adults. J Am Coll Cardiol 1986;7(6):1295–302.

122. Treves S, Cheng C, Samuel A, Fujii A, Lambrecht R. Detection and quantitation of left-right shunting by iridium-191m angiography. In: Medical Radionuclide Imaging, 2nd ed. Vienna: IAEA, 1981:231–41.

123. Treves S, Cheng C, Samuel A, et al. Iridium-191 angiocardiography for the detection and quantitation of left-to-right shunting. J Nucl Med 1980;21(12):1151–7.

124. Treves S, Fyler D, Fujii A, Kuruc A. Low radiation iridium-191m radionuclide angiography: detection and quantitation of left-to-right shunts in infants. J Pediatr 1982;101(2):210–3.

125. Verani MS, Lacy JL, Ball ME, et al. Simultaneous assessment of regional ventricular function and perfusion utilizing iridium-191m and thallium-201 during a single exercise test. Am J Cardiol Imag 1988;2:206–13.

126. Franken PR, Dobbeleir AA, Ham HR, et al. Clinical usefulness of ultrashort-lived iridium-191m from a carbon-based generator system for the evaluation of the left ventricular function. J Nucl Med 1989;30(6):1025–31.

127. Hellman C, Zafrir N, Shimoni A, et al. Evaluation of ventricular function with first-pass iridium-191m radionuclide angiocardiography. J Nucl Med 1989;30(4):450–7.

128. Lacy JL, Verani MS, Ball ME, Roberts R. Clinical applications of a pressurized xenon wire chamber gamma camera utilizing the short lived agent 178Ta. Nucl Inst Meth 1988; A269:369–76.

129. Lacy JL, Layne WW, Guidry GW, Verani MS, Roberts R. Development and clinical performance of an automated, portable tungsten-178/tantalum-178 generator. J Nucl Med 1991;32(11):2158–61.

130. Lacy JL, Verani MS, Ball ME, Boyce TM, Gibson RW, Roberts R. First-pass radionuclide angiography using a multiwire gamma camera and tantalum-178. J Nucl Med 1988;29(3):293–301.

131. Verani MS, Guidry GW, Mahmarian JJ, et al. Effects of acute, transient coronary occlusion on global and regional right ventricular function in humans. J Am Coll Cardiol 1992;20(7):1490–7.

132. Verani MS, Lacy JL, Guidry GW, et al. Quantification of left ventricular performance during transient coronary occlusion at various anatomic sites in humans: a study using tantalum-178 and a multiwire gamma camera. J Am Coll Cardiol 1992;19(2):297–306.

7
Gastroesophageal Reflux, Gastric Emptying, Esophageal Transit, and Pulmonary Aspiration

Zvi Bar-Sever

Gastroesophageal Reflux

Definition, Pathophysiology, and Clinical Manifestations

The definition of gastroesophageal reflux (GER) is the passage of gastric contents into the esophagus. Regurgitation is defined as passage of refluxed gastric contents into the mouth. Vomiting is the expulsion of gastric contents from the mouth. Many episodes of gastroesophageal reflux occur in healthy infants and children and are considered "physiologic." Such episodes are brief and either asymptomatic or cause mild regurgitation or occasional vomiting.[1] Gastroesophageal reflux disease (GERD) occurs when episodes of GER produce symptoms and complications.

The lower esophageal sphincter (LES) is the main barrier preventing retrograde passage of gastric contents into the esophagus. Although the baseline tone of the LES is normal in most children with GER, transient relaxations of the sphincter, unrelated to swallowing, and inadequate adaptation of the sphincter tone to changes in abdominal pressure are the main mechanisms causing GER.[2,3] Distention of the gastric wall can produce transient relaxations of the LES.[4,5] Prolonged distention of the gastric walls due to delayed emptying is a proposed mechanism explaining the relationship between the two conditions. Delayed gastric emptying has been documented in adults with GERD.[6–8] In children this relationship is controversial. Some authors found delayed gastric emptying in children with GERD,[9–11] whereas others did not.[12,13] In one study involving 477 children, delayed gastric emptying was noted only in children with GERD who were older than 6 years.[14] According to another study, GER in children is worsened by increasing the volume and osmolality of meals that affect the LES pressure.[15]

It is not well established why GER is asymptomatic in some children and produces clinical manifestations in others. Multiple factors can contribute to the pathogenesis of GERD, including the frequency and duration of reflux, gastric acidity, gastric emptying, esophageal mucosal barrier, esophageal clearing mechanisms, airway hypersensitivity, etc. Clustering of severe GERD in families and a higher prevalence of acid reflux in monozygotic twins compared with dizygotic twins provide evidence for genetic disposition for GERD. This genetic component, however, accounts for only a small number of GERD cases.[16,17] The prevalence of GER and GERD is not well established. According to some authors it ranges from 20% to 40% in infants and 7% to 20% in older children and adolescents.[18–20] The prevalence of GER may be even higher when determined by clinical symptoms commonly associated with GER, especially vomiting.[21] The higher frequency of GER and GERD in infants is associated with transient immaturity of the esophagus and stomach.[1]

Gastroesophageal reflux disease can affect the gastrointestinal and respiratory systems. Clinical manifestations vary with age. The main GER-related symptom in infants is recurrent vomiting. It occurs in 50% of infants during the first 3 months of life and in 67% of 4-month-old infants. Vomiting resolves spontaneously in the majority of infants and is encountered in only 5% of infants at the age of 10 to 12 months.[21] Severe symptoms of anorexia, dysphagia, painful swallowing, irritability, hematemesis, anemia, and failure to thrive occur only in a small number of infants and are related to complications of esophagitis. Gastroesophageal reflux in infants has been associated with respiratory complications, including apnea and apparent life-threatening events (ALTEs), recurrent pneumonia, hyperactive airway disease, chronic cough, and recurrent stridor. In preschool children, the main manifestation of GER is intermittent vomiting. In older children, common symptoms include heartburn or regurgitation with reswallowing. Rarely, esophageal pain may produce repetitive stretching and arching movements (Sandifer syndrome) commonly mistaken for atypical seizures or dystonia.[22,23] Esophagitis in older children can manifest as dysphagia and in severe cases result in hematemesis, anemia, hypoproteinemia, and melena. Esophageal strictures and circumferential scarring can complicate untreated esophagitis. Erosive esophagitis is encountered in less than 5% of thriving children and is much more common in children with neurologic disabilities. Chronic esophagitis may lead to replacement of the distal esophageal mucosa with Barrett's mucosa, a metaplastic, potentially malignant epithelium.[24] Barrett's esophagus is found in fewer than 2% of children with GERD.[1] Gastroesophageal reflux is prevalent in children with asthma. Recent research suggests that the presence of gastric acid in the esophagus alters bronchial hyperresponsiveness and that effective treatment of GERD can improve respiratory disease in selected asthma patients.[25] Aspiration pneumonia due to GER is mostly encountered in neurologically impaired children. Hoarseness has also been associated with GER in children.

Diagnosis of Gastroesophageal Reflux

Extended Esophageal pH Monitoring

Twenty-four-hour esophageal pH monitoring is the most widely accepted tool for the diagnosis of GER. This technique measures esophageal exposure to gastric acid by detecting the concentration of hydrogen ions (pH) in the distal esophagus. Values under 4 are used to indicate gastric acid exposure due to reflux (the normal esophageal pH varies from 5 to 7). The study has a sensitivity and specificity over 90% for detection of GERD and is considered by many as the gold standard. The electrode is placed a few centimeters above the LES, in the distal esophagus, and records the frequency and duration of reflux episodes and the accumulated exposure times. These parameters are integrated into a composite score that correlates with the degree of esophageal epithelial damage, determined histologically. The percentage of the total time that the esophageal pH is <4 is called the reflux index. Considering the fact that not all episodes of acid reflux are symptomatic or cause complications, the North American Society of Pediatric Gastroenterology and Nutrition recommended that the upper limit of normal for the reflux index is 12% during the first year of life and 6% thereafter.[26]

Esophageal pH monitoring requires introduction of a transnasal pH catheter and is often preceded by esophageal manometry to identify the location of the LES for proper placement of the pH electrode.[27] The main strength of this technique is the 24-hour observation period that provides a true estimate of the frequency of GER and cumulative residence time of acid refluxate in the esophagus. The technique, however, cannot detect nonacidic reflux episodes. It has been shown in infants and children that reflux-associated disturbances such as bronchitis, irritability, sleep disorders, episodes of apnea, oxygen desaturation, and pulmonary aspiration can be induced by both acidic (pH < 4) and nonacidic (pH ? 4) reflux.[28] During the postprandial period, neutralization of gastric acidity of varying duration occurs and is affected by the patient's age, the volume and composition of the meal, and the frequency of feeding.[29] Reflux during these periods may occur in the physiologic esophageal pH (from 5 to 7) and will not be detected with pH monitoring. Antacid therapy for GER can also prevent detection of GER episodes with pH monitoring.[30] The invasive nature of the study and the need to hospitalize young infants for the study are additional important disadvantages. A radiotelemetric, catheter-free, pH capsule secured to the lower esophagus is under investigation as a more comfortable alternative to the pH catheter.

Multiple, Intraluminal Electrical Impedance

Multiple, intraluminal electrical impedance (Imp) is a new, pH-independent, technique for the diagnosis of GER based on changes in electrical impedance during passage of a bolus along an esophageal segment (between two electrodes). The use of multiple segments along a catheter placed in the esophagus enables differentiation between antegrade and retrograde bolus movements in the esophagus and the detection of GER. A pH-sensitive electrode can be attached to the catheter, allowing simultaneous measurements of electrical impedance and changes in esophageal pH.[30] A study of infants with a history of apnea, breathing irregularities, and aspiration that combined IMP with pH monitoring and overnight polysomnography showed that the majority of GER episodes (including many symptomatic episodes) were not associated with pH measurements under 4 and would probably pass undetected by esophageal pH monitoring alone.[31] Currently this promising new technique is not widely available, requires considerable time for analysis of the recordings, and has the same disadvantage of being invasive as extended pH monitoring.

Sonography

Sonographic detection of GER has been attempted and has shown encouraging results in young infants when compared with esophageal pH monitoring. In one study sonographic detection had a sensitivity of 100% and specificity of 87%.[32] Despite these encouraging results, there has been very little experience with this technique, and it is not currently utilized in routine clinical practice.

Barium Contrast Radiography

Upper gastrointestinal (GI) series are often used in the evaluation of GERD, although various studies show this test is neither sensitive nor specific in comparison to 24-hour pH monitoring (sensitivity ranged from 31% to 86% and specificity from 21% to 83%). Imaging is short and intermittent because the radiation dose of cineradiography is prohibitive.[26] The short observation period can result in false-negative studies when reflux is present, while the frequent occurrence of non-pathologic reflux results in false-positive results for GERD. Upper GI series provide high-resolution images that are important in excluding anatomic abnormalities that can produce symptoms of GERD (mainly vomiting). These abnormalities include pyloric stenosis, hiatal hernia, and malrotation. The study is also useful for assessing complications of GERD such as coarse mucosal changes due to esophagitis and esophageal strictures, in more severe cases. In contrast to gastroesophageal scintigraphy, upper GI series cannot be considered a physiologic test because of the usage of barium as a contrast agent and the occasional employment of provocative measures such as abdominal compression.

Endoscopy and Biopsy

Endoscopy with biopsy can evaluate the complications of gastroesophageal reflux in GERD such as esophagitis, strictures, and Barrett's esophagus and exclude other diseases with similar clinical symptoms such as eosinophilic or infectious esophagitis and Crohn's disease. Endoscopy alone is not sufficient because a normal-appearing esophagus does not exclude microscopic esophagitis. Subtle mucosal changes such as erythema and pallor may occur in the absence of esophagitis.[33] The technique is invasive and mostly used in the evaluation of GERD associated esophagitis.

Gastroesophageal Reflux Scintigraphy

Gastroesophageal reflux scintigraphy, also known as the "milk scan," is a radionuclide study for the detection of GER and pulmonary aspiration secondary to reflux. This section focuses on the detection of GER. The ability of this study to detect pulmonary aspiration is discussed later (see Pulmonary Aspiration).

A mixture of milk or milk formula with technetium-99m (^{99m}Tc)–sulfur colloid is introduced into the stomach by oral feeding, gastric tube, or gastrostomy tube. Gastroesophageal reflux episodes can be detected by showing abnormal tracer activity in the esophagus with dynamic scintigraphy of the upper abdomen and thorax over a 60-minute period (Fig. 7.1). Dynamic images are followed by anterior and posterior static images of the chest at 1 and 4 hours postfeeding. Twenty-four-hour images are occasionally obtained as well. The purpose of the static images is to detect abnormal tracer activity in the lungs, indicating pulmonary aspiration. They can demonstrate subtle aspiration that was not evident on the dynamic images and document aspiration that occurred after completion of the dynamic sequence. These images enhance the ability of the study to detect pulmonary aspiration.

There is no single universally accepted protocol for this study. Most techniques, however, share the same basic principles. The protocol for GER scintigraphy, used at Children's Hospital Boston, will be described as a general reference.

^{99m}Tc–sulfur colloid is the radiopharmaceutical of choice for the study because it is not absorbed from the gastrointestinal or pulmonary mucosa and remains stable in the acidic medium of the stomach. Such absorption would increase the background activity and lower the sensitivity of the study for detection of reflux and aspiration.[34] The dose is 0.55 MBq/kg (15 µCi/kg) with a minimum dose of 7.4 MBq (200 µCi) and a maximum dose of 37 MBq (1 mCi).

Older children should fast for at least 4 hours prior to the exam. Young infants should replace a normal scheduled feeding with the radioactive milk or formula. The radiopharmaceutical is added to a portion of the patient's feeding (one third or one half of the normal milk or formula feeding volume). This volume is introduced into the stomach by oral feeding or alternatively by nasogastric tube (which should be removed after feeding) or by gastrostomy tube when used for routine feedings. A second, tracer-free volume is then given to complete the meal. The tracer-free volume has an important role of clearing residual tracer from the oropharynx and esophagus prior to imaging. The volume of the feeding varies according to the patient's age and weight. In most cases the desired volume is similar to the volume the patient is given for regular meals. It is best to wait 48 hours after a barium study to avoid the possibility of inaccuracies in interpretation due the attenuating effect of residual barium in the upper GI tract.

The times of beginning and completing feeding should be recorded. After feeding, the

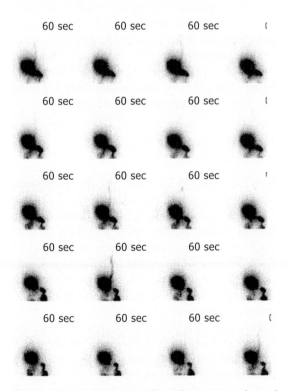

60 sec	60 sec	60 sec	(
60 sec	60 sec	60 sec	(
60 sec	60 sec	60 sec	(
60 sec	60 sec	60 sec	
60 sec	60 sec	60 sec	(

FIGURE 7.1. Several episodes of gastroesophageal reflux up to the proximal esophagus in a 15-year-old girl with recurrent vomiting and rumination.

patient is placed supine on the imaging bed. Young infants should be burped when possible prior to imaging. Restraints may be used to secure young children to the imaging bed and to prevent motion. Dynamic images are carried out from the posterior view with the stomach and chest in the field of view. A low-energy, high-resolution collimator is used, and images are recorded on a 128×128 matrix at a rate of 30 seconds/frame for 60 minutes. The dynamic images are followed by anterior and posterior static images of the chest with the stomach out of the field of view. These images are recorded on a 256×256 matrix over 3 to 5 minutes. A second set of static images is acquired 2 to 4 hours after completion of the meal. Delayed 24-hour images are optional.

Some technical aspects of the study warrant further elaboration. Care should be taken to avoid any form of external contamination due to spillage during feeding or due to vomiting or regurgitation. Contamination artifacts over the lung fields could be mistaken for pulmonary aspiration or prevent detection of such aspiration. Disposable, absorbent sheets, lined on one side with plastic material, may be used to contain contamination over the neck, chest, and upper abdomen during feeding and during imaging. Residual tracer in the mouth or esophagus at the beginning of imaging may limit the ability to detect GER. Using a sufficient volume of nonlabeled milk/formula to complete the meal prevents this problem in most cases.

In some centers imaging is performed with the camera in the anterior position. Anterior imaging has certain advantages. Depending on the camera and imaging table, a closer patient-to-collimator distance can be achieved with anterior imaging. In posterior imaging, counts originating from GER can be attenuated by the superimposed spine and the imaging table. Despite these considerations, we feel that posterior imaging is more practical and does not sacrifice, to any significant extent, the ability to detect reflux and aspiration. Infants and young children are often intimidated by the large camera detector positioned over their head and neck for extended periods and are less likely to lie still. In posterior imaging, with the camera head positioned under the imaging table, there is an unobstructed space over the imaging bed allowing easy communication with the children and access to caregivers. The children are more relaxed and can watch an overhead television.

It is important to perform the dynamic study over 60 minutes. Twenty-five percent of reflux episodes can be missed by limiting the study to 30 minutes.[35] The supine position was found to be more sensitive than the prone, left lateral, and 30-degree right posterior oblique positions for detection of GER.[36]

One study showed that placing the children in the upright position for a few seconds, in the middle of the examination, increased the frequency of GER episodes.[37] Recordings from pH probe monitoring show that reflux episodes may be very brief. Brief episodes of GER can be missed when using a frame time of 30 to 60 seconds during dynamic scintigraphy. Shortening the frame time to 5 to 10 seconds usually allows detection of brief episodes and provides a more accurate estimation of the total number of reflux episodes during the study. The study could later be reformatted to 30 or 60 seconds per frame for more convenient display.

The dosimetry for different ages is shown in Table 7.1.[38] The critical organ is the lower large bowel. The effective dose in this study is among the lowest for nuclear medicine scans.

Interpretation of Gastroesophageal Reflux Scintigraphy

New appearance of tracer in the esophagus indicates a reflux episode (Fig. 7.1). All recorded frames as well as the delayed static images should be inspected. It is best to read the images from a computer screen rather than from films or other forms of hard copy. Computer display allows interactive manipulation of the window as well as count truncation. These measures improve the detectability of subtle reflux episodes. Cinematic playback of the recorded frames is also helpful in detecting reflux and can easily identify patient movement that occurred during the study.

Placing markers over the suprasternal notch and over the xiphoid is helpful in determining the level of reflux in the esophagus or orophar-

TABLE 7.1. Radiation dosimetry

Site	Dose (rads/100 μCi), by age					
	Newborn	1 Year	5 Years	10 Years	15 Years	Adult
Stomach	0.383	0.093	0.0507	0.0308	0.0221	0.0187
SI	0.372	0.164	0.0911	0.0583	0.0361	0.0315
ULI	0.596	0.267	0.164	0.0896	0.0539	0.0518
LLI	0.972	0.380	0.194	0.120	0.0721	0.0329
Ovaries	0.0993	0.0420	0.033	0.0722	0.00149	0.0102
Testes	0.0176	0.00717	0.00334	0.0108	0.0011	0.00029
Thyroid	0.00164	0.00062	0.000215	0.00007	0.00003	0.00002
Whole body	0.0200	0.0107	0.00633	0.00407	0.00268	0.00186

Source: Castronovo,[38] with permission of the Society of Nuclear Medicine.
SI, small intestine; ULI, LLI, upper and lower large intestine.

ynx and in localizing tracer activity over the lung fields. Obtaining a transmission image of the chest, with a cobalt-57 flood source, and overlaying it on the emission image is another technique that can improve localization of tracer activity in the chest.

Interpretation can be enhanced by generating time activity curves from regions of interest (ROIs) placed over the esophagus. Reflux episodes are seen as a sharp spikes in the curves (Fig. 7.2). By placing one ROI over the entire esophagus and a second ROI over the upper esophagus and oropharynx, the proportion of severe reflux episodes from the total number of episodes can be established. Patient motion during the study can introduce significant artifacts in the curves because motion can cause the esophageal region to overlap gastric activity, simulating the appearance of reflux. Images should always be inspected for motion prior to interpretation, and motion correction should be applied when indicated.

Visual inspection of the images in conjunction with curve interpretation is the most

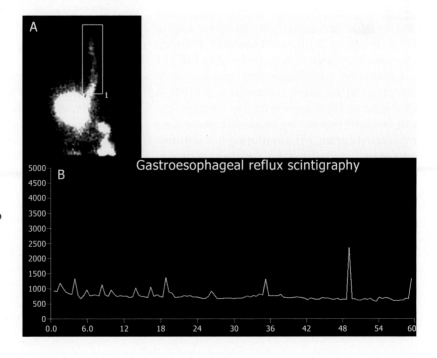

FIGURE 7.2. A region of interest over the entire esophagus (A) is used to generate a time activity curve (B) showing multiple sharp peaks corresponding to episodes of gastroesophageal reflux (same study as in Fig. 7.1).

accurate way to read the study. The number of reflux episodes, the level of reflux (lower esophagus, upper esophagus, pharynx), and the presence of pulmonary aspiration should be documented. Dividing the number of frames showing esophageal reflux by the total number of frames provides a simple index that can roughly estimate the residence time of reflux in the esophagus during the study.

Some authors use more elaborate techniques to quantify GER. These techniques take into account the volume of reflux in each episode, the frequency of reflux, and the rate at which it clears from the esophagus. Some indices normalize esophageal activity during reflux episodes to the initial gastric activity.[35,39,40]

Gastroesophageal reflux scintigraphy is a sensitive, noninvasive, physiologic, and direct technique to demonstrate the presence of GER. It is easy to perform, is well tolerated, and requires minimum patient cooperation. It also entails a relatively low radiation burden. The study can be quantified for better intersubject comparison and for monitoring response to therapy.[41] Additional advantages of GER scintigraphy in comparison to pH monitoring and endoscopy include the ability to detect pulmonary aspiration and to evaluate gastric emptying in the same study. Scintigraphy is considered by many authors to be a safe and reliable screening test for detection of GER. It cannot distinguish, however, between physiologic reflux and reflux related to GERD.

Comparing sensitivities and specificities of the different studies for detection of GER is problematic. Techniques are often compared to extended pH monitoring as a gold standard. As mentioned earlier, pH monitoring is a sensitive and specific study for indirect detection of acid reflux, but not all symptomatic reflux episodes are acidic. Lack of uniform protocols for the various techniques is another confounding factor. Clinical signs and symptoms of GERD are used in some studies to evaluate the sensitivity and specificity of diagnostic methods. This approach is problematic because of significant overlap between signs and symptoms of GERD and those of other conditions.

According to most studies, the sensitivity of gastroesophageal scintigraphy for detection of

GER in comparison to pH monitoring ranges from 60% to 90%.[39,42-48] Specificity is over 90%.[44,47] In a few studies that performed simultaneous esophageal pH monitoring and scintigraphy for 1 to 2 hours, no correlation was found between the total number of reflux episodes detected by scintigraphy and pH monitoring. Scintigraphy, however, detected more reflux episodes than pH monitoring.[49,50] It was concluded that the two tests measure different pathophysiologic phenomena and should be regarded as complementary. Used together they could enhance the sensitivity and specificity of the diagnostic evaluation.[51] The agreement between scintigraphy and esophageal pH monitoring depends to some extent on the acquisition and display parameters used for scintigraphy. The best correlation was achieved when images were reformatted in 60-second frames.[52]

Most authors found gastroesophageal scintigraphy to be more sensitive than barium radiography for the detection of GER.[39,42,45,48,53] The inherent sensitivity of the scintigraphy for detection of small amounts of radioactivity in the esophagus and the longer observation period compared to barium radiography may account for these differences. A combination of diagnostic modalities may be required to diagnose GER in young children.

Treatment

According to the guidelines of the North American Society for Pediatric Gastroenterology and Nutrition, treatment options include the following categories: dietary changes, positioning, life changes in children and adolescents, acid suppressant therapy, prokinetic therapy, and surgical therapy.[26]

Milk and formula thickening agents may decrease the number of vomiting episodes in infants but do not improve the reflux index score on pH monitoring. A trial of hypoallergenic formula in formula-fed infants may reduce vomiting. Twenty-four-hour pH monitoring documented a lower prevalence of GER in the prone versus the supine position. This treatment option, however, is not recommended for most infants under 1 year of age because of the increased risk for sudden infant death in the prone position compared to the supine position. Left-side positioning and elevation of the bed head is probably beneficial for children older than 1 year of age. Lifestyle changes in older children and adolescents include recommendations to avoid caffeine, chocolate, spicy foods, tobacco, and alcohol, and to treat obesity. Acid suppressant therapy is based on histamine-2 receptor antagonists (H2RAs) and on proton pump inhibitors (PPIs). Proton pump inhibitors are more effective in relieving symptoms than H2RAs. Chronic antacid therapy is not indicated because of potential side effects related to increased absorption of aluminum and the presence of better alternatives (H2RAs and PPIs). Prokinetic therapy affects the LES tone, esophageal motility, and gastric emptying. Domperidone and metoclopramide have questionable efficiency and may have adverse effects on the central nervous system. Cisapride, a mixed serotoninergic agent, is more efficient and reduces the frequency of symptoms including vomiting and regurgitation. This drug can cause cardiac arrhythmias, however, and requires proper dosing and proper patient selection and monitoring. Surgical therapy consists of antireflux surgery. The most common surgery is fundoplication. It is indicated when medical therapy fails and in severe life-threatening conditions related to GERD. Surgery should be avoided, if possible, before 2 years of age.[1]

Gastric Emptying

Physiology

The stomach can be divided into three functional regions: proximal stomach (cardia, fundus, and proximal body), distal stomach (distal body, antrum), and the pylorus. The proximal stomach stores and accommodates food. It delivers food to the distal stomach by tonic propulsion. Smooth muscles of the proximal stomach do not exhibit rhythmic or peristaltic contractions but are rather in a state of continual partial contraction. The motor func-

tion of the proximal stomach is to regulate intragastric pressure. This is achieved by receptive relaxation (a reduction in gastric tone in response to swallowing mediated by a vagovagal reflex) and gastric accommodation (a neural mediated reflex triggered by mechanoreceptors in the gastric wall in response to gastric distention). Even large volumes entering the stomach do not cause significant increases in intragastric pressure due to these mechanisms.[41] Receptive relaxation is absent in newborns, which partly explains why GER is more common in newborns than in older infants.[54]

Motor activity of the distal stomach is characterized by peristaltic contractions in response to rhythmic depolarization in muscle cells known as the pacesetter potential. This electrical activity originates from the interstitial cells of Cajal, a network of specialized cells extending from the corpus to the distal antrum.[55] The gastric pacesetter potential has a baseline frequency of three cycles per minute. The motor function of the distal stomach is to mix, grind, and triturate solid food and to propagate the chyme toward the pylorus. Chyme is formed by contact of solids with gastric juices and digestive enzymes. The antropyloric region prevents emptying of particles greater than 1 mm in diameter. Larger particles are repelled back, triturated, and eventually emptied with the liquid phase. During trituration no significant emptying of solids occurs, giving rise to the lag phase that is commonly seen in solid gastric emptying time activity curves.[56] The lag phase is usually absent with emptying of milk. The pylorus regulates the outflow of intraluminal gastric contents. The thickness of the smooth muscle layers and the abundant pyloric mucosa form a mechanical stricture preventing passage of large particles into the duodenum.[41] In general, tonic pressure in the proximal stomach is the main mechanism that regulates emptying of liquids, and the peristaltic motor activity of the distal stomach is the main mechanism that regulates emptying of solids.

Coordinated gastric motor activity in the different functional zones is the end result of complex muscular, neural, and hormonal interactions and is also affected by feedback regulation from the small bowel. Neural regulation of gastric motor activity is largely mediated through the vagus nerve. Gastric emptying rate is influenced by multiple factors. Gastrointestinal hormones such as cholecystokinin, secretin, gastrin, and gastric inhibitory peptide delay gastric emptying. Liquids empty faster than solids.[56] Gastric emptying is delayed by high caloric and high osmolarity meals. High osmolarity delays emptying in adults but was shown to have a smaller influence on emptying rates in premature infants and newborns.[57] Large meals prolong emptying. This is probably due more to the high caloric content of large meals than to the meal size.[58,59] Varying rates of emptying are encountered with different kinds of milk and milk formulas. Human milk empties faster than cow's milk, although both are isocaloric.[60] Whey-based formulas empty more rapidly than casein-based formulas despite similarities in caloric content, osmolarity, and fat content. Acidified milk, however, was found to empty more rapidly.[61] The variability in the emptying rate of different kinds of milk and milk formulas may be related to the formation of solids in the stomach by milk and formulas during digestion. Fatty acids of specific carbon chain lengths, acid solutions, and physiologic concentrations of L-tryptophan have been shown to delay gastric emptying.[62,63] In addition to these factors, gastric emptying in children is influenced by the child's age. Longer emptying times were observed in infants.[64,65] Gastric surgery such as antrectomy and pyloroplasty and prokinetic drugs such as metoclopramide and domperidone shorten the lag phase and can increase gastric emptying rates.[41]

Clinical Manifestations of Abnormal Gastric Emptying

Nausea, vomiting, abdominal discomfort, constipation, and early satiety with long intervals between meals are common clinical manifestations of delayed gastric emptying in children. These manifestations, however, are not specific and can be encountered in many other conditions such as anatomic obstructions (congenital and acquired), GERD, hepatobiliary disease, peptic ulcer, drug effects, infection, etc. Symptoms of delayed gastric emptying may be seen in systemic diseases (e.g., malignancies, dia-

betes) and during drug therapy. Gastric neuromuscular disorders such as visceral hypersensitivity, gastric dysrhythmias, gastric dysrelaxation, antral hypomotility, pylorospasm, and gastroparesis are more often encountered in adults. These conditions manifest as dyspeptic symptoms with early satiety, fullness, gastric discomfort, bloating, nausea, and vomiting, but could also present with ulcer-like symptoms, mainly epigastric pain.[66] Rapid gastric emptying is less frequently encountered and can manifest with signs and symptoms of "dumping" and as diarrhea.[56]

Diagnostic Evaluation of Gastric Emptying

Meaningful quantification of gastric emptying requires standardization of study techniques and standardization of the test meal. Standardization is essential for inter- and intrasubject comparisons.

Gastric emptying scintigraphy is the most widely accepted technique in clinical practice and it is regarded as the gold standard. Non-scintigraphic techniques will be reviewed first, followed by a detailed description of gastric emptying scintigraphy.

Upper GI series with barium contrast provide fine anatomic details and are important for excluding anatomic conditions that can alter gastric emptying such as pyloric stenosis or antral web. Otherwise, the emptying rate of a nonphysiologic substance such as barium does not reflect gastric emptying under native, physiologic conditions.

Gastric ultrasonography can evaluate gastric volume, emptying, and transpyloric flow. It can assess gastric contraction and distention and measure the antral cross-sectional area.[67–69] A high correlation was encountered between ultrasonographic gastric emptying parameters and scintigraphic techniques.[70] Ultrasonography was useful for the detection of motor abnormalities in children with dyspeptic symptoms.[71] Ultrasonography has the advantages of being a widely available, low cost, and a nonradioactive technique. The main limitations of this technique are a short observation period and dependency on operator skills, explaining its limited use in clinical practice.

Electrogastrography measures myoelectrical activity in the gastric antrum during the fasting and postprandial states.[41] Surface recording is usually employed, using cutaneous electrodes placed over the epigastrium.[72] The normal gastric pacesetter potential range is between 2.5 and 3.75 cycles per minute (cpm). This technique can detect bradygastria (<2.5 cpm) or tachygastria (3.75 to 10 cpm). Gastric dysrhythmias have been associated with certain conditions such as diabetes, idiopathic gastric paresis, and motion sickness.[72] This technique, mostly utilized in adults, is not widely available in clinical practice.

Breath tests provide a simple, noninvasive, and nonradioactive technique to evaluate gastric emptying. Most tests today are based on measuring the concentration of the stable isotope carbon-13 (^{13}C) in expired air. ^{13}C-labeled octanoic acid is used as a substrate for solid gastric emptying evaluation and ^{13}C-labeled acetate for liquid emptying. Both substrates are absorbed in the duodenum and transported to the liver. Metabolic degradation in the liver produces $^{13}CO_2$ that is excreted with exhaled air and measured with a mass spectrometer. Breath samples are measured for enrichment with ^{13}C up to 6 hours. The first appearance of $^{13}CO_2$ indicates the beginning of emptying. The slope of the rising time-related ^{13}C enrichment curve is related to the gastric emptying rate.[73,74] Simultaneous performance of gastric emptying scintigraphy with a ^{13}C breath test in 29 children with dyspeptic and respiratory symptoms showed good correlation between the techniques in assessment of gastric emptying times.[75] The reliability of the breath test to accurately reflect gastric emptying can be adversely affected by certain conditions such as malabsorption, pancreatic, liver and lung diseases, and by visceral hemodynamic changes (physical exercise) that can alter the delivery of ^{13}C to the sampled breath air, irrespective of the gastric emptying rate.

Gastric Emptying Scintigraphy

Gastric emptying scintigraphy is a physiologic, noninvasive, low-cost technique to evaluate gastric emptying based on imaging and quantification of a radiolabeled test meal. Several techniques are used in clinical practice for gastric emptying. The techniques vary in the meal content, volume, and imaging technique. The lack of uniformity adversely affects interinstitutional comparison of study results.

Different mechanisms regulate gastric emptying of solids and liquids. A solid test meal is considered more reliable than a liquid meal for measuring gastric emptying. Solid meals are used in adults.[41] In the pediatric population, they are reserved for older children and adolescents. The diet of infants is milk or milk formulas, which makes them the natural and only practical choice for a test meal. This is in keeping with the physiologic nature of the study. Milk or formula is often used in young children too because it is more acceptable to them than standardized solid meals. As mentioned earlier, milk and milk formulas form solids in the stomach due to interactions with digestive enzymes and gastric acid. Their clearance does not truly represent liquid gastric emptying.

Gastric emptying evaluation with milk or formula is often performed simultaneously with evaluation of GER. We use similar preparations and acquisition parameters to those used for gastroesophageal scintigraphy (milk scan). The radiopharmaceutical of choice is ^{99m}Tc–sulfur colloid because it remains stable in an acid medium and is not absorbed from the gastrointestinal mucosa. The dose is 0.55 MBq/kg (15 µCi/kg) with a minimum of 7.4 MBq (200 µCi) and a maximum of 37 MBq (1 mCi). Preparations for the study include fasting for at least 4 hours prior to the test. Young infants should miss a normal feeding just prior to the exam. Medications that affect gastric motility should be discontinued for an appropriate period prior to the exam, depending on the pharmacokinetics of the drugs, unless the scintigraphy is used to evaluate the effect of specific drugs on gastric motility. These drugs include prokinetics, narcotic analgesics, anticholinergic agents, antidepressants, gastric acid suppressants, aluminum-containing antacids, somatostatin, and calcium channel blockers.[41] Barium radiography should not be performed within 48 hours prior to scintigraphy. The volume of the meal is adjusted according to the patient's age or size. For standardization purposes, the feeding period is limited to 10 minutes. The referring physician should indicate the volume of the meal expected to be consumed within this timeframe. The radiopharmaceutical is added to the meal and a second, tracer-free volume is added to complete the desired feeding volume. Oral feeding is preferred, but feeding through a nasogastric tube or gastrostomy tubes is occasionally required. Nasogastric tubes should be removed immediately after feeding. The volume and composition of the meal are recorded for future reference.

After completion of the feeding, the patient is placed in the supine position and continuous dynamic images of the stomach and chest are recorded on a 128 × 128 matrix, 30 seconds per frame for 60 minutes. Images are obtained in the posterior projection using a low-energy, high-resolution collimator. Static images of the abdomen and chest are acquired using a 256 × 256 matrix at 60 minutes. If emptying is delayed, additional images are obtained at 2 hours. Static images of the lung fields are also obtained at 4 hours and occasionally at 24 hours for the detection of late aspiration.

A region of interest (ROI) is placed around the stomach, as seen in the immediate post-feeding image. A time activity curve, corrected for decay, is generated from the stomach ROI. Motion correction should be applied when required. Care should be taken not to include bowel activity in the gastric ROI. An additional gastric ROI derived from the last image is often required for accurate generation of the time activity curve. Another option is to generate separate regions over the stomach every 10 or 15 minutes. Gastric emptying can be expressed as the percentage of the initial activity remaining at a specific time point (residual) or as the activity emptied by the stomach at these times. It can also be expressed as the half emptying time ($t_{1/2}$). We use the 60-minute time point for calculation of the gastric residual; $t_{1/2}$ is more commonly used in adults with solid gastric emptying. The pattern of the emptying curve, including the presence and length of the lag phase (seen in solid gastric emptying), is important because it may provide evidence on abnormalities in gastric motility. Milk usually empties

in an exponential or biexponential manner. A long plateau on the time activity curve may be encountered in intermittent gastric outlet obstruction due to an antral web.

Some features of the protocol are subject to variability and warrant further discussion. The study length is not well standardized. The gastric emptying rate may increase during the second hour postfeeding. In a study that evaluated gastric emptying of a liquid meal for 2 hours in infants and children, the 1-hour measurements did not predict well the 2-hour measurements. It was concluded that gastric emptying measurements in children should be continued until 2 hours after feeding unless rapid emptying is observed during the first hour of the study.[76,77] Extending dynamic acquisition for 2 hours may be difficult to achieve in young children. Serial delayed static images can be used instead. The supine position is best suited for extended imaging in infants and children but can delay gastric emptying. In one study a significant number of children, 1 week to 2 years old, with delayed emptying in the supine position showed significant emptying just by changing position. It was recommended to complement gastric emptying studies with delayed views in the right lateral and upright position.[78]

Physiologic movement of gastric contents from the posteriorly located fundus to the more anteriorly located antrum can produce artifacts in quantitation due to nonuniform attenuation throughout the study. Using a geometrical mean of anterior and posterior counts, acquired simultaneously with a dual detector camera, will correct this problem. It is also possible to use the left anterior oblique projection instead of anterior or posterior projections to minimize this artifact. Nonuniform attenuation mostly pertains to adults and to large and obese older children. Conjugate counting did not significantly change the results compared with anterior imaging alone in a study that evaluated gastric emptying with milk feedings in infants and young children. It was suggested that anterior imaging alone is sufficient in this patient population.[79] We prefer the posterior imaging, which is much more comfortable for the patient. Continuous data recording rather than serial static images is recommended and well suited for small children, who occasionally need to be restrained. Recording data only at discrete time intervals (e.g., every 10 to 30 minutes) is incapable of providing information on the lag phase and may be limited in identifying patterns of rapid gastric emptying.[80]

Occasionally, significant emptying occurs during the feeding period. This emptying is not accounted for when the gastric residual is derived from a region of interest placed over the stomach in the immediate postfeeding image. Calculation of the gastric residual relative to the total dose ingested by the patient can be achieved by comparing the activity in the stomach in the final image to the activity in a ROI that includes the stomach and bowel as seen in the immediate postfeeding image. This value takes into account both the emptying that occurred during imaging and the emptying that occurred before imaging (during feeding). The two methods for calculation of the gastric residual were compared in a study that included 44 children who underwent liquid ^{99m}Tc–sulfur colloid gastric emptying. Sixty-minute gastric residuals from the total ingested dose were significantly lower by 15% to 16% from gastric residuals derived only from the initial stomach activity in the first postfeeding image. It was concluded that emptying that occurs during feeding should be factored into quantitation of liquid gastric emptying in infants and young children to avoid overestimation of gastric residuals and erroneous interpretations of delayed gastric emptying.[81]

A major problem with gastric emptying scintigraphy in children is the lack of age-related normal values derived from large groups of normal controls. Normal children cannot be studied as control subjects due to ethical considerations. Pooling data from different institutions to establish the normal range is problematic due to lack of standardization of the study technique and the test meal. Given these limitations, it is best for individual laboratories to establish their own normal range. The few reports concerning normal values that were published in the literature should serve as a guide. In one study, normal infants were fed with 50 mL milk labeled with indium-111 (^{111}In)

microcolloid. The gastric emptying time activity curve was found to be exponential, and the $t_{1/2}$ was 87 ± 29 minutes. The 1-hour normal gastric residuals extrapolated from these data were 48% to 70%.[82] In another study, normal emptying residuals for young children ranged between 36% and 68% at 1 hour with a sulfur colloid–labeled milk/formula. In a small number of older children, the range was between 42% and 56%.[83] The normal range for liquid gastric emptying residuals with ^{99m}Tc–sulfur colloid–labeled dextrose at 1 hour, in children less than 2 years of age, was 27% to 81% and in children 2 years of age or over, it was 11% to 47%.[64] An example of delayed gastric emptying is shown in (Fig. 7.3).

Gastric emptying with a solid test meal is the preferred method to assess gastric emptying in older children, adolescents, and adults. It is important that the radioactive label remains firmly attached to the solid phase. The best stability is achieved with in vivo labeling of chicken liver using ^{99m}Tc–sulfur colloid[84] (98% bound at 3 hours in gastric juice). This method requires injecting the label into the chicken, harvesting the liver, and cooking the liver. It is therefore impractical for routine clinical use. A stable label can be achieved by mixing and cooking ^{99m}Tc–sulfur colloid with a whole egg (82% bound at 3 hours) or with the egg white (95% bound at 3 hours).[84] A stable label can also be obtained with fat-free egg substitutes. Basing the test meal on radiolabeled eggs is convenient and widely used in clinical practice. Less common alternatives include ^{99m}Tc-labeled bran,[85] pudding,[65] or iodinated fiber.[86] These alternatives may be useful in cases of allergy to eggs. Because liquids affect the emptying of solids, it is common to include unlabeled liquids in the test meal. A suggested test meal includes two eggs as a sandwich and 300 mL of water for a body surface area of 1.73m^2 scaled to the patient's size.[56]

Simultaneous assessment of solid and liquid emptying can be achieved by labeling the solids with ^{99m}Tc–sulfur colloid and the liquid (water) with ^{111}In. Maintaining a ratio of at least 6:1 between the ^{99m}Tc and ^{111}In activities can minimize down-scatter from ^{111}In into the ^{99m}Tc window. A suitable pediatric dose for this dual

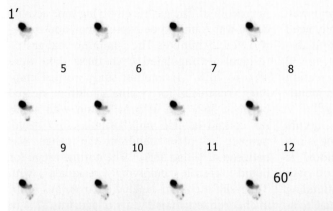

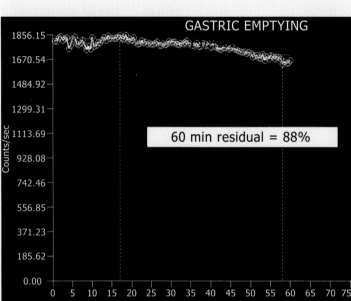

FIGURE 7.3. Delayed gastric emptying in a 2-year-old boy with suspected metabolic disease, hypotonia, psychomotor retardation, and recurrent vomiting. Posterior view images, displayed at 5 minutes per frame, show considerable retention of labeled formula in the stomach. The 60-minute gastric residual calculated from the time activity curve was 88%.

isotope study is 11.1 MBq (300 μCi) for ^{99m}Tc and 1.85 MBq (50 μCi) for ^{111}In.[56] Preparations for solid gastric emptying are similar to those described for liquid emptying. Imaging length should be at least 2 hours. Continuous dynamic imaging can be used. A protocol consisting of 30-second images, acquired in the supine position every 10 minutes for 2 hours, and keeping the patient upright between images can also be used. A gastric emptying time activity curve is constructed from the decay corrected counts in each frame.

The range of normal values for solid gastric emptying in children has not been established. In a small series of 11 normal control children, 5 to 11 years old, solid gastric emptying values corresponded well to those described in adults.[87] Using the anterior imaging projection, normal control values in young adult volunteers can be used as a guide. These values expressed as gastric residuals are 60% to 82% at 1 hour and 25% to 55% at 2 hours.[88]

New Scintigraphic Techniques

Dynamic antral scintigraphy provides information on gastric motility and can be performed in conjunction with standard gastric emptying scintigraphy. A short (4- to 5-minute) dynamic acquisition with 1- to 2-second frames is added at the end of a standard gastric emptying study. Time activity curves are generated from ROIs placed over the proximal, middle, and distal antral areas. The data are corrected for motion artifacts and for translational movement of the stomach. Finally, a refined Fourier transform is performed on the time activity curves to determine the frequency and amplitude of antral contractions. This technique has been investigated in adults.[89–91] The amplitude rather than the baseline frequency of antral contractions (three per minute) was more useful in discriminating various patient groups. Decreased amplitudes have been noted in diabetic patients[91] and increased amplitudes in patients with functional dyspepsia.[92]

Gastric single photon emission computed tomography (SPECT) is a new scintigraphic technique to evaluate gastric accommodation. Impaired postprandial gastric accommodation is responsible for symptoms of bloating, distention, early satiety, and nausea. Abnormal accommodation can be detected with a barostatically controlled balloon in the proximal stomach and by ultrasonography in the distal stomach. The intragastric barostat balloon study is considered the gold standard for measurements of gastric volumes. Gastric SPECT allows evaluation of the entire gastric accommodation reflex by measuring fasting and postprandial gastric volumes. Following an overnight fast, ^{99m}Tc is injected intravenously and localizes in parietal and mucous cells in the gastric mucosa. Sequential gastric SPECTs are performed starting 10 minutes after injection in the fasting state and after ingestion of a test meal without changing the patient's position. Dynamic tomographic acquisition (6-degree steps, 3 seconds per frame 128×128 matrix) has been used for gastric SPECT. Total gastric volumes are measured from the SPECT data with specialized software during the fasting state and in the postprandial state (3 to 12 minutes and 12 to 21 minutes after completion of the meal).[93] Gastric SPECT has been investigated in adults and showed good correlation with invasive barostat balloon studies in determining gastric volumes.[94] Impaired accommodation was found in idiopathic dyspepsia and after fundoplication.[93,95] Simultaneous measurement of gastric emptying and accommodation was reported with dual isotope acquisition (^{111}In for solid or liquid emptying and ^{99m}Tc for accommodation).[96]

Esophageal Transit

Anatomy and Physiology of the Esophagus

The esophagus is a conduit that delivers food from the oropharynx to the stomach with coordinated muscular peristalsis aided by gravity. It begins in the neck, at the lower border of the cricoid cartilage, extends through the diaphragm, and ends at the cardia of the stomach. Circular muscle fibers form sphincters at both ends of the esophagus. The upper esophageal sphincter prevents regurgitation of food from the esophagus back into the oropharynx. The lower esophageal sphincter (LES) controls transit of food from the esophagus into the stomach and prevents retrograde reflux of food from the stomach into the esophagus. The primary peristaltic pump originates in the pharynx and produces signals that propagate through the circular and longitudinal muscles of the esophagus at about 4cm/sec.[41] Esophageal peristalsis is coordinated with the post-swallowing relaxation of the lower esophageal sphincter.[97] The striated muscles of the esophagus are innervated through the vagus and the smooth muscles through sympathetic and parasympathetic nerves.

Esophageal Transit Disorders

Esophageal motor disorders can be primary (e.g., achalasia—failure of relaxation of the LES and loss of esophageal body peristalsis) or secondary to other conditions (e.g., esophagitis, surgery). The occurrence and severity of esophagitis depends on both the severity and the frequency of GER and on esophageal motility. Abnormal clearance of the refluxate contributes to the pathogenesis of esophagitis and can result from decreased amplitude of distal esophageal peristaltic contractions and from an increased frequency of nonperistaltic contractions.

Functional esophageal disorders are determined on the basis of the lack of any identifiable structural or metabolic damage. They are mostly encountered in adults but may also be seen in children and adolescents. They include conditions such as rumination syndrome, globus (sensation of a lump stuck in the throat), functional dysphagia, and functional chest pain.[98] Functional esophageal disorders, in adults, are the second most common functional disorder of the GI tract after irritable bowel syndrome and are sometimes accompanied by psychological and psychiatric disorders.[98,99]

In children and adolescents, esophageal motility disorders are encountered with tracheoesophageal fistula, esophagitis, esophageal strictures, psychomotor retardation, cerebral palsy, and Down syndrome.[100–103] Prolonged esophageal transit was noted in children with familial dysautonomia.[104] Impaired esophageal motility in children is seen following injury to the esophagus from ingestion of caustic materials[105] and following repair of esophageal atresia.[106] Common clinical presentations of esophageal disorders include dysphagia and chest pain.

Evaluation of Esophageal Transit

Nonscintigraphic Techniques

Esophageal endoscopy is the mainstay of the diagnostic procedures for esophageal disorders. It allows direct visualization of the esophageal mucosa and performance of tissue biopsies. Esophagitis, esophageal metaplasia, esophageal diverticula, and fistulas are often evaluated with this technique. Endoscopy is usually extended to evaluate the stomach and duodenum too. It is the first-line diagnostic procedure for patients with complaints of dysphagia or dyspepsia. Endoscopy is an invasive procedure that is not well tolerated by some patients and requires anesthesia in children. It doesn't provide direct information on motility disorders.[41]

Upper GI series with barium contrast provide imaging evaluation of the esophagus stomach and duodenum. The study is commonly used in the diagnosis of esophageal disorders. An upper GI series is useful for the diagnosis of intrinsic or extrinsic anatomic obstructions (e.g., strictures or pressure from mediastinal space-occupying lesions), esophageal fistulas, and diverticula, and can also suggest mucosal changes encountered in esophagitis. It also allows dynamic evaluation of esophageal motility and transit of barium boluses from the mouth to the stomach. The radiation dose during video fluoroscopy is prohibitive. Although noninvasive, the study requires cooperation. Some children refuse to swallow the barium contrast. It is also limited in providing functional data for evaluation of certain motor disorders.

Esophageal manometry is indicated in patients with dysphagia unrelated to structural abnormalities. Manometry provides dynamic pressure measurements that are useful in the diagnosis of primary motor disorders such as achalasia, diffuse esophageal spasm, nutcracker esophagus, and hypertensive LES. It can demonstrate esophageal disorders secondary to systemic diseases such as scleroderma and dermatomyositis.[41] Multichannel intraluminal impedance is a new technique that allows evaluation of bolus movement in the esophagus. The technique was described in the section on GER. When combined with esophageal manometry, simultaneous information on esophageal pressure and bolus movement is recorded. This information is helpful in the diagnosis of motility disorders.

Esophageal Transit Scintigraphy

The study was first introduced in the early 1970s by Kazem[107] and has been adapted for use in children.[108,109] Esophageal transit scintigraphy provides imaging and quantitative data on the transit of a labeled bolus through the esophagus. There are several protocols for the study. The one used at Children's Hospital Boston will be described as a general guide.

Study Protocol

Preparations. Four-hour fasting is recommended for most cases. In infants the study should replace a normal scheduled feeding.

Radiopharmaceutical. ^{99m}Tc–sulfur colloid is mixed with 30 mL of liquid (milk, formula, or

5% dextrose water). The dose range is 7.4 to 37 MBq (200 μCi to 1 mCi). Larger volumes may be used for older patients. Labeled semisolids and solids are used infrequently.

Study Technique. Infants can lie directly on the slightly inclined collimator or be supported on a secured apparatus. Older children can sit up with their back to the collimator. It is important to turn the head of bottle-fed infants to the side to prevent superimposition of the radioactivity in the bottle over the upper esophagus. Older children can be fed with a cup or, preferably, through a straw. Imaging begins at the onset of swallowing. The camera is equipped with a low-energy, high-resolution collimator. Images are recorded on a 128×128 matrix, 2 seconds per frame for 100 seconds. Static images are taken after completion of the dynamic sequence. If a large residual remains in the esophagus, delayed static images are obtained at 30 and 60 minutes. A ^{57}Co transmission image may be taken immediately or at 10 minutes following completion of the dynamic sequence, when the anatomic location (e.g., gastric fundus vs. esophagus) of the tracer is uncertain.

Image Processing and Interpretation

Recorded images are played back in cine mode for visual evaluation of the bolus transit. Oral or pharyngeal retention, esophageal retention, bolus fragmentation, premature swallows (resulting in deglutition inhibition), tracheobronchial aspiration, and GER can be identified by visual inspection. Slow progression or even stopping of the bolus with the craniocaudal direction maintained can be seen in scleroderma and achalasia. Presenting the dynamic data in a single image can enhance visual inspection. The condensed dynamic image shows the profiles of the swallowing event side by side on the y-axis along with time on the x-axis.[110] The condensed image may aid identification of abnormal motility patterns.

Esophageal transit can be measured quantitatively with time and retention parameters. The esophagus is divided into upper, middle, and lower zones. Equal ROIs are placed on each zone, and a fourth ROI is placed over the stomach. Time activity curves are generated from each ROI. The curves allow qualitative and quantitative assessment of the bolus transit. The data from the three zones can be summed for a total esophageal measurement. Normal transit (Fig. 7.4) presents as a sharp peak in the upper esophageal zone followed by sequential sharp peaks in the middle and lower zone and early buildup of activity in the stomach. Deviation from this pattern can suggest esophageal dysmotility (Fig. 7.5). Multiple peaks in the three esophageal time activity curves can be seen in diffuse esophageal spasm. Esophageal transit time (for a single swallow) is defined as the time from initial entry of activity into the esophagus to the time activity drops to less than 10% from the peak. Esophageal transit time is affected by the patient's position and the consistency of the test meal. In adults, transit time for liquids was less than 5 second in the erect position and approximately 8 seconds in the supine position.[111] More complex parameters such as mean transit time, mean time, and retention parameters such as esophageal emptying (10 or 12 seconds after swallowing) as a fraction of the peak activity have been used, mostly in adults.[112–114] Normal quantitative parameters require standardization of techniques and processing algorithms. Such parameters have not been established in children. Characteristic dysmotility patterns can be elicited with esophageal scintigraphy studies in nutcracker esophagus (high amplitude waves in the lower esophagus), diffuse esophageal spasm (multiple simultaneous contractions at different levels induced by wet swallows), scleroderma (retention in the lower esophagus in the supine position that clears after the patient is upright), and achalasia (significant retention in the lower esophagus in the absence of anatomic obstruction that does not clear in the upright position or following a drink of water).[41]

Some aspects of esophageal transit scintigraphy warrant further elaboration. ^{99m}Tc–sulfur colloid is the most commonly used radiopharmaceutical. ^{99m}Tc-nanocolloid and ^{99m}Tc–diethylenetriaminepentaacetic acid (DTPA) have been used too. Radiopharmaceuticals used in transit scintigraphy should not be absorbed by the gastrointestinal mucosa.

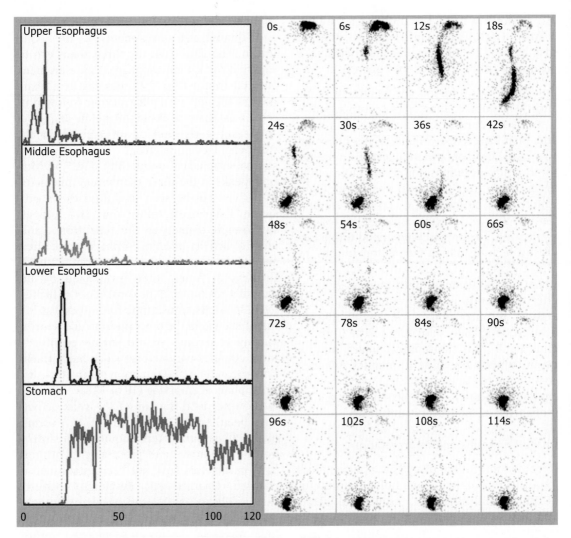

FIGURE 7.4. Normal esophageal motility study. Note the sequential coordinated peaks of the time activity curves derived from the upper, middle and lower esophagus and the complete clearance of activity from the esophagus at the end of the dynamic sequence.

Esophageal transit scintigraphy has also been performed with krypton 81m (^{81m}Kr)-labeled glucose. Glucose 5% in water is infused through a rubidium-81/krypton-81m generator producing several millicuries of ^{81m}Kr solution. In children the solution is delivered into the mouth by syringe.[111] This technique is easy to perform and provides a quantitative assessment of esophageal transit under physiologic conditions. The radiation dose to the patient from ^{81m}Kr is very low compared with other isotopes. High doses can be given to ensure good-quality images, and the study can be repeated as often as necessary. ^{81}Rb/^{81m}Kr generators are not widely available and are more expensive than ^{99m}Tc-based radiopharmaceuticals, which limits the availability of this technique for routine clinical practice.

The patient's position during the study can affect results due to the effect of gravity. Performing the study with the patient in an upright position appears to be more physiologic. Eliminating the force of gravity, however, by performing the study with the patient in the supine position may be more efficient in exposing motility disorders.[115] In infants and young children, the supine or semirecumbent positions are more practical. Most esophageal studies employ a labeled liquid meal. A semisolid bolus requires more intense peristalsis to complete the transport over the distal half of the esophagus[116] and can increase the sensitivity of the test. There is no consensus on the desired viscosity and type of the semisolid. Solids such as radiolabeled gelatin capsules or labeled chicken liver cubes have been used but can remain in the esophagus up to 2 hours even in normal individuals.[117,118] The volume of a liquid bolus may also affect transit rate. Ten-milliliter boluses were shown to travel faster than 20-mL boluses in the upright but not in the supine position.[111] It is obviously difficult to

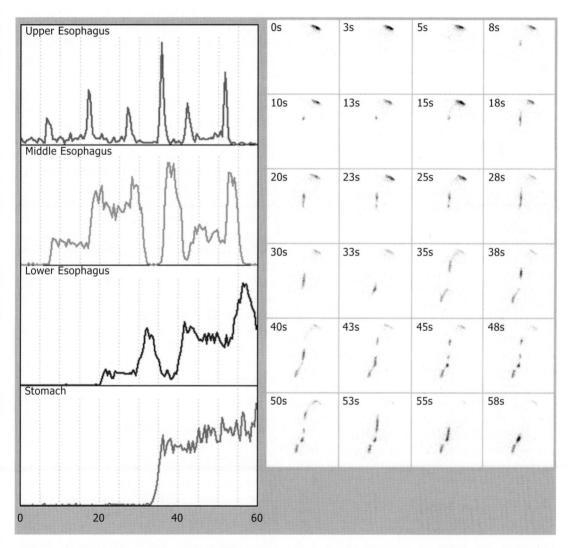

FIGURE 7.5. An esophageal transit study of a young woman with history of renal transplantation and fundoplication surgery for gastroesophageal reflux. The woman presented with complaints of dysphagia and heartburn. Time activity curves obtained from regions of interest placed over the upper, middle, and lower esophagus show multiple uncoordinated spikes and some tracer accumulation in the distal esophagus that clears away on a delayed 10-minute image (not shown). These findings suggest esophageal dysmotility.

control the volume of the swallowed bolus in children and infants. The number and type of swallows is subject to variability. According to one approach, one wet swallow followed by three dry swallows is sufficient for estimation of esophageal residual fraction.[112] According to another approach, the patient is required to perform six independent, wet swallows 30 seconds apart; a summed image of the six swallows is used to analyze time and retention parameters.[114] The number and frequency of swallows in infants and young children in a given timeframe is hard to control.

The sensitivity and specificity of esophageal transit scintigraphy are hard to establish given the lack of technique standardization. They may also differ for different esophageal disorders. Some studies reported sensitivities and specificities of up to 95% and 96%, respectively, compared with the gold standard of esophageal manometry.[114,119] Other studies found esophageal scintigraphy to be more sensitive than esophageal manometry or barium radiography.[120,121] Dosimetry of esophageal transit scintigraphy was calculated for children assuming an ingested dose of 7.4 to 18.5 MBq (200 to 500 μCi). The critical organ was the proximal small bowel. In neonates the proximal small bowel received a dose of 2 to 3 mSv (200 to 300 mrem), and the total body dose was 0.30 mSv (30 mrem).[108]

In summary, esophageal transit scintigraphy is a noninvasive study with low radiation exposure that is well tolerated and easy to perform. It provides quantitative parameters that reflect pathophysiologic processes. It can be used for the diagnosis of organic and functional esophageal disorders and is especially valuable when performed serially to evaluate the effect of medical or surgical therapy.

^{99m}Tc-Sucralfate Scintigraphy

Sucralfate is an aluminum salt of a sulfated disaccharide that binds to proteins exposed in ulcerated mucosal surfaces. Sucralfate has protective and healing properties and has been used therapeutically. ^{99m}Tc-labeled sucralfate adheres to damaged, ulcerated surfaces in the gastrointestinal mucosa.[122–124] In children it was shown to adhere to esophageal mucosal surfaces injured by caustic ingestion. It correlated well with endoscopic findings, providing a simple noninvasive technique to assess esophageal injury after ingestion of caustic substances.[125]

Pulmonary Aspiration

Aspiration is a common cause of pulmonary disease.[126] Risk factors for aspiration include neurologic impairments, congenital malformations of the head and neck (e.g., cleft palate), and surgery of the upper aerodigestive tracts. Traditionally, investigators have emphasized the role of aspiration during feeding or from GER as an important cause of acute, recurrent, and chronic pulmonary disease in children.[126–128] Imaging studies most frequently requested to evaluate children with suspected aspiration include barium swallows, upper GI series, and gastroesophageal scintigraphy ("milk scan"). The barium swallow shows aspiration that occurs during the voluntary ingestion of liquids or, with modified techniques, solids. Aspiration secondary to GER is demonstrated with radionuclide GER studies or with upper GI series. The yield for detecting aspiration from GER has been low in most published series,[129–132] even with the more sensitive radionuclide GER study.[34,133] Aspiration of saliva is not evaluated with any of the studies mentioned.

Gastroesophageal Reflux Scintigraphy for Detection of Pulmonary Aspiration

Recurrent pulmonary infections have been associated with GER. Repeated aspiration of gastric contents following GER has been proposed as a pathogenic mechanism.[134–136] Gastroesophageal reflux scintigraphy ("milk scan"), developed in the late 1970s, can detect pulmonary aspiration secondary to GER.[34,137] The study technique was discussed earlier in the section on GER scintigraphy. The percent of milk scans positive for aspiration ranges from 1% to 25% in different series.[34,130,132,133,137–141] The ability of milk scans to detect pulmonary aspiration is subject to considerable debate.[130,139,142] Some authors report a very low yield in detection of pulmonary aspiration.[130,139] This has been the general experience of many pediatric radiology departments in the United States.[142] It was argued that milk scans are insensitive for detection of pulmonary aspiration. The success of antireflux treatment in lowering the incidence of pulmonary disease in children who failed to demonstrate aspiration on GER scintigraphy was used to support this argument.[130] One study found a higher incidence of aspiration in children with pulmonary disease than in children referred for gastrointestinal symptoms of GER, indicating that detection rates depend on patient selection.[133] The number of children with predisposing risk factors for aspiration such as neurologic impairment, congenital malformations, and surgery of the head and neck varied in different series as well. Differences in study technique may also play a role. Low concentration of radioactivity in the aspirate and rapid clearance of activity from the upper airway by the coughing reflex and the mucociliary transport mechanism could account for low detection rates as well.[143] A phantom study designed to estimate the detectability of different volumes of aspirated gastric contents found a minimal detectable volume of 0.025 mL using a standard concentration of ^{99m}Tc–sulfur colloid (5 µCi/mL).[34] Low detection rates may result from the intermittent nature of pulmonary aspiration even in patients with risk factors for aspiration and recurrent lung infections.[142] Finally, the possibility that infrequent demonstration of aspiration on milk scans indicates that aspiration of gastric contents is not a common mechanism for recurrent pulmonary infections (as traditionally assumed) should also be considered. Figure 7.6 demonstrates pulmonary aspiration secondary to GER.

The radionuclide GER study (milk scan) was found to be more sensitive than upper GI series for demonstrating aspiration of gastric contents.[34,138] This observation was also noted in a study of 120 children referred for scintigraphy and upper GI series due to respiratory disorders, GER, and near-miss sudden infant death syndrome.[133]

Radionuclide Salivagram

Aspiration of saliva is less well recognized as a potential etiology for pulmonary disease, probably due to the lack of methods that could demonstrate aspiration of saliva. Repeated aspiration of oral secretions, as well as failure to adequately clear the aspirate from the respiratory tract, have been proposed as pathogenic mechanisms leading to recurrent pulmonary infections. Bacteriologic studies showing that organisms isolated from the lower respiratory tract in aspiration pneumonia reflect the oropharyngeal flora, with a predominance of anaerobes, support this etiology.[144,145] Aspiration of oral secretions is likely to occur in patients with abnormal laryngeal closure.[146] Aspiration of saliva accounts for ongoing pulmonary infections in neurologically impaired patients despite corrective measures to prevent aspiration, such as antireflux surgery and discontinuation of oral feedings with gastrostomy tube feeding.[147–150] Salivary aspiration warrants consideration and should be evaluated in the context of recurrent lung infections.

The radionuclide salivagram is a technique designed to detect aspiration of saliva. A drop of ^{99m}Tc–sulfur colloid is placed in the oral cavity, mixes with saliva, and is swallowed. Using dynamic scintigraphy, the course of the tracer-saliva mixture is followed as it passes through the esophagus into the stomach. When aspiration occurs, tracer is seen within the tracheobronchial tree (Fig. 7.7).[151]

Study Technique and Interpretation

No specific preparations are required for the test. The patient is placed supine with the camera positioned under the imaging table and centered under the patient's chest. A small drop (100 µL) containing 11.1 MBq (300 µCi) ^{99m}Tc–sulfur colloid is placed on the back of the patient's tongue. Imaging commences immediately after administration. A camera equipped with a low-energy, high-resolution collimator records posterior view dynamic images on a

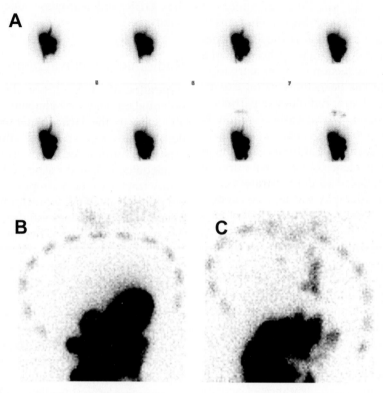

FIGURE 7.6. A "milk scan" of a 1-year-old boy with neurologic impairment due to thiamine deficiency and recurrent pneumonia was obtained due to suspected aspirations. A: Dynamic images show multiple episodes of GER up to the oral cavity. B: An anterior static image of the chest obtained at 1 hour immediately after the dynamic sequence shows clear lung fields. C: A delayed anterior image of the upper abdomen and thorax shows tracer localization in the trachea and right and left main bronchi, indicating late aspiration of gastric contents. The dotted line (B,C) is a radioactive marker outlining the chest boundaries.

128×128 matrix, 30 seconds per frame, for 60 minutes. Static anterior and posterior images of the chest are recorded on a 256×256 matrix immediately after the dynamic sequence. If a significant amount of tracer remains in the oral cavity, additional delayed images are obtained at 120 minutes. A [57]Co transmission image of the chest can improve localization of tracer in the lung fields. Care should be taken to avoid external contamination of clothes by labeled saliva because contamination could be mistaken for aspiration when positioned over the lung fields.

Images are inspected for evidence of tracer penetration into the tracheobronchial tree or into the lung parenchyma. The level of tracer localization in the proximal or distal airways and the persistence or clearance of aspirated tracer are noted. Cinematic display of the dynamic images is helpful.

The effectiveness of this study in demonstrating aspiration of saliva has been reported in several studies. We demonstrated aspiration of saliva in 8 of 31 children (26%) with pulmonary disease and risk factors for aspiration, especially neurologic disorders and birth defects involving the head and neck.[152] Other studies[141,151] performed on children with similar risk factors yielded similar results.

The ability of the radionuclide salivagram to determine the level of aspiration and to determine the clearance of the aspirate from the tracheobronchial tree is important in assessing the

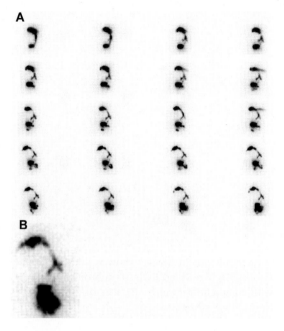

FIGURE 7.7. A: A radionuclide salivagram was performed on a 7-week-old infant with choking episodes and suspected laryngeal cleft. The images are displayed at 60 seconds per frame. Sequential posterior images (left to right, top to bottom) demonstrate transit of tracer from the oral cavity down the esophagus into the stomach. Ectopic activity in the airways, indicating aspiration of saliva, is first noted on the second frame from the left in the top row and becomes more evident as the study progresses. B: An enlarged frame shows more clearly the localization of tracer in the left and right main bronchi.

part of the radiographic barium swallow. The salivagram is a physiologic technique, simple to perform and requiring little patient cooperation. It involves the oral administration of only a tiny volume of saline, often unnoticed by the patient. It provides information on aspiration of oral secretions, unrelated to the conscious ingestion of liquids and solids during feeding. It exposes the patient to minimal radiation [on the order of 0.05 mSv (5 mrem) total body dose].[156] A barium swallow delivers a significantly higher radiation dose to the patient [up to 13 mSv (1300 mrem) for a modified barium swallow in adults],[157] necessitates the ingestion of a larger volume of liquid, the taste of which is unpleasant to some patients, and requires a higher degree of patient cooperation. It provides information on aspiration that occurs during feeding and valuable dynamic anatomic information that is used to assess the integrity of the swallowing mechanism.[158] Information provided by both techniques should be regarded as complementary. Aspiration of oral secretions, detected by salivagrams, was more commonly encountered than aspiration of barium in a study involving 46 children with lung disease, recurrent vomiting, or apnea who underwent scintigraphic and radiographic evaluations for detection of GER and aspiration.[138] Radionuclide salivagrams were more sensitive than barium studies in detecting aspiration in 78 patients with head and neck pathologies and neurologic disorders.[159]

Other Techniques for Detection of Aspiration

Scintigraphic Swallowing Studies

Scintigraphic swallowing techniques are based on swallowing of 10- to 15-mL boluses of liquids labeled with ^{99m}Tc–sulfur colloid. They are designed to detect aspiration that occurs during drinking, unlike the radionuclide salivagram, which is designed to detect aspiration of saliva by using a very small volume of radiotracer (one drop). The majority of such studies were performed in adults with dysphagia.[160,161] The techniques vary in protocols.[132,162,163] Some protocols are similar to esophageal transit

severity of aspiration. In an animal experiment, ^{99m}Tc–sulfur colloid instilled into proximal airways cleared rapidly but the same tracer instilled into distal airways was retained.[34] It is therefore likely that distal aspiration is more ominous than proximal aspiration. In addition, by assessing a patient's ability to clear aspirated secretions, the radionuclide salivagram evaluates the functional integrity of airway protective mechanisms such as the cough reflex and mucociliary transport (Fig. 7.8). Impairment of these protective mechanisms is a significant factor contributing to the development of lung disease in patients who aspirate.[144,153–155]

It should be emphasized that the radionuclide salivagram is not a scintigraphic counter-

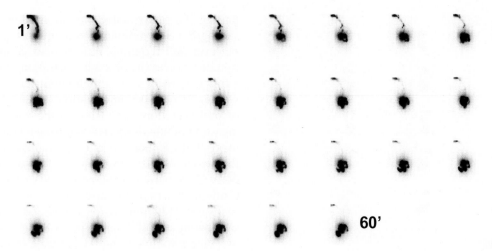

FIGURE 7.8. A radionuclide salivagram of a 4-year-old girl with recurrent lung infections, macrocephalus, psychomotor retardation, and seizure disorder was obtained due to suspected aspiration.

Sequential dynamic images show aspiration of saliva into the right and left main stem bronchi (top row) with complete clearance of tracer from the airways as the study progresses.

scintigraphy, described in the previous section. Aspiration of a swallowed tracer can be volume dependent. This has been shown in a 7-year-old girl with respiratory failure and suspected aspirations. Her radionuclide salivagram was normal; however, when challenged with a 10-mL labeled water bolus, bilateral pulmonary aspiration occurred. It was hypothesized that the swallowing mechanism may be capable of handling small volumes of saliva but malfunctions when challenged with larger volumes. It was recommended to perform a labeled bolus study on patients with suspected aspiration and a normal salivagram.[163]

Nonimaging Techniques for Evaluation of Pulmonary Aspiration

The lipid-laden alveolar macrophage study is a nonimaging technique used as an indicator for recurrent pulmonary aspiration by demonstrating increased lipid content in alveolar macrophages isolated from bronchoalveolar lavage (BAL) fluid. The invasive nature of this study is a disadvantage compared with imaging techniques. Studies assessing the utility of this technique in children yielded conflicting results. Significantly higher lipid-laden alveolar

macrophage (LLAM) scores were found in children with lung disease due to suspected aspirations than in children without lung disease or in children with lung disease from other etiologies.[164–167] Others found elevated LLAM scores in a variety of pulmonary diseases in which there was no clinical evidence of aspiration.[168] In another study, the mean LLAM index of a subgroup of children with both reflux and respiratory symptoms was not significantly different from that of a subgroup that was negative for both conditions.[169] These authors concluded that the low sensitivity and specificity of this test precludes it from becoming a useful indicator of silent pulmonary aspiration in children.

Prevention of Pulmonary Aspiration

Discontinuing oral feedings, substituting gastrostomy tube feedings, and performing antireflux surgeries are effective means to control aspiration that occurs during feeding and aspiration secondary to GER. In contrast, therapy options for children who aspirate saliva are limited, require surgical intervention, and are associated with significant morbidity. Radical surgery is justified in some patients (mostly with severe neurologic impairment and inability to handle oral secretions) in whom intractable aspiration of saliva results in life-threatening respiratory conditions. Tracheotomy is often performed in such patients to allow better respiratory control and the ability to manage secretions, but this doesn't solve the underlying condition of salivary aspirations.

Laryngotracheal separation is a radical, but potentially reversible, surgery that prevents aspiration of oral secretion. Phonation is sacrificed with this procedure. Using this technique, complete control of aspiration was achieved in 19 children with severe neurologic impairment and chronic salivary aspiration.[170] Radionuclide salivagrams proved useful in selecting neurologically impaired children with recurrent respiratory infections and frequent hospitalizations for laryngotracheal separation.[171]

Laryngeal diversion is another radical surgery that achieved stabilization or improvement of pulmonary function in a group of children with life-threatening aspiration.[172] Bilateral submandibular gland excision and parotid duct ligation is a voice-sparing procedure that reduced the incidence of aspiration pneumonia and hospitalization in a select group of neurologically impaired children.[173] A simpler procedure involving bilateral submandibular gland and parotid duct ligation achieved control of salivary aspiration in five children with severe neuromuscular impairment and recurrent aspiration pneumonia.[174]

References

1. Cezard JP. Managing gastro-oesophageal reflux disease in children. Digestion 2004;69(suppl 1):3–8.
2. Werlin SL, Dodds WJ, Hogan WJ, et al. Mechanisms of gastroesophageal reflux in children. J Pediatr 1980;97:244–249.
3. Kawahara H, Dent J, Davidson G. Mechanisms responsible for gastroesophageal reflux in children. Gastroenterology 1997;113:399–408.
4. Omari TI, Barnett CP, Benninga MA, et al. Mechanisms of gastro-oesophageal reflux in preterm and term infants with reflux disease. Gut 2002;51:475–7.
5. Holloway R, Hongo M, Berger K, McCallum R. Gastric distention: a mechanism for postprandial gastroesophageal reflux. Gastroenterology 1985;89:779–84.
6. Velasco N, Hill L, Gannan R, Pope C. Gastric emptying and gastroesophageal reflux. Am J Surg 1982;144:58–62.
7. Fink SM, Barwick KW, DeLuca V, Sanders FJ, Kandathil M, McCallum RW. The association of histologic gastritis with gastroesophageal reflux and delayed gastric emptying. J Clin Gastroenterol 1984;6:301–9.
8. Buckles DC, Sarosiek I, McMillin C, McCallum RW. Delayed gastric emptying in gastroesophageal reflux disease: reassessment with new methods and symptomatic correlations. Am J Med Sci 2004;327:1–4.
9. Hillemeier AC, Lange R, McCallum R, Seashore J, Grybosky J. Delayed gastric emptying in infants with gastroesophageal reflux. J Pediatr 1981;98:190–3.
10. Hillemeier AC, Grill BB, McCallum R, Grybosky J. Esophageal and gastric motor abnormalities in gastroesophageal reflux during infancy. Gastroenterology 1983;84:742–6.
11. Cucchiara S, Salvia G, Borrelli O, et al. Gastric electrical dysrhythmias and delayed gastric emptying in gastroesophageal reflux disease. Am J Gastroenterol 1997;92:1077–8.
12. Rosen PR, Treves S. The relationship of gastroesophageal reflux and gastric emptying in infants and children: concise communication. J Nucl Med 1984;25:571–4.
13. Jolley SG, Leonard JC, Tunell WP. Gastric emptying in children with gastroesophageal reflux. An estimate of effective gastric emptying. J Pediatr Surg 1987;22:923–6.
14. Di Lorenzo C, Piepsz A, Ham H, Cadranel S. Gastric emptying with gastroesophageal reflux. Arch Dis Child 1987;2:449–53.
15. Salvia G, De Vizia B, Manguso F, et al. Effect of intragastric volume and osmolality on mechanisms of gastroesophageal reflux in children with gastroesophageal reflux disease. Am J Gastroenterol 2001;96:1725–32.
16. Cameron AJ, Lagergren J, Henriksson C, Nyren O, Locke GR, Pedersen NL. Gastroesophageal reflux disease in monozygotic and dizygotic twins. Gastroenterology 2002;122:55–9.
17. Orenstein SR, Shalaby TM, Barmada MM, Whitcomb DC. Genetics of gastroesophageal reflux disease: a review. J Pediatr Gastroenterol Nutr 2002;34:506–10.

18. Shepherd RW, Wren J, Evans S, Lander M, Ong TH. Gastroesophageal reflux in children. Clinical profile, course and outcome with active therapy in 126 cases. Clin Pediatr (Phila) 1987;26:55–60.

19. Treem WR, Davis PM, Hyams JS. Gastroesophageal reflux in the older child: presentation, response to treatment and long-term follow-up. Clin Pediatr (Phila) 1991;30:435–40.

20. Vandenplas Y. Hiatal hernia and gastroesophageal reflux. In: Buts JP, Sokal EM, eds. Management of Digestive and Liver Disorders in Infants and Children. New York: Elsevier Science, 1993:103–16.

21. Nelson SP, Chen EH, Syniar GM, et al. Prevalence of symptoms of gastroesophageal reflux during infancy. A pediatric practice based survey. Pediatric Practice Research Group. Arch Pediatr Adolesc Med 1997;151:569–72.

22. Werlin SL, D'Souza BJ, Hogan WJ, et al. Sandifer syndrome: an unappreciated clinical entity. Dev Med Child Neurol 1980;22:374–8.

23. Gorrotxategi P, Reguilon MJ, Arana J, et al. Gastroesophageal reflux in association with the Sandifer syndrome. Eur J Pediatr Surg 1995;5:203–5.

24. Hassall E. Barrett's esophagus: new definitions and approaches in children. J Pediatr Gastroenterol Nutr 1993;16:345–64.

25. Harding SM. Recent clinical investigations examining the association of asthma and gastroesophageal reflux. Am J Med. 2003;18:39S–44S.

26. Rudolph CD, Mazur LJ, Liptak GS, et al. Guidelines for the evaluation and treatment of gastroesophageal reflux in infants and children. Recommendations of the North American Society for Pediatric Gastroenterology and Nutrition. J Pediatr Gastroenterol Nutr 2001;32(suppl 2):S1–S31.

27. Streets CG, DeMeester TR. Ambulatory 24–hour esophageal pH monitoring: why, when, and what to do. J Clin Gastroenterol 2003;37:14–22.

28. Thomson M. The pediatric esophagus comes of age. J Pediatr Gastroenterol Nutr 2002;34(suppl 1):S40–5.

29. Mitchell DJ, McClure BG, Tubman TRJ. Simultaneous monitoring of gastric and oesophageal pH reveals limitations of conventional oesophageal pH monitoring in milk fed infants. Arch Dis Child 2001;84:273–6.

30. Wenzl TG. Evaluation of gastroesophageal reflux events in children using multichannel intraluminal electrical impedance. Am J Med 2003;18:115(suppl 3A):161S–5S.

31. Wenzl TG, Silny J, Schenke S, et al. Gastroesophageal reflux and respiratory phenomena in infants: status of the intraluminal impedance technique. J Pediatr Gastroenterol Nutr 1999;28:423–8.

32. Riccabona M, Maurer U, Lackner H, Uray E, Ring E. The role of sonography in the evaluation of gastro-oesophageal reflux-correlation to pH-metry. Eur J Pediatr 1992;151:655–7.

33. Biller JA, Winter HS, Grand RJ, et al. Are endoscopic changes predictive of histologic esophagitis in children? J Pediatr 1983;103:215–18.

34. Heyman S, Kirkpatrick JA, Winter HS, Treves S. An improved radionuclide method for the diagnosis of gastroesophageal reflux and aspiration in children (milk scan). Radiology 1979;131:479–82.

35. Piepsz A, Georges B, Perlmutter N, Rodesch P, Cadranel S. Gastro-oesophageal scintiscanning in children. Pediatr Radiol 1981;11:71–4.

36. Piepsz A, Georges B, Rodesch P, Cadranel S. Gastroesophageal scintiscanning in children. J Nucl Med 1982;23:631–2.

37. Braga FJ, De Miranda JR, Arbex MA, et al. A physiological manoeuvre to improve the positivity of the gastro-oesophageal reflux scintigraphic test. Nucl Med Commun 2001;22:521–4.

38. Castronovo FP. Gastroesophageal scintigraphy in a pediatric population: dosimetry. J Nucl Med 1986;27:1212–14.

39. Fisher RS, Malmud LS, Roberts GS, Lobis IF. Gastroesophageal (GE) scintiscanning to detect and quantitate GE reflux. Gastroenterology 1976;70:301–8.

40. Devos PG, Forget P, DeRoo M, Eggermont E. Scintigraphic evaluation of gastrointestinal reflux (GER). J Nucl Med 1979;20:636(abstr).

41. Mariani G, Boni G, Barreca M, et al. Radionuclide gastroesophageal motor studies. J Nucl Med 2004;45:1004–28.

42. Arasu TS, Wyllie R, Fitzgerald JF, et al. Gastroesophageal reflux in infants and children: comparative accuracy of diagnostic methods. J Pediatr 1980;96:798–803.

43. Blumhagen JD, Rudd TG, Christie DL. Gastroesophageal reflux in children: radionuclide gastroesophagography. AJR 1980;135:1001–4.

44. Seibert JJ, Byrne WJ, Euler AR, Latture T, Leach M, Campbell M. Gastroesophageal reflux—the acid test: scintigraphy or the pH probe? AJR 1983;140:1087–90.

45. Laudizi L, Zaniol P, Venuta A, Pantusa M, Sturloni N, Laudizi Z. Gastroesophageal reflux in children. A combined radiologic and scintigraphic study. Radiol Med (Torino) 1990;79:381–3.

46. Kashyap R, Sharma R, Madan N, Sachdev G, Chopra MK, Chopra K. Evaluation of radionuclide gastroesophagography as a suitable screening test for detection of gastroesophageal reflux. Indian Pediatr 1993;30:625–8.

47. Patwari AK, Bajaj P, Kashyp R, et al. Diagnostic modalities for gastroesophageal reflux. Indian J Pediatr 2002;69:133–6.

48. Ozcan Z, Ozcan C, Erinc R, Dirlik A, Mutaf O. Scintigraphy in the detection of gastrooesophageal reflux in children with caustic oesophageal burns: a comparative study with radiography and 24–h pH monitoring. Pediatr Radiol 2001;31:737–41.

49. Tolia V, Kuhns L, Kauffman RE. Comparison of simultaneous esophageal pH monitoring and scintigraphy in infants with gastroesophageal reflux. Am J Gastroenterol 1993; 88:661–4.

50. Vandenplas Y, Derde MP, Piepsz A. Evaluation of reflux episodes during simultaneous esophageal pH monitoring and gastroesophageal reflux scintigraphy in children. J Pediatr Gastroenterol Nutr 1992;14:256–60.

51. Tolia V, Calhoun JA, Kuhns LR, Kauffman RE. Lack of correlation between extended pH monitoring and scintigraphy in the evaluation of infants with gastroesophageal reflux. J Lab Clin Med 1990;115:559–63.

52. Orenstein SR, Klein HA, Rosenthal MS. Scintigraphy versus pH probe for quantification of pediatric gastroesophageal reflux: a study using concurrent multiplexed data and acid feedings. J Nucl Med 1993;34:1228–34.

53. Jona JZ, Sty JR, Glicklich M. Simplified radioisotope technique for assessing gastroesophageal reflux in children. J Pediatr Surg 1981;16:114–7.

54. DiLorenzo C, Mertz H, Alvarez S, Mori C, Mayer E, Hyman PE. Gastric receptive relaxation is absent in newborn infants. Gastroenterology 1993;104:A498(abstr).

55. Huisinga JD. Physiology and pathophysiology of interstitial cells of Cajal: from bench to bedside. II. Gastric motility lessons from mutant mice on slow waves and innervation. Am J Physiol 2001;281:G1129–34.

56. Heyman S. Gastric emptying in children. J Nucl Med 1998;39:865–9.

57. Siegel M, Lebenthal E, Topper W, Krantz B, Li PK. Gastric emptying in prematures of isocaloric feedings with differing osmolalities. Pediatr Res 1982;16:141–7.

58. Christian PE, Moore JG, Brown F, et al. Effect of caloric content and meal size in gastric emptying. J Nucl Med 1982;23(suppl):P20(abstr).

59. Maes BD, Ghoos YF, Geypens BJ, Hiele MI, Rutgeerts PJ. Relation between gastric emptying rate and energy intake in children compared with adults. Gut 1995;36:183–8.

60. Cavell B. Gastric emptying in infants fed human milk or infant formula. Acta Paediatr Scand 1981;70:639–41.

61. Billeaud C, Guillet J, Sandler B. Gastric emptying in infants with or without gastrooesophageal reflux according to the type of milk. Eur J Clin Nutr 1990;44:577–83.

62. Hunt JN, Knox MT. A relation between the chain length of fatty acids and the slowing of gastric emptying. J Physiol 1968;194:327–36.

63. Cooke AR, Moulang J. Control of gastric emptying by amino acids. Gastroenterology 1972; 62:528–32.

64. Rosen PR, Treves S. The relationship of gastroesophageal reflux and gastric emptying in infants and children: concise communication. J Nucl Med 1984;25:571–4.

65. Di Lorenzo C, Piepsz A, Ham H, Cadranel S. Gastric emptying with gastro-oesophageal reflux. Arch Dis Child 1987;62:449–53.

66. Koch KL. Diagnosis and treatment of neuromuscular disorders of the stomach. Curr Gastroenterol Rep 2003;5:323–30.

67. Portincasa P, Colecchia A, Di Ciaula A, et al. Standards for diagnosis of gastrointestinal motility disorders. Section: ultrasonography. A position statement from the Gruppo Italiano di Studio Motilita' Apparato Digerente (GISMAD). Dig Liver Dis 2000;32:160–72.

68. Bolondi L, Bortolotti M, Santi V, Caletti T, Gaiani S, Labo G. Measurement of gastric emptying time by real-time ultrasonography. Gastroenterology 1985;89:752–9.

69. Berstad A, Hausken T, Gilja OH, Hveem K, Nesje LB, Odegaard S. Ultrasonography of the human stomach. Scand J Gastroenterol. 1996;220:75–82.

70. Benini L, Sembenini C, Heading RC, et al. Simultaneous measurement of gastric emptying of a solid meal by ultrasound and by scintigraphy. Am J Gastroenterol 1999;94:2861–5.

71. Cucchiara S, Minella R, Iorio R, et al. Real-time ultrasound reveals gastric motor abnormalities

in children investigated for dyspeptic symptoms. J Pediatr Gastroenterol Nutr. 1995;21:446–53.

72. Kock KL. Electrogastrography. In: Schuster M, Crowell MD, Koch KL, eds. Schuster Atlas of Gastrointestinal Motility in Health and Disease. Hamilton, Canada: BC Decker, 2002:185–201.

73. Ghoos YF, Maes BD, Geypens BJ, et al. Measurement of gastric emptying rate of solids by means of a carbon-labeled octanoic acid breath test. Gastroenterology 1993;104:1640–7.

74. Kim DY, Camilleri M. Stable isotope breath test and gastric emptying. In: Schuster M, Crowell MD, Koch KL, eds. Schuster Atlas of Gastrointestinal Motility in Health and Disease. Hamilton, Canada: BC Decker, 2002:203–18.

75. Braden B, Peterknecht A, Piepho T, et al. Measuring gastric emptying of semisolids in children using the 13C-acetate breath test: a validation study. Dig Liver Dis 2004;36:260–4.

76. Gelfand MJ, Wagner GG. Gastric emptying in infants and children: limited utility of 1–hour measurement. Radiology 1991;178:379–81.

77. Heyman S. Radionuclide transit studies In: Hyman PE, DiLorenzo CD, eds. Pediatric Gastrointestinal Motility Disorders, 1st ed. New York: Academy Professional Information Services, 1994:291–304.

78. Villanueva-Meyer J, Swischuk LE, Cesani F, Ali SA, Briscoe E. Pediatric gastric emptying: value of right lateral and upright positioning. J Nucl Med 1996;37:1356–8.

79. Heyman S, Reich H. Gastric emptying of milk feedings in infants and young children: anterior vs conjugate counting. J Nucl Med 1995;36(suppl):259P(abstr).

80. Halkar KR, Paszkowski A, Jones M. Two point, timesaving method for measurement of gastric emptying with diagnostic accuracy comparable to that of the conventional method. Radiology 1999;213:599–602.

81. Lin E, Connolly LP, Drubach L, et al. Effect of early emptying on quantitation and interpretation of liquid gastric emptying studies of infants and young children. J Nucl Med 2000;41:596–9.

82. Signer E. Gastric emptying in newborns and young infants. Measurement of the rate of emptying using indium-113m-microcolloid. Acta Paediatr Scand 1975;64:525–30.

83. Seibert JJ, Byrne WJ, Euler AR. Gastric emptying in children: unusual patterns detected by scintigraphy. Am J Roentgenol 1983;141:49–51.

84. Knight LC. Radiopharmacy aspects of gastrointestinal imaging. In: Henkin RE, Boles MA, Dillehay GL, et al., eds. Nuclear Medicine, vol 2. St. Louis: Mosby, 1996:922–32.

85. Sagar S, Grime JS, Little W, et al. ^{99m}Tc labelled bran: a new agent for measuring gastric emptying. Clin Radiol 1983;34:275–8.

86. Malagelada JR, Carter SE, Brown ML, Carlson GL. Radiolabeled fiber: a physiologic marker for gastric emptying and intestinal transit of solids. Dig Dis Sci 1980;25:81–7.

87. Montgomery M, Escobar-Billing R, Hellstrom PM, Karlsson KA, Frenckner B. Impaired gastric emptying in children with repaired esophageal atresia: a controlled study. J Pediatr Surg 1998;33:476–80.

88. Malmud LS, Fisher RS, Knight LC, Rock E. Scintigraphic evaluation of gastric emptying. Semin Nucl Med 1982;12:116–25.

89. Urbain JLC, Van Custem E, Sirgel JA, et al. Visualization and characterization of gastric contractions using a radionuclide technique. Am J Physiol 1990;259:G1062–7.

90. Ham HR, Muls V, Cadiere G-B, et al. Radionuclide study of regional gastric motility. Nucl Med Commun 1995;16:827–33.

91. Urbain JLC, Vekemans MC, Bouillon R, et al. Characterization of gastric antral motility disturbances in diabetes using the scintigraphic technique. J Nucl Med 1993;34:576–81.

92. Urbain JLC, Vekemans MC, Parkman H, et al. Dynamic antral scintigraphy to characterize antral motility in functional dyspepsia. J Nucl Med. 1995;36:1579–86.

93. Kuiken SD, Samson M, Camilleri M, et al. Development of a test to measure gastric accommodation in humans. Am J Physiol 1999;277:G1217–21.

94. Bouras EP, Delgado-Aros S, Camilleri M, et al. SPECT imaging of the stomach: comparison with barostat, and effects of sex, age, body mass index, and fundoplication. Single photon emission computed tomography. Gut 2002;51:781–6.

95. Kim D-Y, Delgado-Aros S, Camilleri M, et al. Noninvasive measurement of gastric accommodation in patients with idiopathic nonulcer dyspepsia. Am J Gastroenterol 2001;96:3099–105.

96. Simonian HP, Maurer AH, Knight LC, et al. Simultaneous assessment of gastric accommodation and emptying: studies with liquid and solid meals. J Nucl Med 2004;45:1155–60.

97. Bonapace ES, Parkman HP. Normal esophageal physiology. In: Brandt LJ, ed. Clinical Practice

of Gastroenterology Philadelphia: Churchill Livingstone, 1999:2–12.

98. Clouse RE, Richter JE, Heading RC, Janssens J, Wilson JA. Functional esophageal disorders. Gut 1999;45:31–6.

99. Dekel R, Fass R. Current perspectives on the diagnosis and treatment of functional esophageal disorders. Curr Gastroenterol Rep 2003;5:314–22.

100. Hillemeir C, Buchin P, Gryboski J. Esophageal dysfunction in Down's syndrome. J Pediatr Gastroenterol Nutr 1983;1:101–4.

101. Staiano A, Cucchiara S, Del Giudice E, Andreotti MR, Minella R. Disorders of oesophageal motility in children with psychomotor retardation and gastro-oesophageal reflux. Eur J Pediatr 1991;150:638–41.

102. Del Giudice E, Staiano A, Capano G, et al. Gastrointestinal manifestations in children with cerebral palsy. Brain Dev 1999;21:307–11.

103. Gustafsson PM Tibbling L. Gastroesophageal reflux and esophageal dysfunction in children and adolescents with brain damage. Acta Paediatr 1994;83:1081–5.

104. Krausz Y, Maayan C, Faber J, Marciano R, Mogle P, Wynchank S. Scintigraphic evaluation of esophageal transit and gastric emptying in familial dysautonomia. Eur J Radiol 1994; 18(1):52–6.

105. Genc A, Mutaf O. Esophageal motility changes in acute and late periods of caustic esophageal burns and their relation to prognosis in children. J Pediatr Surg 2002;37:1526–8.

106. Engum SA, Grosfeld JL, West KW, Rescorla FJ, Scherer LR 3rd. Analysis of morbidity and mortality in 227 cases of esophageal atresia and/or tracheoesophageal fistula over two decades. Arch Surg 1995;130:502–8.

107. Kazem I. A new scintigraphic technique for the study of the esophagus. AJR 1972;115: 681–8.

108. Guillet J, Wynchank S, Basse-Cathalinat B, Christophe E, Ducassou D, Blanquet P. Pediatric esophageal scintigraphy. Results of 200 studies. Clin Nucl Med 1983;8:427–33.

109. Heyman S. Esophageal scintigraphy (milk scans) in infants and children with gastroesophageal reflux. Radiology 1982;144:891–3.

110. Svedberg JB. The bolus transport diagram: a functional display method applied to esophageal studies. Clin Phys Physiol Meas 1982;3:267–72.

111. Ham HR, Piepsz A, Georges B, Verelst J, Guillaume M, Cadranel S. Quantitation of

esophageal transit by means of 81mKr. Eur J Nucl Med 1984;9:362–5.

112. Klein HA, Wald A. Computer analysis of radionuclide esophageal transit studies. J Nucl Med 1984;25:957–64.

113. Tatsch K. Multiple swallow test for quantitative and qualitative evaluation of esophageal motility disorders. J Nucl Med. 1991;32: 1365–70.

114. Tatsch K, Voderholzer WA, Weiss MJ, Schrottle W, Hahn K. Reappraisal of quantitative esophageal scintigraphy by optimizing results with ROC analyses. J Nucl Med 1996;37: 1799–805.

115. Lamki L. Radionuclide esophageal transit study: the effect of body posture. Clin Nucl Med 1985;10:108–10.

116. Buthpitiya AG, Stroud D, Russell CO. Pharyngeal pump and esophageal transit. Dig Dis Sci 1987;32:1244–8.

117. Kjellen G, Svedberg JB, Tibbling L. Solid bolus transit by esophageal scintigraphy in patients with dysphagia and normal manometry and radiology. Dig Dis Sci 1984;29:1–5.

118. Fisher RS, Malmud LS, Applegate G, Rock E, Lorber SH. Effect of bolus composition on esophageal transit: concise communication. J Nucl Med 1982;23:878–82.

119. Mughal MM, Marples M, Bancewicz J. Scintigraphic assessment of esophageal motility: what does it show and how reliable is it? Gut 1986;27:946–53.

120. Russell CO, Hill LD, Holmes ER 3rd, Hull DA, Gannon R, Pope CE 2nd. Radionuclide transit: a sensitive screening test for esophageal dysfunction. Gastroenterology 1981;80:887–92.

121. Kjellen G, Svedberg JB, Tibbling L. Solid bolus transit by esophageal scintigraphy in patients with dysphagia and normal manometry and radiology. Dig Dis Sci 1984;29:1–5.

122. Van Zyl JH, Nel MG, Otto AC, et al.: Evaluation of reflux oesophagitis with technetium-99m labelled sucralfate. S Afr Med 1996;86: 1422–4.

123. Mearns AJ, Hart GC, Cox JA: Dynamic radionuclide imaging with 99m Tc-sucralfate in the detection of oesophageal ulceration. Gut 1989;30:1256–9.

124. Dawson DJ, Khan AN, Nuttall P, Shreeve DR: Technetium-99m-labelled-sucralphate isotope scanning in the detection of peptic ulceration. Nucl Med Commun 1985;6:319–25.

125. Millar AJ, Numanoglu A, Mann M, Marven S, Rode H. Detection of caustic oesophageal

injury with technetium-99m-labelled sucralfate. J Pediatr Surg 2001;36:262–5.

126. Cameron JL, Zuidema GD. Aspiration pneumonia: magnitude and frequency of the problem. JAMA 1972;219:1194–6.

127. Euler AR, Byrne WJ, Ament ME et al. Recurrent pulmonary disease in children: a complication of gastroesophageal reflux. Pediatrics 1979;63:47–51.

128. Berquist WE, Rachelefsky GS, Kadden M, et al. Gastroesophageal reflux associated recurrent pneumonia and chronic asthma in children. Pediatrics 1981;68:29–35.

129. Heyman S. Evaluation of gastroesophageal reflux and gastrointestinal bleeding. In: Freeman LM, Weissmann HS. eds. Nuclear Medicine Annual. New-York: Raven Press, 1985:133–69.

130. Fawcett HD, Hayden CK, Adams JC, et al. How useful is gastroesophageal reflux scintigraphy in suspected childhood aspiration? Pediatr Radiol 1988;18:311–13.

131. Berdon WE, Mellins RB, Levy J. Commentary: On the following paper by H.D. Fawcett, C.K. Hayden, J.C. Adams and L.E. Swischuk: How useful is gastroesophageal reflux scintigraphy in suspected childhood aspiration? Pediatr Radiol 1988;18:309–10.

132. Miller JH. How useful is gastroesophageal reflux scintigraphy in suspected childhood aspiration? Letter to the editor. Pediatr Radiol 1988;19:70.

133. McVeagh P, Howman-Giles R, Kemp A. Pulmonary aspiration studies by radionuclide milk scanning and barium swallow roentgenography. Am J Dis Child 1987;141:917–21.

134. Berquist WE, Rachelefsky GS, Kadden M, et al. Gastroesophageal reflux-associated recurrent pneumonia and chronic asthma in children. Pediatrics 1981;68:29–35.

135. Euler AR, Byrne WJ, Ament ME, et al. Recurrent pulmonary disease in children: a complication of gastroesophageal reflux. Pediatrics 1979;63:47–51.

136. Christie DL, O'Grady LR, Mack DV. Incompetent lower esophageal sphincter and gastroesophageal reflux in recurrent acute pulmonary disease of infancy and childhood. J Pediatr 1978;93:23–7.

137. Boonyaprapa S, Alderson PO, Garfinkel DJ, Chipps BE, Wagner HN Jr. Detection of pulmonary aspiration in infants and children with respiratory disease: concise communication. J Nucl Med 1980;21:314–18.

138. Bar-Sever Z, Steinberg T, Connolly LP, et al. Scintigraphic and radiographic imaging of aspiration and gastroesophageal reflux in young children. J Nucl Med 1999;40:13P(abstr).

139. MacFadyen UM, Hendry GM, Simpson H. Gastro-oesophageal reflux in near-miss sudden infant death syndrome or suspected recurrent aspiration. Arch Dis Child 1983;58:87–91.

140. Berger D, Bischof-Delaloye A, Reinberg O, Roulet M. Esophageal and pulmonary scintiscanning in gastroesophageal reflux in children. Prog Pediatr Surg 1985;18:68–77.

141. Levin K, Colon A, DiPalma J, Fitzpatrick S. Using the radionuclide salivagram to detect pulmonary aspiration and esophageal dysmotility. Clin Nucl Med 1993;18:110–14.

142. Berdon WE, Mellins RB, Levy J. On the following paper by H.D. Fawcett, C.K. Hayden, J.C. Adams and L.E. Swischuk: How useful is gastroesophageal reflux scintigraphy in suspected childhood aspiration? Pediatr Radiol 1988;18:309–10.

143. Heyman S, Eicher PS, Alavi A. Radionuclide studies of the upper gastrointestinal tract in children with feeding disorders. J Nucl Med 1995;36:351–4.

144. Lorber B, Swenson RM. Bacteriology of aspiration pneumonia: a prospective study of community and hospital acquired cases. Ann Intern Med 1974;81:329–31.

145. Bartlett JG, Gorbach SL, Finegold SM. The bacteriology of aspiration pneumonia. Am J Med 1974;56:202–7.

146. Russin SJ, Adler AG. Pulmonary aspiration: the three syndromes. Postgrad Med 1989;85:155–61.

147. Heyman S. The radionuclide salivagram for detecting the pulmonary aspiration of saliva in an infant. Pediatr Radiol 1989;19:208–9.

148. Martinez DA, Ginn-Pease ME, Caniano DA. Sequelae of antireflux surgery in profoundly disabled children. J Pediatr Surg 1992;27:267–71.

149. Bauer ML, Figueroa-Colon R, Georgeson K, Young DW. Chronic pulmonary aspiration in children. South Med J 1993;86:789–95.

150. Bui HD, Dang CV, Chaney RH, Vergara LM. Does gastrostomy and fundoplication prevent aspiration pneumonia in mentally retarded persons? Am J Ment Retard 1989;94:16–19.

151. Heyman S, Respondek M. Detection of pulmonary aspiration in children by radionuclide "salivagram." J Nucl Med 1989;30:697–9.

152. Bar-Sever Z, Connolly LP, Treves ST. The radionuclide salivagram in children with pulmonary disease and a high risk of aspiration. Pediatr Radiol 1995;25(suppl 1):S180–3.

153. Huxley EJ, Viroslav J, Gray WR, et al. Pharyngeal aspiration in normal adults and patients with depressed consciousness. Am J Med 1978;64:565–7.

154. Green GM. Pulmonary clearance of infectious agents. Annu Rev Med. 1968;19:315–36.

155. Green GM. Lung defense mechanisms. Med Clin North Am 1973;57:547–62.

156. Siegel JA, Wu RK, Knight LC, Zelac RE, Stern HS, Malmud LS. Radiation dose estimates for oral agents used in upper gastrointestinal disease. J Nucl Med 1983;24:835–7.

157. Crawley MT, Savage P, Oakley F. Patient and operator dose during fluoroscopic examination of swallow mechanism. Br J Radiol 2004;77: 654–6.

158. Dodds WJ, Stewart ET, Logemann JA. Physiology and radiology of the normal oral and pharyngeal phases of swallowing. Am J Roentgenol 1990;154:953–63.

159. Muz J, Mathog RH, Miller PR, Rosen R, Borrero G. Detection and quantification of laryngotracheopulmonary aspiration with scintigraphy. Laryngoscope 1987;97:1180–5.

160. Silver KH, Van Nostrand D. The use of scintigraphy in the management of patients with pulmonary aspiration. Dysphagia 1994;9:107–15.

161. Shaw DW, Williams RB, Cook IJ, et al. Oropharyngeal scintigraphy: a reliable technique for the quantitative evaluation of oral-pharyngeal swallowing. Dysphagia 2004;19:36–42.

162. Miller JH. Upper gastrointestinal tract evaluation with radionuclides in infants. Radiology 1991;178:326–7.

163. Heyman S. Volume-dependent pulmonary aspiration of a swallowed radionuclide bolus. J Nucl Med 1997;38:103–4.

164. Bauer ML, Lyrene RK. Chronic aspiration in children: evaluation of the lipid-laden macrophage index. Pediatr Pulmonol 1999;28:94–100.

165. Ahrens P, Noll C, Kitz R, Willigens P, Zielen S, Hofmann D. Lipid-laden alveolar macrophages (LLAM): a useful marker of silent aspiration in children. Pediatr Pulmonol 1999; 28:83–8.

166. Nussbaum E, Maggi JC, Mathis R, Galant SP. Association of lipid-laden alveolar macrophages and gastroesophageal reflux in children. J Pediatr 1987;110:190–4

167. Colombo JL, Hallberg TK. Recurrent aspiration in children: lipid-laden alveolar macrophage quantitation. Pediatr Pulmonol 1987;3: 86–9.

168. Knauer-Fischer S, Ratjen F. Lipid-laden macrophages in bronchoalveolar lavage fluid as a marker for pulmonary aspiration. Pediatr Pulmonol 1999;27:419–22.

169. Krishnan U, Mitchell JD, Tobias V, Day AS, Bohane TD. Fat laden macrophages in tracheal aspirates as a marker of reflux aspiration: a negative report. J Pediatr Gastroenterol Nutr 2002;35:309–13.

170. Cook SP, Lawless ST, Kettrick R. Patient selection for primary laryngotracheal separation as treatment of chronic aspiration in the impaired child. Int J Pediatr Otorhinolaryngol 1996; 38:103–13.

171. Cook SP, Lawless S, Mandell GA, Reilly JS. The use of the salivagram in the evaluation of severe and chronic aspiration. Int J Pediatr Otorhinolaryngol 1997;41:353–61.

172. De Vito MA, Wetmore RF, Pransky SM. Laryngeal diversion in the treatment of chronic aspiration in children. Int J Pediatr Otorhinolaryngol. 1989;18:139–45.

173. Gerber ME, Gaugler MD, Myer CM 3rd, Cotton RT. Chronic aspiration in children. When are bilateral submandibular gland excision and parotid duct ligation indicated? Arch Otolaryngol Head Neck Surg 1996;122: 1368–71.

174. Klem C, Mair EA. Four-duct ligation: a simple and effective treatment for chronic aspiration from sialorrhea. Arch Otolaryngol Head Neck Surg 1999;125:796–800.

8
Gastrointestinal Bleeding

S.T. Treves and Richard J. Grand

Gastrointestinal bleeding is a relatively common problem in pediatric patients. Multiple disease processes lead to this complication, and many of these are age dependent. In patients of all ages, it is important to remember that while bright red blood in vomitus nearly always signifies bleeding proximal to the ligament of Treitz, this is not always so. Conversely, bright red bleeding per rectum may actually be from a source in the upper gastrointestinal tract. Thus the urgent evaluation of patients with either upper or lower gastrointestinal bleeding should always include the use of nasogastric tube sampling of gastric contents. Common causes of upper and lower gastrointestinal bleeding are listed in Tables 8.1 and 8.2.

Methods for the detection and localization of gastrointestinal bleeding in children include technetium-99m pertechnetate (^{99m}Tc-O$_4^-$) scintigraphy and ^{99m}Tc-labeled red blood cell (^{99m}Tc-RBC) scintigraphy. Of these two methods, the most frequently used for the detection of Meckel's diverticulum is ^{99m}Tc-O$_4^-$ abdominal scintigraphy. This method relies on the detection of pertechnetate uptake by functioning ectopic gastric mucosa. Gastrointestinal bleeding from any source can be detected by ^{99m}Tc-RBC scintigraphy, which relies on the visualization of extravasated labeled red blood cells from the blood pool.

Meckel's Diverticulum

The first recorded observation of an ileal diverticulum has been attributed to Fabricius Hildamus in 1650,[1] and the first comprehensive embryologic and pathologic description of the lesion was made by Johan Friedrick Meckel, the younger, in 1809. Ileal (Meckel's) diverticulum is a noninherited congenital abnormality of the antimesenteric side of the small intestine, resulting from incomplete closure of the embryonic vitelline or omphalomesenteric duct. Meckel's diverticuli may measure from 1 to 56 cm in length, and 1 to 50 cm in diameter. Most Meckel's diverticuli are found within the ileum approximately 90 cm proximal to the ileocecal valve.[2]

A Meckel's diverticulum usually contains ileal mucosa but may contain gastric, duodenal, jejunal, colonic mucosa, or pancreatic tissue. Heterotopic tissue in a diverticulum of the pancreatic type was reported by Zonkel in 1861 and of the gastric type by Tillmans in 1882. The relationship of aberrant gastric mucosa to the ulcer of a diverticulum was considered by Deetz in 1907. Gastric mucosa is present in Meckel's diverticulum in approximately 50% of cases.[3,4]

Meckel's diverticulum is the most common cause of lower gastrointestinal hemorrhage in previously healthy infants, and more than 50% of

TABLE 8.1. Principal causes of lower gastrointestinal bleeding in relation to age

Newborn (birth–1 month)	Infant (1 month–2 years)	Preschool age (2–5 years)	School age (>5 years)
Necrotizing enterocolitis	Anal fissure	Anal fissure	Anal fissure
Malrotation with volvulus	Infectious colitis	Infectious colitis	Infectious colitis
Allergic proctocolitis	Allergic proctocolitis	Polyp	Polyp
Hirschsprung disease enterocolitis	Intussusception	Meckel diverticulum	Henoch-Schönlein purpura
Hemorrhagic disease of the newborn	Meckel diverticulum	Henoch-Schönlein purpura	Inflammatory bowel disease
	Lymphonodular hyperplasia	Hemolytic uremic syndrome	
	Malrotation with volvulus	Lymphonodular hyperplasia	
	Hirschsprung disease enterocolitis		
	Intestinal duplication		

infants with the remnant have symptoms before the second year of life.[5] Clinical symptoms occur in 25% to 30% of all the patients. Estimates of the probable incidence of Meckel's diverticulum in the general population range from approximately 1% to 3%, with a frequency three times greater in males than females.[3] The most common symptom of Meckel's diverticulum is gross rectal bleeding with or without associated abdominal complaints. The bleeding apparently results from mucosal ulceration in the diverticulum or adjacent ileum caused by hydrochloric acid secreted by the ectopic gastric mucosa. Nearly all diverticula of patients with symptoms of gastrointestinal bleeding contain ectopic gastric mucosa.[3,5–8] Other pathologic conditions associated with Meckel's diverticulum include intestinal obstruction caused by bands, knots, volvulus, inflammation, or intussusception; regional enteritis; hernia; enterolith; calcification; diverticulitis; tuberculosis; and foreign body.[5,9]

Several years ago, we reviewed the records of all patients with Meckel's diverticulum less than 2 years of age undergoing surgery at Children's Hospital Boston between 1951 and 1972. Among 60 infants less than age 2, 32 had painless rectal bleeding. Of these 32, 56% presented before 1 year of age and the remaining 44% before age 2. Among those symptomatic patients, 91% (29 of 32 patients) had ectopic gastric mucosa in their Meckel's diverticula.[10] The differential diagnosis of rectal bleeding in infants less than age 2 years includes Meckel's diverticulum, anal fissure, volvulus, intussusception, peptic ulcer, and colonic polyp. Of these disorders, only colonic polyp and Meckel's diverticulum usually cause painless bleeding.

^{99m}Tc-O$_4^-$ Abdominal Scintigraphy

Technetium-99m pertechnetate abdominal scintigraphy was initially proposed by Harden

TABLE 8.2. Etiologies of upper gastrointestinal bleeding in children by age group, in relative order of frequency

Newborn	Infant	Child–adolescent
Swallowed maternal blood	Stress gastritis or ulcer	Mallory-Weiss tear
Vitamin K deficiency	Acid–peptic disease	Acid–peptic disease
Stress gastritis or ulcer	Mallory-Weiss tear	Varices
Acid–peptic disease	Vascular anomaly	Caustic ingestion
Vascular anomaly	Gastrointestinal duplications	Vasculitis (Henoch-Shönlein purpura)
Coagulopathy	Gastric/esophageal varices	Crohn's disease
Milk-protein sensitivity	Duodenal/gastric webs	Bowel obstruction
	Bowel obstruction	Dieulafoy lesion, hemobilia

and Alexander[11] in 1967 and was subsequently introduced into clinical practice by Jewett et al.[12] in 1970. Since then, many reports have demonstrated the safety and effectiveness of this examination in the detection of functioning ectopic gastric mucosa in a Meckel's diverticulum, as well as other sites.[13–20] A comprehensive review of the topic has been written by Sfakianakis and Conway.[18,21] Meckel's diverticulum cannot be diagnosed as simply and reliably by other imaging modalities,[10,22–24] and at present pertechnetate abdominal scintigraphy is the best nonoperative method of definite diagnosis of this condition. It is easy to perform, and the radiation exposure to the patient is equivalent to only 20 seconds of fluoroscopy.[25]

Indications

Asymptomatic gross rectal bleeding (bright red stools) in a young child is a frequent indication for pertechnetate scintigraphy. A pediatric patient presenting with rectal bleeding suspected to be caused by ulceration of a Meckel's diverticulum requires a complete physical examination, which may include a careful examination of the anal area, rectoscopy, or sigmoidoscopy to exclude distal colonic disease, and, when indicated, a hematologic examination to exclude a systemic bleeding disorder. Pertechnetate abdominal scintigraphy should then be performed.

Radiopharmaceutical

For the detection of Meckel's diverticulum, $^{99m}Tc\text{-}O_4^-$ is injected intravenously in a dose of 0.1 mCi (3.7 MBq)/kg of body weight [minimum dose 0.2 mCi (7.4 MBq), maximum dose 10 mCi (370 MBq)]. It should be obvious that abdominal scintigraphy ($^{99m}Tc\text{-}O_4^-$) does not detect a Meckel's diverticulum per se but reveals uptake of radiopertechnetate by functioning ectopic gastric mucosa in the diverticulum or elsewhere. To give a sense of the intensity of pertechnetate uptake in gastric mucosa, normally, approximately 25% of the intravenously administered dose of $^{99m}Tc\text{-}O_4^-$ localizes in the wall of the stomach. The gastric uptake of pertechnetate is rapid and increases in intensity over time.

A number of authors have investigated the cellular localization of pertechnetate in the stomach. Keramidas et al.[26] found no significant differences in the concentration of pertechnetate in the body and antrum of the stomach in dogs. Using microautoradiography, Meier-Ruge and Fridrich[27] demonstrated that pertechnetate is selectively taken up by the parietal cells of the stomach, whereas iodine-131 as sodium iodide is absorbed and secreted by the gastric chief and mucosal cells.[27,28] Wine et al.,[28,29] using Heidenhain pouches and denervated antral pouches in dogs, suggested that parietal cells are not essential for $^{99m}Tc\text{-}O_4^-$ concentration and that both acid output and volume output relate to the amount of $^{99m}Tc\text{-}O_4^-$ output. Priebe et al.,[30] using contact autoradiographs of canine gastric mucosa, demonstrated that $^{99m}Tc\text{-}O_4^-$ concentrated in surface mucous cells of the gastric pits but not in the gastric glands. Using autoradiography, Berquist et al.[3] showed pertechnetate concentration in the superficial cells only. These authors also had six cases of histologically proven Barrett's esophagus, all with abnormal scintigraphy. Biopsy material revealed complete absence of parietal cells in all but one.[31,32] In contrast, the gastric type of surface epithelial cells was present in every case. The pertechnetate anion is believed to be accumulated selectively by surface cells of gastric mucosa and then secreted into the bowel lumen.[33–36] Approximately 20% of the injected dose of $^{99m}Tc\text{-}O_4^-$ is rapidly eliminated by the kidneys. Organs that also normally concentrate radiopertechnetate include the choroid plexus, the thyroid, and the salivary glands.[37–40] The blood disappearance rate of $^{99m}Tc\text{-}O_4^-$ may be prolonged in infants because of renal immaturity, a normally low gastric mucosal uptake, or both. Slow blood disappearance and low gastric uptake of pertechnetate in older children with normal renal function may be caused by hormonal, vascular, or stress-related factors.

A variety of drugs and hormones affect the gastric uptake of pertechnetate. Perchlorate suppresses uptake of pertechnetate by the gastric mucosa two- to fourfold.[28,41–44] Although administration of perchlorate has not been known to result in failure to identify a Meckel's diverticulum, this is theoretically possible.

Consequently, premedication with perchlorate in patients undergoing radiopertechnetate abdominal scintigraphy is not recommended. Pentagastrin increases gastric mucosal uptake of pertechnetate, and it has been used to enhance imaging on patients and animals.[41,45–48] Cimetidine, a histamine H_2-receptor antagonist, inhibits release of pertechnetate by the intraluminal cells.[49–51] Glucagon slightly reduces gastric activity of pertechnetate and suppresses peristaltic activity.[52] Other agents that have been investigated include histamine, which has a lesser effect than pentagastrin, and secretin. Secretin has little effect on pertechnetate localization.[30,41]

Imaging

As mentioned above, the patient should not be premedicated with perchlorate. Barium in the abdomen can cause false negative results, so one must ensure that scintigraphy is performed in the absence of barium in the abdomen. All metallic and other radiation-absorbing objects (belt buckles, coins, etc.) must be removed from the patient prior to imaging. The patient should fast for approximately 4 hours before the examination to reduce the size of the gastric silhouette. When available, we routinely use subcutaneous pentagastrin (6 μg/kg) a half hour prior to the administration of pertechnetate to increase its uptake by the gastric mucosa. During imaging, the patient lies supine with the gamma camera viewing the entire abdomen. A high-resolution or ultrahigh-resolution parallel-hole collimator should be used. First, a radionuclide angiogram (1- to 5-second frames for 60 seconds, 128×128 matrix format) is obtained to diagnose vascular malformations and attempt to localize a site of rapid bleeding. Second, a series of 1-minute images is obtained in the anterior projection for 30 minutes (Figs. 8.1 to 8.5). The study should be monitored on the display as it progresses. In cases of strong

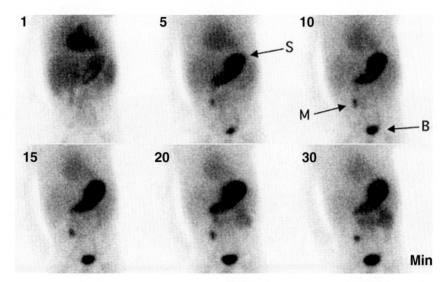

FIGURE 8.1. Meckel's diverticulum. Study from a 21-month-old boy with a recent history of abdominal cramps and large blood clots in the stool 5 days prior to this examination. The patient had an air enema and a barium enema, which were both negative. Selected anterior images taken at 5-minute intervals are shown. In the first image, tracer is seen in the cardiac blood pool, liver, spleen, stomach, and in the vascular and extravascular compartment. Sequential images reveal increasing concentration of tracer in the stomach (S) and decreasing blood pool and background activity. Beginning on the second image, there is a small, intense and well-defined region (M) in the right lower quadrant that concentrates pertechnetate. This area reveals gradual increase of tracer uptake with time that is characteristic of ectopic gastric mucosa in a Meckel's diverticulum. Note tracer accumulating in the bladder (B) and in the small bowel. A Meckel's diverticulum containing gastric mucosa was removed at surgery.

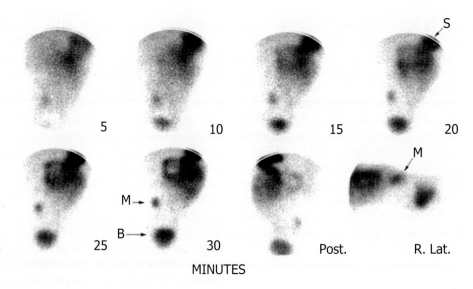

MINUTES

FIGURE 8.2. Meckel's diverticulum. Study from a 4-year-old boy who presented with lower abdominal cramps and guaiac-positive stools. A barium enema demonstrated no evidence of intussusception or polyp. An abnormal accumulation of pertechnetate can be seen in the right lower quadrant (M) that appears at the same time as the gastric activity (S) and increases in intensity with time. The urinary bladder (B) is visible at 10 minutes and increased in intensity during the observation period. A cross-table image reveals the abnormal tracer accumulation to be located anteriorly in the abdomen. At surgery, a Meckel's diverticulum containing gastric mucosa was removed.

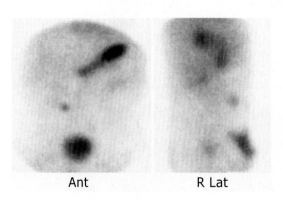

FIGURE 8.3. Meckel's diverticulum. This 2-year-old boy presented with a 3-month history of bloody stools. Selected images at 10 (Ant.) and 15 (R. Lat.) minutes postinjection reveal a small, well-localized area of increased pertechnetate uptake in the right lower quadrant anteriorly.

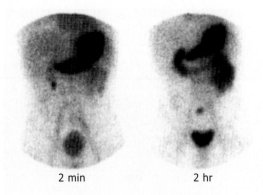

FIGURE 8.4. Meckel's diverticulum. Two selected images from a 2.5-year-old boy with a history of rectal bleeding. The image at 2 minutes did not reveal a clear abnormality. Tracer in the right upper quadrant could have been the duodenum or a highly placed Meckel's diverticulum. The image at 2 hours postinjection reveals a well-defined and focal region of increased pertechnetate concentration that suggests a Meckel's diverticulum containing gastric mucosa.

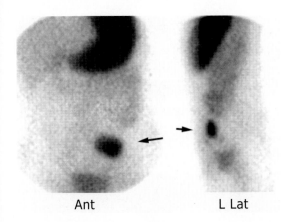

Ant   L Lat

FIGURE 8.5. Meckel's diverticulum, left lower quadrant. Selected anterior (Ant.) and left lateral (L. Lat.) pertechnetate images revealing a rather large and well-defined area of intense pertechnetate concentration in the left lower quadrant anteriorly.

Single photon emission computed tomography (SPECT) has been used to help identify tracer uptake in Meckel's diverticulum obscured by the bladder. Upright anterior and oblique images may assist in differentiating duodenal activity, which will not change position, from ectopic gastric mucosa, which may move more in response to the altered direction of gravitational pull.[18,21,53]

Background activity in the abdomen reflecting blood levels of pertechnetate usually decreases with time and in most cases allows for identification of ectopic gastric mucosa within 30 minutes after injection of pertechnetate. If blood disappearance and gastric uptake of the tracer are slow, as in infants or anemic patients, the scanning time should be prolonged in order to increase the chance for identification of a lesion not visible early in the study.

clinical suspicion, prolonged imaging (images at 1 and/or 2 hours postinjection) may be necessary if the study appears normal.

A lateral image is helpful in determining the anterior position of uptake in a Meckel's diverticulum and to exclude uptake in the genitourinary system. This image should be obtained as soon as a suspicious area of increased activity is visualized on the anterior view to avoid the possibility of being unable to define the abnormal uptake in three dimensions at a later time, because of the possibility of overlap with radiopertechnetate within the intestine. Laterals or posterior images should be obtained at any time after the injection to help localize abnormal tracer uptake. This may confuse untrained observers, especially if the left renal pelvis is obscured by the gastric outline, as it often is. Similarly, tracer in the right renal pelvis should be recognized. Later images, hydration, moving the patient to the upright position to help empty the renal pelvis, posterior and lateral images, and diuretic administration are often helpful maneuvers to help identify potentially confusing concentration of the tracer. Some Meckel's diverticula lie very close to the urinary bladder, preventing detection. Obtaining images with an empty bladder or even after bladder catheterization should be considered part of the routine practice.

Prior Bleeding Study

Yen and Lanoie[54] warned that a pertechnetate study should not be performed after a bleeding study with in vivo labeled red blood cells using [99mTc] and stannous pyrophosphate. These authors reported a case showing blood pool distribution of pertechnetate with absent gastric uptake in a 1-week-old patient who had a recent bleeding study with in vivo stannous pyrophosphate. The scan was considered uninterpretable.

However, Kwok et al.[55] reported a successful Meckel's scan done 26 hours after a labeled RBC study using a commercial in vitro labeling kit, UltraTag (Mallinckrodt Medical, Inc., St. Louis, MO). Normal distribution of [99mTc] was observed. This case demonstrates that it is feasible to perform an in vitro labeled RBC study and to follow-up with a Meckel's scan if necessary. However, the reverse sequence is preferred.

In the in vivo labeling method, the amount of stannous ion in the pyrophosphate kit injected into the patient is quite large (0.4 to 0.9 mg). If pertechnetate is injected afterward, it will be rapidly and efficiently attached to the red blood cells and render a blood pool scan. This effect may last for days. In contrast, the in vitro kit has a very small amount of tin (50 to 96 μg of tin),

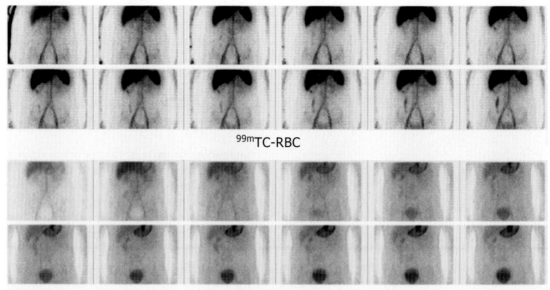

^{99m}TC-RBC

^{99m}TC-Pertechnetate

FIGURE 8.6. Pertechnetate scan following ^{99m}Tc–red blood cell (RBC) study for the detection of bleeding using an in vitro labeling technique. A 15-year-old boy presented with rectal bleeding. A blood pool scan using an in vitro technique demonstrates gas-trointestinal bleeding along the ascending colon (upper panel). A pertechnetate scan performed a day later reveals normal distribution of the tracer (lower panel).

and this factor may explain he differences reported.

In our practice, we have confirmed that a pertechnetate scan can be performed effectively following a bleeding study using the commercially available kit for in vitro RBC labeling. The pertechnetate biodistribution appears not be affected by the prior blood pool study (Fig. 8.6).

Clinical Applications

Normal Pertechnetate Abdominal Scintigraphy

A normal ^{99m}Tc-O$_4^-$ abdominal series reveals rapid gastric uptake followed by a gradual increase of tracer in the wall of the stomach. Some pertechnetate is eliminated into the gastric cavity and transported into the lumen of the duodenum and small intestine. The speed of this transit is variable. In some patients with rapid gastric emptying, tracer in the duodenum

and intestine could interfere with interpretation, but this is rare. The intense gastric outline usually shows a central area of relatively lower concentration of pertechnetate corresponding to the gastric cavity. This area of decreased uptake can be quite large if the patient has eaten before the examination. The bladder (if full) initially contains less tracer activity than background. As radiopertechnetate is eliminated by the kidneys, progressively increasing levels of tracer are evident in the bladder.

Meckel's Diverticulum

A scintigraphic abdominal survey revealing ectopic gastric mucosa is almost unmistakable; in addition to the normal uptake pattern, one can observe a well-defined area of increased radiopertechnetate uptake anteriorly, usually in the right lower quadrant. This abnormal uptake of tracer in the ectopic gastric mucosa appears at the same time as the stomach and persists with increasing intensity as the study progresses

(Figs. 8.1 to 8.5). Rarely, tracer activity in the lesion may fluctuate if intestinal secretions or hemorrhage carry the radiotracer away from the diverticulum.[18] Observation for 30 minutes after injection of the radiopertechnetate is usually sufficient to detect most cases of Meckel's diverticulum containing functioning gastric mucosa.

In questionable cases or cases in which the gastric uptake or the gastric-to-background ratio is low, one should delay the imaging by 1 hour or longer. A potential problem with delayed images is migration of radioactive gastric contents into the duodenum, small bowel, and even large bowel, obscuring uptake within the ectopic gastric mucosa. An alternative is to restudy the patient on another day using pentagastrin (Fig. 8.7).

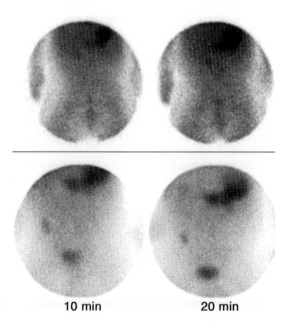

10 min   20 min

FIGURE 8.7. Meckel's diverticulum, use of pentagastrin. Selected images at 10 and 20 minutes of two consecutive pertechnetate studies on the same patient. The study in the upper panel reveals no abnormality. The study following administration of pentagastrin reveals a clearly defined abnormality of pertechnetate uptake in the right lower quadrant corresponding to Meckel's diverticulum containing gastric mucosa (lower panel).

A Meckel's diverticulum may appear to shift in position caudally if the patient is raised or has voided. Only rarely does more than one area of ectopic gastric mucosa occur in the intestine, or does the ectopic mucosa extend beyond the diverticulum, producing a larger area of uptake.[21,32]

Abnormal Uptake Due to Other Causes

Other conditions in the abdomen that accumulate pertechnetate include intestinal obstruction or intussusception,[56] inflammation,[56-58] vascular malformations,[59] ulcers,[57] some tumors,[60,61] and various urinary tract abnormalities that interrupt urinary excretion of the pertechnetate. Certain drugs, such as ethosuximide (Zarontin) or laxatives, may also cause variable uptake of tracer in the intestine. The nature of these findings should be recognized during evaluation of the images, and such findings not be considered falsely positive. They are true abnormalities in the distribution of radiopertechnetate in the abdomen, and experienced physicians will recognize their appearance as different from that of Meckel's diverticulum.

Blood pool tracer activity, as in vascular malformations or hemangiomas, should be apparent on the radionuclide angiogram and initial images and may or may not fade with time.[18,21] However, these lesions do not exhibit a response to pentagastrin.

Other abnormalities that may contain ectopic gastric mucosa include otherwise normal bowel,[32] enteric duplication,[57,62] duplication cysts,[57,63,64] and gastrogenic cysts.[65] As in Meckel's diverticulum, the complications and symptoms in these conditions are due to hydrochloric acid secretion by the gastric mucosal cells, and the treatment is surgical excision.

In Barrett's esophagus, the esophageal mucosa may be lined with gastric epithelium rather than normal squamous epithelium and it takes up pertechnetate, yielding scans with uptake above the stomach.[66] Gastric mucosa that has been moved surgically to an ectopic site in the body will also take up pertechnetate (Fig. 8.8).

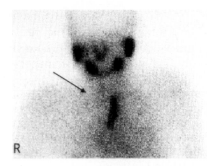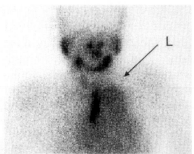

FIGURE 8.8. Gastric mucosal remnant in the mediastinum. These unusual pertechnetate images are from a 12-year-old boy who swallowed caustic material at 2 years of age, damaging his esophagus. He had an esophagectomy and a gastric pull-through at that age. More recently, he underwent a colonic interposition, complicated by mediastinal fluid collection that eventually drained through the neck causing severe local pain. In addition, there was fluid collection in the left chest. The patient had multiple imaging examinations in an attempt to elucidate the problem, without much success. The image obtained at 5 minutes following intravenous administration of pertechnetate reveals exquisite tracer uptake in the region of the mediastinum (left panel, arrow). This was a residual gastric remnant from the surgery to place the colonic interposition. The image on the right panel reveals, in addition, tracer in the left hemithorax, due to gastric secretion from the remnant. The gastric remnant was removed surgically.

Accuracy

Among the surgically proven cases of Meckel's diverticulum in the literature, the accuracy of ^{99m}Tc-O$_4^-$ scintigraphy is 90%. The overall sensitivity among published accounts is 85%, and the specificity is 95%.[21] With meticulous attention to technique, and in the appropriate clinical setting, pertechnetate scintigraphy is an effective method for the detection of Meckel's diverticulum containing functioning gastric mucosa. Prior to use of pertechnetate scintigraphy for Meckel's diverticulum, the lesion was diagnosed at laparotomy in approximately 60% of the symptomatic patients.[67,68]

A normal pertechnetate study does not rule out the presence of a Meckel's diverticulum, however, as ectopic gastric mucosa must be functioning in order to take up pertechnetate. Hypofunction, necrosis, fibrosis, ischemia, or other causes can reduce or even prevent scintigraphic detection.[29,41,69] Low pertechnetate uptake by gastric mucosa in infants may be a cause of false-negative examinations. As the child matures, normal ^{99m}Tc-O$_4^-$ uptake should allow detection of ectopic gastric mucosa. Drug effects and normal structures may obscure ^{99m}Tc-O$_4^-$ uptake by the gastric mucosa in the diverticulum. Because peptic ulceration of the intestinal mucosa is usually responsible for the bleeding, most of the Meckel's diverticula that bleed contain ectopic gastric mucosa. Experiments on animals show that at least 1 to 2 cm^2 of such tissue may be required for the lesion to be visible on scintigraphy.[21,30,70,71] One reported patient whose scan was negative had considerable scarring of the diverticulum and little intact gastric mucosa.[32] In one of our patients, the pertechnetate survey was normal in the presence of a cystic Meckel's diverticulum with fluid within the cyst and necrotic gastric mucosa.

^{99m}Tc-RBC Scintigraphy

Diagnosis of gastrointestinal bleeding from any cause (including bleeding from a Meckel's diverticulum) can be detected and often localized using ^{99m}Tc-labeled RBC scintigraphy. Following intravenous injection, this radiopharmaceutical remains largely within the blood pool and can be visualized with scintigraphy.

Because of their long residence time in the blood pool, ^{99m}Tc-RBCs allow the possibility of localizing intermittent bleeding, as the observation period can be extended for several hours. Bleeding rates detected with ^{99m}Tc-RBC are lower than those detectable by angiography. The bleeding rates detectable with ^{99m}Tc-RBC are 0.4 mL/min in areas of high background and 0.1 mL/min in areas of low background.[72] The sensitivity of this technique, however, depends not only on bleeding rate but also on bowel motility.[73] Another approach to the detection of bleeding employs ^{99m}Tc–sulfur colloid. The advantages of ^{99m}Tc-RBC over ^{99m}Tc–sulfur colloid have been recognized.[74]

Radiopharmaceutical

Red blood cells can be labeled with ^{99m}Tc using an in vivo or an in vitro method. We routinely employ the in vitro method, in which 1 to 3 mL of the patient's blood are drawn and anticoagulated with heparin or acid-citrate dextrose (ACD). Ethylenediaminetetraacetic acid (EDTA) or oxalate must not be used as an anticoagulant. The red blood cells are labeled using a commercial preparation (Ultratag®RBC, Mallinckrodt, St. Louis, Mo.). Technetium-[99m]-labeled RBCs are given in a dose of 0.2 mCi (7.4 MBq)/kg of body weight with a minimum dose of 1.0 mCi (37 MBq) and a maximum dose of 20 mCi (740 MBq). *The labeled red blood cells are reinjected slowly into the patient and only the patient from whom the blood was drawn.*

Imaging

For this method to be most effective, it must be performed while the patient is actually bleeding. Barium within the abdomen as well as photon-absorbing objects on the patient can cause false-negative results, and their presence should be avoided. The patient is positioned supine with the gamma camera equipped with a high-resolution collimator viewing the entire abdomen. The tracer is injected, and a radionuclide angiogram is obtained at a rate of one frame per second for 60 seconds (128 × 128 matrix). The angiogram is immediately followed by serial imaging of the abdomen at one frame per minute for 60 to 90 minutes (128 × 128 matrix). Additional images are obtained at various intervals as needed, up to approximately 24 hours. The radionuclide angiogram and the following serial imaging should be evaluated using a cinematic mode. This is more effective than reviewing series of static images.

Clinical Application

A normal ^{99m}Tc-RBC study will demonstrate tracer within the blood pools of the aorta, inferior vena cava, and other vessels (iliac, portal, mesenteric, renal). Tracer activity can also be seen in the blood pool of the kidneys and penile blood pool. If present in sufficient amount, free pertechnetate can be seen in the kidneys, ureters, and urinary bladder. The observer should be aware of these normal scintigraphic features and not confuse them with bleeding (Fig. 8.9). None of the areas mentioned above changes in location with time, while abnormal tracer concentration associated with bleeding usually shows changes in location.

Bleeding sites are detected by a focal intraluminal accumulation of the radiotracer with a characteristic pattern of increasing tracer in bowel. Blood entering the bowel causes altered motility, and blood may be seen moving forward and backward in the intestine.[75,76] Even massive bleeding can be intermittent. Sometimes bleeding occurs after the initial hour of continuous observation and can only be detected on delayed images. Bleeding in these cases may have occurred during the interval while the patient was not being imaged. If bleeding is detected on delayed imaging and the clinical impression is of active bleeding, a second tracer injection may be of value.[77] Administration of heparin has been suggested as a method of enhancing detection of bleeding sites.[78,79] Reported correct localization of bleeding sites varies from 40% to 90%.[80–84] In most cases, surgery should not be based on scintigraphic appearance alone. There is a need for randomized studies comparing scintigraphy and angiography performed within close proximity of each other.[85] Examples of gastrointestinal bleeding detected with radiolabeled RBCs are illustrated in Figures 8.10 to 8.14).

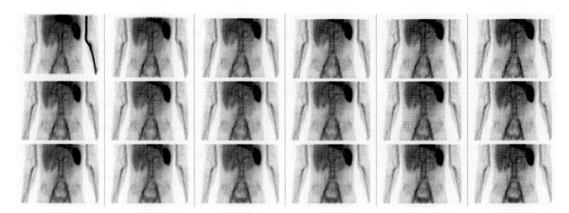

FIGURE 8.9. Normal ^{99m}Tc-RBC blood pool scan. The study reveals no evidence of gastrointestinal bleeding. The patient had hemophilia; the spleen is visualized.

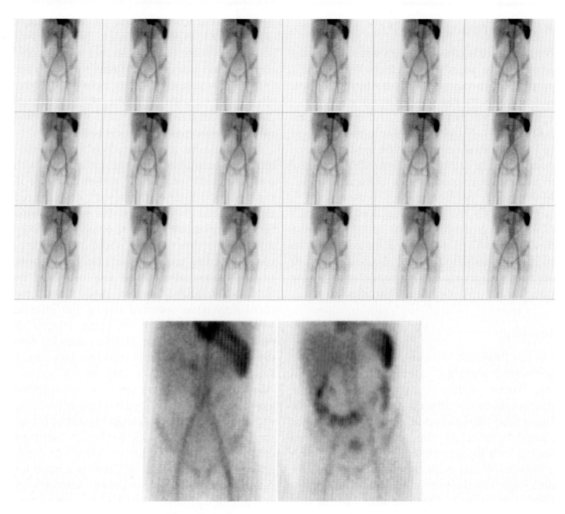

FIGURE 8.10. A 10-year-old with rectal bleeding. Compressed display of initial 60-minute recording (upper panel) reveals no evidence of bleeding. An image at 1.5 hours (lower left) doesn't show bleed-ing. Bleeding into the large bowel is visible; the actual site of bleeding could not be pinpointed, however.

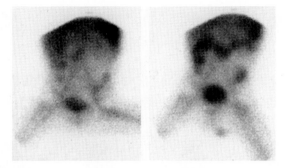

FIGURE 8.11. Massive lower gastrointestinal bleeding. Technetium-99m-RBC scintigraphy from an 18-month-old boy with acute leukemia on treatment presenting with a falling hematocrit and increasingly severe gastrointestinal bleeding. The sequential anterior images reveal abnormal tracer accumulation first at the level of the epigastrium followed by tracer migrating into both the proximal and distal colon. The bleeding was thought to be secondary to chemotherapy-induced enterocolitis. The patient underwent surgery for the removal of part of his colon. At surgery, a swollen colon with marked inflammation with multiple deep linear mucosal ulcerations was noted.

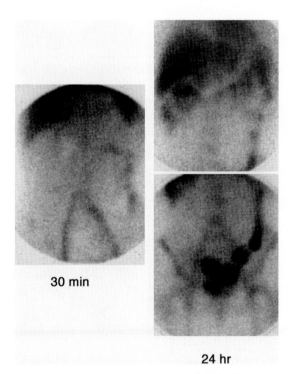

30 min

24 hr

FIGURE 8.12. Massive gastrointestinal bleeding. Technetium-99m-RBC scintigraphy from a teenage girl with uncontrollable gastrointestinal bleeding for several years. The image on the left (30 minutes postinjection) reveals bleeding in a portion of the small bowel. Images 24 hours later (right panel) reveal tracer within the entire course of the colon. The patient had a small bowel resection in which a cluster of veins was found.

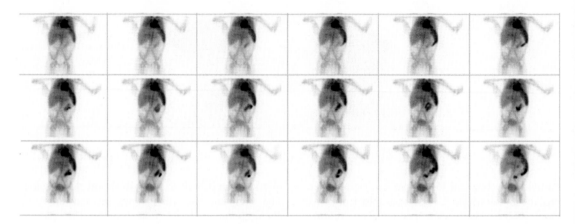

FIGURE 8.13. A ^{99m}Tc-RBC scan from a 6-year-old girl with leukemia and melena. There is rapid accumulation of RBCs in the spleen, and tracer appears in the small bowel in the left upper quadrant near the midline.

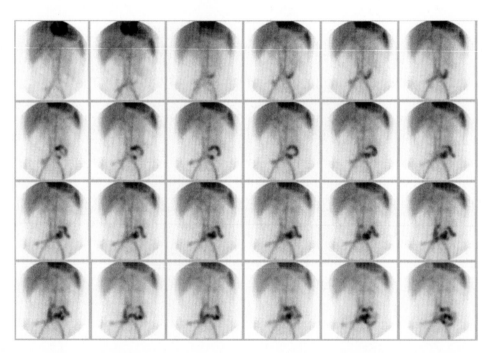

FIGURE 8.14. A ^{99m}Tc-RBC scan from a 16-year-old with severe pulmonary hypertension and a hypercoagulable state treated with anticoagulants. The patient presented with a second episode of massive gastrointestinal bleeding with a hematocrit decrease from 42 to 26 during one day. Bleeding is detected in the small bowel in the left lower quadrant.

Indium-111 (^{111}In) RBC scintigraphy has also been proposed for the detection of gastrointestinal bleeding.[86] The potential advantage of this method is that it permits evaluation beyond 24 hours. The disadvantages are the relatively lower photon flux of ^{111}In than of ^{99m}Tc and the relatively high radiation exposure for the patient.

^{99m}Tc-Sulfur Colloid Scintigraphy

Another scintigraphic method to localize bleeding employs ^{99m}Tc–sulfur colloid. After intravenous injection, ^{99m}Tc–sulfur colloid is extracted rapidly from the blood by cells of the reticuloendothelial system with a normal half-time in blood of 2.5 to 3.5 minutes.

The patient is examined supine with the gamma camera, which is equipped with a high-resolution collimator viewing the entire abdomen. Technetium-^{99m}–sulfur colloid is given in a dose of 0.05 mCi/kg (1.85 MBq/kg) with a minimum total dose of 0.1 mCi (3.7 MBq) and a maximum total dose of 3.0 mCi (111 MBq). The study is recorded at 1 frame per minute for 30 minutes on a 128×128 matrix format.

If bleeding occurs during the tracer's presence in the blood pool, it extravasates, and this can be detected scintigraphically. Because of the high bleeding-to-background activity ratio achievable with this tracer, small amounts of bleeding may be detected. In the gastrointestinal tract, this technique has detected bleeding at rates as low as 0.05 to 0.1 mL/min.[87–89] Bleeding rates of 0.1 to 0.2 mL/min have been detected in dogs.[90] In patients who have intermittent bleeding, the "window of opportunity" for the detection of bleeding with colloid is very small. Another disadvantage of this method is the intense accumulation of sulfur colloid in the liver and spleen, which may obscure bleeding in this region.

References

1. Neff G. Sas Meckelsche Divertikel. Ergeb Chir Orthop 1937;30:227–315.
2. DeBartolo HM Jr, van Heerden JA. Meckel's diverticulum. Ann Surg 1976;183:30–3.
3. Berquist TH, Nolan NG, Carlson HC, et al. Diagnosis of Barrett's esophagus by pertechnetate scintigraphy. Mayo Clin Proc 1973;48:276–9.
4. Rosenthall L, Henry JN, Murphy DA, et al. Radiopertechnetate imaging of the Meckel's diverticulum. Radiology 1972;105:371–3.
5. Rutherford RB, Akers DR. Meckel's diverticulum: a review of 148 pediatric patients, with special reference to the pattern of bleeding and to mesodiverticular vascular bands. Surgery 1966;59:618–26.
6. Kilpatrick JM. Scanning in diagnosis of Meckel's diverticulum. Hosp Pract 1974;9:131–8.
7. Kilpatrick ZM, Aseron CA, Jr. Radioisotope detection of Meckel's diverticulum causing acute rectal hemorrhage. N Engl J Med 1972;287:653–4.
8. Martin GI, Kutner FR, Moser L. Diagnosis of Meckel's diverticulum by radioisotope scanning. Pediatrics 1976;57:11–12.
9. Canty T, Meguid MM, Eraklis AJ. Perforation of Meckel's diverticulum scan (letter to the editor). Surgery 1972;71:313.
10. Meguid MM, Wilkinson RH, Canty T, et al. Futility of barium sulfate in diagnosis of bleeding Meckel diverticulum. Arch Surg 1974;108:361–2.
11. Harden R, Alexander WD. Isotope uptake and scanning of stomach in man with ^{99m}Tc-pertechnetate. Lancet 1967;1:1305–7.
12. Jewett TC, Jr., Duszynski DO, Allen JE. The visualization of Meckel's diverticulum with ^{99m}Tc-pertechnetate. Surgery 1970;68:567–70.
13. Bauer R, van de Flierdt E, Schroter G, et al. [Scintigraphic detection of gastrointestinal hemorrhage and ectopic mucosa.] Z Gastroenterol Verh 1991;26:117–24.
14. Datz FL, Christian PE, Hutson WR, et al. Physiological and pharmacological interventions in radionuclide imaging of the tubular gastrointestinal tract. Semin Nucl Med 1991;21:140–52.
15. Giorgetti R, Dottorini M, Cazzani M, et al. [Meckel's diverticulum: the usefulness of ^{99m}Tc pertechnetate scintigraphy.] Minerva Pediatr 1990;42:349–50.
16. Joseph K. [Nuclear medicine methods for the detection of gastrointestinal hemorrhages.] Dtsch Med Wochenschr 1993;118:109–12.
17. Sfakianakis GN, Conway JJ. Detection of ectopic gastric mucosa in Meckel's diverticulum and in other aberrations by scintigraphy: I. Pathophysiology and 10-year clinical experience. J Nucl Med 1981;22:647–54.

18. Sfakianakis GN, Conway JJ. Detection of ectopic gastric mucosa in Meckel's diverticulum and in other aberrations by scintigraphy: II. Indications and methods—a 10-year experience. J Nucl Med 1981;22:732–8.

19. Tauscher JW, Bryant DR, Gruenther RC. False positive scan for Meckel diverticulum. J Pediatr 1978;92:1022–3.

20. Valenza V, Salvatori M, Calisti A, et al. [Scintigraphic diagnosis of Meckel's diverticulum using Tc-^{99m}-pertechnetate.] Minerva Dietol Gastroenterol 1990;36:139–43.

21. Sfakianakis GN, Anderson GF, King DR, et al. The effect of gastrointestinal hormones on the pertechnetate imaging of ectopic gastric mucosa in experimental Meckel's diverticulum. J Nucl Med 1981;22:678–83.

22. Bree RL, Reuter SR. Angiographic demonstration of a bleeding Meckel's diverticulum. Radiology 1973;108:287–8.

23. Dalinka MK, Wunder JF. Meckel's diverticulum and its complications, with emphasis on roentgenologic demonstration. Radiology 1973;106:295–8.

24. Faris HC, Whitley JE. Angiographic demonstration of Meckel's diverticulum. Case report and review of the literature. Radiology 1973;108:285–6.

25. Conway JJ. Radionuclide diagnosis of Meckel's diverticulum. Gastrointest Radiol 1980;5:209–13.

26. Keramidas DC, Coran AG, Zaleska RW. An experimental model for assessing the radiopertechnetate diagnosis of gastric mucosa in Meckel's diverticulum. J Pediatr Surg 1974;9:879–83.

27. Meier-Ruge W, Fridrich R. [Distribution of technetium-99m and iodine-131 in the gastric mucosa. Microhistoautoradiography method using water-soluble isotopes.] Histochemie 1969;19:147–54.

28. Wine CR, Nahrwold DL, Waldhausen JA. Role of the technetium scan in the diagnosis of Meckel's diverticulum. J Pediatr Surg 1974;9:885–8.

29. Wine CR, Nahrwold DL, Rose RC, et al. Effect of histamine on technetium-99m excretion by gastric mucosa. Surgery 1976;80:591–4.

30. Priebe CJ Jr, Marsden DS, Lazarevic B. The use of 99m technetium pertechnetate to detect transplanted gastric mucosa in the dog. J Pediatr Surg 1974;9:605–13.

31. Berquist TH, Nolan NG, Stephens DH, et al. Radioisotope scintigraphy in diagnosis of Barrett's esophagus. AJR Radium Ther Nucl Med 1975;123:401–11.

32. Berquist TH, Nolan NG, Stephens DH, et al. Specificity of ^{99m}Tc-pertechnetate in scintigraphic diagnosis of Meckel's diverticulum: review of 100 cases. J Nucl Med 1976;17:465–9.

33. Chaudhuri TK. Letter: Cellular site of secretion of ^{99m}TcO$_4$ in the stomach—a controversial point. J Nucl Med 1975;16:1204–5.

34. Chaudhuri T, Polak JJ. Autoradiographic studies of distribution in the stomach of ^{99m}Tc-pertechnetate. Radiology 1977;123:223–4.

35. Taylor AT Jr, Alazraki N, Henry JE. Intestinal concentration of ^{99m}Tc-pertechnetate into isolated loops of rat bowel. J Nucl Med 1976;17:470–2.

36. Winter PF. Letter: Cellular site of ^{99m}TcO$_4$ secretion in the stomach. J Nucl Med 1976;17:756–7.

37. Harper PV, Andros G, Lathrop K. Preliminary observations on the use of six-hour Tc99m as a tracer in biology and medicine. Semiannual Reports to the U.S. Atomic Energy Commission, Vol. 4, Parts 16–20, 1961 to 1963. Chicago: Argonne Cancer Research Hospital, 1962:76–88.

38. Harper PV, Lathrop KA, Jiminez F, et al. Technetium-99m as a Scanning Agent. Radiology 1965;85:101–9.

39. Lathrop KA, Harper PV. Biologic behavior of 99m Tc from ^{99m} Tc-pertechnetate ion. Prog Nucl Med 1972;1:145–62.

40. Loken MK, Telander GT, Salmon RJ. Technetium-99m compounds for visualization of body organs. JAMA 1965;194:152–6.

41. Khettery J, Effmann E, Grand RJ, et al. Effect of pentagastrin, histalog, glucagon, secretin, and perchlorate on the gastric handling of 99mTc pertechnetate in mice. Radiology 1976;120:629–31.

42. Marsden DS, Priebe CJ, Jr. Preliminary appraisal of present ^{99m}Tc-pertechnetate techniques for detecting ectopic gastric mucosa. Radiology 1974;113:459–60.

43. Oldendorf WH, Sisson WB, Lisaka Y. Compartmental redistribution of ^{99m}Tc-pertechnetate in the presence of perchlorate ion and its relation to plasma protein binding. J Nucl Med 1970;11:85–8.

44. Seltzer MH, Conte PJ Jr, Rickert RR, et al. Diagnosis of a bleeding Meckel's diverticulum using radiopertechnetate. Am J Gastroenterol 1977;67:235–9.

45. Holder LE, Ashare AB, Smith W, et al. Pentagastrin: a new drug for stimulating gastric secretion of pertechnetate. J Nucl Med 1975;16:535–6(abstr).

46. Jewett TJ, Lebowitz R, Treves S. Search for Meckel's diverticulum (letter to the editor and response). Surgery 1972;72:492–3.

47. Johnson LR. The trophic action of gastrointestinal hormones. Gastroenterology 1976;70:278–88.

48. Treves S, Grand RJ, Eraklis AJ. Pentagastrin stimulation of technetium-99m uptake by ectopic gastric mucosa in a Meckel's diverticulum. Radiology 1978;128:711–12.

49. Diamond RH, Rothstein RD, Alavi A. The role of cimetidine-enhanced technetium-99m-pertechnetate imaging for visualizing Meckel's diverticulum. J Nucl Med 1991;32:1422–4.

50. Petrokubi RJ, Baum S, Rohrer GV. Cimetidine administration resulting in improved pertechnetate imaging of Meckel's diverticulum. Clin Nucl Med 1978;3:385–8.

51. Sagar VV, Piccone JM. The gastric uptake and secretion of Tc-99m pertechnetate after H2 receptor blockage in dogs. J Nucl Med 1980; 21:67(abstr).

52. Necheles H, Sporn J, Walker L. Effect of glucagon on gastrointestinal motility. Am J Gastroenterol 1966;45:34–9.

53. Singh PR, Russell CD, Dubovsky EV, et al. Technique of scanning for Meckel's diverticulum. Clin Nucl Med 1978;3:188–92.

54. Yen CK, Lanoie Y. Effect of stannous pyrophosphate red blood cell gastrointestinal bleeding scan on subsequent Meckel's scan. Clin Nucl Med 1992;17:454–6.

55. Kwok CG, Lull RJ, Yen CK, et al. Feasibility of Meckel's scan after RBC gastrointestinal bleeding study using in-vitro labeling technique. Clin Nucl Med 1995;20:959–61.

56. Duszynski DO, Jewett TC, Allen JE. Tc 99m Na pertechnetate scanning of the abdomen with particular reference to small bowel pathology. AJR Radium Ther Nucl Med 1971;113:258–62.

57. Ho JE, Gleason WA, Thompson JS. The expanding spectrum of disease demonstrable by Tc-99m pertechnetate. J Nucl Med 1978;19:691(abstr).

58. Lunia S, Lunia C, Chandramouly B, et al. Radionuclide Meckelogram with particular reference to false-positive results. Clin Nucl Med 1979;4:285–8.

59. Chaudhuri TK, Christie JH. False positive Meckel's diverticulum scan. Surgery 1972;71:313.

60. Polga JP. Nasogastric suction to improve gastrointestinal scanning. J Nucl Med 1974;15:374.

61. Smith RK, Arterburn G. Detection and localization of gastrointestinal bleeding using Tc-99m-pyrophosphate in vivo labeled red blood cells. Clin Nucl Med 1980;5:55–60.

62. Wilson JP, Wenzel WW, Campbell JB. Technetium scans in the detection of gastrointestinal hemorrhage. Preoperative diagnosis of enteric duplication in an infant. JAMA 1977; 237:265–6.

63. Rodgers BM, Youssef S. "False positive" scan for Meckel diverticulum. J Pediatr 1975;87:239–40.

64. Winter PF. Sodium pertechnetate Tc 99m scanning of the abdomen. Diagnosis of an ileal duplication cyst. JAMA 1977;237:1352–3.

65. Mark R, Young L, Ferguson C, et al. Diagnosis of an intrathoracic gastrogenic cyst using ^{99m}Tc-pertechnetate. Radiology 1973;109:137–8.

66. Berquist TH, Nolan NG, Adson MA, et al. Diagnosis of Meckel's diverticulum by radioisotope scanning. Mayo Clin Proc 1973;48:98–102.

67. Jaros R, Schussheim A, Levy LM. Preoperative diagnosis of bleeding Meckel's diverticulum utilizing 99m technetium pertechnetate scintiimaging. J Pediatr 1973;82:45–9.

68. Seitz W, Keim HJ, Hahn K. Abdominal scintigraphy for diagnosis of intestinal bleeding. World J Surg 1978;2:613–18.

69. Moss AA, Kressel HY. Intestinal infarction: current problems and new methods of diagnosis using radionuclide scans. Appl Radiol Nucl Med 1976:156–60.

70. Anderson GF, Sfakianakis G, King DR, et al. Hormonal enhancement of technetium-99m pertechnetate uptake in experimental Meckel's diverticulum. J Pediatr Surg 1980;15:900–5.

71. Conway JJ. The sensitivity, specificity and accuracy of radionuclide imaging of Meckel's diverticulum. J Nucl Med 1976;17:553(abstr).

72. Chandeysson PD, Hanson RJ, Watson CE, et al. Minimum gastrointestinal bleeding detectable by abdominal scintigraphy. J Nucl Med 1983; 24:97(abstr).

73. Smith RK, Arterburn JG. The advantages of delayed imaging and radiographic correlation in scintigraphic localization of gastrointestinal bleeding. Radiology 1981;139:471–2.

74. Bunker SR, Lull RJ, Tanasescu DE, et al. Scintigraphy of gastrointestinal hemorrhage: superiority of ^{99m}Tc red blood cells over 99mTc sulfur colloid. AJR 1984;143:543–8.

75. Starshak RJ, Sty JR. Trends in physiologic and pharmacologic interventions in pediatric nuclear medicine. Pediatr Ann 1992;21:101–9.

76. Wise PA, Saga W. Retrograde flow pattern on a gastrointestinal bleeding scan. Clin Nucl Med 1982;23:315–18.

77. Jacobson AF, Cerqueira MD. Prognostic significance of late imaging results in technetium-99m-

labeled red blood cell gastrointestinal bleeding studies with early negative images. J Nucl Med 1992;33:202–7.

78. Chaudhuri TK, Brantly M. Heparin as a pharmacologic intervention to induce positive scintiscan in occult gastrointestinal bleeding. Clin Nucl Med 1984;9:187–8.

79. Murphy WD, Di Simone RN, Wolf BH, et al. The use of heparin to facilitate bleeding in technetium-99m RBC imaging. J Nucl Med 1988;29:725–6.

80. Bentley DE, Richardson JD. The role of tagged red blood cell imaging in the localization of gastrointestinal bleeding. Arch Surg 1991;126:821–4.

81. Gupta S, Luna E, Kingsley S, et al. Detection of gastrointestinal bleeding by radionuclide scintigraphy. Am J Gastroenterol 1984;79:26–31.

82. Nicholson ML, Neoptolemos JP, Sharp JF, et al. Localization of lower gastrointestinal bleeding using in vivo technetium-99m-labelled red blood cell scintigraphy. Br J Surg 1989;76:358–61.

83. Orecchia PM, Hensley EK, McDonald PT, et al. Localization of lower gastrointestinal hemorrhage. Experience with red blood cells labeled in vitro with technetium Tc 99m. Arch Surg 1985;120:621–4.

84. Winzelberg GG, McKusick KA, Strauss HW, et al. Evaluation of gastrointestinal bleeding by red blood cells labeled in vivo with technetium-99m. J Nucl Med 1979;20:1080–6.

85. Zuckerman DA, Bocchini TP, Birnbaum EH. Massive hemorrhage in the lower gastrointestinal tract in adults: diagnostic imaging and intervention. AJR 1993;161:703–11.

86. Ferrant A, Dehasque N, Leners N, et al. Scintigraphy with In-111-labeled red cells in intermittent gastrointestinal bleeding. J Nucl Med 1980;21:844–5.

87. Alavi A. Scintigraphic demonstration of acute gastrointestinal bleeding. Gastrointest Radiol 1980;5:205–8.

88. Alavi A. Detection of gastrointestinal bleeding with 99mTc-sulfur colloid. Semin Nucl Med 1982;12:126–38.

89. Alavi A, Dann RW, Baum S, et al. Scintigraphic detection of acute gastrointestinal bleeding. Radiology 1977;124:753–6.

90. Barry J, Alazraki NP, Heaphy JH. Scintigraphic detection of intrapulmonary bleeding using technetium-99m sulfur colloid: concise communication. J Nucl Med 1981;22:777–80.

9
Liver and Spleen

S.T. Treves and A.G. Jones

This chapter discusses hepatobiliary scintigraphy, reticuloendothelial system (RES) scintigraphy, and splenic scintigraphy. Hepatobiliary scintigraphy employs intravenously injected radiopharmaceuticals that are rapidly taken up by the parenchymal cells of the liver and eliminated through the biliary system into the intestine. Reticuloendothelial system scintigraphy employs technetium-99m (^{99m}Tc)–sulfur colloid, which permits static imaging-planar scintigraphy and single photon emission computed tomography (SPECT) of functional hepatic parenchyma by its localization in cells of the RES. It permits evaluation of size, position, displacement, and replacement of functional hepatic and splenic tissue. At present, hepatobiliary scintigraphy is used in pediatric practice more frequently than static RES scintigraphy.

Ultrasonography, computed tomography (CT), and magnetic resonance imaging (MRI) have largely replaced RES scintigraphy for the morphologic evaluation of the liver. The spleen can be imaged with ^{99m}Tc–sulfur colloid scintigraphy, but the method of choice for splenic scintigraphy is with ^{99m}Tc-labeled denatured red blood cells (^{99m}Tc–denatured RBC scintigraphy). Indications for hepatic and splenic scintigraphy in pediatrics are listed in Tables 9.1 and 9.2.

Methods

Hepatobiliary Scintigraphy

Radiopharmaceuticals

The knowledge that organic dyes are localized in the liver led to the first successful hepatobiliary imaging agent, iodine-131 (^{131}I)–rose bengal, devised by Taplin et al.[1] in 1955. Modern hepatobiliary agents are labeled with ^{99m}Tc (Fig. 9.1).

Administered Doses

Technetium-99m disofenin (Hepatolite, CIS-US, Bedford, MA) is given in a dose of 0.05 mCi/kg (1.85 MBq) with a minimum total dose of 0.25 mCi (9.25 MBq) and a maximum total dose of 3.0 mCi (111 MBq).

Imaging Method

The patient should fast for 3 to 4 hours prior to the examination to facilitate visualization of the gallbladder. In infants the principal indication is determination of the patency of the biliary tract and not the visualization of the gallbladder. Therefore, fasting prior to hepatobiliary scintigraphy is not absolutely necessary in most infants.

TABLE 9.1. Indications for hepatobiliary scintigraphy in pediatric patients

Biliary atresia versus neonatal hepatitis
Right upper quadrant pain/cholecystitis
Postoperative/Kasai operation
Choledochal cyst
Liver transplantation
Right upper quadrant mass
Trauma
Congenital malformations

TABLE 9.2. Indications for splenic scintigraphy in pediatric patients

Heterotaxia (polysplenia, asplenia)
Functional asplenia
Abdominal trauma
Accessory spleen(s)
Splenosis
Infarction

Patients are studied in the supine position with the gamma camera equipped with high-resolution, parallel-hole collimator viewing the entire abdomen including the liver. Intravenous access is gained using a butterfly-type needle that is securely fastened to the skin with tape and kept patent with normal saline until the time of radiopharmaceutical administration. After the patient is positioned under the gamma camera, the radiopharmaceutical is injected as a bolus and flushed with normal saline. Recording begins simultaneously with the start of the injection.

The hepatobiliary study is recorded with serial 0.5-minute frames for 60 minutes using a 128×128 matrix (Fig. 9.1). Additional images are obtained at later intervals (i.e., 2, 4, 6, and 24 hours) or until radiotracer appears in the bowel. If the gallbladder fails to empty significantly during the initial 60-minute period, an additional series of images (one frame per minute for 60 minutes) is obtained following the administration of a cholecystokinin analogue or a standard fatty meal. If a biliary leak is suspected, additional images in various projections are obtained in order to identify any abnormal collection of tracer.

Pharmacologic Interventions

A cholecystokinin analogue (Kinevac, sincalide; Bracco Diagnostics, Princeton, NJ)[2] or a

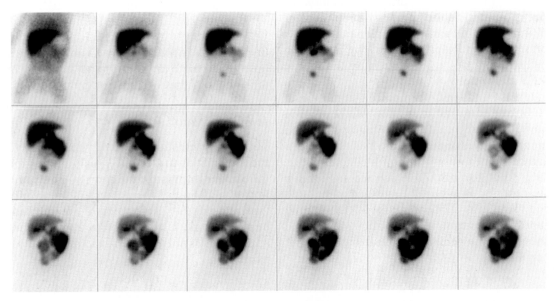

FIGURE 9.1. Normal ^{99m}Tc-disofenin hepatobiliary scintigraphy in a young infant. There is normal blood clearance and hepatic uptake of the tracer. Tracer appears in the bowel within 10 minutes. The gallbladder is visualized at approximately 30 minutes. Each image represents 3 minutes, anterior projection.

fatty meal (Lipomul; Roberts Laboratories, Eatontown, NJ) may be given to stimulate gallbladder contraction. Sincalide (0.02 µg/kg, 1.4 µg/70 kg) given intravenously over a 30- to 60-second interval causes prompt contraction of the gallbladder that becomes maximum in 5 to 15 minutes.

In jaundiced neonates pretreatment with phenobarbital is frequently used to increase bile secretion and, therefore, to help improve differentiation of neonatal hepatitis and biliary atresia (phenobarbital 5 mg/kg/day divided into two equal doses for 3 to 5 days prior to hepatobiliary scintigraphy).

Evaluation

The physician should evaluate the study on a computer monitor in a cinematic mode. Varying the playback speed and contrast are helpful for assessment of bile flow. Evaluation of the later static images directly on the computer monitor is useful to ascertain the presence and nature of any extrahepatic tracer activity. Evaluation of time-activity curves from regions of interest over the cardiac blood pool, liver, and abdomen complements assessment of the images.

Reticuloendothelial System Scintigraphy

Although rarely used at present, RES scintigraphy is discussed for the sake of completeness. All metallic and other photon-absorbing objects are removed from the patient's clothing before imaging. It should be noted that barium in the abdomen from previous radiographic procedures causes artifacts on ^{99m}Tc-sulfur colloid imaging.

Radiopharmaceutical

Technetium-99m–sulfur colloid in a dose of 0.05 mCi/kg (1.85 MBq), with a minimal total dose of 0.1 mCi (3.7 MBq) and a maximum total dose of 3.0 mCi (111 MBq) is administered intravenously 10 to 15 minutes prior to imaging. After intravenous injection, ^{99m}Tc–sulfur colloid is rapidly absorbed by cells of the RES in the liver (Kupffer's cells), spleen, and bone marrow. The normal circulating half-time of

this radiotracer in adults is approximately 2.5 minutes. The size of colloidal particles is 0.01 to 1.0 µm. Approximately 80% to 90% of the radiocolloid is taken up by the liver, 5% to 10% by the spleen, and the remainder by the bone marrow. Once absorbed, the colloidal particles have an effective half-life equal to the physical half-life of ^{99m}Tc.[3]

Imaging Method

Patients are imaged in the supine position. For planar studies, imaging is carried out using a parallel-hole, high- or ultrahigh-resolution collimator. Electronic magnification (zoom) is used for small children. Images of 500,000 counts are obtained in the anterior, posterior, right and left lateral, right and left posterior oblique, and right and left anterior oblique projections (256 × 256 matrix). Magnification scintigraphy with the pinhole collimator (2 mm) is useful for evaluating small children's organs and questionable areas on planar scintigraphy. Single photon emission computed tomography is carried out with the patient in the supine position. The same dose of ^{99m}Tc–sulfur colloid as above is given. SPECT recording consists of images 360 degrees around the body on a 128 × 128 matrix format. It is evaluated using volume- and surface-rendered images, as well as through transverse, coronal, and sagittal slices (Fig. 9.2).

Splenic Scintigraphy (^{99m}Tc-Denatured RBCs)

Splenic scintigraphy is done using ^{99m}Tc-labeled denatured RBCs. A specimen (1 to 3 mL) of the patient's blood is drawn and anticoagulated with heparin or acid-citrate dextrose (ACD). Do not use ethylenediaminetetraacetic acid (EDTA) or oxalate as an anticoagulant. Red blood cells are labeled using a commercial preparation (Ultratag RBC, Mallinckrodt, Maryland Heights, MO). After the labeling procedure, the RBCs are denatured by incubating the tube containing the blood in a constant-temperature bath at 49.5°C for 12 to 15 minutes. The denatured RBCs are reinjected slowly into the patient. *The labeled blood cells*

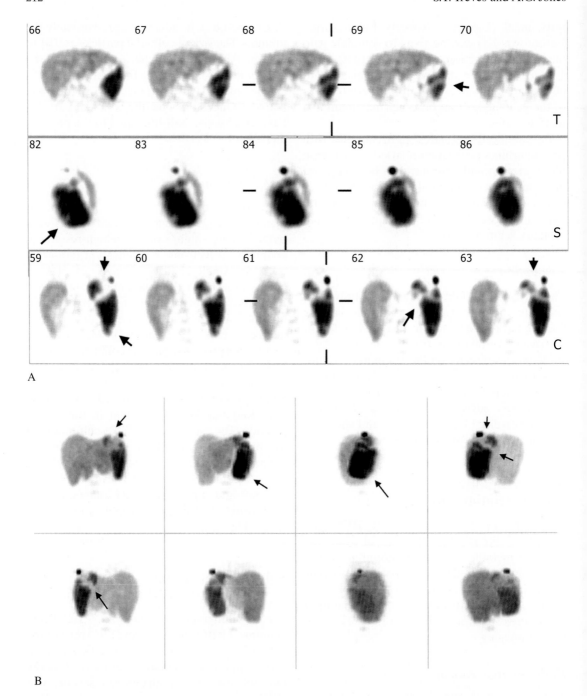

FIGURE 9.2. Splenic infarction. Technetium-99m–sulfur colloid study in a 12-year-old boy with subbacterial endocarditis and recent episode of septic emboli to the brain, kidneys, and spleen. A: Single photon emission computed tomography (SPECT) reveals splenomegaly with several splenic defects presumably due to infarcts (arrows). B: Volume-rendered images from the same study.

must be reinjected only into the patient from whom the blood was drawn. Splenic imaging can begin 15 minutes after injection.

Anterior, posterior, left and right posterior obliques, and left lateral projections are obtained using the high- or ultrahigh-resolution collimator. Images are recorded for 300,000 to 500,000 counts each on a 256 × 256 matrix. The pinhole collimator (2mm) or SPECT is helpful in some patients for obtaining more detailed assessment.

Clinical Applications

Neonatal Jaundice

Neonatal hepatitis is difficult to differentiate from biliary atresia because these two conditions have similar clinical, biochemical, and histologic features (Figs. 9.3 to 9.7). Early diagnosis of biliary atresia is important because the results of surgical intervention are most successful during the first 2 weeks of life. In contrast, surgery is not indicated in patients with neonatal hepatitis.[4]

Clinical Characteristics

Neonatal hepatitis is almost four times more common in male infants, and biliary atresia is encountered twice as often in females. A wide variation and overlap of these two diseases must be kept in mind. Clinical criteria provide some help in differentiation of neonatal hepatitis from biliary atresia. Biliary atresia is accompanied by familial incidence, low birth weight for gestational age, associated anomalies, hemolytic anemia, and splenomegaly.

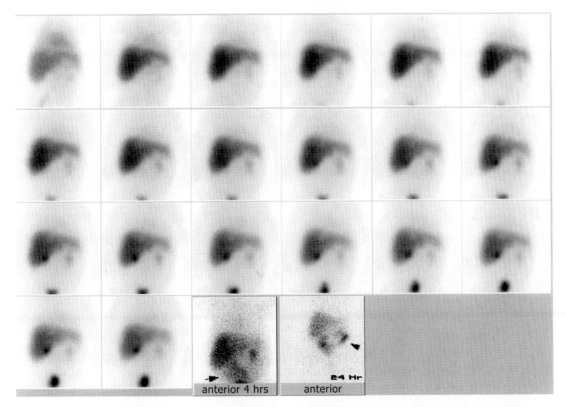

FIGURE 9.3. Hepatocellular disease in a 2-week-old boy with jaundice (^{99m}Tc-disofenin 60-minute dynamic study, each image represents 3 minutes). Hepatic uptake of the tracer is lower than normal, and renal excretion (9–12 minutes) of the radio- pharmaceutical into the bladder (15 minutes) is evident. The gallbladder is visible at approximately 25 minutes; however, no evidence of intestinal tracer activity is detected at 1 hour. Images at 4 and 24 hours demonstrate tracer in the bowel (arrows).

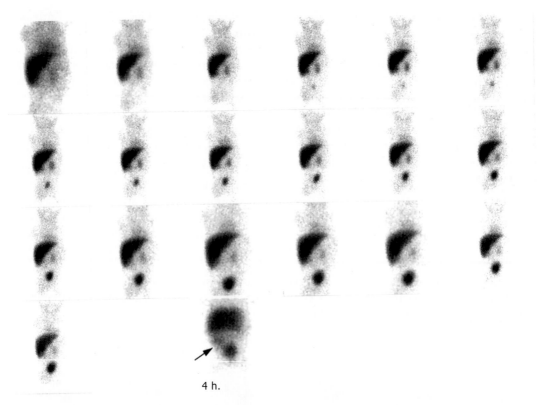

4 h.

FIGURE 9.4. Hepatocellular disease in a 3-month-old boy with jaundice (^{99m}Tc-disofenin, 60-minute dynamic study, each image represents 3 minutes). Hepatic uptake of the radiopharmaceutical appears adequate. Renal excretion of the tracer into the bladder is visible early (12 minutes) in the study. The image at 4 hours reveals tracer in the bowel (arrow).

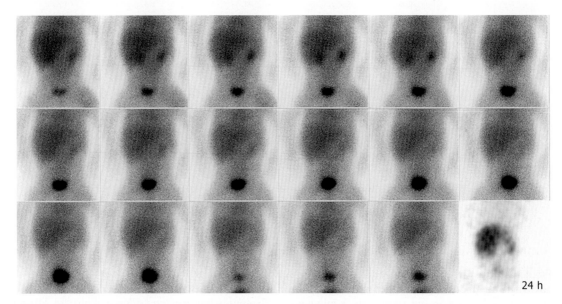

24 h

FIGURE 9.5. Severe hepatocellular disease in a 1-month-old boy with severe jaundice and high bilirubin level. The ^{99m}Tc-disofenin study reveals poor extraction by the liver, high blood level, and significant urinary excretion of the tracer. An anterior image at 24 hours reveals tracer in the liver, kidneys, and bladder without evidence of tracer in the bowel.

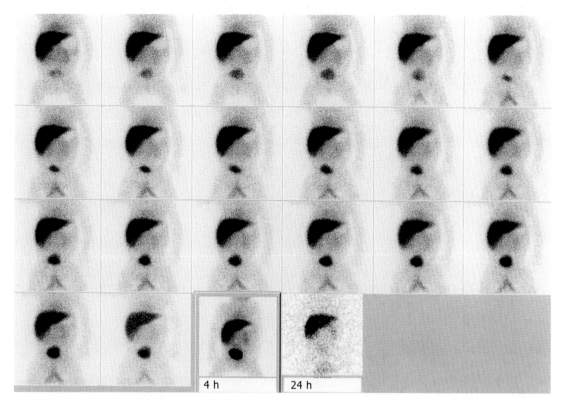

4 h

24 h

FIGURE 9.6. Biliary atresia. A ^{99m}Tc-disofenin study in a 1-month-old boy with conjugated hyperbilirubinemia. Tracer is rapidly taken up by the liver. Renal excretion of the radiotracer is high. However, there is no evidence of tracer in the intestine during the initial hour of the study, nor at 4 or 24 hours.

These factors are not usually encountered in patients with neonatal hepatitis, which tends to occur in otherwise healthy infants between 1 and 4 weeks of age.[5] Patients with hepatitis have splenomegaly and jaundice, and with time they may develop cirrhosis. The pathologic findings vary, but in general multinucleated giant cells are present (as they are in some other liver diseases). The canaliculi are free of bile, and there is parenchymal disorganization.

Etiology

Neonatal hepatitis has been associated with a number of entities affecting the liver during the neonatal period: infectious agents (cytomegalovirus, hepatitis A and B, rubella, toxoplasma, spirochetes) and metabolic factors (α_1-antitrypsin deficiency, inborn errors of metabolism). With neonatal hepatitis the intrahepatic and extrahepatic biliary system is patent but small. Biliary atresia and neonatal hepatitis are most likely variations of the same process.[6] With biliary atresia there is sclerosing cholangitis of the extrahepatic biliary system and sometimes progressive occlusion of bile ducts after birth. In patients with biliary atresia, the major biliary ducts are partially or totally absent. Periportal fibrosis and intrahepatic proliferation of small bile ducts are characteristic, but there is no dilation of these intrahepatic ducts. Cirrhosis of the liver ultimately develops unless surgical correction is successful.

Differential Diagnosis

Clinical and laboratory diagnosis of biliary atresia is difficult and often impossible. Morphologic imaging can be useful if it demonstrates a patent biliary tree, and hepatobiliary scintigraphy can rule out biliary atresia when it demonstrates passage of the radiotracer into the bowel. If passage of tracer into the bowel cannot be demonstrated, scinti-

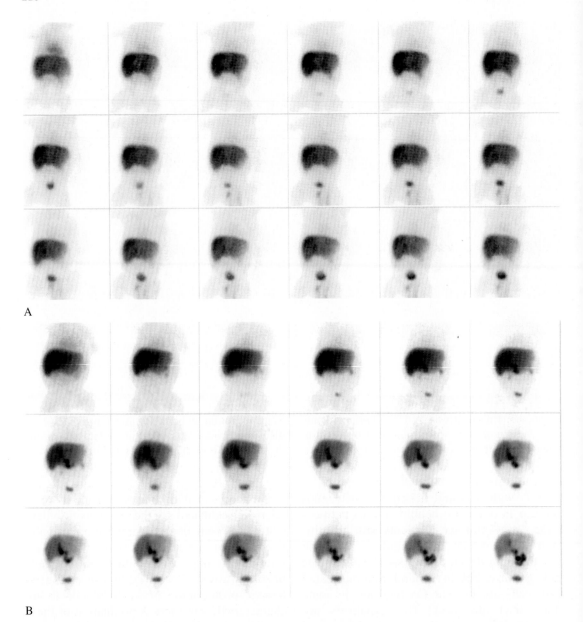

A

B

FIGURE 9.7. Biliary atresia. A: ^{99m}Tc-disofenin study in a 2-month-old boy with jaundice. The study reveals hepatomegaly, renal excretion of the tracer, and no evidence of bowel activity up to 24 hours (image not shown). B: Same patient after surgery for a choledo-chojejunal anastomosis (Kasai procedure). There is greater initial ^{99m}Tc-disofenin uptake by the liver, less renal excretion of the tracer, and passage of radiolabeled bile though the anastomosis into the bowel.

graphic distinction between biliary atresia and severe hepatocellular disease cannot be made with certainty.[7-10] Repeat hepatobiliary scintigraphy after a few days may be helpful in those patients in whom excretion of tracer in the bowel is not demonstrated in a single examination. A definitive diagnosis can be made by percutaneous transhepatic cholangiography, laparotomy, laparoscopy, or analysis of duodenal fluids.[11-14]

Gerhold et al.[15] have demonstrated the accuracy (91%), sensitivity (97%), and specificity (82%) of hepatobiliary imaging in the diagnosis of biliary atresia. They proposed a visual grading that includes the assessment of hepatocyte clearance and timing of radiotracer appearance in the intestine or extrahepatic biliary system. Hepatocyte clearance was graded by visually comparing hepatic activity with cardiac blood pool activity on the 5-minute image. The studies were categorized as normal when hepatocyte clearance was normal and radiotracer appeared in the biliary tract or intestine (or both) within 15 minutes after injection. The scintigraphic diagnosis of biliary atresia was made when there was no intestinal activity through 24 hours and hepatocyte clearance was relatively preserved. Studies were interpreted as compatible with neonatal hepatitis when there was impairment in hepatocyte clearance and hepatobiliary transit time and the radiotracer reached the intestine. The interpretation was intrahepatic cholestasis when hepatocyte clearance was relatively preserved compared with hepatobiliary transit time but radiotracer eventually reached the intestine. Indeterminate studies were classified as those in which there was no intestinal radiotracer and hepatocellular function was severely impaired.[15] In another study of neonatal jaundice, Majd et al.[16] concluded that hepatobiliary scintigraphy after 3 to 7 days of phenobarbital therapy (see above) is highly accurate for differentiating biliary atresia from other causes of neonatal jaundice.

Arteriohepatic dysplasia (Alagille syndrome) is an uncommon cause of neonatal jaundice. This syndrome is characterized by typical facial features, pulmonary artery stenosis, and a liver disorder that presents as neonatal jaundice. We have obtained hepatobiliary scintigraphy in two neonates who were later found to have Alagille syndrome. In both cases the initial scintigraphic patterns were similar to those found in biliary atresia, and both patients required surgical exploration. Bile plug syndrome in patients with cystic fibrosis, dehydration, sepsis, or on total parenteral nutrition (TPA) may also appear similar to biliary atresia on scintigraphy.

Biliary Obstruction and Cholecystitis

Obstruction of the cystic duct is a major factor in the development of acute cholecystitis. The obstruction may be partial or complete and may or may not be associated with cholelithiasis. Scintigraphic visualization of the gallbladder rules out the diagnosis of acute cholecystitis with a high degree of accuracy in adults. Among 296 patients, Weissmann et al.[17-19] found an accuracy of 98%, a specificity of 100%, a falsenegative rate of 5%, and a false-positive rate of 0% for hepatobiliary scintigraphy in the diagnosis of acute cholecystitis.

In children, however, visualization of the gallbladder on hepatobiliary scintigraphy does not exclude cholecystitis (Fig. 9.8). The gallbladder can be visualized in acalculous cholecystitis or toxic cholecystitis. Some patients affected by these conditions may have only partial obstruction of the cystic duct, and the gallbladder may not be visualized because of edema of the cystic duct. When acalculous cholecystitis is present, a fatty meal or injection of cholecystokinin usually results in failure of the gallbladder to contract effectively. This failure suggests partial cystic duct obstruction, chronic cholecystitis, or acalculous cholecystitis. With chronic cholecystitis there may be a delay in gallbladder filling in the presence of normal liver function.

Cholecystitis in pediatric patients is infrequently associated with cholelithiasis and is usually a complication of another infection (e.g., scarlet fever, other streptococcal infections, Kawasaki disease).[20-22] Children with acute cholecystitis generally present with abdominal pain localized to the right upper quadrant several days after a systemic infection or a streptococcal pharyngitis. The gallbladder may be enlarged and palpable, and jaundice may be present.

Cholelithiasis can be observed in patients with cystic fibrosis who may be asymptomatic or present with symptoms of cholecystitis or

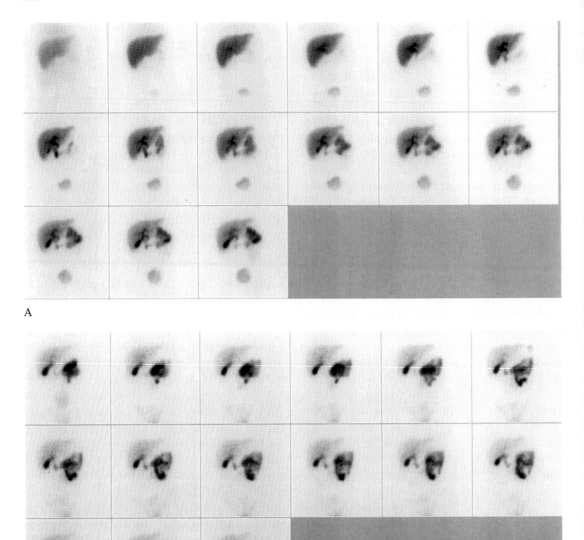

A

B

FIGURE 9.8. Acalculous cholecystitis. A hepatobiliary study (^{99m}Tc-disofenin, 3-minute frames) was done in a 14-year-old girl with a 3-week history of right upper quadrant pain and intermittent chills. A: Initial 60-minute study reveals adequate hepatic uptake of the tracer and transhepatic transit time. Tracer is visual-ized in the gallbladder at 15 minutes into the study and reveals ever-increasing concentration. Some tracer is seen in the bladder beginning at 6 minutes. B: Gallbladder fails to contract adequately after intravenous administration of cholecystokinin analogue.

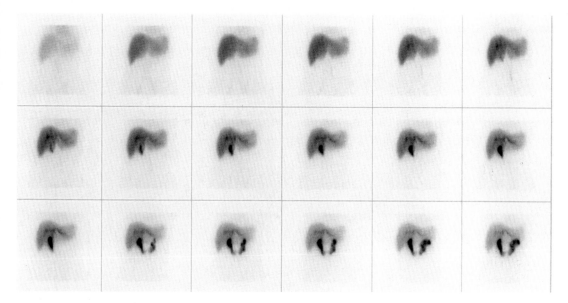

FIGURE 9.9. Cholelithiasis. Hepatobiliary study in a 19-year-old woman with cystic fibrosis and gallstones. Adequate hepatic uptake of the ^{99m}Tc-disofenin without tracer entering the gallbladder. Bile flow is patent but sluggish.

obstruction (Fig. 9.9). Ultrasonography is an essential diagnostic modality for evaluating the biliary tract and should be performed in conjunction with hepatobiliary imaging. A large gallbladder with a thickened wall may be apparent on ultrasonography in patients with cholecystitis, although this is a nonspecific finding. Usually, there is no concomitant dilatation of the biliary tree.

Choledochal Cyst

Choledochal cyst is a congenital dilatation of the extrahepatic biliary tree. There are three types of choledochal cyst. The most common one is a dilatation of the common bile duct, which may be accompanied by dilatation of the hepatic ducts. With this type of cyst, the cystic duct and the gallbladder are usually not dilated. Approximately 15% of these patients also have biliary atresia. In a review by Kim,[23] dilatation of the common bile duct accounted for 93% of 188 cases of choledochal cyst reviewed. The second type of choledochal cyst is a diverticulum of the common bile duct, with the biliary tree being otherwise normal (diverticulum).

The third type is a dilatation of the duodenal intramural portion of the common bile duct (choledochocele).

Ninety percent of the patients with choledochal cyst present before 12 years of age, 70% before age 6, and approximately 40% before age 1. The lesion occurs two to three times more frequently in female than in male children. The symptoms at presentation, in order of decreasing frequency, include jaundice (70%), abdominal pain (55%), dark urine (50%), hepatomegaly (45%), acholic stools (45%), abdominal mass (40%), and fever (35%). Other symptoms include splenomegaly, anemia, cholecystitis, and vomiting. Ultrasonography and hepatobiliary scintigraphy (with cholecystokinin or fatty meal) can make the diagnosis of choledochal cyst in most cases (Figs. 9.10 to 9.12).

Caroli's Disease

Caroli's disease is characterized by a saccular dilatation of the intrahepatic biliary ducts without biliary obstruction.[24,25] This rare disease

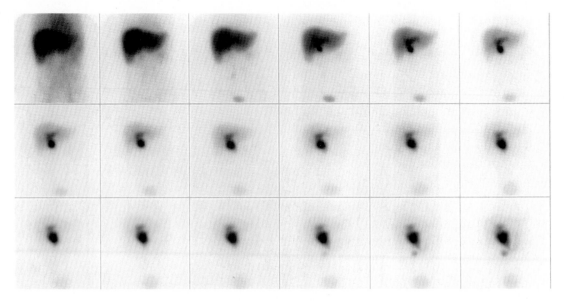

FIGURE 9.10. Choledochal cyst in a 6-year-old girl with right upper quadrant pain. There is adequate uptake of tracer by the liver, with normal parenchy- mal transit time. ^{99m}Tc-disofenin is held in a localized dilatation of the hepatic duct (choledochal cyst).

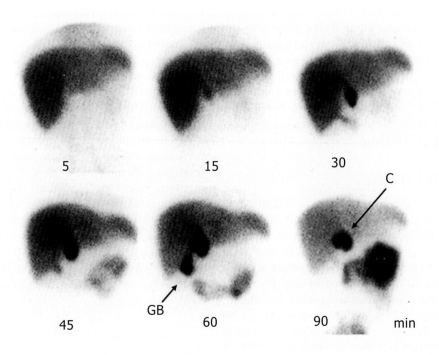

FIGURE 9.11. Choledochal cyst in a 12-year-old patient. The liver takes up the tracer adequately, and it delineates a dilated common duct on the images at 15, 30, and 45 minutes. At 60 minutes tracer is seen in the gallbladder (GB). The image at 90 minutes demonstrates complete drainage of the gallbladder while the tracer is retained in the cyst (C).

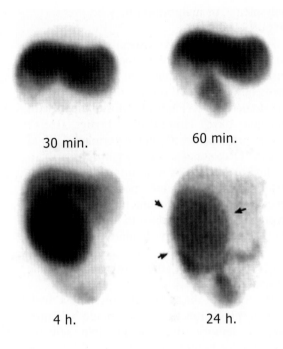

FIGURE 9.12. Choledochal cyst. Hepatobiliary scintigraphy shows a large defect in the posterior margin of the hepatic silhouette (30 minutes), which corresponds to a large choledochal cyst that slowly fills with the tracer.

30 min.   60 min.

4 h.   24 h.

is sometimes associated with congenital hepatic fibrosis.[26] Infection of the dilated ducts may result in cholangitis, calculi, and cirrhosis. Ultrasonography and transhepatic cholangiography play a major part in the diagnosis of this rare disease by demonstrating widespread dilatation of the biliary ducts. Hepatobiliary scintigraphy demonstrates dilatation of the biliary ducts, normal transhepatocyte transit time, and, sometimes, delay in transit of tracer into the intestine without obstruction.

Biliary Leak

Biliary leak secondary to trauma or as a surgical complication can be readily demonstrated with hepatobiliary scintigraphy. This technique demonstrates leakage of radiotracer into the peritoneal cavity. Resultant bile collections are usually contained by the hepatic capsule or localized adjacent to the liver, although free bile ascites may also occur. Advantages of the tracer method include its inherent high contrast and lack of interference from adjacent structures or bowel gas. Ultrasonography and CT can define biliary collections, but cannot easily

determine if there is an active leak. A radiotracer study can establish the integrity of the capsule and determine the presence of an active leak.[27]

Congenital Anomalies

Congenital abnormalities, such as organ malposition, symmetric liver, asplenia, polysplenia, and accessory spleens can be diagnosed by ^{99m}Tc–denatured RBCs or radiocolloid scintigraphy. Hepatobiliary agents are useful in identifying an abnormal position of the gallbladder.

The heterotaxia syndrome includes complex congenital heart disease, visceral heterotaxia, bronchopulmonary abnormalities, a common gastrointestinal mesentery (often with malrotation), nonretroperitoneal location of the pancreas, and often asplenia or polysplenia. This syndrome may be accompanied by abnormalities, such as double inferior vena cava or absence of the hepatic portion of the inferior vena cava. The liver may have a symmetric or "horizontal" appearance, or it may be located in the left upper quadrant. In this syndrome the spleen may be normal or abnormal; asplenia, polysplenia, or malposition may be present[28,29] (Figs. 9.13 to 9.16).

Asplenia is usually associated with other congenital abnormalities, including complex cardiac anomalies, isomerism of the liver and lungs, bowel malrotation, and dextroposition of the stomach[28,30–33] (Fig. 9.17). Most patients with asplenia have Howell-Jolly bodies, Heinz bodies, and siderocytes on the peripheral blood smear. Occasionally, the erythrocytes of a normal premature or term infant also demonstrate these abnormalities, possibly because of splenic immaturity. Documentation of splenic hypofunction in patients with congenital cyanotic heart disease by hematologic findings is highly suggestive of the congenital asplenia syndrome and the associated cardiac anomalies.

The specific diagnosis of polysplenia with normal splenic function can be made by scintigraphic demonstration of multiple spleens. Associated abnormalities include absence of the proximal portion of the inferior vena cava and bilateral hyperarterial bronchi. Polysplenia can also occur without significant heart disease. Absence of the renal-to-hepatic portion of the inferior vena cava is accompanied by azygos or hemiazygos extension. In some cases patients also may have a persistent left superior vena

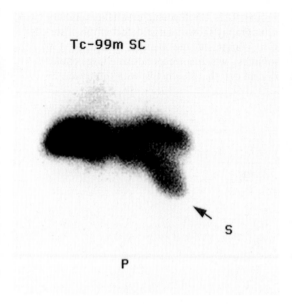

FIGURE 9.13. Symmetric ("horizontal") liver and right-sided spleen. A posterior (P) ^{99m}Tc–sulfur colloid image reveals the spleen in the right upper quadrant (S). The liver has a symmetric appearance.

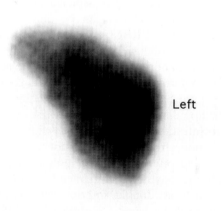

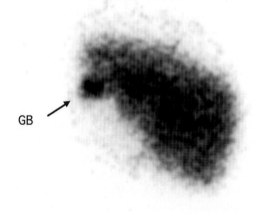

FIGURE 9.14. Heterotaxia. Anterior image of the abdomen using ^{99m}Tc–sulfur colloid shows the liver in the left upper quadrant (left). ^{131}I–rose bengal imaging demonstrates the abnormal location of the gallbladder (GB, right).

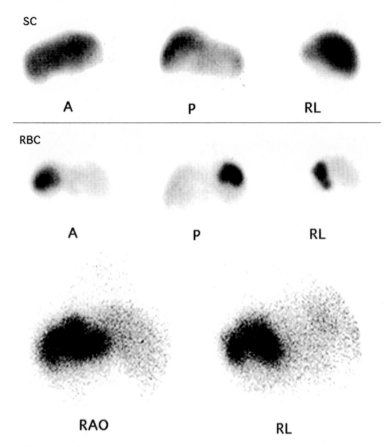

FIGURE 9.15. Polysplenia in the heterotaxia syndrome. Top: ^{99m}Tc–sulfur colloid images (SC) reveal a rather uniform distribution of the tracer. Bottom: The same patient imaged with ^{99m}Tc–denatured red blood cells (RBCs) demonstrates the spleen in the right upper quadrant. Magnification (pinhole) scintigraphy in the right anterior oblique (RAO) and right lateral (RL) projections with ^{99m}Tc–denatured RBCs reveal polysplenia.

cava. Radionuclide venography can detect patency of the inferior vena cava and facilitate cardiac catheterization.[28]

Diffuse and Focal Liver Disease

Enlargement of the liver can be due to homogeneous involvement, such as in glycogen storage disease, biliary obstruction, congestive heart failure, infection, leukemia, Hodgkin's disease, or diffuse tumor. The usual appearance in glycogen storage disease is a diffuse reduction in the concentration of tracer within the liver. Diffuse parenchymal processes, such as cirrhosis (α_1-antitrypsin deficiency, congenital hepatic fibrosis, cystic fibrosis) may reveal hepatomegaly or reduction of liver size depending on the stage of the disease. Often these patients have increased uptake of radiocolloid in the spleen and vertebral marrow. With diffuse lung disease (cystic fibrosis, asthma), the hepatic silhouette may be depressed inferiorly by the expanded lungs.

Single or multiple space-occupying lesions of the liver, for example, hematoma (Fig. 9.18), abscess, cyst, tumors (hepatoma, hepatoblastoma, metastatic Wilms' tumor, neuroblastoma, hemangioma, lymphoma), can occur with or without hepatomegaly. In cirrhosis (primary, cystic fibrosis, α_1-antitrypsin deficiency)

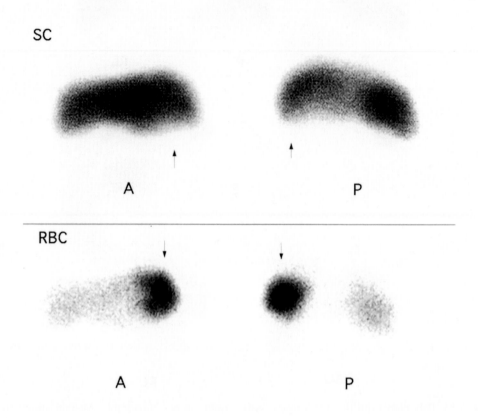

FIGURE 9.16. Heterotaxia. Top: Anterior (A) and posterior (P) images obtained with ^{99m}Tc–sulfur colloid reveal uniform distribution of the tracer. The spleen cannot be identified. Bottom: Images obtained with ^{99m}Tc–denatured RBCs demonstrate the location of the spleen in the left upper quadrant.

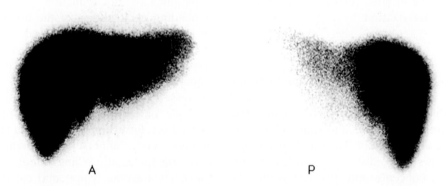

FIGURE 9.17. Asplenia. Anterior (A) and posterior (P) ^{99m}Tc–sulfur colloid images reveal no evidence of functioning splenic tissue in the left upper quadrant. The hepatic silhouette appears normal.

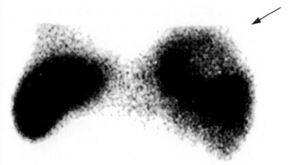

FIGURE 9.18. Posttraumatic hepatic hematoma. Posterior ^{99m}Tc–sulfur colloid scintigraphy reveals a well-defined area of decreased to absent uptake posteriorly and superiorly (arrow) corresponding to a subcapsular hematoma.

multiple hepatic defects can be seen. Liver metastases from lymphoma, leukemia, or neuroblastoma can be diffuse and infiltrative and can cause hepatomegaly with or without defects. Focal space-occupying lesions usually appear on hepatic scintigraphy as areas of reduced to absent radiocolloid uptake. A scintiscan using a ^{99m}Tc-labeled hepatobiliary agent can occasionally demonstrate uptake in a hepatoma. Hepatic adenomas and focal nodular hyperplasia may contain a sufficient concentration of Kupffer cells to allow for colloidal uptake. Areas of increased normal or decreased radiocolloid uptake within the liver may be detected in patients with focal nodular hyperplasia.[34,35]

Enlargement, tumors, or abscesses of neighboring structures can produce abnormal scintiscans. For example, a gallbladder cyst, renal mass or renal hypertrophy, pancreatic tumor or cyst, gastric or mesenteric tumors or cysts, the diaphragm, the aorta, the paraaortic nodes, and pulmonary pathology may cause impressions on the hepatic or splenic image that can be indistinguishable from intrahepatic or intrasplenic disease.[36,37]

The course of hepatic regeneration after partial hepatectomy or radiation therapy can be followed by means of hepatic scintigraphy. Radiation directed to an area of normal hepatic tissue produces a defect with well-defined margins corresponding to the radiotherapy port. Sometimes radiation injury to the liver is

reversible, and the liver scan returns to normal. In other cases fibrosis leads to atrophy of the involved area of the liver. The intact portion of the liver hypertrophies in these patients, and the normal portion of the liver rapidly becomes hyperplastic and assumes a globular shape. Portions of the liver within a radiation therapy portal may not be visible by ^{99m}Tc–sulfur colloid scintigraphy, or with ^{99m}Tc-labeled hepatobiliary agents. After partial hepatectomy, the liver usually undergoes rapid regeneration and resumes a normal size and shape.

Focal liver defects can also be seen with intrahepatic gallbladder, choledochal cysts, and Caroli's disease. Hepatobiliary scintigraphy confirms the biliary nature of these lesions. Reticuloendothelial system scintigraphy can easily assist with the diagnosis of eventration or herniation of the liver (Fig. 9.19). In the presence of a mass in the left lower lung field, splenic scintigraphy with ^{99m}Tc–denatured RBCs rapidly and effectively identifies misplaced splenic tissue.

Multiple intrahepatic defects can be found with polycystic liver disease, which is associated with renal cysts. Single or multiple focal defects may be seen in patients with hydatid cysts. Primary tumors of the liver may be solitary or multifocal, avascular or hypervascular, but scintigraphy does not permit differentiation of malignant and benign lesions of the liver. Tumors with high blood flow within the liver show an arterial blush on radionuclide angiography. Conventional hepatic scintigraphy reveals those tumors as areas of decreased to

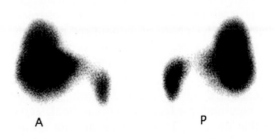

A   P

FIGURE 9.19. Hepatic eventration. Anterior (A) and posterior (P) ^{99m}Tc–sulfur colloid images demonstrate part of the hepatic substance within the right lower hemithorax.

absent radiotracer uptake. Liver abscesses are uncommon in children, but when they occur they are usually a complication of an underlying process. For example, abscesses can be seen in chronic granulomatous disease, leukemia, and other diseases. These lesions show no radiocolloid concentration and can be seen on gallium-67, thallium-201 scintigraphy, or fluorine-18 fluorodeoxyglucose positron emission tomography (^{18}F-FDG-PET) as areas of increased uptake.

Patients with superior vena caval obstruction and the Budd-Chiari syndrome[38] may exhibit increased focal uptake of radiocolloid within the liver. With superior vena caval obstruction, systemic-to-portal venous shunting occurs through the internal thoracic and periumbilical venous channels. After intravenous injection (within a vein of an upper extremity), part of the radiotracer reaches the liver in high concentrations, bypassing the systemic circulation. It results in an area of increased radiocolloid concentration in the medial segment of the left lobe of the liver. If tracer is injected in a vein of the lower extremities, it reaches the liver through the normal pathways, and the distribution of colloid in the liver is normal. With inferior vena caval obstruction, the reverse is true.[39] The typical pattern of Budd-Chiari is preserved ^{99m}Tc–sulfur colloid uptake in the caudate lobe with diminished uptake by the remainder of the liver.

Hepatic scintigraphy in patients with lymphoma or leukemia usually reveals hepatosplenomegaly without focal defects, although sometimes defects are found. Hepatotoxicity due to chemotherapy in leukemia and other disorders may result in hepatomegaly with or without uniform distribution of tracer within the liver with or without splenomegaly. If severe hepatocellular damage occurs, a shift of colloid uptake to the spleen may be apparent. In other cases, when chemotherapeutic agents are given together with radiation therapy, multiple focal defects can be detected within the liver. These defects are not always metastatic tumors, and they may represent local congestion, atrophy, or necrosis.

Children with Wilms' tumor treated with radiation therapy and chemotherapy may develop sudden enlargement of the liver with intrahepatic defects resembling metastases. Temporary withdrawal of chemotherapy may result in resolution of the intrahepatic abnormalities and normalization of the liver size. Awareness of this effect of chemotherapy and radiation on the liver may prevent the erroneous diagnosis of metastatic disease.

Splenomegaly can be seen with a variety of conditions, including portal hypertension (cirrhosis, cystic fibrosis, α_1-antitrypsin deficiency), Gaucher's disease, leukemia, lymphoma, anemia, congestive heart failure, bacterial endocarditis, pyelonephritis, metastatic disease, hepatitis, granulomatous disease, hemolytic disease, glycogen storage disease, and systemic infections. Increased uptake of ^{99m}Tc–sulfur colloid in the spleen without an increase in the size of the organ can be found in children suffering from any of a large variety of infectious diseases or in children with splenic congestion following trauma. Relatively increased ^{99m}Tc–sulfur colloid uptake in the spleen with or without splenomegaly is found with severe liver dysfunction, including hepatic cirrhosis, chemotoxicity, trauma with edema of the liver, and storage disease of the liver.

Focal splenic defects can be found with splenic rupture, subcapsular hematoma, tumor, lymphoma, abscess, cyst, leukemia, infarction (Fig. 9.2), and histiocytosis.[40,41] Positional changes may affect the shape of the spleen or simulate focal splenic defects. Likewise, gastric dilation caused by food or carbonated liquids may change the shape of the spleen. Sometimes it is difficult to distinguish the left lobe of the liver from the spleen. In these cases one may consider using oral carbonated beverages to induce gastric dilatation for better separation of these organs.[42,43] Single photon emission computed tomography using ^{99m}Tc–sulfur colloid improves assessment of hepatic disease.[44]

Trauma

With blunt abdominal trauma, both liver and spleen may be damaged, with other abdominal organs involved as well. In large medical centers, blunt abdominal trauma is usually evaluated initially with CT, which enables the diagnosis of multiple organ involvement in one examination.

Hepatic trauma can be effectively detected by RES scintigraphy. Multiple projections (or preferably SPECT) and awareness of anatomic variants are essential for correct interpretation. Hematoma or rupture of the liver appears as an area of reduced or absent uptake of variable size or shape within the organ (Fig. 9.18).[45]

The spleen comprises 25% of the total lymphoid mass of the body and functions to clear the body of particulate antigens. An increased risk of septicemia, often fatal in children, after splenectomy has been reported. The risk of overwhelming, lethal infection following splenectomy is approximately 0.1% in otherwise normal individuals.[22,46-50] The risk of overwhelming sepsis is greatest in patients who require splenectomy as part of the therapy for an underlying debilitating disease, such as portal hypertension or thalassemia. This risk appears to be greatest in children, especially those under age 1. Approximately 75% of infections occur within 2 years after surgery.[50] Fifty percent of these infections are due to *Diplococcus pneumoniae* and the remainder to *Haemophilus influenzae*, *Staphylococcus aureus*, group A streptococci, and *Neisseria meningitidis*. The explanation for the increased incidence of infection is not known. One theory attributes the susceptibility to the low serum opsonin levels and defective production of immunoglobulin M (IgM).[51] The total incidence of postsplenectomy mortality from sepsis in all groups is estimated to range from 0.25% to 0.58%.[22,48] Nonoperative management of patients with splenic injury has become the treatment of choice. If surgery is required, alternatives to total splenectomy include oversuturing splenic lacerations or partial splenectomy.[52,53] Potential risks or complications associated with the failure to excise a damaged spleen include delayed rupture and the development of a splenic pseudocyst. Delayed rupture of the spleen is a controversial subject.[54-56] We have not seen a single case of delayed rupture among our patients. Splenic pseudocysts are non–epithelium-lined cystic structures that contain bloody material.[57,58] They can present as an abdominal mass at a time when the episode of trauma may not even be remembered.

With ^{99m}Tc–sulfur colloid and multiple projections (or preferably SPECT), splenic scintigraphy is a reliable, simple, safe, and convenient method for diagnosing splenic injury and, if necessary, following its resolution[59-62] (Figs. 9.20 and 9.21). Splenic injury may be seen on

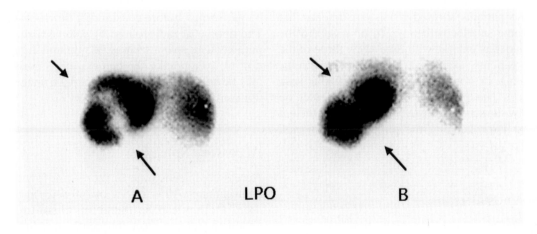

A   LPO   B

FIGURE 9.20. Splenic injury. Two ^{99m}Tc–sulfur colloid images in the left posterior oblique projection (LPO) obtained 20 months apart. The first image (left), obtained shortly after blunt abdominal trauma, reveals a discrete defect extending across the spleen. The second image (right) obtained 20 months later, reveals significant reduction of the defect.

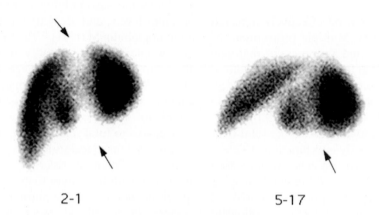

2-1   5-17

FIGURE 9.21. Splenic injury. Two consecutive ^{99m}Tc–sulfur colloid images obtained 3 months apart reveal resolution of a splenic defect (arrows) after blunt abdominal trauma.

scintigraphy as a focal defect, a band of decreased to absent activity, apparent amputation of a portion of the spleen, a T- or Y-shaped defect or band, or a very small or absent spleen. After the diagnosis of splenic trauma has been made, scintigraphy can show that the laceration or hematoma is resolving and that a posttraumatic cyst is not developing. Scintigraphic follow-up should be done if pain develops or a left upper quadrant mass appears. Fischer et al.[60] at our institution followed 20 patients with splenic trauma for 2 months to 1 year. Most of these patients showed persistent defects that became smaller with time. In no case did the scan defect enlarge with time. Only three of the 20 patients examined showed scintigraphic healing or total disappearance of the scan defect. The presence of a residual defect on follow-up scintigraphy is probably not sufficient reason for keeping the patient on restricted activity.

Splenosis

Splenosis is autotransplantation of splenic tissue after splenic trauma.[63–66] It does not have a characteristic clinical picture and is not commonly encountered. Splenic scintigraphy using either ^{99m}Tc–sulfur colloid or ^{99m}Tc–denatured RBCs makes the specific diagnosis of splenosis. When evaluating liver and spleen scans in patients with previous abdominal trauma who may or may not be splenectomized, the possibility of splenosis should be kept in mind. Splenosis can also occur in the thorax.[63,67] Radionuclide scintigraphy is useful for making the diagnosis of splenosis in any pediatric patient with an unexplained thoracic mass who has a prior history of splenic trauma and should be performed before considering thoracotomy. The uptake of radiocolloid by splenic tissue in patients with splenosis may be minimal in relation to liver uptake. To recognize splenosis, it may be necessary to shield the hepatic image or use contrast enhancement (Fig. 9.22).

Accessory Spleen

Accessory spleens (one or more) are found in approximately 10% to 15% of autopsies in children.[65,68] They can be found anywhere in the abdomen but are most frequently seen in the left upper quadrant. Usually, accessory spleens are not visible on routine imaging with

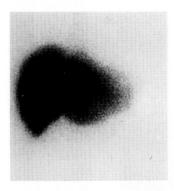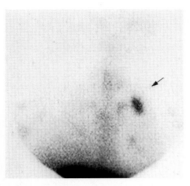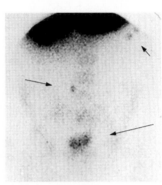

FIGURE 9.22. Splenosis. A conventional anterior image of the liver using ^{99m}Tc–sulfur colloid is normal, and the spleen is not visible (left). There are three foci of selective radiocolloid concentration in the left hemithorax (center). In addition, there are three or more foci of colloid uptake in the abdomen (right).

^{99m}Tc–sulfur colloid or ^{99m}Tc–denatured RBCs. Accessory spleens are more likely to be seen by scintigraphy after splenectomy[67] (Figs. 9.23 and 9.24).

Splenic Torsion and Wandering Spleen

The main support of the spleen is provided by its various ligaments and vessels. The surrounding organs and the intraabdominal pressure also help keep the spleen in its normal position and limit its mobility.

Torsion of the spleen, which is a rare condition, can present with a varied clinical picture, such as acute intestinal obstruction.[69] Radiographically, torsion of the spleen may not be apparent or may appear as a mass lesion on plain films. Scintigraphically, splenic torsion can cause nonvisualization of the spleen. Acute torsion of the spleen reportedly has caused

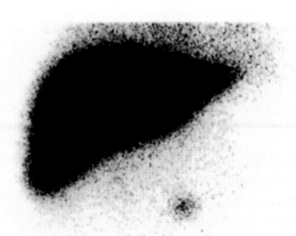

FIGURE 9.23. Accessory spleen. Abnormal concentration of ^{99m}Tc–sulfur colloid below the hepatic silhouette corresponds to an accessory spleen seen after splenectomy.

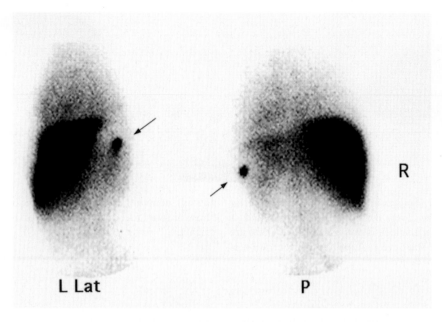

FIGURE 9.24. Accessory spleen. Images obtained with ^{99m}Tc–denatured RBCs demonstrate accessory splenic tissue (arrows).

gastric varices that subsequently bleed.[70] In this instance chronic splenic vein occlusion probably leads to retrograde filling of the short gastric and gastroepiploic veins, which rupture in response to the increased pressure.

Wandering spleen is a rare condition characterized by unusual mobility of this organ and is usually discovered when torsion of the splenic pedicle occurs. The patient usually presents with an acute abdomen. On scintigraphy, the spleen may appear in its normal position or be displaced inferiorly or medially. Repeated views with the patient in various positions may help diagnose the unusual mobility of the spleen.[71]

Nonvisualization of the Spleen ("Functional Asplenia")

Nonvisualization of the spleen on ^{99m}Tc–sulfur colloid images was first described in patients with sickle cell disease.[72–74] The spleen in these patients can be identified with a ^{99m}Tc bone-seeking radiopharmaceutical[75] (Fig. 9.25). Dhawan et al.[76] published a tentative classifica-

tion of disorders associated with reversible functional asplenia, including certain cyanotic congenital heart diseases (treated), sickle cell disease, hemoglobin sickle cell disease, and combined immunodeficiency. Functional asplenia of patients with sickle cell disease can be reversed by transfusion of normal RBCs, with the circulating level of normal RBCs required for visualization of the spleen being approximately 50%. Functional asplenia can be observed in some patients with no circulating Howell-Jolly bodies.[77] Kevy et al.[78] reported a small number of children with hereditary splenic hypoplasia who had extraordinary susceptibility to infection and showed little or no evidence of significant splenic function by scintigraphy.

Splenic Abscess

Abscesses of the spleen are rare. They are most often found in patients with a preexisting hematologic disorder, primary infection elsewhere, or trauma to the spleen. Trauma is responsible

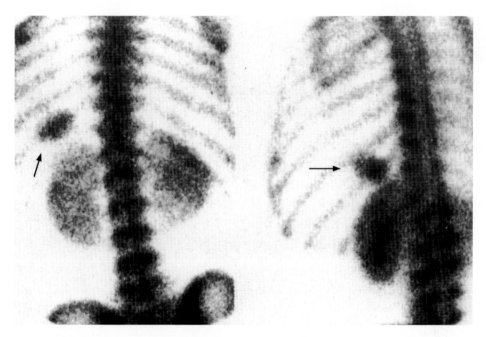

FIGURE 9.25. Sickle cell disease. The spleen (arrows) is visualized after administration of ^{99m}Tc–methylene diphosphonate (^{99m}Tc-MDP) for skeletal scintigra- phy in a patient suffering from sickle cell disease. ^{99m}Tc–sulfur colloid scintigraphy (not shown) did not reveal splenic uptake.

for approximately 15% of cases of splenic abscess. Brown et al.[79] reported a *Salmonella* splenic abscess detected on a ^{99m}Tc–sulfur colloid study that also appeared as a defect surrounded with a halo of increased uptake on gallium-67 (^{67}Ga) scintigraphy.[79]

addition to the initial evaluation, hepatobiliary scintigraphy is useful at any time after transplantation when clinical or laboratory findings indicate that a complication may be present (Figs. 9.26 and 9.27). Bile leaks can be detected with remarkable sensitivity (Fig. 9.28).

Liver Transplantation

Hepatobiliary scintigraphy is useful for evaluating recipients of liver transplants.[44,80–83] This technique provides an overall view of the transplant's functional parenchyma and of bile drainage. Typically, and unless there is a suspicion of surgical complication, a baseline study is obtained within 24 hours of the transplant. This study is useful for detecting regional hepatic flow, global hepatic function, and biliary drainage. The presence of focal defects caused by vascular damage that may have occurred during harvesting can be detected early. In

Liver and Spleen Sizes

In practice, the size of the liver and spleen are estimated by the physician after physical examination with consideration of the patient's overall size and body proportions and sometimes with the aid of imaging. Comments on the size of the liver and spleen on diagnostic images must be evaluated with caution because these organs grow and change size relatively rapidly in children. Furthermore, it is difficult to establish precise normal hepatic and splenic sizes in children. Information on these sizes by scintigraphy must be refined in terms of distribution

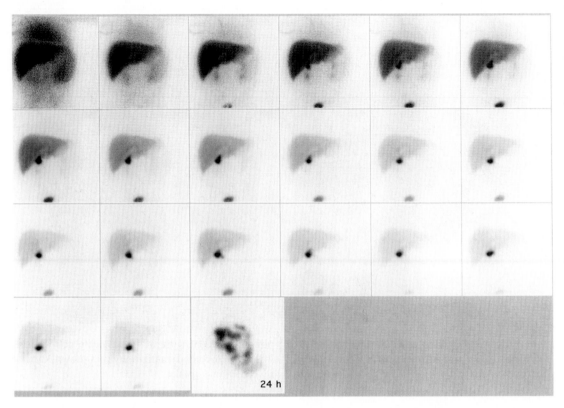

FIGURE 9.26. Liver transplant. Hepatobiliary scintigraphy 1 day after liver transplantation. There is rapid
uptake of the radiotracer (^{99m}Tc-disofenin) by the
liver with adequate blood clearance. Minimal tracer
activity is visualized in the kidneys and bladder.
Throughout the 60-minute study, the tracer appears
to be retained in a region just below the inferior
margin of the hepatic silhouette, presumably corresponding to the biliary anastomosis. An image
obtained at 24 hours demonstrates hepatic clearance
and tracer within several bowel loops.

by sex, weight percentile, age, body surface
area, nutritional status, and other factors.

The maximum vertical dimension (MVD) in
centimeters of the hepatic silhouette on hepatic
scintigrams has been related to age in years (A)
in 66 children from 0 to 19 years of age by the
formula: MVD = 8.8 + 0.46A. The correlation
coefficient was 0.89. Similarly, the maximum
splenic dimension (MSD) on posterior splenic
scintigraphy was related to age in 45 children
by the formula: MSD = 5.7 + 0.31A. The
liver/spleen ratio of lengths was found to be
independent of age: 1.55 at birth, 1.52 at 10
years of age, and 1.52 at 18 years of age.[84,85] It
may be possible to compare the calculated
weights or dimensions of the liver or spleen
(from height, weight, body surface area, or
other measurements) with that suggested by
the scans.[37,86] Markisz and associates[87] from our
institution found a reasonably good correlation
between the maximum vertical dimension on
the liver scan and the age and body weight in

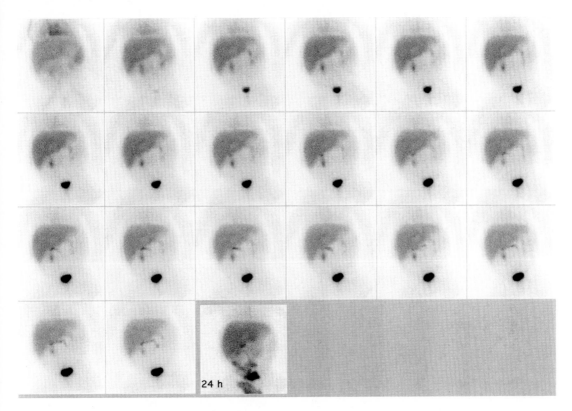

FIGURE 9.27. Liver transplant with failure. Hepatobiliary study reveals poor blood clearance and poor liver uptake of the tracer. A large proportion of the tracer is excreted by the kidneys. There is no evidence of biliary obstruction as the tracer slowly appears in the bowel, and at 24 hours it can be seen within several bowel loops.

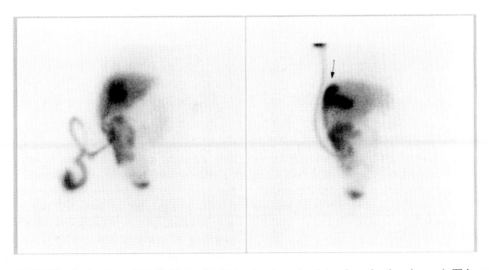

FIGURE 9.28. Bile leak. Anterior (left) and right lateral (right) images demonstrating a bile leak over the posterior and superior aspects of the liver seen best on the lateral projection (arrow). This study is from a recipient of a liver transplant.

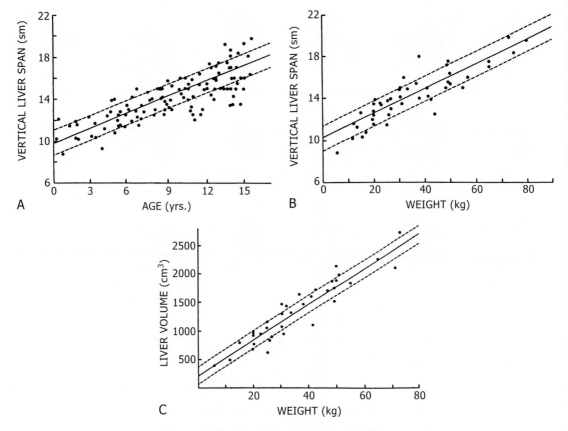

FIGURE 9.29. Normal hepatic sizes in children.

children with normal liver function. Good correlation was also found between estimated liver volume and patient weight. In addition, they found a good correlation of spleen measurements and age and weight in normal children (Figs. 9.29 and 9.30).

Normal Variants

Scintigraphic recognition of normal anatomic variants of the liver and spleen is difficult at times. Prominent notches or separation of the left and right lobes of the liver or impressions by surrounding organs or the costal margins may produce irregularities in the hepatic or splenic image. An accentuated porta hepatis may simulate intrahepatic disease. A kidney situated in a high position can produce impressions on either the liver or the spleen. Gastric dilatation may produce an impression on the splenic silhouette or the left lobe of the liver that mimics a lesion.[88,89]

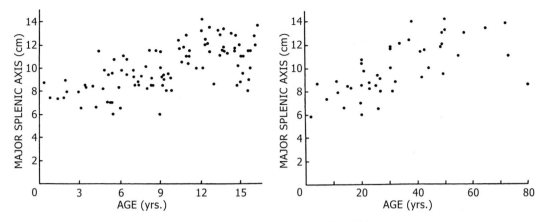

FIGURE 9.30. Normal splenic sizes in children.

References

1. Taplin GV, Meredith OM Jr, Kade H. The radioactive (I131 tagged) rose bengal uptake-excretion test for liver function using external gamma-ray scintillation counting techniques. J Lab Clin Med 1955;45(5):665–78.

2. Ziessman HA, Fahey FH, Hixson DJ. Calculation of a gallbladder ejection fraction: advantage of continuous sincalide infusion over the three-minute infusion method. J Nucl Med 1992;33(4): 537–41.

3. Atkins HL, Richards P, Schiffer L. Scanning of the liver, spleen, and bone marrow with colloidal Tc-99m. Nucl Appl 1966;2:27.

4. Kasai M, Watanabe I, Ohi R. Follow-up studies of long term survivors after hepatic portoenterostomy for "noncorrectible" biliary atresia. J Pediatr Surg 1975;10(2):173–82.

5. Odell GBN, Boitnott JK. Evaluation of jaundice. In: James AE, Wagner HN, Cooke RE, eds. Pediatric Nuclear Medicine. Philadelphia: Saunders, 1974.

6. Hays DM, Woolley MM, Snyder WH Jr, Reed GGJ, Landing BH. Diagnosis of biliary atresia: relative accuracy of percutaneous liver biopsy, open liver biopsy, and operative cholangiography. J Pediatr 1967;71(4):598–607.

7. Johnston GS, Rosenbaum RC, Hill JL, Diaconis JN. Differentiation of jaundice in infancy: an application of radionuclide biliary studies. J Surg Oncol 1985;30(4):206–8.

8. Majd M, Reba RC, Altman RP. Hepatobiliary scintigraphy with 99mTc-PIPIDA in the evaluation of neonatal jaundice. Pediatrics 1981;67(1): 140–5.

9. Picozzi R, Bossi MC, Arosio M, et al. Value of hepatobiliary scintigraphy and ultrasonography in the differential diagnosis of jaundice. Nucl Med Commun 1985;6(2):97–108.

10. Spivak W, Sarkar S, Winter D, Glassman M, Donlon E, Tucker KJ. Diagnostic utility of hepatobiliary scintigraphy with 99mTc-DISIDA in neonatal cholestasis. J Pediatr 1987;110(6): 855–61.

11. Franken EA Jr, Smith WL, Smith JA, Fitzgerald JF. Percutaneous cholangiography in infants. AJR 1978;130(6):1057–8.

12. Greene HL, Helinek GL, Moran R, O'Neill J. A diagnostic approach to prolonged obstructive jaundice by 24–hour collection of duodenal fluid. J Pediatr 1979;95(3):412–4.

13. Hashimoto T, Yura J. Percutaneous transhepatic cholangiography (PTC) in biliary atresia with special reference to the structure of the intrahepatic bile ducts. J Pediatr Surg 1981;16(1): 22–5.

14. Hirsig J, Rickham PP. Early differential diagnosis between neonatal hepatitis and biliary atresia. J Pediatr Surg 1980;15(1):13–5.

15. Gerhold JP, Klingensmith WC 3rd, Kuni CC, et al. Diagnosis of biliary atresia with radionuclide hepatobiliary imaging. Radiology 1983; 146(2):499–504.

16. Majd M, Reba RC, Altman RP. Effect of phenobarbital on 99mTc-IDA scintigraphy in the evaluation of neonatal jaundice. Semin Nucl Med 1981;11(3):194–204.

17. Weissmann HS, Frank MS, Bernstein LH, Freeman LM. Rapid and accurate diagnosis of acute cholecystitis with 99mTc-HIDA cholescintigraphy. AJR 1979;132(4):523–8.

18. Weissmann HS, Rosenblatt R, Sugarman LA, Freeman LM. The role of nuclear imaging in evaluating the patient with cholestasis. Semin Ultrasound CT MR 1980;1:134–42.

19. Weissmann HS, Sugarman LA, Freeman LM. The clinical role of technetium-99m iminodiacetic acid cholescintigraphy. In: Freeman LM, Weissmann HS, eds. Nuclear Medicine Annual. New York: Raven Press, 1981:v.

20. Crystal RF, Fink RL. Acute acalculous cholecystitis in childhood. Clin Pediatr (Phila) 1971; 10(7):423–6.

21. Dickinson SJ, Corley G, Santulli TV. Acute cholecystitis as a sequel of scarlet fever. Am J Dis Child 1971;121(4):331–3.

22. Walker W. Splenectomy in childhood: a review in England and Wales, 1960–4. Br J Surg 1976; 63(1):36–43.

23. Kim SH. Choledochal cyst: survey by the surgical section of the American Academy of Pediatrics. J Pediatr Surg 1981;16(3):402–7.

24. Caroli J. Diseases of intrahepatic bile ducts. Isr J Med Sci 1968;4(1):21–35.

25. Caroli J, Soupault R, Kossakowski J, Plocker L, Paradowska. [Congenital polycystic dilation of the intrahepatic bile ducts; attempt at classification.] Sem Hop 1958;34(8/2):488–95/SP.

26. Wechsler RL, Thiel DV. Fibropolycystic disease of the hepatobiliary system and kidneys. Am J Dig Dis 1976;21(12):1058–69.

27. Weissmann HS, Chun KJ, Frank M, Koenigsberg M, Milstein DM, Freeman LM. Demonstration of traumatic bile leakage with cholescintigraphy and ultrasonography. AJR 1979;133(5): 843–7.

28. Freedom RM, Treves S. Splenic scintigraphy and radionuclide venography in the heterotaxy syndrome. Radiology 1973;107(2):381–6.

29. Treves ST. Spleen. In: Treves ST, ed. Pediatric Nuclear Medicine. New York: Springer-Verlag, 1985:141–56.

30. Chandra RS. Biliary atresia and other structural anomalies in the congenital polysplenia syndrome. J Pediatr 1974;85(5):649–55.

31. Ivemark BI. Implications of agenesis of the spleen on the pathogenesis of conotruncus anomalies in childhood; an analysis of the heart malformations in the splenic agenesis syndrome, with fourteen new cases. Acta Paediatr 1955; 44(suppl 104):7–110.

32. Roberts WC, Berry WB, Morrow AG. The significance of asplenia in the recognition of inoperable congenital heart disease. Circulation 1962;26:1251–3.

33. Rose V, Izukawa T, Moes CA. Syndromes of asplenia and polysplenia. A review of cardiac and non-cardiac malformations in 60 cases with special reference to diagnosis and prognosis. Br Heart J 1975;37(8):840–52.

34. Atkinson GO Jr, Kodroff M, Sones PJ, Gay BB Jr. Focal nodular hyperplasia of the liver in children: a report of three new cases. Radiology 1980;137(1 pt 1):171–4.

35. Rosenthall L. Gastrointestinal imaging: imaging the liver in pediatrics. In: James AE, Wagner HN, Cooke RE, eds. Pediatric Nuclear Medicine. Philadelphia: Saunders, 1974.

36. Freeman LM, Meng CH, Johnson PM, Bernstein RG, Bosniak MA. False positive liver scans caused by disease processes in adjacent organs and structures. Br J Radiol 1969;42(501):651–6.

37. Rollo FD, DeLand FH. The determination of liver mass from radionuclide images. Radiology 1968;91(6):1191–4.

38. Meindok H, Langer B. Liver scan in Budd-Chiari syndrome. J Nucl Med 1976;17(5):365–8.

39. Gooneratne NS, Buse MG, Quinn JL 3rd, Selby JB. "Hot spot" on hepatic scintigraphy and radionuclide venacavography. AJR 1977;129(3): 447–50.

40. Freeman MH, Tonkin AK. Focal splenic defects. Radiology 1976;121(3 pt 1):689–92.

41. Treves ST. Unpublished data, 1984.

42. Landgarten S, Spencer RP. Splenic displacement due to gastric dilatation. J Nucl Med 1972;13(3): 223.

43. Parker JD, Bennett LR. Effect of water ingestion on spleen size as determined by radioisotope scans. Acta Radiol Diagn (Stockh) 1971;11(4): 385–92.

44. Van Heertum RL, Yudd AP, Brunetti JC, Pennington MR, Gualtieri NM. Hepatic SPECT imaging in the detection and clinical assessment of hepatocellular disease. Clin Nucl Med 1992;17(12):948–53.

45. Froelich JW, Simeone JF, McKusick KA, Winzelberg GG, Strauss HW. Radionuclide imaging and ultrasound in liver/spleen trauma: a prospective comparison. Radiology 1982;145(2): 457–61.

46. Eraklis AJ, Kevy SV, Diamond LK, Gross RE. Hazard of overwhelming infection after splenectomy in childhood. N Engl J Med 1967; 276(22):1225–9.

47. King H, Shumacker HB Jr. Splenic studies. I. Susceptibility to infection after splenectomy performed in infancy. Ann Surg 1952;136(2): 239–42.

48. Singer DB. Postsplenectomy sepsis. In: Rosenberg HS, Bolande RP, eds. Perspectives in Pediatric Pathology. Chicago: Year Book, 1973.

49. Smith CH, Erlandson M, Schulman I, Stern G. Hazard of severe infections in splenectomized infants and children. Am J Med 1957;22(3):390–404.

50. Winter ST. Editorial: trauma, splenectomy and the risk of infection. Clin Pediatr (Phila) 1974;13(12):1011–2.

51. Likhite VV. Immunological impairment and susceptibility to infection after splenectomy. JAMA 1976;236(12):1376–7.

52. Douglas GJ, Simpson JS. The conservative management of splenic trauma. J Pediatr Surg 1971;6(5):565–70.

53. Mishalany H. Repair of the ruptured spleen. J Pediatr Surg 1974;9(2):175–8.

54. Ayala LA, Williams LF, Widrich WC. Occult rupture of the spleen: the chronic form of splenic rupture. Ann Surg 1974;179(4):472–8.

55. Benjamin CI, Engrav LH, Perry JF Jr. Delayed rupture or delayed diagnosis of rupture of the spleen. Surg Gynecol Obstet 1976;142(2):171–2.

56. Olsen WR. Editorial: delayed rupture of the spleen as an index of diagnostic accuracy. Surg Gynecol Obstet 1974;138(1):82.

57. Topilow AA, Steinhoff NG. Splenic pseudocyst: a late complication of trauma. J Trauma 1975;15(3):260–3.

58. Wright FW, Williams EW. Large post-traumatic splenic cyst diagnosed by radiology, isotope scintigraphy and ultrasound. Br J Radiol 1974;47(560):454–6.

59. Bethel CA, Touloukian RJ, Seashore JH, Rosenfield NS. Outcome of nonoperative management of splenic injury with nuclear scanning. Clinical significance of persistent abnormalities. Am J Dis Child 1992;146(2):198–200.

60. Fischer KC, Eraklis A, Rossello P, Treves S. Scintigraphy in the followup of pediatric splenic trauma treated without surgery. J Nucl Med 1978;19(1):3–9.

61. Gilday DL, Alderson PO. Scintigraphic evaluation of liver and spleen injury. Semin Nucl Med 1974;4(4):357–70.

62. Solheim K, Nerdrum HJ. Radionuclide imaging of splenic laceration and trauma. Clin Nucl Med 1979;4(12):528–33.

63. Ahmadi A, Faber LP, Milloy F, Jensik RJ. Intrathoracic splenosis. J Thorac Cardiovasc Surg 1968;55(5):677–81.

64. Albrecht H. Ein Fall von sehr Zahlreichen uber ganze Peritoneum versprentgen nebenmilzen. Beitr Pathol Anat 1918;20:513–27.

65. Buchbinder JH, Lipkoff CJ. Splenosis: multiple peritoneal splenic implants following abdominal injury. Surgery 1939;6:927–34.

66. Jacobson SJ, De Nardo GL. Splenosis demonstrated by splenic scan. J Nucl Med 1971;12(8):570–2.

67. Ehrlich CP, Treves ST. Unpublished data, 1981.

68. Eraklis AJ, Filler RM. Splenectomy in childhood: a review of 1413 cases. J Pediatr Surg 1972;7(4):382–8.

69. Broker FH, Khettry J, Filler RM, Treves S. Splenic torsion and accessory spleen: a scintigraphic demonstration. J Pediatr Surg 1975;10(6):913–5.

70. Sorgen RA, Robbins DI. Bleeding gastric varices secondary to wandering spleen. Gastrointest Radiol 1980;5(1):25–7.

71. Broker FH, Fellows K, Treves S. Wandering spleen in three children. Pediatr Radiol 1978;6(4):211–4.

72. Pearson HA, Cornelius EA, Schwartz AD, Zelson JH, Wolfson SL, Spencer RP. Transfusion-reversible functional asplenia in young children with sickle-cell anemia. N Engl J Med 1970;283(7):334–7.

73. Pearson HA, Schiebler GL, Spencer RP. Functional hyposplenia in cyanotic congenital heart disease. Pediatrics 1971;48(2):277–80.

74. Pearson HA, Spencer RP, Cornelius EA. Functional asplenia in sickle-cell anemia. N Engl J Med 1969;281(17):923–6.

75. Fischer KC, Shapiro S, Treves S. Visualization of the spleen with a bone-seeking radionuclide in a child with sickle-cell anemia. Radiology 1977;122(2):398.

76. Dhawan VM, Spencer RP, Sziklas JJ. Reversible functional asplenia in chronic aggressive hepatitis. J Nucl Med 1979;20(1):34–6.

77. Dhawan VM, Spencer RP, Pearson HA, Sziklas JJ. Functional splenia in the absence of circulating Howell-Jolly bodies. Clin Nucl Med 1977;2:395–6.

78. Kevy SV, Tefft M, Vawier GF, Rosen FS. Hereditary splenic hypoplasia. Pediatrics 1968;42(5):752–7.

79. Brown JJ, Sumner TE, Crowe JE, Shaffner LD. Preoperative diagnosis of splenic abscess by ultrasonography and radionuclide scanning. South Med J 1979;72(5):575–7, 580.

80. Gelfand MJ, Smith HS, Ryckman FC, et al. Hepatobiliary scintigraphy in pediatric liver

transplant recipients. Clin Nucl Med 1992; 17(7):542–9.

81. Hawkins RA, Hall T, Gambhir SS, et al. Radionuclide evaluation of liver transplants. Semin Nucl Med 1988;18(3):199–212.

82. Klingensmith WC 3rd, Fritzberg AR, Koep LJ, Ronai PM. A clinical comparison of ^{99m}Tc-diethyl-iminodiacetic acid, ^{99m}Tc-pyridoxyli-deneglutamate, and 131I-rose bengal in liver transplant patients. Radiology 1979;130(2): 435–41.

83. Scott-Smith W, Raftery AT, Wraight EP, Calne RY. Tc-99m labeled HIDA imaging in suspected biliary leaks after liver transplantation. Clin Nucl Med 1983;8(10):478–9.

84. Salvo AF, Schiller A, Athanasoulis C, Galdabini J, McKusick KA. Hepatoadenoma and focal nodular hyperplasia: pitfalls in radiocolloid imaging. Radiology 1977;125(2):451–5.

85. Spencer RP, Banever C. Growth of the human liver: a preliminary scan study. J Nucl Med 1970;11(11):660–2.

86. DeLand FH, North WA. Relationship between liver size and body size. Radiology 1968; 91(6):1195–8.

87. Markisz JA, Treves ST, Davis RT. Normal hepatic and splenic size in children: scintigraphic deter-mination. Pediatr Radiol 1987;17(4):273–6.

88. Treves S, Spencer RP. Liver and spleen scintig-raphy in children. Semin Nucl Med 1973;3(1): 55–68.

89. Treves ST, Markisz JA. Liver. In: Treves ST, ed. Pediatric Nuclear Medicine. New York: Springer-Verlag, 1985:129–40.

10
Kidneys

S.T. Treves, William E. Harmon, Alan B. Packard, and Alvin Kuruc

Nuclear medicine techniques are of primary importance in the initial diagnosis and follow-up of many renal diseases in children. These techniques are highly sensitive, enabling early detection of disease, often before structural changes are apparent. Nuclear medicine provides unique functional and anatomic information with negligible risk to the patient. These techniques are physiologic and minimally invasive, requiring only a very small amount of tracer material (0.02 to 0.08mg range) in a very small volume of solution delivered by intravenous injection (0.1 to 0.5mL). The radiation exposures to the patients are very low, well below conventional radiography and computed tomography (CT) techniques. Sedation for these studies is not needed in the vast majority of patients. Motion correction techniques can be applied and are quite effective. Radionuclide techniques can be used safely in all pediatric age groups and in severely ill patients, including those with renal insufficiency. The well-known advantages of radiopharmaceuticals include their lack of toxic or pharmacologic effects (e.g., osmotic effect, hemodynamic overload) and the fact that they do not provoke allergic reactions, even in patients allergic to iodinated contrast agents.

Ultrasonography has provided a clear indication of the incidence of renal disease during the prenatal and neonatal periods.[1] The complementary nature of radionuclide and other diagnostic imaging methods of the pediatric urinary tract, especially ultrasonography, should be emphasized. In many instances, a combined approach allows anatomic-functional correlations, which often provide additional insight into the nature and severity of the problem under investigation.

Collectively, congenital abnormalities account for approximately 42% of cases of chronic renal failure.[2] The incidence of end-stage renal disease in children in the United States is approximately 11 new cases per 1 million total population per year.[3] Koenigsberg et al.[4] reported that the incidence of preexisting lesions is 15% to 23% in children showing serious renal injury following relatively minor trauma.

Associated anomalies of other organs are not uncommon, especially when the kidney is involved. For example, infections of the urinary tract affect 3% to 5% of all children. During the neonatal period, male infants are more commonly affected, but after 3 months of age, female infants are affected approximately three times more often than their male counterparts.[5]

Approximately 10% of the population is affected by renal anomalies, but many of these problems are minor and of no clinical significance. Excluding polycystic kidneys, the incidence of major malformations has been estimated at 4 per 1000 to 7 per 1000.[6] An ultrasonography screening study conducted in China on slightly more than 132,000 schoolchildren of both sexes, revealed renal abnormalities in approximately 0.5% of the subjects.[7]

Early diagnosis and treatment of abnormalities of the urinary tract in children can reduce morbidity and mortality.[8] The high sensitivity of diagnostic nuclear medicine has placed it in a central role in the diagnosis of renal disorders and the evaluation of renal function in pediatric patients.

Methods

Radiopharmaceuticals

Radiopharmaceuticals used for evaluation of the kidneys may be classified into two groups. The first group includes radiopharmaceuticals that are rapidly eliminated by the kidneys and thus enable evaluation of renal function and urine drainage. This group includes technetium-99m-disodium [N-[N-N-(mercaptoacetyl) glycyl]-glycinate(2-)-N,N',N'',S]oxotechnetate(2-) (^{99m}Tc-MAG$_3$), ^{99m}Tc-diethylenetriaminepentaacetic acid complex (^{99m}Tc-DTPA), ^{99m}Tc-glucoheptonate, and ^{123}I-OIH (^{123}I-orthoiodohippurate). These agents (except for ^{99m}Tc-glucoheptonate) are not appropriate for static renal scintigraphy because just after intravenous injection they appear only briefly in the renal parenchyma.

The second group includes radiopharmaceuticals that concentrate in the renal parenchyma for a sufficiently long period so that detailed scintigraphic mapping of regional functioning renal parenchyma is possible. ^{99m}Tc–dimercaptosuccinic acid (^{99m}Tc-DMSA) and ^{99m}Tc-glucoheptonate. Note that glucoheptonate is included in both groups because, while approximately 65% of the injected dose is eliminated in the urine within 6 hours after injection, 10% to 15% is retained in the renal parenchyma.[9]

Selection of the renal agent depends largely on the problem to be investigated and on the practitioner's experience and preference. In general, however, it is best to become familiar with one agent for dynamic renal scintigraphy and one for static renal scintigraphy and to use them consistently. Many pediatric patients affected with renal disease require follow-up evaluations, and the use of the same radiopharmaceutical and technique facilitates assessment of change.

Estimates of radiation absorbed doses for these agents are found in Chapter 20.

^{99m}Tc-MAG_3

Technetium-99m-MAG$_3$ (Mallinckrodt, St Louis, MO) is the current agent of choice for dynamic renal scintigraphy. The agent is excreted principally through active renal tubular transport. It is more extensively protein-bound than ^{123}I-OIH (88% versus 65%);[10] therefore, its volume of distribution is lower than that of ^{123}I-OIH. The plasma clearance of this tracer is on the order of 300 mL/min, approximately 60% that of ^{123}I-OIH,[11-14] and after 3 hours, approximately 90% of the injected dose can be recovered in urine.[15] Because ^{99m}Tc-MAG$_3$ is eliminated by tubular secretion and has a high initial renal uptake, it provides high kidney/background ratios. Its rapid excretion provides good temporal resolution.

^{99m}Tc-$DTPA$

Technetium-99m-DTPA (CIS-US, Bedford, MA) has been used for dynamic renal scintigraphy for more than three decades. It has been replaced in many centers by ^{99m}Tc-MAG$_3$ for the reasons stated above. In contrast to ^{99m}Tc-MAG$_3$, ^{99m}Tc-DTPA is excreted primarily by glomerular filtration, albeit at a slightly lower rate than inulin.[16-27] The lower rate of glomerular filtration compared with inulin is probably due to protein binding, the amount of which varies with the formulation.[28] A maximum concentration of 5% in each kidney is achieved 2 to 3 minutes after injection.[29]

^{99m}Tc-$DMSA$

Technetium-99m-DMSA is the agent of choice for renal cortical imaging by planar or pinhole scintigraphy, or by single photon emission computed tomography (SPECT). This agent is 90% bound to plasma proteins, and 0% to 5% is associated with red cells.[30] Enlander and coworkers[30] investigated the biokinetics of ^{99m}Tc-DMSA and found that in most normal individuals the blood disappearance of ^{99m}Tc-DMSA follows a single exponential with a mean half-time of 56 minutes with 6% to 9% of the dose present in the blood at 14 hours after injection. The renal uptake of ^{99m}Tc-DMSA is 50% of the injected dose at 1 hour after injection and 70% at 24 hours,[30] which is in relatively good agreement with the results of Kawamura et al.,[31] who found 48% ± 5% of the injected dose in the kidneys 2 hours after injection. The manufacturer's package insert states that total renal uptake at 6 hours is approximately 40% (GE Healthcare, Arlington Heights, IL).

Enlander et al.[30] reported that the cumulative urinary excretion of ^{99m}Tc-DMSA was 6% at 1 hour, 10% to 12% at 2 hours, and 25% at 14 hours. The package insert reports that the cumulative renal excretion in 2 hours is 16%. At 1 hour or more after injection, the activity is found principally in the proximal convoluted tubules, with minimal activity elsewhere in the kidney (Fig. 10.1).[32]

Several studies demonstrate a correlation between ^{99m}Tc-DMSA uptake and renal blood flow or renal mass (or both). For example, the fractional distribution of ^{99m}Tc-DMSA in the right and left kidneys was shown to correlate well with renal blood flow as determined by strontium-85 microsphere distribution (r = 0.95).[33] In our laboratory at Children's Hospital Boston, a study in rats with normal and obstructed kidneys showed a good correlation in the split renal uptake of ^{99m}Tc-DMSA and cobalt-57 microspheres (DiPietro M, Caldicott W, Treves S, unpublished data). In dogs, changes in renal mass showed a high degree of correlation with changes in ^{99m}Tc-DMSA distribution.[34] In patients, good correlation was observed between the relative renal accumulation of ^{99m}Tc-DMSA at 24 hours and relative effective renal plasma flow to each kidney as measured with ^{131}I-OIH.[34,35]

In most patients, excellent images of renal cortex can be obtained at approximately 4 hours after injection of ^{99m}Tc-DMSA. In patients with obstruction, tracer retained within the pelvicaliceal system can interfere with mapping of functioning renal parenchyma and may lead to the wrong estimate of split renal function. It is therefore important to evaluate the images at 4 hours postinjection to determine that there is no tracer in the pelvicaliceal system. If tracer is retained, later images, up to 24 hours after injection, is recommended to allow tracer in the urine to be eliminated and to permit a better assessment (Figs. 10.2 and 10.3).

[99m]Tc-Glucoheptonate

Technetium-99m-glucoheptonate (Drax Image, Montreal, Canada) is promptly taken up by the kidneys and rapidly eliminated in the urine. By 1 hour after injection, 8% to 10% of the initial tracer activity is present in the kidneys and almost 40% of the administered dose has been eliminated in the urine.[9] This renal uptake permits static renal scintigraphy at approximately 2 or more hours after injection of the agent. The tracer retained within the kidney is associated with the cells of the proximal convoluted tubules. Renal handling of ^{99m}Tc-glucoheptonate appears to occur principally by active renal tubular transport and, to a lesser extent, by glomerular filtration.[36]

Technetium-99m-glucoheptonate permits adequate dynamic renal imaging with rapid

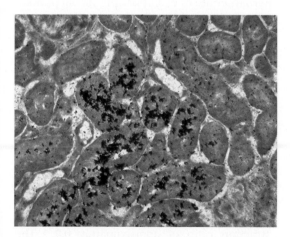

FIGURE 10.1. ^{99m}Tc-DMSA. Frozen section autoradiography from a rat kidney 1 hour after intravenous injection of ^{99m}Tc-DMSA. Tracer concentrates principally in the proximal convoluted tubules. Minimal or no tracer activity is seen elsewhere.

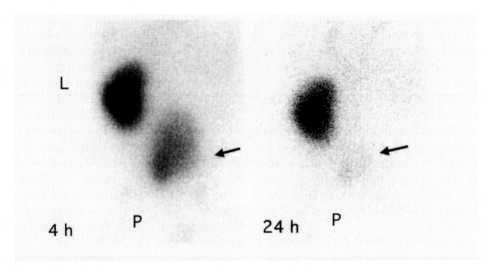

FIGURE 10.2. ^{99m}Tc-DMSA. Four- and 24-hour imags in a 3-month-old boy with nonvisualization of the right kidney by ultrasonography. This study was performed to look for any evidence of right renal function. Left: Scintigraphy at 4 hours revealed normal tracer accumulation in the left kidney (L). Tracer accumulation in the right side could correspond to an ectopic right kidney or tracer in the bladder (arrow). Right: Image at 24 hours clearly demonstrates that tracer had accumulated in the bladder (arrow), and there was no evidence of an ectopic right kidney.

visualization of renal parenchyma, collecting system, pelvis, ureters, and bladder. The observation made in the case of ^{99m}Tc-DMSA in children with renal obstruction also applies to

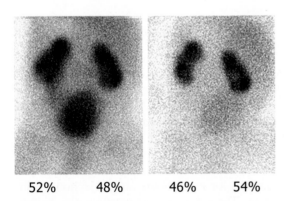

52%   48%   46%   54%

FIGURE 10.3. A 4-day-old infant with bilateral hydronephrosis, hydroureters and severe bilateral reflux. Left: The 4-hour image estimates a 52% to 48% differential ^{99m}Tc-DMSA uptake. However, high levels of tracer in the pelves and ureters interfere with assessment. Right: An image at 24 hours postinjection is clear of urinary activity and best represents the split renal function.

^{99m}Tc-glucoheptonate; tracer retained within the pelvicaliceal system may interfere with imaging of the functioning renal parenchyma and can lead to false interpretation of the study. Therefore, late imaging should be considered in these cases. The hepatobiliary system is an alternate route of excretion for glucoheptonate and in patients with severe renal failure; images at 4 to 6 hours may show activity in the bowel.

^{123}I-Orthoiodohippurate (OIH)

Iodine-123-OIH is useful for dynamic renal scintigraphy because of its high uptake by the renal tubules and rapid excretion into the urine. This radiopharmaceutical is excreted by the kidneys similarly to para-aminohippuric acid (PAH), the standard for the measurement of effective renal plasma flow.[37] Approximately 80% of PAH is eliminated by tubular secretion and 20% by glomerular filtration, with an extraction ratio of approximately 0.9.[38] The extraction ratio (ER) quantifies the efficiency with which a compound is extracted by the kidney. It is defined as

$$ER = (A - V)/A,$$

where A is the arterial concentration of the substance and V is the venous concentration. The extraction ratio of ^{131}I-OIH is approximately 85% that of PAH.[39]

Because of the well-known limitations of ^{131}I, ^{131}I-OIH is not used for renal scintigraphy. The availability of ^{123}I-OIH is limited in the U.S.; currently, most pediatric nuclear medicine practitioners opt for one of the ^{99m}Tc-labeled agents.

Imaging Techniques

Precaution: Recent intravascular administration of radiographic contrast agents may result in a reduction of renal uptake of dynamic renal tracers accompanied by a prolongation of their renal transit times. This effect lasts approximately 24 hours. Dynamic radionuclide studies of the kidneys should be performed either before or 24 hours after the administration of contrast agents.

Dynamic Renal Scintigraphy

Dynamic renal scintigraphy refers to rapid serial imaging following the intravenous injection of one of the following radiotracers: ^{99m}Tc-MAG$_3$, ^{99m}Tc-DTPA, ^{99m}Tc-glucoheptonate, or ^{123}I-OIH. Dynamic renal scintigraphy encompasses three phases: (1) radionuclide angiography, (2) dynamic renal scintigraphy per se, and (3) diuretic renography. The methodology for diuretic renography is discussed below (see Hydronephrosis/Obstruction). Captopril renography with ^{99m}Tc-MAG$_3$ is also reviewed below (see Hypertension).

Radionuclide Angiography

Radionuclide angiography consists of rapid imaging of the initial appearance of the radiotracer in the kidneys following a rapid intravenous of a bolus of tracer. No special patient preparation is necessary. Patients are studied in the supine position on the imaging table with the gamma camera viewing the renal region.

The usual dose of ^{99m}Tc-MAG$_3$ (or other ^{99m}Tc-labeled radiopharmaceutical) for radionuclide angiography is 0.1 mCi (3.7 MBq)/kg body weight with a minimum total dose of 0.5 mCi (18.5 MBq). Typically, the angiogram is recorded on serial 0.25- to 1.0-second frames for 60 seconds. The radionuclide angiogram can be viewed as a series of sequential images or preferably in a cinematic mode. The series of images depict tracer activity as it initially circulates within the aorta and the arteriocapillary territories of the kidneys. Because of inherently limited spatial resolution of imaging systems, the dilution of tracer as it reaches the kidneys, and the relatively low administered dose, it is difficult or impossible to differentiate the arterial, capillary, and venous phases. Radionuclide angiography only reveals major abnormalities in renal blood flow. In practice, radionuclide angiography rarely provides information not available from 20-minute dynamic renal scintigraphy.

Dynamic Renal Scintigraphy Per Se

Patient Preparation

Patients should be encouraged to drink fluids approximately 1 hour prior to the study. In pediatric practice, however, it is difficult to implement a standard prestudy hydration method; therefore, many patients are examined in their normal state of hydration. When possible, patients are asked to empty their bladder before the examination begins. A vesical catheter (Foley type) should be inserted if urinary tract obstruction is suspected and the patient cannot or will not void. The bladder should be allowed to drain through the catheter during the entire duration of the study. Intravenous access is established using a butterfly needle (23 to 25 gauge) or a short intravenous catheter that is securely fastened to the skin with tape. Before proceeding, one must ensure that intravenous access is reliable and stable. Next, an intravenous infusion of normal saline (10 to 15 mL/kg) is begun and should be maintained during the entire examination, including diuretic renography when this is indicated. The saline infusion maintains a satisfactory level of hydration and provides a convenient route for the administration of furosemide. Complete extravasation of the tracer could ruin the examination. Partial extravasation will severely

TABLE 10.1. Usual radiopharmaceutical doses for dynamic scintigraphy*

Radiopharmaceutical	Dose		Minimum dose		Maximum dose	
	(mCi/kg)	(MBq/kg)	(mCi/kg)	(MBq/kg)	(mCi/kg)	(MBq/kg)
^{99m}Tc-MAG$_3$	0.100	3.7	0.5	18.5	10.0	370
^{99m}Tc-DTPA	0.100	3.7	0.5	18.5	8.0	296
[99m]Tc-glucoheptonate	0.100	3.7	0.5	18.5	8.0	296
^{123}I-OIH	0.01	0.37	0.1	3.7	0.5	18.5

*Excluding radionuclide angiography.

compromise the quality of the study and if not recognized, yield erroneous interpretation. Avoiding extravasation of tracer is, therefore, extremely important.

Radiopharmaceutical

As mentioned above, dynamic renal scintigraphy can be performed with ^{99m}Tc-MAG$_3$, ^{99m}Tc-DTPA, ^{99m}Tc-glucoheptonate, or ^{123}I-OIH. Usual administered doses for dynamic renal radiopharmaceuticals are listed in Table 10.1.

Imaging Technique

Children are usually examined in the supine position with the gamma camera placed underneath the examining table, viewing the area of the kidneys and bladder. In the supine position, the distance from the skin to each of the kidneys is approximately the same, and for the calculation of the left-to-right renal uptake ratio, depth correction is not critical. Recipients of renal transplants are examined in the supine position with the gamma camera viewing the kidney and the bladder from the anterior projection.

Appropriate immobilization equipment should be used to reduce patient motion. The gamma camera is equipped with a parallel-hole, low-energy, high-resolution collimator. Electronic magnification is employed according to the patient's size.

After the patient is positioned, the tracer is injected as a rapid intravenous bolus, and recording of the study is begun simultaneously with the injection. Our protocol records the study as serial 0.25-minute frames for 20 minutes (128×128 matrix format). If the study includes a radionuclide angiogram, recording is begun at one frame per 0.25 second for 60 seconds, immediately followed by one frame per 0.25 minute for a total of 20 minutes.

Interpretation

Interpretation of a dynamic renal study should include evaluation of the parenchymal phase, the cortical transit time, and the urine drainage phase.

Careful evaluation of the *parenchymal phase* is critical. During the first minutes of the ^{99m}Tc-MAG$_3$ dynamic study, after the initial vascular distribution and before the first appearance of tracer in the renal collecting system, the tracer concentrates in the renal parenchyma. During this period, the blood level of tracer is decreasing and the parenchymal concentration is at its maximum. The parenchymal phase is usually visualized 60 to 120 seconds following intravenous injection and provides important information: (1) relative and absolute size of the functional renal parenchyma, (2) total renal function (kidney/background ratio), (3) relative or split renal function (right versus left), (4) overall renal morphology and distribution of functioning parenchyma, and (5) position of the kidneys.

The *relative renal size* can be estimated by simple visual observation of the parenchymal image. The maximum renal dimensions in the longitudinal and transverse planes can be measured with a calibrated system or by imaging a radioactive ruler placed to the side of the patient. In addition, the *functional size of the kidneys* can be estimated by comparing the kidneys with the body outline and relative proportions of visible organs on early images.

The parenchymal phase shows the *position of the kidneys*. If a pelvic kidney is suspected, it is important to include the pelvic area within the field of view of the camera.

By visually evaluating the ratio of the total renal uptake of ^{99m}Tc-MAG$_3$ and the background activity from the blood pool and the liver, one can obtain a qualitative estimate of *total renal function*. During the normal parenchymal phase, little tracer activity should be present in the body background, the blood pool, and the liver. The higher the level of tracer activity within these regions and the lower the renal uptake, the poorer is the renal function and vice versa.

A quantitative estimate of the total renal uptake of the injected dose helps in the assessment of total renal function. This is especially useful in the serial evaluation of individual patients. Total renal uptake can be estimated using the following procedure. The syringe containing the tracer to be injected is placed at 15 cm from the face of the collimator using a specially made plastic holder and is recorded on the computer as the initial dose. All materials used for the injection of the tracer (e.g., syringe, butterfly needle) are saved for later counting. The dynamic study is recorded as described above. At the end of the dynamic study, the saved materials are placed in front of the collimator using the same holder, and another image (residual dose) is recorded. The total renal counts are determined in regions of interest (ROIs) drawn around the kidneys on the parenchymal phase (60 to 120 seconds). All measurements are corrected for background and radioactive decay. Results are expressed as percentage of the administered dose (initial minus residual) in the kidney(s) during the parenchymal phase.

The higher the renal function, the higher is the renal uptake, and vice versa. As this approach does not correct for tissue attenuation and depth, only an estimate of the total renal uptake is obtained, not an absolute value. Meticulous attention to detail and study-to-study consistency are essential to avoid errors that may lead to inadequate assessment of renal function.

The parenchymal phase provides information about *relative renal function* (split renal function). This can be assessed visually and by calculating individual renal uptake as a fraction of the total renal uptake from renal ROIs. Placement of ROIs over the kidneys without including extraparenchymal sources of activity may be difficult, especially in cases of poor renal function and in hydronephrosis. Careful attention to detail and consistency during selection of background ROIs is essential. This step is usually done manually, and different sizes and positions of background regions can produce different results, a particular problem when the renal function is low or hydronephrosis is present. It is crucial to verify any semiquantitative results with visual assessment. Until highly reliable methodology to provide precise renal uptake values is available, visual assessment should govern the final assessment of split renal function.

The parenchymal phase can provide some information about *intrarenal distribution of radiotracer*. It can reveal hydronephrosis by showing a photon-deficient area within the renal pelvis. The cortical uptake appears as a rim of variable size depending on the severity of the hydronephrosis. Larger defects, and some renal scars can be idenified. Reduced or absent uptake of tracer in a relatively large portion of the kidney or larger defects, such as a malfunctioning upper pole in a duplex kidney, trauma, tumor, or cyst, can be detected. The parenchymal phase does not allow detection of small cortical defects, however.

A very useful parameter that can be measured from the dynamic renal study is the *cortical transit time*. For the purpose of this discussion, cortical transit time is defined as the time between the intravenous injection of the tracer and the first appearance of tracer within the renal collecting system. Normally, radiotracer appears within the renal collecting system 3 to 5 minutes after intravenous injection. The presence of normal cortical transit time indicates that renal parenchymal function is not compromised, even in the presence of dilatation of the pelvicaliceal system. The poorer the renal function, the slower is the cortical transit time. As the tracer is eliminated into the renal pelvis, the parenchymal activity decreases gradually. Even if the cortical transit time appears to be within the normal range, it is important to determine if it is associated with a decrease of tracer activity in the renal cortex. Prolonged cortical transit time indicates renal dysfunction. Cortical transit time may be prolonged in several conditions including renal immaturity, ureteral obstruction, hydronephrosis, renal insufficiency, acute tubular necrosis, renal artery stenosis, renal vein thrombosis, acute and chronic pyelonephritis, transplant rejection, nephrotoxicity, and trauma.

As the study progresses to the *drainage phase*, the tracer is gradually eliminated through the pelvicaliceal system and the ureters into the bladder. Normally, at the end of 20 minutes, a large proportion of the tracer has left the renal parenchyma. At this time, minimal or no tracer should be visible in the renal collecting system(s). Time-activity curves generated from regions of interest over an entire kidney usually reveal peak activity at 4 to 7 minutes

with subsequent decrease to approximately 30% to 50% of the peak activity at 20 minutes. These time-activity curves must not be interpreted alone, but along with careful evaluation of the parenchymal phase, the cortical transit time, and the series of images during the drainage phase. It is possible to see normal cortical transit time with complete cortical clearance of the tracer from the cortex at 20 minutes accompanied with a renal time-activity curve that reveals a delayed peak and high residual value. This pattern indicates delayed urine drainage without parenchymal dysfunction and is, in most cases, without clinical significance. Best results are obtained when both serial imaging and time-activity curves are utilized in the interpretation. This point cannot be overemphasized.

A *normal dynamic renal study* reveals relatively rapid and intense concentration of the tracer in the renal parenchyma at 1 to 2 minutes after injection (Fig. 10.4). Passage of the tracer into the renal calyces and the renal pelvis occurs at 3 to 5 minutes. Under normal condi-

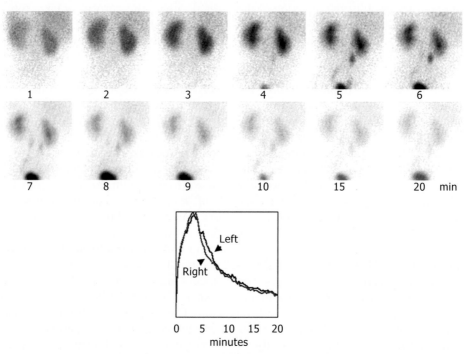

FIGURE 10.4. Normal ⁹⁹ᵐTc-MAG₃ study. A 4-week-old girl with a question of renal obstruction. Top: Serial images for 20 minutes. Bottom: Time activity curves. At frames at 5 and 6 minutes, tracer is transiently seen in the right upper ureter.

tions, visualization of tracer in the ureters is variable. The ureter may be visualized in some normal patients and those with slow ureteral transit time. Ureteral dilatation, with or without obstruction, is usually associated with ureteral visualization. By 20 minutes after injection the radiotracer has usually almost completely cleared the renal parenchyma. Small residual amounts of tracer persisting in the pelvicaliceal system at 20 minutes may be normal and are usually of no clinical significance. Minimal residual tracer tends to clear spontaneously, with a change in the patient's position, or after voiding. Tracer appears within the bladder 3 to 6 minutes after injection, and its level increases with time as more of it is excreted by the kidneys. In the patient with normal renal function, background (which reflects blood clearance of the tracer and therefore total renal function) rapidly decreases with time. If there is no retention of tracer within the pelvicaliceal system or the ureter(s), the study is terminated at 15 to 20 minutes. If at the end of the initial 20 minutes tracer is retained within the pelvicaliceal system, the patient should be encouraged to get up and walk around for a few minutes if possible (a small child should be picked up for a few minutes) to promote postural drainage. An additional image is then obtained to determine if drainage has occurred. Kidneys that drain with a change in patient position should not be considered obstructed.[40] If urinary obstruction is suspected, a diuretic renogram may be indicated (see below).

Static Renal Scintigraphy

Technetium-99m-DMSA is administered intravenously with a usual dose of 0.05 mCi/kg (1.85 MBq/kg) [minimum 0.3 mCi (11.1 MBq); maximum 3.0 mCi (111 MBq)]. Imaging should begin approximately 4 hours after injection. Three techniques are available: planar, pinhole magnification, and SPECT.

Planar Renal Scintigraphy

Conventional planar renal scintigraphy provides the following information: (1) number, position, size, and overall morphology of the

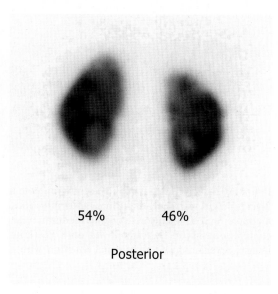

54%   46%

Posterior

FIGURE 10.5. ^{99m}Tc-DMSA planar scintigraphy in an 8-year-old girl with pyelonephritis. Focal decrease of ^{99m}Tc-DMSA uptake in the right upper pole. Split renal uptake is shown.

functioning kidneys; (2) split renal function; and (3) an assessment of regional parenchymal function. The patient is examined in the supine position, and a posterior image containing 300,000 to 500,000 counts is recorded using a high-resolution or, preferably, ultrahigh-resolution collimator on a 256 × 256 matrix format. Left and right posterior oblique projections may be useful for identifying cortical defects. A calibrated system enables measurement of the size of the functional renal parenchyma. The ROIs of each kidney and background areas are outlined on the image. The split renal uptake corrected for body background is then calculated. Normally, the split renal uptake varies from 50%/50% to 45%/55% (Fig. 10.5).

In cases of renal duplication, it is sometimes desirable to outline the upper and lower poles and to estimate the distribution of functioning renal parenchyma in the affected kidney. With severe obstruction some ^{99m}Tc-DMSA activity may be present in the collecting system, which can be confusing and can contribute to an overestimation of renal uptake. Later images (up to

Parallel hole collimator | Pinhole collimator

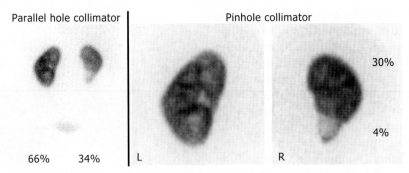

66%   34%   L   R

FIGURE 10.6. ^{99m}Tc-DMSA pinhole scintigraphy in a 2-year-old girl with repeated urinary tract infections, a double right collecting system, and moderate vesicoureteric reflux in the right lower pole. Posterior images reveal reduced right renal function with a defect in the right lower pole (left panel). Pinhole images reveal greater detail with a clear delineation of the focal reduction of tracer uptake in the right lower pole. (Right panel, L = left, R = right).

24 hours after the injection), allowing drainage of retained tracer, allow better measurement of split and regional renal function. More comprehensive assessment of regional parenchymal function (e.g., scar, inflammation, infarct, duplex) is best done with SPECT or with pinhole magnification in patients less than 1 year-of-age.

Magnification Renal Scintigraphy

Pinhole magnification is very effective for examining the kidneys not only in infants, in whom magnification should be considered mandatory, but can also be useful in older children and adolescents. Cortical functional defects in pyelonephritis, infarction, scarring, duplication, and fetal lobations can be discerned better with pinhole magnification than parallel-hole, high-resolution collimators. A pinhole collimator with an internal diameter of 2 to 3 mm provides images of higher spatial resolution than parallel-hole or converging collimators. Posterior and posterior-oblique projections are useful to detect and outline cortical abnormalities. Each pinhole image is obtained for approximately 150,000 counts using a 256×256 matrix (Figs. 10.6 to 10.8).

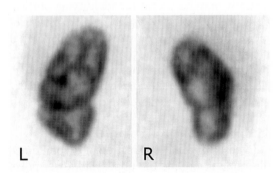

L   R

FIGURE 10.7. Fetal lobations. Posterior pinhole ^{99m}Tc-DMSA images in a 1-month-old infant with right vesicoureteral reflux. There is relatively lower right renal function without focal cortical defects. The normal fetal lobations are visualized.

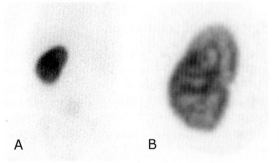

A   B

FIGURE 10.8. Right multicystic dysplastic kidney. The right kidney is not visualized. Planar (A) and pinhole images (B) are shown. Note the detailed visualization of renal cortex on the pinhole image.

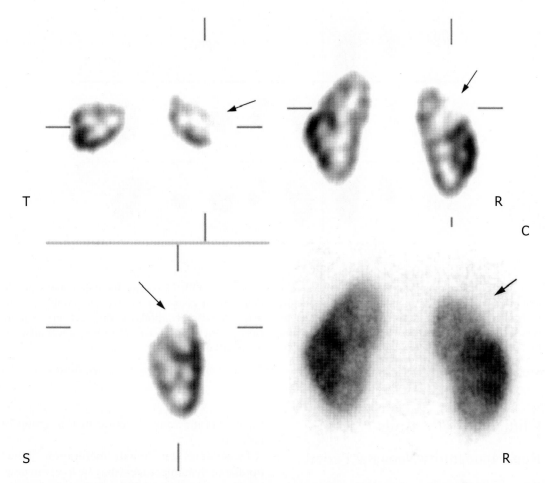

FIGURE 10.9. Single photon emission computed tomography (SPECT) and conventional planar scintigraphy in pyelonephritis. This 16-year-old girl with a history of repeated urinary tract infections and vesicoureteric reflux presented with acute onset of right flank pain and fever. Selected slices transverse (T), coronal (C), and sagittal (S) slices reveal focal cortical defect in the right upper pole (arrows). Conventional planar scintigraphy does not show the defect (arrow) as clearly as SPECT.

Single Photon Emission Computed Tomography

Technetium-99m-DMSA single photon emission computed tomography (SPECT) is superior to conventional planar scintigraphy for mapping regional functioning renal parenchyma (Figs. 10.9 and 10.10). By defini-tion, SPECT permits simultaneous evaluation of images in the transverse, coronal, or sagittal plane, or in any plane. The ability to evaluate rotating volume rendered images permits a superior overall view of the functional anatomy of the kidneys. Using modern systems, SPECT acquisition requires 15 to 20 minutes.

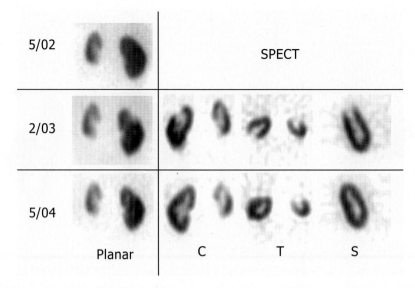

FIGURE 10.10. Pyelonephritis and recovery. Planar and SPECT ^{99m}Tc-DMSA images of a 7-year-old girl with bilateral vesicoureteral reflux. Planar images reveal the left kidney has lower renal function and that on 2/03 a cortical defect was present in the right upper pole. SPECT reveals the defect more clearly. Following a course of intravenous antibiotics, the defect has largely resolved. This recovery is more clearly seen on SPECT. C = Coronal, T = Transverse, S = Sagittal.

Clinical Applications

Renal Immaturity/Neonatal Period

When evaluating newborn infants, nuclear medicine clinicians should recognize normal renal immaturity and its effect on the renal handling of radiotracers. The glomerular filtration rate (GFR) per unit of surface area in the newborn is approximately 30% of the adult rate. During the first few days of life, there is a dramatic rise in the GFR, followed by a more gradual increase with adult levels (normalize to BSA) reached at 6 months to 1 year of age. Studies of very low birth weight (VLBW) premature infants have revealed dramatically lower GFRs (10% of normal) with a much slower rise to normal levels.[41] PAH clearance is typically lower in the newborn.

Most newborns are able to urinate within 24 hours. In problem cases, radionuclide imaging is useful to assess renal function, even in the absence of diuresis. The combination of ultrasonography and scintigraphy has proved useful for evaluating renal function in this group of patients.

Depending on renal maturation, renal uptake of dynamic tracers may be lower in newborns than in older children and adults. In addition, intrarenal transit time and excretion of these tracers may be slow at this age. A normal dynamic radionuclide study in newborns during the first or second week of life may demonstrate faint, delayed renal uptake of the tracer with or without bladder activity at the expected times. If tracer is seen in the bladder within 2 to 5 minutes, the amount present may be lower than in older children. Background may be high throughout the study, reflecting low plasma clearance of the tracer. As renal function matures, renal uptake, intrarenal transit time, and excretion of tracers reach normal values. Some normal newborns, however, show apparently normal handling of dynamic renal tracers.

Renal function immaturity may also be reflected on ^{99m}Tc-DMSA studies. In normal newborns, images may show relatively low kidney/background ratio or may be normal.

Intravenous urography is not the initial method of choice in this age group because of the poor concentration of contrast agents by the kidneys and the relatively high doses of contrast agents that must be used.[42–44]

Hydronephrosis/Obstruction

Hydronephrosis is one of the most common indications for radionuclide evaluation of the kidneys in pediatric patients. Findings on renal scintigraphy vary depending on hydration, age, type and severity of the disease, site of obstruction, unilateral or bilateral pathology, presence or absence of reflux, and recent surgery. In cases of hydronephrosis caused by obstruction at the ureteropelvic junction or ureterovesical junction, dynamic renal scintigraphy demonstrates abnormalities in structure and function on the involved side. In posterior urethral valves, there is bilateral renal involvement, and patients who present during early infancy may have severe obstruction with impaired renal function. In young children, the evaluation of function in the presence of obstruction does not give a reliable indication of the potential for recovery. It does indicate, however, the minimal function

that may be expected. In the young, even poor renal function caused by chronic obstruction is potentially reversible.[45] In these patients, ultrasonography should be done to search for surgically correctable lesions. Serial renal scintigraphy can be used to assess recovery as renal function may improve once the obstruction has been relieved. In newborn hydronephrosis without obvious obstruction, the hydronephrosis may resolve spontaneously, suggesting that some hydronephrosis in neonates and infants is a manifestation of physiologic change during development.[46–50] Thus, in a young child with hydronephrosis, one should not arrive at the diagnosis of obstruction based on a single examination. A single study does not have prognostic value: It provides only a "snapshot" of a changing situation. Serial studies over time may provide a better indication of the natural progression of the hydronephrosis and help determine the presence of an obstruction (Figs. 10.11 to 10.15).

On dynamic studies, the hydronephrotic kidney initially appears as a rim of tracer concentration in the renal parenchyma surrounding an area devoid of tracer, corresponding to the renal pelvis and collecting system. The size

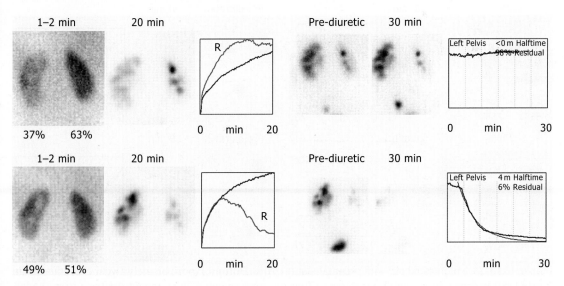

FIGURE 10.11. Left hydronephrosis with ureteropelvic junction obstruction in a 2-month-old boy. Top: Preoperative study reveals prolonged retention of tracer in the left renal pelvis with a clearly obstructive pattern after diuretic challenge. The differential function is left, 37%, and right, 63%. Following left pyeloplasty, there is a dramatic improvement in left pelvic drainage and an improvement in split renal function (left, 49%; right, 51%).

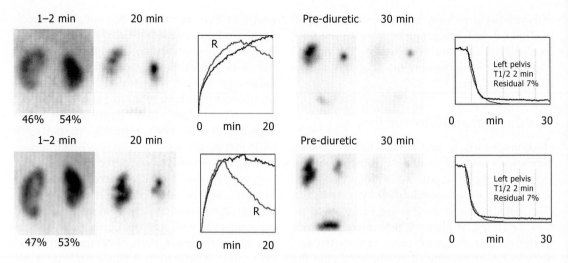

FIGURE 10.12. Prenatal diagnosis of left hydronephrosis in a 2-month-old with mild uretero-pelvic junction obstruction by intravenous urography. Top: Preoperative ^{99m}Tc-MAG$_3$ study reveals lack of spontaneous drainage from the left kidney. However, there was rapid washout of tracer following diuretic challenge with a half-time $t_{1/2}$ of 2 minutes and a 30-minute residual of 7%. Bottom: ^{99m}Tc-MAG$_3$ study 3 months after left pyeloplasty. There is no change in split renal function and better spontaneous drainage from the left kidney. The diuretic phase is unchanged from the preoperative study. Ultrasonography and intravenous urogram revealed mild postoperative improvement.

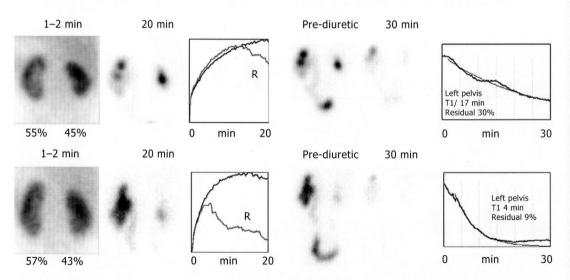

FIGURE 10.13. A 1-month-old girl with prenatal diagnosis of left hydronephrosis and no treatment. Top: ^{99m}Tc-MAG$_3$ study shows lack of significant spontaneous drainage from the left kidney. The washout half-time is 17 minutes with a 30-minute residual of 30%. Bottom: Approximately 1 year later, there is an improvement in spontaneous drainage from the left kidney, a postdiuretic washout half-time of 4 minutes, and a 30-minute residual of 9%.

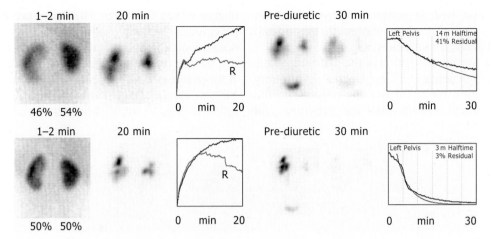

FIGURE 10.14. A 2-month-old boy with congenital left hydronephrosis ^{99m}Tc-MAG$_3$ study. Top: Lack of significant spontaneous drainage from the left kidney. Following diuretic challenge, there was a washout half-time of 14 minutes with a high (41%) 30-minute residual. Bottom: Following left pyeloplasty, there is an improvement on the split renal function to 50% and a rapid washout following diuretic challenge ($t_{1/2}$ = 3 minutes, 30-minute residual = 3%).

of this photon-deficient area depends on the degree of dilatation. As the study progresses in time, the pelvicaliceal system fills with radiotracer that leaves the renal parenchyma. The rate of appearance and the amount of the tracer in the pelvicaliceal system depends on the function of the hydronephrotic kidney. Depending on the severity and duration of the obstruction, tracer may begin to accumulate in the renal pelvis within 3 to 6 minutes despite severe

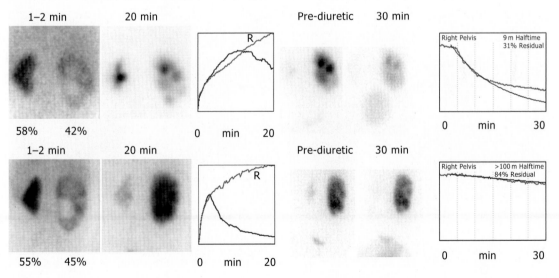

FIGURE 10.15. Worsening ureteropelvic junction obstruction. A 6-month-old boy with prenatal diagnosis of right hydronephrosis. Top: Baseline ^{99m}Tc-MAG$_3$ study showing right hydronephrosis, lack of spontaneous drainage from the right kidney, and washout following diuretic challenge (washout $t_{1/2}$ = 9 minutes and 31% residual). Bottom: Six months later there is no significant spontaneous drainage from the right kidney and the diuretic renogram is grossly abnormal ($t_{1/2}$ > 100 minutes with a 30-minute residual of 84%). There is an apparent increase in right renal function. The patient underwent right pyeloplasty to relieve the obstruction.

dilatation; with prolonged severe obstruction, however, tracer accumulation in the dilated renal pelvis is much slower.

The apparent function of the hydronephrotic kidney depends on the degree of urinary obstruction that increases the pressure in the pelvicaliceal system and the presence and degree of renal damage. High pressure in the pelvicaliceal system results in a reduction of renal blood flow and function that in the young, can be reversed after relief of the obstruction. A more accurate assessment of renal functional capacity can be attained after the obstruction is relieved (Fig. 10.16).[51,52] The amount of radio-

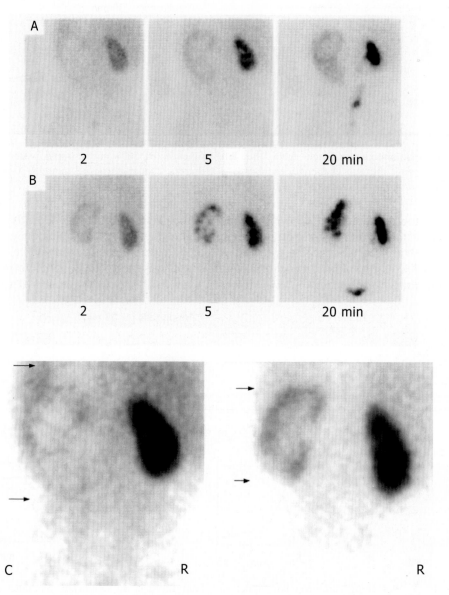

FIGURE 10.16. Left ureteropelvic junction obstruction, preoperative and postoperative ^{99m}Tc-MAG$_3$ studies. Selected ^{99m}Tc-MAG$_3$ images at 2, 5, and 20 minutes in a 2-year-old patient with left ureteropelvic junction obstruction, before and after left pyeloplasty. A: The preoperative study reveals a large left kidney with low tracer uptake and severe hydronephrosis. The cortical transit time of the tracer is prolonged. B: The postoperative study shows a smaller left renal kidney with improved tracer uptake and cortical transit time. C: Parenchymal images (2 minutes) before (left) and after (right) surgery show the reduction of size (arrows) and improvement in renal function of the left kidney.

tracer uptake in the renal parenchyma is directly related to the functional capacity of the kidney in question. We studied the effect of minute-to-minute changes in renal blood flow following acute increases in renal pelvic pressure in New Zealand white rabbits. We employed ultrashort-lived iridium-191m ($t_{1/2}$ = 5 seconds). A nonobstructive constant renal pelvic pressure model with bilateral ureteral catheters was used. Unilateral pressure increases of 16, 25, 30, and 35 cm H^2O were applied, using the contralateral kidney as control. Three sequential radionuclide angiograms at each pressure level were obtained. At baseline, the experimental side showed a differential flow of 47.5% [standard deviation (SD) 7.3]. With increasing pressure, flow was reduced to 42.3% (SD 2.6). Return to normal pressures increased the flow back to near baseline levels or 51.0% (SD 4.0). There was no significant difference between baseline and postcompression values (p = .4807). This study suggests that there can be reversible changes in renal blood flow responding to acute changes in pelvic pressure (Fig. 10.17).[53] In studies of hydronephrosis due to obstruction, the obstructed kidney may take up more tracer than the contralateral side. This may be secondary to the kidney trying to provide more urine to overcome the obstruction (stressed kidney) (Fig. 10.5). Over time, renal function in the obstructed kidney may be reduced.

It has been suggested that in preoperative patients in whom the cortical time-activity curves appear more nearly normal than the total kidney curve, there is a strong likelihood of improvement after the obstruction is relieved. Conversely, abnormal cortical curves may be associated with a poor prognosis for functional improvement.[54] It is possible to identify the site of obstruction at the ureterovesical or the pelvicaliceal junction. In cases where there is obstruction at both the pelvicaliceal and ureterovesical junctions, it may be difficult to detect the ureterovesical obstruction. Detection of the level of obstruction depends on adequate renal function and the presence or absence of dilatation of the pelvicaliceal system and ureter.[55] Differentiating obstructed from dilated nonobstructed systems can be achieved by serial imaging after

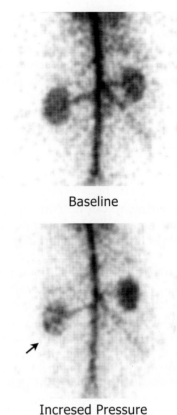

Baseline

Incresed Pressure
in Left Kdney

FIGURE 10.17. Effect of acute increases in hydrostatic pelvic pressure on renal blood flow. Iridium-191m radionuclide angiograms, 2-second frames. Top: Baseline study reveals symmetric renal blood flow. Bottom: Decreased left renal blood flow (arrow) during acute increase of hydrostatic pressure.

intravenous administration of furosemide (diuretic renography).

Diuretic Renography

Intravenous administration of furosemide is followed by a rapid diuretic response that displaces tracer from dilated unobstructed systems. In significantly obstructed kidneys, radiotracer in the renal area decreases slowly, fails to decrease, or even increases in response to the induced diuresis.

In diuretic renography, drainage is directly proportional to urine flow and inversely proportional to the volume of the renal pelvis and ureter. Urine flow depends on the function and amount of renal parenchyma present, as well as the ability of the parenchyma to respond to the diuretic. There are a set of factors that, when present, limit the ability of diuretic renography to determine if there is obstruction or not. These include poor renal function; parenchymal loss; large, flaccid, and compliant renal pelvis and/or ureter; infiltration of the diuretic; bladder overdistention; prune belly syndrome; and complex surgeries.[56-58]

Technique

Diuretic renography can be performed using the dynamic renal radiopharmaceuticals mentioned above. Prior to administration of the diuretic, it is important to ensure that radiotracer has filled the renal pelvis and postural drainage has not occurred. Many practitioners administer furosemide after the completion of the initial dynamic renal study, approximately 30 to 40 minutes after intravenous injection of the radiotracer (see Dynamic Renal Scintigraphy, above). Others administer the diuretic simultaneously with the radiotracer (F-0) with a total recording time of 20 to 30 minutes. Others give the diuretic 10 to 15 (F-10, F-15) minutes before tracer administration. Forced hydration has been suggested as a means to improve the diagnosis of obstruction versus nonobstruction by diuretic renography.[59-61]

Although the method of diuretic renography is relatively simple, it is not standardized. There are several variations in the technique and interpretation. For simplicity, we describe the method used at Children's Hospital Boston, in which furosemide is administered 30 to 40 minutes after injection of the radiotracer.* Because the patient is usually hydrated intravenously (10 to 15 mL/kg) and a bladder catheter is in place for the preceding dynamic renal study, no additional preparation is needed. The saline infusion is continued, and the bladder is allowed to drain through the catheter during the study.

The computer is set to record at one frame per 0.25 minute for 30 minutes (128 × 128 matrix format). The dose of furosemide (1.0 mg/kg, maximum dose 40 mg) is prepared and readied for injection. Recording is begun 1 minute prior to the administration of the diuretic; the images serve as a baseline. The furosemide then is injected through the intravenous line. The diuretic effect is usually seen within 1 to 2 minutes after administration of the furosemide.

In some patients, the forced diuresis causes or reproduces flank pain, especially in those with hydronephrosis who complain of intermittent pain. In some cases, rapid overdistention of the renal pelvis may disrupt the status of a system in which urine flow and drainage are otherwise balanced. In many cases, even with dilatation, rapid increased diuresis causes no pain or discomfort.

Interpretation

Interpretation of the diuretic study should incorporate knowledge gained from both the initial dynamic renal study and the diuretic renogram. Relevant information includes the parenchymal phase (total and split renal function; size, morphology, and position of functioning renal parenchyma; and dilatation of the renal pelvis), the cortical transit time, and the drainage phase.

In general terms, diuretic renography is relatively easy to interpret where results fall at the two extremes. In the absence of obstruction, rapid and almost complete washout of radiotracer from the pelvicaliceal system occurs. In obstructed systems, drainage of tracer following administration of the diuretic is slow and there is tracer retention at the end of the study. Interpretation of intermediate diuretic renographic patterns is more difficult.

A comparison is made of images obtained prior to the administration of the diuretic and at the end of the diuretic study. The study is displayed on cinematic mode to verify that the patient did not move during the procedure. If the patient moved, motion correction is applied. ROIs are drawn over the region of the pelvicaliceal system(s) showing tracer

---

*Preferences on technical detail(s) and idiosyncrasies vary, and it would be impractical to discuss all of them here.

retention, as well as background region(s). If a kidney drained satisfactorily during the initial dynamic renal study, $t_{1/2}$ is not calculated. In normal kidneys, there is not much tracer remaining to be drained; the $t_{1/2}$ may, therefore, be long and could possibly be misleading. We estimate the diuretic washout $t_{1/2}$ using mono exponential interpolation between a point on the initial descent of the time-activity curve and another point on the downslope while the curve is decaying monotonically. In addition, we estimate the percentage of pre-diuretic tracer activity remaining at 30 minutes. A rapid initial $t_{1/2}$ can be followed by significant retention of tracer in the renal pelvis. Reporting an initially short $t_{1/2}$ without mentioning significant retention of tracer in the pelvicaliceal system at 30 minutes may be misleading does not provide a complete assessment.[†]

[†] A few comments on diuretic half-time ($t_{1/2}$) may be appropriate. Estimation of the diuretic half-time is a useful adjunct to the assessment of urinary obstruction. Unfortunately, over the past several years, the value of the diuretic half-time has been overemphasized. Washout half-time has been used by some clinicians as the only factor in the assessment of possible kidney obstruction. This approach frequently leads to oversimplification of a rather complex condition. The diuretic half-time is only one of several factors considered when assessing urinary obstruction. This point cannot be emphasized enough.

Adding to the problem is the fact that the calculation method of the diuretic half-time is not standardized. Conceptually, most would agree that the diuretic half-time is the time at which the time-activity curve generated from a renal pelvis containing radionuclide decreases to half of its initial activity. However, there are at least four methods used to calculate this half-time. One method uses a linear interpolation of the washout curve with the initial point at recording and the last point at 30 minutes. A second method interpolates a straight line between the first point of the diuretic downslope and another point in the downslope where tracer activity is decreasing monotonically. Another method uses an exponential interpolation of the washout curve with the initial point at recording and the last point at 30 minutes. Finally, some use an exponential interpolation of the first point on the diuretic downslope and another point down the time-activity curve where the decline is monotonic. Diuretic half-time values vary therefore from method to method and

Pyelonephritis

Clinical Features

Urinary tract infection (UTI) is a common problem in children. Presenting signs and symptoms of children with UTI are varied and sometimes confusing. Infection may be confined to the bladder (cystitis); it may involve the upper collecting systems (ureteritis, pyelitis); or the renal parenchyma (pyelonephritis). This differentiation is very difficult to make on clinical grounds alone.[63] Patients may present with fever, flank pain or tenderness, malaise, irritability, leukocytosis, and bacteriuria, but there may be no indication that there is renal parenchymal infection. Other patients with pyelonephritis may present with puzzling fevers of unknown origin. Neonates and infants in particular present with nonspecific clinical findings. Prospective clinical studies have shown that commonly used clinical and laboratory findings are unreliable in differentiating acute pyelonephritis from lower UTI in children.[64] Acute pyelonephritis can result in irreversible renal damage (scarring), which in the long term leads to hypertension and/or chronic renal failure.[65] Experimental and clinical studies have shown that renal scarring can be prevented or reduced by early effective antimicrobial therapy.[66–68] Clearly, early and accurate diagnosis of acute pyelonephritis has clinical relevance.

Vesicoureteral Reflux and Pyelonephritis

Although the coexistence of vesicoureteral reflux and pyelonephritis is well documented, a large propotion of cases of pyelonephritis occur in the absence of vesicoureteral reflux. Furthermore, once acute pyelonephritis occurs, the subsequent development of renal scarring is independent of the presence of vesicoureteric reflux.[64,69–75] Therefore, it seems unwise to limit evaluation of cortical integrity in UTI only to

---

from observer to observer. Despite these variations in technique, the overall sensitivity of diuretic renography for the detection of obstruction in children has been estimated at 93%.[62]

those patients who present with a history of vesicoureteral reflux.

Cortical Scintigraphy

Renal cortical scintigraphy is the most reliable, simplest, and most practical imaging technique for routine use in the initial evaluation and follow-up of children with febrile UTI. It has provided us with many insights into the pathophysiology of pyelonephritis and its consequences. Technetium-99m-DMSA scintigraphy is useful to identify the degree of renal damage and to assess recovery or residual renal damage. The high sensitivity of ^{99m}Tc-DMSA scintigraphy for the early diagnosis and localization of acute pyelonephritis is well established.[76–78] Technetium-99m-DMSA planar scintigraphy has been shown to have both sensitivity and specificity of better than 90% in the diagnosis of experimentally induced acute pyelonephritis in piglets, using strict histopathologic criteria as the standard of reference.[33,34] The sensitivity of ^{99m}Tc-DMSA scintigraphy for pyelonephritis is 96% and the specificity 98%.[79] Imaging strategies in patients suspected of pyelonephritis or patients with sudden onset of fever, flank pain, and pyuria or bacteriuria should include ^{99m}Tc-DMSA scintigraphy.[80–82]

Images should be obtained in the posterior and posterior oblique projections using a parallel-hole, ultrahigh-resolution collimator. Pinhole magnification provides greater diagnostic sensitivity than the parallel-hole collimator for the detection of focal cortical defects. Technetium-99m-DMSA SPECT provides additional sensitivity and specificity over planar imaging in the evaluation of patients suspected of having pyelonephritis (Figs. 10.9 and 10.10).[77,83,84]

In normal kidneys, ^{99m}Tc-DMSA scintigraphy shows a pattern of tracer distribution reflecting the morphology of the renal cortex. No tracer uptake is seen in the medulla or in the collecting system. Flattening of the superolateral aspect of the left cortex may be due to splenic impression. Irregularities in the contour of the renal image may be due to fetal lobations (Fig. 10.7). In these instances, cortical thickness and

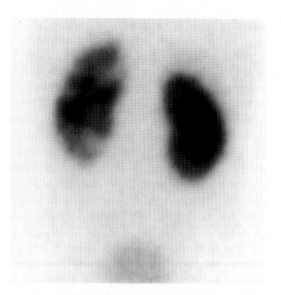

FIGURE 10.18. Acute multifocal pyelonephritis in a 2-year-old boy who presented with recurrent fever and left flank pain. The patient had no evidence of vesicoureteric reflux. Conventional ^{99m}Tc-DMSA planar scintigraphy reveals several cortical defects in the left kidney.

tracer uptake are normal. Acute pyelonephritis usually appears as a single or as multiple focal areas of reduced or absent uptake with a soft edge, without deformity of the renal outline or apparent loss of volume (Figs. 10.9, 10.10, and 10.18 to 10.21). In some cases, however, this reduced uptake is accompanied by an increase in volume of the affected area. Although the majority of lesions occur in the upper or lower

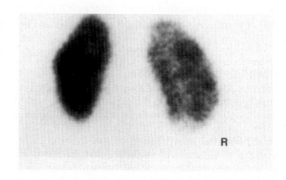

FIGURE 10.19. Diffuse acute pyelonephritis. Diffuse and focal pattern of decreased ^{99m}Tc-DMSA uptake in an enlarged (swollen) right kidney.

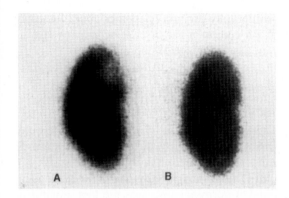

FIGURE 10.20. Resolution of acute pyelonephritis. A: Magnified image of a 3-month-old infant at the time of acute urinary tract infection shows focal decreased uptake of ^{99m}Tc-DMSA in the medial aspect of the left upper pole. B: Corresponding image 6 months later shows complete resolution (right image).

poles, the mid-zone of the kidney is also frequently involved. Renal scars show loss of cortical volume with relatively sharp edges. A less common scintigraphic pattern is one of diffuse decreased tracer uptake in an enlarged kidney. Acute pyelonephritis may resolve completely and scintigraphic images become normal within a few months (Fig. 10.22). Alternatively, a permanent scar(s) or damage may develop. A mature cortical scar is usually associated with contraction and loss of volume of the involved cortex. This may manifest as cortical thinning, flattening of the renal contour, or a wedge-shaped defect. The defect resulting from a mature scar may gradually become more prominent due to growth of the surrounding normal renal cortex. The scintigraphic pattern of a maturing scar varies according to the severity, age, and location of the lesion as well as the rate of growth of surrounding normal tissue.

Mechanisms of ^{99m}Tc-DMSA Renal Uptake

The pathophysiologic mechanisms that account for the decrease of ^{99m}Tc-DMSA uptake in acute pyelonephritis are probably multifactorial. Cortical ^{99m}Tc-DMSA uptake is dependent on renal blood flow and proximal tubular cell membrane transport function. Any pathologic process that alters either or both of these factors may result in focal or diffuse decreased uptake of ^{99m}Tc-DMSA. In our laboratory at Children's Hospital Boston we have shown using frozen section autoradiography that ^{99m}Tc-DMSA uptake in the kidney is largely associated with the regions of the brush border of cells of the proximal convoluted tubules (Fig. 10.1).[32] During acute inflammation, intratubular neutrophils release toxic enzymes and produce superoxide, causing direct damage not only to bacteria but to renal tubular cells as well.[85] In an experimental study in primates, it has been demonstrated that ischemia, as

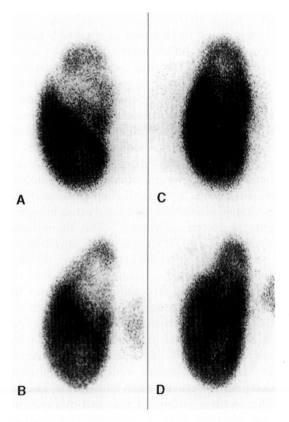

FIGURE 10.21. Progression of acute pyelonephritis to cortical scar. Posterior (A) and posterior oblique (B) images of the left kidney from a 5-year-old child at the time of acute febrile urinary tract infection demonstrate focally decreased ^{99m}Tc-DMSA uptake in the upper pole with preserved renal outline and without evidence of volume loss. Corresponding images obtained 1 year later (C,D) show contraction and loss of volume of the upper pole.

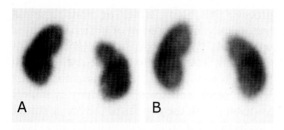

FIGURE 10.22. Pyelonephritis of the right upper pole before and after 2 weeks of antibiotic therapy. ^{99m}Tc-DMSA. A: Focal cortical defects in the right upper and lower poles. B: Normalization of cortical scintigraphy. The patient had complained of 2 weeks of right flank pain and fever. Two ultrasonograms were normal, and an intravenous urogram did not reveal reflux.

demonstrated by elevation of renal vein renin, occurs early in inflammatory response to acute pyelonephritis. This was attributed to intravascular granulocyte aggregation leading to arteriolar or capillary occlusion.[86] In another study, microvascular changes in experimental acute pyelonephritis in pigs were studied using combined stereomicroscopic and microradiographic techniques. Focal ischemia in areas involved by the acute inflammatory response was evidenced by compression of glomeruli, peritubular capillaries, and vasa rectae, presumably by interstitial edema.[87] This diminished uptake of ^{99m}Tc-DMSA in areas of acute inflammation probably reflects both focal tubular cell dysfunction and ischemia. Evaluation of focal renal blood flow using microspheres in experimentally induced acute pyelonephritis in piglets revealed significant focal ischemia in almost all of the pyelonephritic lesions. In approximately 40% of the lesions, the decrease in ^{99m}Tc-DMSA uptake was proportional to a decrease in regional renal blood flow. Therefore, in these lesions, tubular cell dysfunction may not have been a significant contributing factor for the decreased ^{99m}Tc-DMSA uptake. In the remaining 60% of the lesions, ^{99m}Tc-DMSA uptake was much more severely reduced than the corresponding decrease in blood flow, indicating the presence of regional tubular dysfunction. This study suggests that ischemia is an early event that precedes tubular cell dysfunction. Therefore, ^{99m}Tc-DMSA

scintigraphy probably becomes abnormal early in the course of the disease before any significant tissue damage has occurred.[73]

Intravenous Urography and Renal Ultrasonography

The low sensitivities of intravenous urography and ultrasonography in the demonstration of early renal infection are well known.[79,80,88–90] Ultrasonography is very useful in diagnosing renal or perirenal abscesses, but less valuable in acute pyelonephritis in which renal enlargement may be the only abnormal finding. Intravenous urograms are abnormal in only 24% to 26% of patients with acute pyelonephritis.[88,90] Possible abnormal urographic findings include a renal pelvis of small volume, dilated and distorted pelvicaliceal structures, renal enlargement, delayed pyelogram, reduced concentration of urographic material, and dilatation of the ureter without obstruction. In contrast to urography, cortical scintigraphy can detect cortical defects that do not deform the renal outline or the collecting system.[89,91] Computed tomography is an effective technique for documenting the nature of parenchymal involvement, particularly for the evaluation of the perinephric space. Concern about CT radiation exposures limits its use; therefore, routine use in the initial and follow-up evaluation of children with UTI is not practical, and CT should be reserved for complicated cases.[92,93] The role of magnetic resonance imaging (MRI) in the diagnosis of acute pyelonephritis remains to be defined.[94]

In the diagnosis of pyelonephritis, the combination of ultrasonography and cortical scintigraphy is useful. Changes secondary to pyelonephritis may be recognized on ultrasonography as hyperechoic or hypoechoic foci, loss of corticomedullary differentiation, focal or diffuse renal enlargement, and mild or moderate dilatation of the renal pelvis. However, renal ultrasonography has proved to have a low sensitivity for the detection of acute focal inflammatory changes of the renal cortex. In a prospective study, ultrasonographic changes consistent with acute pyelonephritis were found in only 39% of the children with scintigraphically documented acute pyelonephritis. When abnormal, ultrasonography under-estimated the number and extent of the pyelonephritic lesions.[69] Ultrasonography should not, therefore, be regarded as the primary imaging technique for the diagnosis of acute pyelonephritis. Ultrasonography is, however, highly reliable for the detection of hydronephrosis and of the congenital abnormalities that may be associated with UTI in some patients.

Renal Venous Thrombosis

Most types of acquired renal disease in newborns are due to circulatory disturbances, such as renal arterial or venous thrombosis. Renal vein thrombosis in infants is probably related to venous stasis secondary to shock, septicemia, or dehydration. The diagnosis of renal vein thrombosis may be suggested by the presence of oliguria, mild hematuria, and proteinuria. Renal vein thrombosis is also seen in infants of diabetic mothers and children with congenital heart disease. Consumptive coagulopathy or intravascular coagulation may be present in some of these patients.[70,95–101] The infant presents with a flank mass, oliguria, and hematuria. Hypertension, which is not frequent in this condition, has been seen in several patients we have studied.

Approximately two-thirds of all cases of renal vein thrombosis occur in the pediatric age group, with most seen during the neonatal period. In older children, renal vein thrombosis may develop as a consequence of nephrotic syndrome or severe illness (nephrotic syndrome is a very frequent cause of large-vessel thrombosis because of urinary losses of antithrombin III, protein C, protein S, and other factors.)

Renal vein thrombosis has been described as a bilateral disease, with asymmetric involvement. Because of this characteristic, a minor lesion in the apparently noninvolved kidney may be missed. Most frequently, the thrombus originates in the interlobar or arcuate veins and less commonly in the main renal vein. The thrombus may extend into the main renal vein and the inferior vena cava, or in a retrograde fashion, it may involve the renal cortex. The venous obstruction then leads to infarction and hemorrhage. Blood leaking into the interstitium and renal tubules may ultimately result in fibrosis. Most patients with renal vein thrombosis are treated medically with maintenance of normal fluid and electrolyte balance.[99]

There is considerable variability in the urographic identification of renal vein thrombosis. In most patients with this condition, the kidney involved is not visualized by intravenous urography. Before modern nuclear medicine techniques were widely employed, it was thought that affected renal units not visible on initial urographic examination virtually ensured an atrophic, functionless kidney later.[102] Ultrasonography or inferior vena cavagraphy may be normal, or it may show evidence of venous thrombosis. Ultrasonography may also demonstrate a normal or enlarged kidney and reveal thrombi in the inferior vena cava. Doppler ultrasonography may show decreased or absent flow in the affected kidney.

Renal scintigraphy using ^{99m}Tc-MAG$_3$ or ^{99m}Tc-DMSA is a sensitive method for screening patients with renal vein thrombosis[103] because the findings on serial renal scintigraphy that show the evolution of renal function correlate well with the ultimate outcome.

In severe cases there may be no perfusion or apparent function in the involved side (Figs. 10.23 and 10.24). A follow-up study may be useful to demonstrate the residual renal function after recovery. Radionuclide studies may reveal information of prognostic significance, with a normal study predicting a rapid and complete recovery.

Renal Infarction

Renal infarction can occur in patients with cyanotic congenital heart disease, polycythemia, atrial fibrillation, dehydration, or trauma. Aortic thrombosis and renal infarction are also well-recognized complications of prolonged umbilical artery catheterization. Treatment with thrombolytic agents has produced resolution of the clot and recovery of renal function in some cases. Technetium-99m DMSA scintigraphy demonstrates focal perfusion defect(s) in the affected kidney(s) (Fig. 10.25).

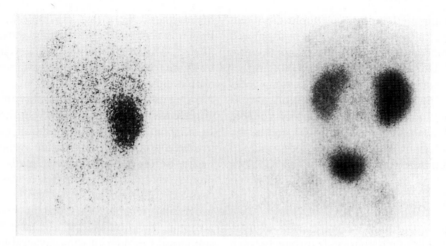

FIGURE 10.23. Renal vein thrombosis. This ^{99m}Tc-DMSA study was done in a premature, 1400-g female infant who developed hypertension after withdrawal of an umbilical artery catheter. Ultrasonography showed two kidneys of normal size. On the initial study (left) the kidney is not visualized. After treatment with hydralazine the patient became normotensive, and another study 3 weeks later showed return of left renal function (right).

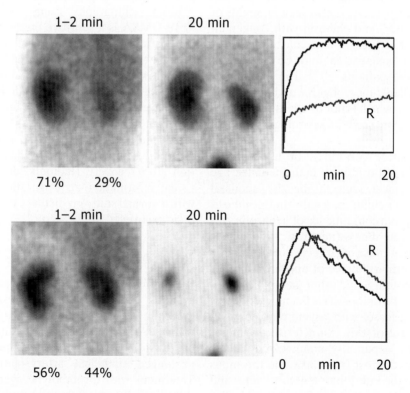

FIGURE 10.24. Renal vein thrombosis (^{99m}Tc-MAG$_3$). A 1-week-old girl presenting with oliguria, cardiomegaly, and hypertension. Top: First study shows asymmetric renal function (L > R) with bilateral delay in transit time and cortical retention. Bottom: One month later there is more symmetric renal function (L = 56%, R = 44%) and a normalization of transit times. There is some retention of tracer in the right pelvis accounting for a longer time-to-peak.

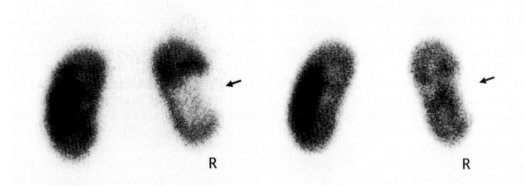

FIGURE 10.25. Renal infarct. A 16-year-old boy with cyanotic congenital heart disease had undergone several surgical interventions and presented with acute right flank pain. Left: Initial ^{99m}Tc-DMSA scintigraphy shows a well-defined defect in the right kidney due to an infarct. Right: A follow-up study 1.5 months later shows considerable resolution of the defect.

Hypertension

The incidence of hypertension in children is 1.4% to 2.3%.[104] The reported incidence of secondary hypertension varies, however, with the source of patients.[105–107] The younger the child, the more common is secondary hypertension, and the most common cause of secondary hypertension in children is renal disease. Renal disease associated with hypertension is frequently caused by diseases that involve the renal arteries or the renal parenchyma. In a study of 563 pediatric patients with secondary hypertension, 78% had a renal abnormality and 12% were diagnosed with renal artery disease.[106] Less frequently, secondary hypertension may be caused by disorders of the endocrine, cardiovascular, or nervous systems. Radionuclide renal studies play an important role in the evaluation and treatment of hypertension in infants and children.

Some of the renal causes of hypertension, such as infarction, postpyelonephritic scarring, and posttraumatic lesions, are easily diagnosed by conventional renal scintigraphy. Both dynamic and static scintigraphy have been found to be very sensitive for the identification of renovascular hypertension.[87,108,109] On dynamic scintigraphy, the affected kidney is usually smaller and shows less uptake than the contralateral kidney. The more severe the renal artery stenosis, the lower the renal uptake of the tracer. Excretion of the tracer into the pelvicaliceal system may not be impaired with mild degrees of stenosis. When stenosis is severe, however, excretion of tracer in the collecting system is delayed or even absent during the 20-minute observation period. Parenchymal retention of the tracer increases with severity of stenosis. Technetium-99m DMSA scintigraphy in patients with renovascular hypertension typically reveals renal asymmetry; the affected kidney is smaller and has less tracer uptake. This method can also demonstrate focal cortical defects.

Conventional radionuclide imaging may show evidence of reduced renal perfusion and function on the affected side. The kidney with a stenotic artery, however, may remain adequately perfused; owing to the autoregulation mechanism, and the radionuclide renal study may therefore, appear normal in a significant number of patients. Radionuclide studies in the presence of bilateral or segmental renal artery stenosis may not be helpful. The efficacy of renal scintigraphy for the diagnosis of renovascular hypertension, however, is markedly improved by the use of angiotensin-converting enzyme (ACE) inhibitors, such as captopril, which block the formation of angiotensin II, resulting in dilatation of the efferent arterioles and a decrease in the transcapillary pressure gradient. This situation leads to a significant decrease in GFR of the kidney in the presence of renal artery stenosis that can be detected by renal scintigraphy and renography.[110–114]

The choices of radiopharmaceutical, ACE inhibitor, and examination technique vary among investigators. In the original studies in pediatric patients, ^{99m}Tc-DTPA was used.[111] Subsequent experience has shown that either glomerular or tubular agents can be used. ^{99m}Tc-MAG$_3$ captopril renography appears to be effective.

The radiopharmaceutical of choice for detecting focal parenchymal abnormalities such as infarcts and pyelonephritic scars is ^{99m}Tc-DMSA.[35,80,108,109] Administration of captopril may cause decrease in the renal ^{99m}Tc-DMSA uptake in patients with renovascular hypertension.[115]

Either captopril or enalaprilat can be used as the ACE inhibitor. To ensure better absorption of captopril, the patient should not eat solids for approximately 4 hours before the study. The advantage of enalaprilat is that it is administered intravenously and, unlike oral captopril, its effect does not depend on variable rate of absorption through the gastrointestinal tract.

A significant fall in blood pressure can be observed even after a single dose of captopril. Therefore, the patient should be well hydrated, well monitored, and an intravenous access maintained throughout the study. The blood pressure should be monitored every 5 to 15 minutes. The probability of severe hypotensive crisis is even higher with intravenous enalaprilat. The routine use of enalaprit is not recommended. Diuretics may exaggerate the hypotensive effect of ACE inhibitors and should not be used in conjunction with captopril renography.

Ideally, a baseline study is obtained followed by another examination 1 hour after oral administration of captopril (1 mg/kg up to 50 mg). An alternative approach is to obtain the initial study performed with the use of ACE inhibitor and repeat the study without the use of ACE inhibitor (only if the first study is abnormal).

The scintigraphic manifestations of decreased renal function induced by ACE inhibitor in the presence of hemodynamically significant renal artery stenosis depend on which radiopharmaceutical is used. The primary effect of ACE inhibitor is decreased GFR. Therefore, the effect of an ACE inhibitor on a ^{99m}Tc-DTPA study will, therefore, be observed as a varying degree of decreased extraction of tracer and delayed visualization of the collecting system, whereas with the use of tubular agents, prolonged retention of the tracer is seen. ^{99m}Tc-MAG$_3$ scintigraphy is effective in identifying focal renal ischemia (Fig. 10.26). The typical findings of a positive captopril study include an increase in the differential renal uptake, an increase in cortical transit time, a prolongation of time to peak, and retention of tracer in the renal parenchyma. An important parameter is split renal uptake. Other parameters that can be abnormal in renovascular hypertension include time to peak, time to half-peak, relative excretion delay, and residual cortical activity. Scintigraphic abnormalities in unilateral renal artery stenosis can be appreciated visually by inspection of the images and the renal time-activity curves. Numerical or semiquantitative evaluation of time-activity curves have been utilized.

In the presence of bilateral renal artery stenosis, narrowing is usually asymmetrical, as is the effect of captopril on each kidney.

In adult patients, scintigraphic abnormalities induced by the administration of captopril in hypertensive adults appear to be strongly associated with cure or improvement in blood pressure control following revascularization or nephrectomy. Cases in which captopril does not induce scintigraphic changes are associated with failure of revascularization or nephrectomy.[116–119] Such failure appears to be due to a high prevalence of atherosclerosis and its possible coexistence with essential hypertension. Angiographic demonstration of renal artery narrowing in older patients does not, therefore, necessarily indicate renovascular hypertension, and revascularization may fail to cure hypertension. In hypertensive children, however, a negative captopril renogram is rarely associated with angiographic evidence of renal artery stenosis.

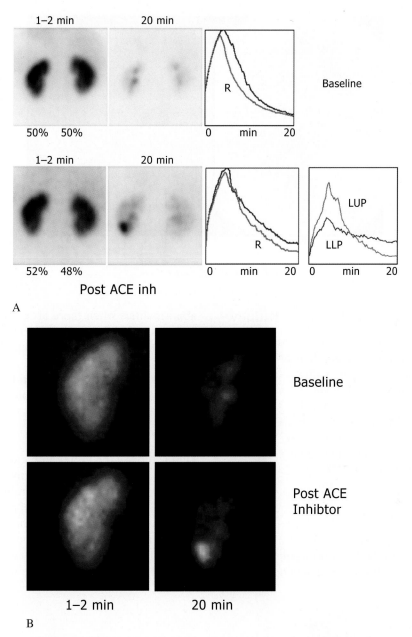

A

B

FIGURE 10.26. A: Hypertension. Baseline and post–angiotensin-converting enzyme (ACE) inhibitor ^{99m}Tc-MAG$_3$ studies. On the baseline study (top), the left renal time-activity curve shows a delayed time-to-peak. Renal function is symmetric, and there is no retention of tracer in the renal parenchyma. On the post-ACE inhibitor study (bottom), relative renal function appears normal. However, there is focal parenchymal retention of tracer in the left lower pole. The time-activity curve of the left lower pole (LLP) shows less amplitude and high residual at 20 minutes than the left upper pole (LUP). B: Baseline study (top): 1- to 2-minute and 20-minute images reveal normal intrarenal distribution of tracer. Similar images (bottom) after administration of ACE inhibitor reveal a focal reduction of tracer uptake in the left lower pole (1–2 minutes) and focal parenchymal tracer retention in the same region (20 minutes). C: Renal angiography reveals arterial stenosis to the involved segment of the left lower pole. Following selective balloon angioplasty, the patient's blood pressure dropped from 170/110 to 120/60 mm Hg.

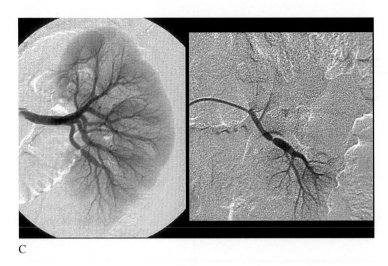

C

FIGURE 10.26. *Continued*

Ectopic Kidney and Solitary Kidney

One or both kidneys may be displaced in association with or independent of other renal malformations. Ectopic kidneys situated in the pelvis may be difficult to visualize on intravenous urography, partly because of interference by surrounding bony structures. Scintigraphy with ^{99m}Tc-DMSA or ^{99m}Tc-MAG$_3$ are helpful for diagnosing renal ectopia or a solitary kidney (Fig. 10.27).

Horseshoe Kidney

With horseshoe-shaped kidneys, fusion is usually between the two lower poles. Radionuclide studies are useful for assessing functional abnormalities when there are symptoms referable to the kidney, such as infection, hypertension, and hematuria. Technetium-99m-DMSA images (including anterior views) show whether the kidneys are joined by functioning renal tissue or by a fibrous band (Fig. 10.28).

Duplication

Duplication of the ureter and renal pelvis is one of the most common abnormalities of the urinary tract. It occurs bilaterally in 25% to 30% of affected patients. The upper pole ureter tends to insert more caudally and medially than the normally placed lower pole ureter. The ureter from the lower pole is more often affected by reflux, whereas the upper ureter is

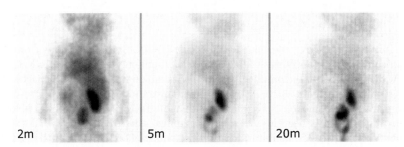

2m   5m   20m

FIGURE 10.27. Ectopic left kidney. ^{99m}Tc-MAG$_3$ study reveals tracer uptake in the pelvis on the 2 minute image. By 5 minutes, tracer appears in the renal pelvis of the ectopic kidney. By 20 minutes bladder activity overlaps with the pelvic kidney. The right kidney reveals a mild ureteropelvic junction obstruction.

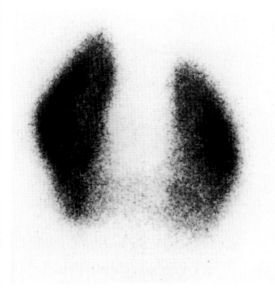

FIGURE 10.28. Horseshoe-shaped kidney. ^{99m}Tc-DMSA scintigraphy in a 15-year-old girl.

more often obstructed. When surgery is contemplated, ^{99m}Tc-DMSA is used to evaluate the relative function of the upper and lower renal segments (Fig. 10.29).

Polycystic Renal Disease

There are two types of polycystic renal disease. Autosomal dominant polycystic kidney disease is the more common type, but usually does not present until adulthood. Autosomal recessive polycystic kidney disease usually presents during infancy and is an inherited cystic disorder affecting both kidneys. It is twice as frequent in male infants as in female infants. Scintigraphy with ^{99m}Tc-DMSA often reveals large renal silhouettes and outlines of renal parenchymal uptake surrounding the cysts. The appearance of the scan in polycystic renal disease depends on the degree of renal involvement. In more severe cases, there may be no evidence of renal uptake.

Multicystic Dysplastic Kidneys

Multicystic dysplasia of the kidney (MCDK) is the most frequent cystic disorder of infants and

children.[120] There is marked variation in the size of the lesions and extent of involvement. The multicystic dysplastic kidney can be of varying sizes and shapes and contains cortical and medullary cysts. Classically, MCDK has been described as a mass of noncommunicating cysts resembling a bunch of grapes with no discernible renal parenchyma or pelvis.[121,122] Urogenital abnormalities are frequently associated with MCDK. In approximately 75% of the cases, scintigraphy with ^{99m}Tc-DMSA does not demonstrate tracer uptake in the involved kidney. In some instances, however, some tracer uptake can be seen in small regions of distorted renal parenchyma. Often it can be demonstrated only with computer enhancement (Fig. 10.30). Sometimes scintigraphic images of newborns with MCDK appear similar to the images seen with hydronephrosis.

Prune-Belly Syndrome

Prune-belly syndrome occurs in male infants and manifests as dilatation of the urinary bladder and ureters with a bizarre, wrinkled, flabby abdominal wall.[123–126] The cause of the abdominal muscular deficiency is not known. The most severely affected patients die soon after birth or may be stillborn. Abnormalities associated with this syndrome include pulmonary hypoplasia, renal dysplasia, urethral obstruction, weak chest wall muscles, vesicoureteric reflux, and undescended testes. Dynamic renal scintigraphy reveals a spectrum of findings. Scintigraphy may show dilatation of the pelvicaliceal systems without obstruction; yet others reveal dilatation with apparent obstruction. Technetium-99m-DMSA scintigraphy can help assess regional distribution of functioning renal parenchyma, detect renal scarring, and evaluate the course of the renal disease. Frequently, ^{99m}Tc-DMSA imaging at 24 hours is necessary to allow drainage of the tracer activity in the dilated ureters.

Renal Trauma

Radionuclide imaging is used infrequently in these patients. In some cases, ^{99m}Tc-DMSA scintigraphy can be helpful for detecting

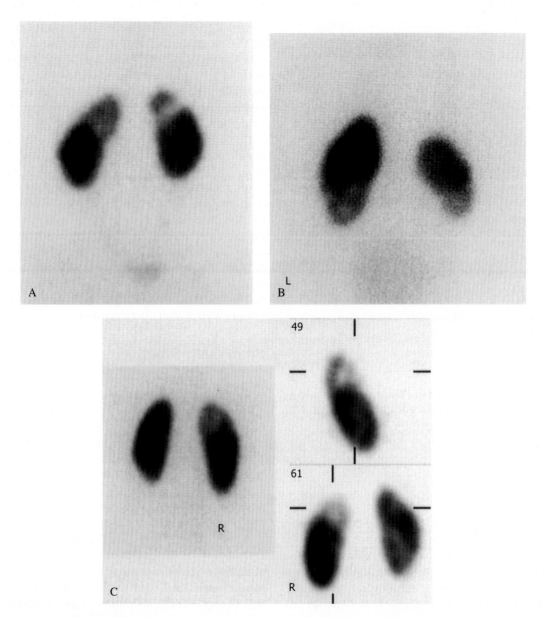

FIGURE 10.29. Duplication. Three examples of ^{99m}Tc-DMSA scintigraphy in duplication. A: Bilateral duplication with relatively poor function in both upper poles. B: Bilateral duplication with less function in the left kidney and in both lower poles.

C: Conventional planar scintigraphy (left) and selected sagittal and transverse SPECT slices (right) in unilateral duplication with relatively poor function of the right upper pole, anteriorly.

nonobvious functional or structural damage to the kidney. Renal scintigraphy can be used to assess recovery or residual damage (Figs. 10.31 and 10.32). Studies using ^{99m}Tc-MAG$_3$ or ^{99m}Tc-DTPA can effectively detect urinary leaks following trauma.

Acute Renal Failure

With acute renal failure, radionuclide studies have a predictive value. Improvements in function detected on such studies usually precede biochemical changes by 1 to 2 days. Similarly,

FIGURE 10.30. Multicystic dysplastic kidneys (MCDK), ^{99m}Tc-DMSA scintigraphy. A: Right MCDK showing a thin region of tracer uptake over the posterior aspect of a photon-deficient region. The left renal image was computer-enhanced to show the right uptake. B: Three other examples of ^{99m}Tc-DMSA appearance in MCDK: 0, no evidence of uptake; 1, minimal uptake detected only by computer enhancement; 2, minimal uptake without computer enhancement.

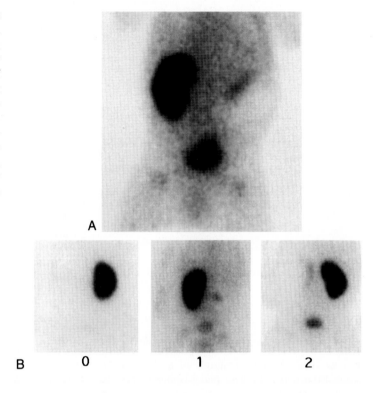

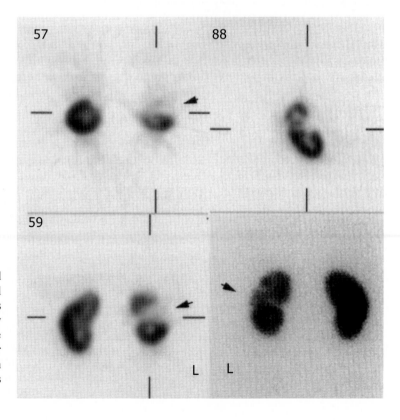

FIGURE 10.31. Trauma. Selected transverse, sagittal, and coronal ^{99m}Tc-DMSA SPECT slices as well as planar scintigraphy reveal cortical damage of the left kidney (arrows) after trauma. These images are from a follow-up study to assess recovery.

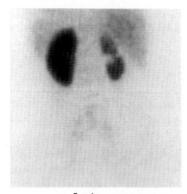

2 min.

Uptake 10% of Injected Dose

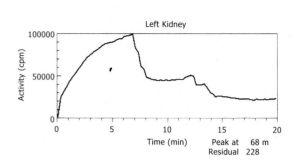

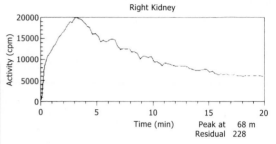

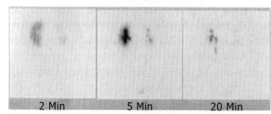

2 Min   5 Min   20 Min

FIGURE 10.32. Trauma. Example of a ^{99m}Tc-MAG$_3$ study from a patient who had sustained previous renal trauma. The parenchymal phase (top left) reveals a hypertrophic left kidney and a small right kidney with cortical defect in its midportion. Cortical transit time and drainage are normal bilaterally.

radionuclide studies have been used to follow functional changes in patients with acute glomerulonephritis.

Tumors

Renal scintigraphy is very infrequently used in the investigation of renal tumors. Diagnosis and further evaluation of renal and perirenal masses and tumors are carried out with ultrasonography, MRI, and CT. Hypertrophy of a renal column of Bertin may appear as a mass that at times is difficult to distinguish from neoplasm or cyst on urography. Cortical radionuclide imaging can firmly establish the diagnosis of normal renal cortex and absence of tumor.[127-129]

Effect of Radiotherapy

Radiation therapy can cause transient or permanent functional defect(s) in the irradiated kidney. This effect can be seen as one or more regions in the kidney with reduced to absent uptake of ^{99m}Tc-DMSA and ^{99m}Tc-MAG$_3$. Radiation therapy can cause delayed uptake and retention of dynamic renal tracers.

Renal Transplantation

Living Renal Donors

Living donors comprise approximately 60% of all donors for renal transplants in children.[2] Renal scintigraphy is useful for assessing both renal function and the anatomy in living donors. For example, if previously undetected renal abnormalities are seen, a donor may be considered unsuitable. If a radionuclide study on a living donor reveals renal function asymmetry, the surgeon may elect to transplant the kidney showing less function. Finally, detection of anatomic variants (e.g., an extrarenal pelvis), prior to transplantation can prevent unnecessary investigation in the recipient after the transplant procedure.

Recipients of Renal Transplants

Radionuclide studies are useful during the early and late periods after renal transplantation to assess surgical results and detect complications.[130-136] As mentioned above, radiopharmaceuticals produce no osmotic load and no pharmacologic effects and therefore can be used safely even in the presence of severe renal transplant dysfunction. Radionuclide techniques can predict rejection and recovery of function 24 to 48 hours before changes in the clinical course or blood chemistries occur. It is possible with scintigraphic methods to assess perfusion of the transplant during the early and late postoperative periods and assist in the differential diagnosis of diminished graft function, which includes rejection, obstruction, and urinary leak (Fig. 10.33).

If there are no suspected surgical complications, a baseline evaluation of the transplant is often obtained during the first 24 hours following transplantation. Subsequent studies are performed depending on the patient's progress. Renal transplants from living donors that have had short cold and warm ischemia times will often function immediately after transplantation. The initial uptake of the tracers in these transplants is normal and occasionally more intense than in a normally functioning kidney. In addition, the intrarenal transit time is normal or even faster than normal (Fig. 10.34). After a few days, in the absence of complications, the handling of tracers by the transplant becomes identical to that of normal kidneys.

As many as one third of grafts, particularly those from deceased donors, are affected by acute tubular necrosis (ATN), which can persist for just a few days or for as long as 2 months after the procedure. In patients with ATN, delayed images obtained with ^{99m}Tc-MAG$_3$ several hours after administration of the tracer

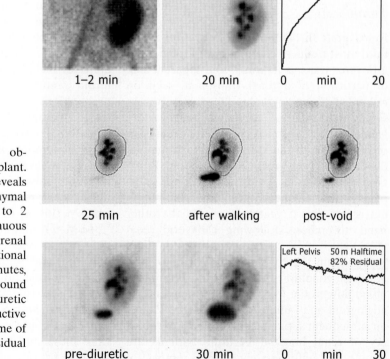

FIGURE 10.33. Ureteropelvic obstruction in a renal transplant. The ^{99m}Tc-MAG$_3$ study reveals somewhat diminished parenchymal uptake of the tracer at 1 to 2 minutes followed by continuous accumulation of tracer in the renal pelvis by 20 minutes. Additional images were obtained at 25 minutes, after the patient walked around and following voiding. Diuretic renography reveals an obstructive pattern with a washout half-time of 50 minutes and a 30-minute residual of 82%.

1–2 min   20 min   0   min   20

25 min   after walking   post-void

pre-diuretic   30 min   0   min   30

Left Pelvis   50 m Halftime
82% Residual

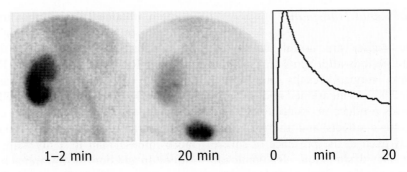

1–2 min   20 min   0   min   20

FIGURE 10.34. Kidney from a living donor. ^{99m}Tc-DMSA a few hours posttransplantation. Tracer uptake is brisk at 1 to 2 minutes, and there is no parenchymal or urinary retention at 20 minutes. The renal time-activity curve shows a time-to-peak of only 2 minutes and less than 35% residual at 20 minutes.

reveal retention of the radionuclide within the renal parenchyma with little if any accumulation or passage of activity into the renal pelvis, ureter, or bladder. If tracer activity within the transplant is similar to background on radionuclide angiography and later images, it indicates severe depression of renal function. However, the kidney should not be assumed nonviable. The patient usually recovers from ATN unless rejection or other complications appear.

Thrombosis

Renal graft thrombosis and infarction is the third most frequent cause of graft loss in pediatric renal transplantation.[137] The apparent lack of perfusion of a renal transplant, seen on radionuclide angiography, does not always signify occlusion of the main renal artery leading to the transplant but reflects actual lack of blood flow to the kidney. This lack may be due to renal or hyperacute rejection. Renal graft thrombosis in a living related donor transplant is most frequently seen when the recipient is less than 5 years of age. On the other hand, thrombosis following cadaveric renal transplant is most common when the donor is young, again usually less than 5 years of age. All these conditions present as a lack of renal blood flow to the transplant on a radionuclide angiogram and failure to visualize the kidney on subsequent serial images. Chances of recovery of renal function in these patients are remote, and unfortunately surgical removal of the graft may be indicated.

Rejection

The most common cause of renal graft dysfunction during the first several months following transplantation is an acute rejection episode. As many as 25% of deceased transplants and 15% of living-related-donor transplant recipients have acute rejection episodes during the first year after transplantation. Rejection is often suspected on the basis of nonspecific clinical findings (fever, tenderness over the graft site) or specific clinical findings (decreased urine output, increased serum urea nitrogen and creatinine). A renal biopsy is frequently obtained to confirm the diagnosis of rejection. Treatment for acute rejection episodes includes high-dose "pulse" corticosteroid treatment or the use of antilymphocyte preparations. Complications associated with these therapies, particularly opportunistic infections, are sometimes severe.

Renal scintigraphy is generally performed during the evaluation of an apparent acute rejection episode. The scintigraphic findings during acute rejection episodes include diminished perfusion of the graft, poor uptake of ^{99m}Tc-MAG$_3$, and, occasionally, increased size of the renal silhouette. There are no specific findings in renal scintigraphy to confirm renal transplant rejection. The major value of the study is to rule out other conditions (e.g., renal obstruction, vascular comprise or urinary leak) that could cause diminished graft function. These studies are particularly important, as they provide the basis for avoiding unnecessary therapy when processes other than rejection account for the diminished graft function.

Virtually all acute rejection episodes are reversible with treatment. With many episodes, however, return of graft function to prerejection levels may be delayed for up to several weeks, possibly related to renal interstitial edema secondary to the infiltrating lymphocytes and their subsequent destruction. Serial follow-up radionuclide studies may be helpful for assessing the returning renal function, as these studies often predict the recovery of function 24 to 48 hours before the blood chemistry values improve.

Obstruction

Urinary obstruction is a very rare complication following renal transplantation and may be difficult to diagnose in the presence of depressed renal function, such as occurs in acute tubular necrosis or after a rejection episode. Obstruction soon after surgery may be due to edema and/or inflammation in the region of the ureterovesical junction; it may be temporary. Later, obstruction may be due to external compression, which may be caused by (1) a lymphocele or scarring secondary to previous surgery or (2) internal obstruction, such as that caused by a ureteral stone or stenosis at the ureteral anastomosis site. In most cases, the transplant ureter is implanted directly into the bladder. In some cases, however, the native ureter may be used as a ureterostomy or, by

anastomosis, connected directly to the pelvis of the graft. Because the transplant's ureter obtains its blood supply only from the graft, the distal ureter may be poorly perfused and may result in distal ureteral scarring and obstruction. Partial or even total obstruction of a transplant kidney may be relatively asymptomatic, as the graft is not innervated. Diagnosis of partial obstruction is sometimes difficult, and the use of furosemide after injection of the tracer may aid in the diagnosis. In cases of diminished graft function, ^{99m}Tc-MAG$_3$ sometimes demonstrates urinary obstruction, even in the presence of severe renal failure.

Urinary Leak

Urinary leak usually occurs in the first few months following transplantation. It can occur at the site of anastomosis of the transplant ureter or through necrosis of the distal transplant ureter related to diminished perfusion of that section. The presence of urinary leak is detected with serial scintigraphy with greater sensitivity than other methods because of the high contrast of the radiotracer technique.[138] Multiple images at several minutes to several hours after the injection tracer may be necessary to detect urinary leakage. On the series of scintigrams, the leakage appears as a focal or diffuse area of increasing tracer accumulation outside the confines of the transplant, the ureter, or the bladder (Fig. 10.35). Urinoma

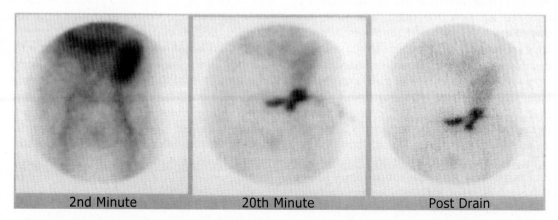

| 2nd Minute | 20th Minute | Post Drain |

FIGURE 10.35. Urinary leak. Postoperatively, this recipient of a renal transplant developed a urinary leak. Selected images of a ^{99m}Tc-MAG$_3$ study (left to right: 2 minutes, 20 minutes, and after drain) reveal an abnormal accumulation of radiotracer inferior to the left-sided transplant, which corresponded to a urine leak through the transplanted ureter.

usually appears as a photon-deficient area on early images (5 to 10 minutes). On later images, tracer accumulates within this region. If the area that is photon-deficient on early images does not concentrate radiotracer on later images, this region may represent a hematoma or a lymphocele.

Appendix: Quantitative Analysis of Renal Function

Nuclear medicine is unique among medical imaging modalities in that it is capable of providing detailed quantitative physiologic information about the kidneys. In large part, this is due to the availability of radiotracers whose properties approximate those of the classic tracers PAH and inulin.

Although quantitative physiologic information is useful in monitoring patients, producing it in a consistent and accurate way requires close attention to detail. In what follows, we have tried to emphasize the assumptions that are made in some common approaches to the quantitative analysis of the renogram.

Correction for Tissue Attenuation and Detection of Extrarenal Activity

In quantitative analysis of dynamic renal scintigraphy, one is attempting to measure the amount of activity in each kidney as a function of time. These functions are approximated by time-activity curves obtained from ROIs over the kidneys. The resulting time-activity curves have components that are due to the detection of extrarenal (i.e., background) activity. In addition, there is attenuation of photons from the kidney due to the intervening tissue. Thus in order to estimate the activity in each kidney, it is desirable to attempt to correct for background activity and attenuation.

Background and attenuation correction for renography is a somewhat controversial subject that is an area of ongoing research. We limit ourselves here to describing some simple first-order corrections that illustrate the general ideas involved and that are adequate except in the case of extremely poor renal function. For

more sophisticated approaches, we refer the reader to the literature.

Background correction is usually based on the time-activity curve obtained from an ROI adjacent to the kidneys. This ROI is termed the background region. Various background regions have been proposed: an area between the kidneys,[139] an area around the kidneys,[140] an area superior to the kidneys, and an area inferolateral to the kidneys[141] have been used.

A simple approach to *background correction* is as follows: Let $K(t)$ and $B(t)$ denote the kidney and background time-activity curves, respectively. Let A_K and A_B denote the area in pixels of the renal and background ROIs, respectively. The background-corrected kidney time-activity curve, $K_c(t)$, is computed using the formula

$$K_c(t) = K(t) - S(A_K/A_B)B(t)$$

where S is a scaling factor (usually equal to 1).[139]

More sophisticated techniques for background correction take into account such factors as kidney volume and differences in kinetics between the kidney and background curves.[142,143] The use of such techniques reportedly results in more accurate quantification of renal function.[143]

A simple approach to *attenuation correction* is based on the mean distance of the kidney from the surface of the body. This distance may be measured by the gamma camera using a lateral view or by ultrasonography. Alternatively, this distance may be estimated from the patient's height and weight using a nomogram.[144] Attenuation correction is done by multiplying the background-corrected renal time-activity curve by e^{ux}, where u is the linear attenuation coefficient of the radiotracer in soft tissues and x is the mean distance of the kidney from the surface of the body.[141,145] A more sophisticated approach may be found in the paper by Takaki et al.[143]

Deconvolution Analysis

After background and attenuation correction, the renal time-activity curve approximates the amount of tracer in the kidney as a function of time. It is intuitively clear that this time-activity curve depends on how much radiotracer enters the kidney from the bloodstream as a function of time, which we refer to as the input function, as well as the handling of the radiotracer by the kidney. The input function, and hence the observed renal time-activity curve, are affected by factors that have no bearing on the function of a particular kidney, such as the function of the other kidney, loss of radiotracer from the intravascular space, and, occasionally, continued input of radiotracer from a partially extravasated injection.[146] The purpose of deconvolution analysis is to describe the handling of the tracer by the kidney in a way that is independent of the input function.

One way to describe the handling of radiotracer by the kidney is to construct a curve showing the fraction of radiotracer entering the kidney at time 0, that remains in the kidney at time t. We call this curve the retention function. The retention function is of direct clinical significance. For example, prolonged retention of radiotracer suggests obstruction. It is intuitively clear that the observed renal curve is determined by the input function and the retention function. To make this statement mathematically precise, the kidney is modeled as a linear, time-invariant system whose input is the input function discussed above and whose unit impulse response is equal to the retention function. With this model, the observed renal curve is given by the mathematical operation of convolution of the input function and the retention function. Denoting the input, retention, and kidney functions by $I(t)$, $R(t)$, and $K(t)$, respectively, we can write it as

$$K(t) = I(t) * R(t),$$

where * denotes the mathematical operation of convolution. Given $I(t)$ and $K(t)$, one can solve this equation for $R(t)$. This is known as deconvolution. The concepts of linear, time-invariant system, unit impulse response, convolution, and so forth are discussed in more detail by Oppenheim et al.[147]

The input function is commonly assumed to be proportional to the plasma tracer concentration in the blood entering the kidney. This function is difficult to measure directly. In practice, the input function may be approximated as being proportional to a time-activity curve obtained from the abdominal aorta, heart, liver, or brain.[146,148] There are two possible sources of error in this approximation: temporal differences in tracer concentration between the plasma in the pool being monitored and the renal artery, and possible contamination of the observed blood-pool curve by detection of extravascular activity. However, this approximation of the input function by externally detected time-activity curves has been found to work well in practice.[149]

Several investigators have reported using deconvolution to estimate the renal retention function.[41,139,146,150] One difficulty with deconvolution is that small observation errors may lead to physiologically unrealistic negative values and high-frequency oscillations in the computed retention function.[151] To prevent this, we have found it useful to introduce constraints derived from physiologic considerations of the renal system into the deconvolution process. Specifically, the computed retention function is constrained to be nonnegative and nonincreasing. Retention functions computed using this technique have been shown to be relatively insensitive to random data errors.[152]

Interpretation of the Renal Retention Function

The computed retention function is an estimate of the renal time-activity curve that would be obtained after an instantaneous intraarterial injection of a radiotracer without recirculation. Consider such a curve obtained with a PAH-like substance that is handled primarily by tubular secretion (e.g., ^{123}I-OIH). All of the tracer arriving in the kidney subsequently enters the tubular space by either glomerular filtration or tubular secretion and leaves via the ureter. The corresponding retention function, shown in Figure 10.36A, consists of a tubular plateau phase (from time 0 to the minimal tubular transit time) followed by a tubular washout phase. In contrast, consider such a curve obtained with a substance like inulin, that is handled primarily by glomerular filtration

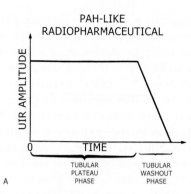

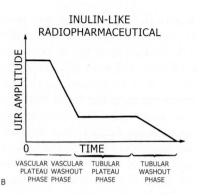

FIGURE 10.36. A: Deconvoluted renal time-activity histogram from a substance behaving like para-aminohippuric acid (PAH). B: Deconvoluted renal time-activity curve from a substance behaving like inulin.

(e.g., ^{99m}Tc-DTPA). A fraction of the tracer, equal to the filtration fraction, enters the tubular space by glomerular filtration and leaves via the ureter. The remainder of tracer stays in the vascular space and leaves the kidney via the renal vein. The corresponding retention function, shown in Figure 10.36B, consists of a vascular plateau phase (from time 0 until the minimal vascular transit time), a vascular washout phase (until the maximal vascular transit time), a tubular plateau phase (until the minimal tubular transit time), and a tubular washout phase. The amplitude of the tubular plateau divided by the amplitude of the vascular plateau is equal to the filtration fraction. The vascular phase occurs quite rapidly, however, and is difficult to delineate at the frame rates commonly used for dynamic renal imaging. It is sometimes useful for interpretation to eliminate the vascular phase of the retention function by setting the retention function values prior to a set time (chosen to be greater than the maximal vascular transit time and less than the minimal tubular transit time) equal to the retention function value at that time. The resulting curve is termed the tubular retention function.

Computed retention functions may be used to calculate indices of relative renal function (i.e., left versus right). Relative effective renal plasma flow (ERPF) may be estimated from the relative initial amplitudes of the retention functions obtained using a tracer that is handled like PAH.[139,150] Relative GFR may be estimated from the relative initial amplitudes of the tubular retention functions obtained using a tracer that is handled like inulin.[146] Relative GFR calculated by this method has been shown to correlate well with individual kidney creatinine clearance.[153] Computed retention functions are also useful for quantifying transit times of radiotracer through the kidney. The mean tubular transit time (MTTT) (i.e., the mean time that filtered or secreted radiotracer remains in the kidney) has been shown to be of value for distinguishing obstructive from nonobstructive renal disease.[148] The MTTT may be computed using the formula

$$MTTT = \int_0^\infty t\left(-dR(t)/dt\right)dt$$

where $R(t)$ is the tubular retention function.[143]

Glomerular Filtration Rate

The GFR may be estimated following intravenous injection of a radiotracer that is handled like inulin. The substance most commonly used for this purpose is ^{99m}Tc-DTPA. There are two basic approaches to the estimation of GFR. The first approach is based on clearance of the radiotracer from the plasma, and the second approach is based on the rate of tracer uptake by the kidney. Both approaches are reasonable, and the choice between them is a matter of convenience.

With the plasma clearance method, it is assumed that the radiotracer leaves the body solely through the urine. Single-injection techniques have largely replaced the classic, but tedious, constant-infusion techniques and have been shown to correlate well with inulin,[154] iothalamate, and creatinine[155] clearances obtained using the constant-infusion technique. The concentration of the tracer in the plasma as a function of time may be monitored by counting a series of blood samples. Alternatively, plasma concentration of the tracer may be recorded by an external detector over the heart or head. The resulting time-activity curve must be calibrated by one or more blood samples. External detection introduces a possible source of error because activity outside of the intravascular space may be detected.[156] In practice, however, it results in similar estimates of GFR[157,158] and has the advantage of reducing the number of blood samples needed.

Equations for calculating the clearance of a radiotracer after a single injection are derived from either a single- or multiple-compartment model.[159,160] The parameters of the model are estimated by fitting a single or multiple exponential curve to the plasma concentration curve.[154,155,158,161] More generally, it can be shown that GFR may be calculated from the dose injected (D) and the total area under the plasma concentration curve (interpolated and extrapolated to infinity) (A) using the formula[162]

$$GFR = D/A.$$

From this point of view, exponential curve fitting is merely a method for interpolating and extrapolating the plasma concentration curve (Fig. 10.37).

There has been a great deal of interest in procedures for estimating GFR that require no external counting and only a single blood sample. Essentially, these procedures use an empirically derived approximation for the effective volume of distribution of the radiotracer. Although this approximation introduces some additional error,[152] it has nevertheless been shown to result in good estimates of GFR in children.[163] The elimination of prolonged

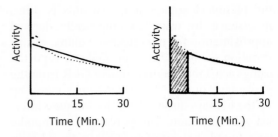

FIGURE 10.37. Calculation of glomerular filtration rate (GFR) using the equation $GFR = D/A$ required an estimate of the area under the tracer disappearance curve. Left: The area may be estimated as an exponential fit to the data curve. Right: Greater accuracy may be obtained by numerically integrating the first 5 minutes of the data curve and adding the area under an exponential fit to the remainder.

monitoring and multiple blood sampling make it an attractive approach, particularly in children.

The other approach to estimation of GFR, based on the uptake of the tracer by the kidney, assumes that the radiotracer remains in the kidney for at least some fixed period of time after it enters (typically 2 to 3 minutes). It also assumes that the amount of intravascular activity is negligible relative to the amount of intratubular activity during the time of measurement. Under these conditions, GFR may be calculated using the formula

$$GFR = (dR(t)/dt)/P(t),$$

where $R(t)$ and $P(t)$ denote total renal activity and plasma activity concentration as functions of time. Piepsz et al.[164] reported using such a method to estimate GFR, where $R(t)$ and $P(t)$ were estimated from the renal and cardiac time-activity curves obtained during the first 3 minutes after injection of ^{99m}Tc-DTPA, and $P(t)$ was calibrated using a blood sample. The method was found to correlate with 24-hour creatinine clearances in a series of 45 children.[165]

As in the case of plasma-clearance approach, there has been much interest in developing simplified procedures for estimating GFR by the renal-uptake approach. One goal has been to eliminate the need for blood sampling. As with the plasma-clearance approach, this is done, in essence, by using an empirically derived approximation for the effective volume of distribution of the radiotracer. Gates[141] reported using such a method to estimate GFR from the percentage of the ^{99m}Tc-DTPA dose taken up by the kidneys during the 2- to 3-minute interval after injection. The percentage of uptake was found to correlate well with 24-hour creatinine-clearance values in a series of 31 adults. More recently, Gordon et al.[166] have reported using such a method in children.

For many years, we have measured the percent uptake of ^{99m}Tc-DTPA during the 1- to 2-minute interval after injection. This measurement has been helpful for estimating global and individual renal function. With this method, it is possible to monitor changes in renal function in patients undergoing surgical or medical treatment for a variety of renal diseases. It is also possible to estimate differential GFR from the relative percentage of uptake by the two kidneys. This method for estimating differential GFR has been shown to correlate well with separate kidney iothalamate[155] and chromium-51–ethylenediaminetetraacetic acid (^{51}Cr–EDTA)[167] clearance values obtained by ureteral catheterization.

Effective Renal Plasma Flow

The ERPF may be estimated in the same manner as GFR if a radiotracer is used that is handled as PAH rather than as inulin. The most commonly used radiotracers for this purpose are ^{99m}Tc-MAG$_3$[163] and ^{123}I-OIH. In practice, ERPF measured with tracers such as ^{123}I-OIH is always slightly lower than the actual renal plasma flow because no substance is completely extracted in a single pass.[168] The plasma clearance and renal uptake approaches have both been used. The techniques used are essentially the same as those used for estimating GFR from inulin-like radiopharmaceuticals.

As with estimation of GFR, the concentration of the tracer in plasma may be followed by either multiple blood samples or external detection. The two methods have been found to produce similar results. Blaufox et al.[159] found a good correlation in the measurement of ERPF using ^{131}I-OIH with serial blood sampling and external detection using a scintillation probe over the patient's head. Similarly, Ram et al.[169] and Razzak et al.[170] found good agreement in the values of ERPF calculated by serial blood sampling and external detection over the precordium. Ram et al. reported a strong correlation between ERPF estimates obtained by single-exponential extrapolation of ^{125}I-OIH time-activity curves obtained from over the precordium and PAH clearance. Mackay et al.[171] reported the estimation of ERPF from a ^{123}I-OIH time-activity curve obtained over the abdomen and a single blood sample using single-exponential extrapolation. The ERPF estimates were found to correlate closely with PAH clearances but tended to be slightly lower. The average value was 89% of the PAH clearance values. Heidenreich et al.[172] reported their clinical experience in the estimation of ERPF from the clearance of ^{123}I-OIH in 153 children.

As in the case of estimating GFR, there has been much interest in procedures for estimating ERPF that require no external counting and only a single blood sample. Again, these procedures work by using an empirically derived approximation for the effective volume of distribution of the radiotracer. Such simplified techniques have been shown to produce good estimates of ERPF in children.[28]

The renal uptake approach to ERPF estimation has also been used.[144] Thompson et al.[173] reported the renal uptake of ^{131}I-OIH in the 1- to 2-minute interval after injection correlated with PAH clearances.

Relative ERPF may also be estimated from the relative percentage of uptake of the two kidneys.[145,172,174] Relative uptake of ^{123}I-OIH in the 0.5- to 2.5-minute interval following injection has been shown to correlate with separate kidney PAH clearance values obtained by ureteral catheterization.[114]

References

1. Moretti M, Magnani C, Calzolari E, Roncarati E. Genitourinary tract anomalies: neonatal medical problems. Fetal Ther 1986;1(2–3): 114–5.

2. Seikaly M, Ho PL, Emmett L, Tejani A. The 12th Annual Report of the North American Pediatric Renal Transplant Cooperative Study: renal transplantation from 1987 through 1998. Pediatr Transplant 2001;5(3):215–31.

3. National Institute of Diabetes and Digestive and Kidney Diseases (U.S.). Division of Kidney Urologic and Hematologic Diseases: United States renal data system. 1993 annual data report. In: Bethesda, MD: National Institutes of Health, National Institute of Diabetes and Digestive and Kidney Diseases, Division of Kidney, Urologic, and Hematologic Diseases, Urban Institute, Renal Research Program, University of Michigan, USRDS Coordinating Center, 1993.

4. Koenigsberg M, Blaufox MD, Freeman LM. Traumatic injuries of the renal vasculature and parenchyma. In: Freeman LM, Blaufox MD, eds. Radionuclide Studies of the Genitourinary System. New York: Grune & Stratton, 1975.

5. Burko H, Rhamy RK. Lower urinary tract problems related to infection: diagnosis and treatment. Pediatr Clin North Am 1970;17(2): 233–53.

6. Bois E, Feingold J, Benmaiz H, Briard ML. Congenital urinary tract malformations: epidemiologic and genetic aspects. Clin Genet 1975;8(1):37–47.

7. Sheih CP, Liu MB, Hung CS, Yang KH, Chen WY, Lin CY. Renal abnormalities in schoolchildren. Pediatrics 1989;84(6):1086–90.

8. Barakat AJ, Drougas JG. Occurrence of congenital abnormalities of kidney and urinary tract in 13,775 autopsies. Urology 1991;38(4): 347–50.

9. Arnold RW, Subramanian G, McAfee JG, Blair RJ, Thomas FD. Comparison of 99mTc complexes for renal imaging. J Nucl Med 1975; 16(5):357–67.

10. Taylor A Jr, Eshima D, Fritzberg AR, Christian PE, Kasina S. Comparison of iodine-131 OIH and technetium-99m MAG3 renal imaging in volunteers. J Nucl Med 1986;27(6):795–803.

11. Bubeck B, Brandau W, Steinbacher M, et al. Technetium-99m labeled renal function and imaging agents: II. Clinical evaluation of 99mTc MAG3 (99mTc mercaptoacetylglycylglycylclycine). Int J Rad Appl Instrum B 1988;15(1):109–18.

12. Jafri RA, Britton KE, Nimmon CC, et al. Technetium-99m MAG3, a comparison with iodine-123 and iodine-131 orthoiodohippurate, in patients with renal disorders. J Nucl Med 1988;29(2):147–58.

13. Russell CD, Thorstad B, Yester MV, Stutzman M, Baker T, Dubovsky EV. Comparison of technetium-99m MAG3 with iodine-131 hippuran by a simultaneous dual channel technique. J Nucl Med 1988;29(7):1189–93.

14. Russell CD, Thorstad BL, Yester MV, Stutzman M, Dubovsky EV. Quantitation of renal function with technetium-99m MAG3. J Nucl Med 1988;29(12):1931–3.

15. Taylor A Jr, Eshima D, Alazraki N. 99mTc-MAG3, a new renal imaging agent: preliminary results in patients. Eur J Nucl Med 1987; 12(10):510–4.

16. Atkins HL, Cardinale KG, Eckelman WC, Hauser W, Klopper JF, Richards P. Evaluation of 99mTc-DTPA prepared by three different methods. Radiology 1971;98(3): 674–7.

17. Cohen ML, Smith FG Jr, Mindell RS, Vernier RL. A simple, reliable method of measuring glomerular filtration rate using single, low dose sodium iothalamate I-131. Pediatrics 1969; 43(3):407–15.

18. Elwood CM, Sigman EM. The measurement of glomerular filtration rate and effective renal plasma flow in man by iothalamate 125-I and iodopyracet 131-I. Circulation 1967;36(3): 441–8.

19. Elwood CM, Sigman EM, Treger C. The measurement of glomerular filtration rate with 125I-sodium iothalamate (Conray). Br J Radiol 1967;40(476):581–3.

20. Gagnon JA, Schrier RW, Weis TP, Kokotis W, Mailloux LU. Clearance of iothalamate-125 I as a measure of glomerular filtration rate in the dog. J Appl Physiol 1971;30(5):774–8.

21. Hauser W, Atkins HL, Nelson KG, Richards P. Technetium-99m DTPA: a new radiopharmaceutical for brain and kidney scanning. Radiology 1970;94(3):679–84.

22. Houwen B, Donker A, Woldring MG. Simultaneous determination of glomerular filtration rate with 125I-iothalamate and effective renal plasma flow with 131I-hippuran. In: Dynamic Studies with Radioisotopes in Medicine: Proceedings of the Symposium Organized by the International Atomic Energy Agency, and held in Rotterdam, August 31 to September 4, 1970 and 1971. Vienna: International Atomic Energy Agency, 1971.

23. Klopper JF, Hauser W, Atkins HL, Eckelman WC, Richards P. Evaluation of 99m Tc-DTPA

for the measurement of glomerular filtration rate. J Nucl Med 1972;13(1):107–10.

24. Kountz SL, Yeh SH, Wood J, Cohn R, Kriss JP. Technetium-99m(V)-citrate complex for estimation of glomerular filtration rate. Nature 1967;215(108):1397–9.

25. Maher FT, Nolan NG, Elveback LR. Comparison of simultaneous clearances of 125–I-labeled sodium lothalamate (Glofil) and of inulin. Mayo Clin Proc 1971;46(10):690–1.

26. Oester A, Wolf H, Madsen PO. Double isotope technique in renal function testing in dogs. Invest Urol 1969;6(4):387–92.

27. Sigman EM, Elwood C, Reagan ME, Morris AM, Catanzaro A. The renal clearance of I-131 labelled sodium iothalamate in man. Invest Urol 1965;15:432–8.

28. Russell CD, Bischoff PG, Rowell KL, et al. Quality control of Tc-99m DTPA for measurement of glomerular filtration: concise communication. J Nucl Med 1983;24(8):722–7.

29. McAfee JG, Gagne G, Atkins HL, et al. Biological distribution and excretion of DTPA labeled with Tc-99m and In-111. J Nucl Med 1979;20(12):1273–8.

30. Enlander D, Weber PM, dos Remedios LV. Renal cortical imaging in 35 patients: superior quality with 99mTc-DMSA. J Nucl Med 1974;15(9):743–9.

31. Kawamura J, Hosokawa S, Yoshida O. Renal function studies using 99mTc-dimercaptosuccinic acid. Clin Nucl Med 1979;4(1):39–46.

32. Willis KW, Martinez DA, Hedley-Whyte ET, Davis MA, Judy PF, Treves S. Renal localization of 99mTc-stannous glucoheptonate and 99mTc-stannous dimercaptosuccinate in the rat by frozen section autoradiography. The efficiency and resolution of technetium-99m. Radiat Res 1977;69(3):475–88.

33. Daly MJ, Jones WA, Rudd TG, Tremann JA. Differential 99mTc dimercaptosuccinic acid (DMSA) renal localization: correlation with renal function. J Nucl Med 1977;18:594–5.

34. Daly MJ, Jones W, Rudd TG, Tremann J. Differential renal function using technetium-99m dimercaptosuccinic acid (DMSA): in vitro correlation. J Nucl Med 1979;20(1):63–6.

35. Taylor A, Jr. Quantitation of renal function with static imaging agents. Semin Nucl Med 1982;12(4):330–44.

36. Lee HB, Blaufox MD. Mechanism of renal concentration of technetium-99m glucoheptonate. J Nucl Med 1985;26(11):1308–13.

37. Tubis M, Posnick E, Nordyke RA. Preparation and use of I 131 labeled sodium iodohippurate in kidney function tests. Proc Soc Exp Biol Med 1960;103:497–8.

38. Chervu LR, Freeman LM, Blaufox MD. Radiopharmaceuticals for renal studies. Semin Nucl Med 1974;4(1):3–22.

39. Mailloux LU, Gagnon JA. Measurement of effective renal plasma flow. In: Blaufox MD, ed. Progress in Nuclear Medicine. Baltimore: University Park Press, 1972.

40. Shore RM, Uehling DT, Bruskewitz R, Polcyn RE. Evaluation of obstructive uropathy with diuretic renography. Am J Dis Child 1983;137(3):236–40.

41. Vanpee M, Blennow M, Linne T, Herin P, Aperia A. Renal function in very low birth weight infants: normal maturity reached during early childhood. J Pediatr 1992;121(5 pt 1): 784–8.

42. Dunbar JS, Nogrady B. Excretory urography in the first year of life. Radiol Clin North Am 1972;10(2):367–91.

43. Martin DJ, Gilday DL, Reilly BJ. Evaluation of the urinary tract in the neonatal period. Radiol Clin North Am 1975;13(2):359–68.

44. Slutsky LJ, Golimbu M, Braunstein P, Al-Askari S, Genieser N, Golimbu C. Urographic imaging in neonatal period: radionuclide scan and x-ray. Urology 1977;10(2):169–72.

45. Sherman RA, Blaufox MD. Obstructive uropathy in patients with nonvisualization on renal scan. Nephron 1980;25(2):82–6.

46. Chung YK, Chang PY, Lin CJ, Wang NL, Sheu JC, Shih BF. Conservative treatment of neonatal hydronephrosis. J Formos Med Assoc 1992;91(1):75–80.

47. Gordon I, Dhillon HK, Peters AM. Antenatal diagnosis of renal pelvic dilatation—the natural history of conservative management. Pediatr Radiol 1991;21(4):272–3.

48. Homsy YL, Saad F, Laberge I, Williot P, Pison C. Transitional hydronephrosis of the newborn and infant. J Urol 1990;144(2 pt 2):579–83; discussion 593–4.

49. Ransley PG, Dhillon HK, Gordon I, Duffy PG, Dillon MJ, Barratt TM. The postnatal management of hydronephrosis diagnosed by prenatal ultrasound. J Urol 1990;144(2 pt 2):584–7; discussion 593–4.

50. Samuelson U, Granerus G, Bjures J, Hagberg S, Hjalmas K. Renal function in idiopathic hydronephrosis in children. Follow-up after

conservative and surgical treatment. Scand J Urol Nephrol 1984;18(2):135–41.

51. Djurhuus JC, Dorph S, Christiansen L, Ladefoged J, Nerstrom B. Predictive value of renography and i.v. urography for the outcome of reconstructive surgery in patients with hydronephrosis. Acta Chir Scand Suppl 1976;472:37–41.

52. McAfee JG, Singh A, O'Callaghan JP. Nuclear imaging supplementary to urography in obstructive uropathy. Radiology 1980;137(2):487–96.

53. Treves ST, Packard AB, Fung LC. Assessment of rapid changes in renal blood flow with (191m)Ir, an ultra-short-lived radionuclide. J Nucl Med 2004;45(3):508–11.

54. Kalika V, Bard RH, Iloreta A, Freeman LM, Heller S, Blaufox MD. Prediction of renal functional recovery after relief of upper urinary tract obstruction. J Urol 1981;126(3):301–5.

55. Jamar F, Piret L, Wese FX, Beckers C. Influence of ureteral status on kidney washout during technetium-99m-DTPA diuresis renography in children. J Nucl Med 1992;33(1):73–8.

56. Koff SA, Thrall JH, Keyes JW Jr. Assessment of hydroureteronephrosis in children using diuretic radionuclide urography. J Urol 1980;123(4):531–4.

57. Mesrobian HG, Perry JR. Radionuclide diuresis pyelography. J Urol 1991;146(2 pt 2):601–4.

58. Thrall JH, Koff SA, Keyes JW Jr. Diuretic radionuclide renography and scintigraphy in the differential diagnosis of hydroureteronephrosis. Semin Nucl Med 1981;11(2):89–104.

59. Howman-Giles R, Uren R, Roy LP, Filmer RB. Volume expansion diuretic renal scan in urinary tract obstruction. J Nucl Med 1987;28(5):824–8.

60. Nauta J, Pot DJ, Kooij PP, Nijman JM, Wolff ED. Forced hydration prior to renography in children with hydronephrosis. An evaluation. Br J Urol 1991;68(1):93–7.

61. Sukhai RN, Kooy PP, Wolff ED, Scholtmeijer RJ. Predictive value of 99mTc-DTPA renography studies under conditions of maximal diuresis for the functional outcome of reconstructive surgery in children with obstructive uropathy. Br J Urol 1986;58(6):596–600.

62. Meller ST, Eckstein HB. Renal scintigraphy: quantitative assessment of upper urinary tract dilatation in children. J Pediatr Surg 1981;16(2):126–33.

63. Busch R, Huland H. Correlation of symptoms and results of direct bacterial localization in patients with urinary tract infections. J Urol 1984;132(2):282–5.

64. Majd M, Rushton HG, Jantausch B, Wiedermann BL. Relationship among vesicoureteral reflux, P-fimbriated Escherichia coli, and acute pyelonephritis in children with febrile urinary tract infection. J Pediatr 1991;119(4):578–85.

65. Jacobson SH, Eklof O, Eriksson CG, Lins LE, Tidgren B, Winberg J. Development of hypertension and uraemia after pyelonephritis in childhood: 27 year follow up. BMJ 1989;299(6701):703–6.

66. Glauser MP, Lyons JM, Braude AI. Prevention of chronic experimental pyelonephritis by suppression of acute suppuration. J Clin Invest 1978;61(2):403–7.

67. Miller T, Phillips S. Pyelonephritis: the relationship between infection, renal scarring, and antimicrobial therapy. Kidney Int 1981;19(5):654–62.

68. Slotki IN, Asscher AW. Prevention of scarring in experimental pyelonephritis in the rat by early antibiotic therapy. Nephron 1982;30(3):262–8.

69. Bjorgvinsson E, Majd M, Eggli KD. Diagnosis of acute pyelonephritis in children: comparison of sonography and 99mTc-DMSA scintigraphy. AJR 1991;157(3):539–43.

70. Farnsworth RH, Rossleigh MA, Leighton DM, Bass SJ, Rosenberg AR. The detection of reflux nephropathy in infants by 99m-technetium dimercaptosuccinic acid studies. J Urol 1991;145(3):542–6.

71. Jantausch BA, Wiedermann BL, Hull SI, et al. Escherichia coli virulence factors and 99mTc-dimercaptosuccinic acid renal scan in children with febrile urinary tract infection. Pediatr Infect Dis J 1992;11(5):343–9.

72. Kass EJ, Fink-Bennett D, Cacciarelli AA, Balon H, Pavlock S. The sensitivity of renal scintigraphy and sonography in detecting nonobstructive acute pyelonephritis. J Urol 1992;148(2 pt 2):606–8.

73. Majd M, Rushton HG. Renal cortical scintigraphy in the diagnosis of acute pyelonephritis. Semin Nucl Med 1992;22(2):98–111.

74. Rushton HG, Majd M, Jantausch B, Wiedermann BL, Belman AB. Renal scarring following reflux and nonreflux pyelonephritis in children: evaluation with 99m-technetium-

dimercaptosuccinic acid scintigraphy. J Urol 1992;147(5):1327–32.

75. Verber IG, Meller ST. Serial 99mTc dimercaptosuccinic acid (DMSA) scans after urinary infections presenting before the age of 5 years. Arch Dis Child 1989;64(11):1533–7.

76. Goldraich NP, Ramos OL, Goldraich IH. Urography versus DMSA scan in children with vesicoureteric reflux. Pediatr Nephrol 1989; 3(1):1–5.

77. Itoh K, Asano Y, Tsukamoto E, et al. Single photon emission computed tomography with Tc-99m-dimercaptosuccinic acid in patients with upper urinary tract infection and/or vesicoureteral reflux. Ann Nucl Med 1991;5(1): 29–34.

78. Verboven M, Ingels M, Delree M, Piepsz A. 99mTc-DMSA scintigraphy in acute urinary tract infection in children. Pediatr Radiol 1990;20(7):540–2.

79. Merrick MV, Uttley WS, Wild SR. The detection of pyelonephritic scarring in children by radioisotope imaging. Br J Radiol 1980; 53(630):544–56.

80. Handmaker H. Nuclear renal imaging in acute pyelonephritis. Semin Nucl Med 1982;12(3): 246–53.

81. Jakobsson B, Nolstedt L, Svensson L, Soderlundh S, Berg U. 99m-Technetium-dimercaptosuccinic acid scan in the diagnosis of acute pyelonephritis in children: relation to clinical and radiological findings. Pediatr Nephrol 1992;6(4):328–34.

82. Tappin DM, Murphy AV, Mocan H, et al. A prospective study of children with first acute symptomatic E. coli urinary tract infection. Early 99m-technetium dimercaptosuccinic acid scan appearances. Acta Paediatr Scand 1989;78(6):923–9.

83. Applegate KE, Connolly LP, Davis RT, Zurakowski D, Treves ST. A prospective comparison of high-resolution planar, pinhole, and triple-detector SPECT for the detection of renal cortical defects. Clin Nucl Med 1997;22(10):673–8.

84. Joseph DB, Young DW, Jordon SP. Renal cortical scintigraphy and single proton emission computerized tomography (SPECT) in the assessment of renal defects in children. J Urol 1990;144(2 pt 2):595–7; discussion 606.

85. Roberts JA, Roth JK Jr, Domingue G, Lewis RW, Kaack B, Baskin G. Immunology of pyelonephritis in the primate model. V. Effect of superoxide dismutase. J Urol 1982;128(6): 1394–400.

86. Kaack MB, Dowling KJ, Patterson GM, Roberts JA. Immunology of pyelonephritis. VIII. E. coli causes granulocytic aggregation and renal ischemia. J Urol 1986;136(5):1117–22.

87. Androulakakis PA, Ransley PG, Risdon RA, Sorger K, Hohenfellner R. Microvascular changes in the early stage of reflux pyelonephritis. An experimental study in the pig kidney. Eur Urol 1987;13(4):219–23.

88. Elink M. Emergency uroradiology for the nontraumatized patient. Radiol Clin North Am 1978;16(1):135–46.

89. Handmaker H, Young BW, Lowenstein JM. Clinical experience with 99mTc-DMSA (dimercaptosuccinic acid), a new renal-imaging agent. J Nucl Med 1975;16(1):28–32.

90. Silver TM, Kass EJ, Thornbury JR, Konnak JW, Wolfman MG. The radiological spectrum of acute pyelonephritis in adults and adolescents. Radiology 1976;118(1):65–71.

91. Kahn PC. Renal imaging with radionuclides, ultrasound, and computed tomography. Semin Nucl Med 1979;9(1):43–57.

92. June CH, Browning MD, Smith LP, et al. Ultrasonography and computed tomography in severe urinary tract infection. Arch Intern Med 1985;145(5):841–5.

93. Montgomery P, Kuhn JP, Afshani E. CT evaluation of severe renal inflammatory disease in children. Pediatr Radiol 1987;17(3):216–22.

94. Raynaud C, Tran-Dinh S, Bourguignon M, et al. Acute pyelonephritis in children. Preliminary results obtained with NMR imaging. Contrib Nephrol 1987;56:129–34.

95. Arneil GC, MacDonald AM, Sweet EM. Renal venous thrombosis. Clin Nephrol 1973;1(3): 119–31.

96. Avery ME, Oppenheimer EH, Gordon HH. Renal-vein thrombosis in newborn infants of diabetic mothers; report of 2 cases. N Engl J Med 1957;256(24):1134–8.

97. Kaufmann HJ. Renal vein thrombosis. 1. Age incidence in infancy and childhood. 2. Sex incidence. 3. Incidence of unilateral and bilateral involvement. Am J Dis Child 1958;95(4): 377–84.

98. Rasoulpour M, McLean RH. Renal venous thrombosis in neonates. Initial and follow-up abnormalities. Am J Dis Child 1980;134(3): 276–9.

99. Stark H. Renal vein thrombosis in infancy. Recovery without nephrectomy. Am J Dis Child 1964;108:430–5.

100. Takeuchi A, Benirschke K. Renal venous thrombosis of the newborn and its relation to maternal diabetes. Report of 16 cases. Biol Neonat 1961;3:237–56.

101. Verhagen AD, Hamilton JP, Genel M. Renal vein thrombosis in infants. Arch Dis Child 1965;40:214–7.

102. Duncan RE, Evans AT, Martin LW. Natural history and treatment of renal vein thrombosis in children. J Pediatr Surg 1977;12(5):639–45.

103. Quigley JM, Druy EM, Rich JI. Acute renal vein thrombosis with a diagnostic renal scintigram. AJR 1981;137(5):1066–8.

104. Blaufox MD. Systemic arterial hypertension in pediatric practice. Pediatr Clin North Am 1971;18(2):577–93.

105. Ingelfinger JR. Pediatric hypertension. Philadelphia: Saunders, 1982.

106. Londe S. Causes of hypertension in the young. Pediatr Clin North Am 1978;25(1):55–65.

107. Olson DL, Lieberman E. Renal hypertension in children. Pediatr Clin North Am 1976; 23(4):795–805.

108. Rosen PR, Treves S. The efficacy of 99mTc screening of pediatric patients for renal etiologies in hypertension. J Nucl Med 1983;24(5):22.

109. Vivan G, Stringer D, DeBruyn R, et al. 99mTc DMSA in renovascular hypertension in children. In: Raynaud C, ed. Nuclear Medicine and Biology Advances: Proceedings of the Third World Congress of Nuclear Medicine and Biology, August 29 to September 2, 1982, Paris, France. Oxford, New York: Pergamon Press, 1983:4.

110. Geyskes GG, Oei HY, Puylaert CB, Dorhout Mees EJ. Renography with captopril. Changes in a patient with hypertension and unilateral renal artery stenosis. Arch Intern Med 1986; 146(9):1705–8.

111. Majd M, Potter BN, Guzzeta PC, Ruley EJ. Effect of captopril on efficacy of renal scintigraphy in detection of renal artery stenosis abstract. J Nucl Med 1983;24:23.

112. Sfakianakis GN, Sfakianaki E, Bourgoignie J. Lasix captopril renography in the diagnosis of renovascular hypertension. Contrib Nephrol 1990;79:219–27.

113. Siegel MJ, St Amour TE, Siegel BA. Imaging techniques in the evaluation of pediatric hypertension. Pediatr Nephrol 1987;1(1):76–88.

114. Wenting GJ, Tan-Tjiong HL, Derkx FH, de Bruyn JH, Man in't Veld AJ, Schalekamp MA. Splint renal function after captopril in unilateral renal artery stenosis. Br Med J (Clin Res Ed) 1984;288(6421):886–90.

115. Minty I, Lythgoe MF, Gordon I. Hypertension in paediatrics: can pre- and post-captopril technetium-99m dimercaptosuccinic acid renal scans exclude renovascular disease? Eur J Nucl Med 1993;20(8):699–702.

116. Dondi M. Captopril renal scintigraphy with 99mTc-mercaptoacetyltriglycine (99mTc-MAG3) for detecting renal artery stenosis. Am J Hypertens 1991;4(12 pt 2):737S–40S.

117. Dondi M, Fanti S, De Fabritiis A, et al. Prognostic value of captopril renal scintigraphy in renovascular hypertension. J Nucl Med 1992;33(11):2040–4.

118. Oei HY. Captopril renography. Early observations and diagnostic criteria. Am J Hypertens 1991;4(12 pt 2):678S–84S.

119. Setaro JF, Chen CC, Hoffer PB, Black HR. Captopril renography in the diagnosis of renal artery stenosis and the prediction of improvement with revascularization. The Yale Vascular Center experience. Am J Hypertens 1991; 4(12 pt 2):698S–705S.

120. Hildebrandt. Anatomie der Nierengeschwulste. Arch Klin Chir 1894;48:343.

121. Bernstein J. The morphogenesis of renal parenchymal maldevelopment (renal dysplasia). Pediatr Clin North Am 1971;18(2):395–407.

122. Zerres K, Volpel MC, Weiss H. Cystic kidneys. Genetics, pathologic anatomy, clinical picture, and prenatal diagnosis. Hum Genet 1984; 68(2):104–35.

123. Berdon WE, Baker DH, Wigger HJ, Blanc WA. The radiologic and pathologic spectrum of the prune belly syndrome. The importance of urethral obstruction in prognosis. Radiol Clin North Am 1977;15(1):83–92.

124. Guthrie L. Case of congenital deficiency of the abdominal muscles with dilatation and hypertrophy of the bladder ureters. Trans Pathol Soc Lond 1918;47:139–45.

125. Parker RW. Case of an infant in whom some of the abdominal muscles were absent. Trans Clin Soc Lond 1895;28:201–3.

126. Williams DI, Burkholder GV. The prune belly syndrome. J Urol 1967;98(2):244–51.

127. Leonard JC, Allen EW, Goin J, Smith CW. Renal cortical imaging and the detection of renal mass lesions. J Nucl Med 1979;20(10): 1018–22.

128. Older RA, Korobkin M, Workman J, et al. Accuracy of radionuclide imaging in distinguishing renal masses from normal variants. Radiology 1980;136(2):443–8.

129. Parker JA, Lebowitz R, Mascatello V, Treves S. Magnification renal scintigraphy in the differential diagnosis of septa of Bertin. Pediatr Radiol 1976;4(3):157–60.

130. Awad W, Bennett LR, Martin DC. Detection of renal homograft rejection reaction with a single dose of radiohippuran. J Urol 1968;100(3): 233–7.

131. Awad W, Boake RC, Bennett LR, Martin DC. Double isotope scan in kidney transplantation. Am Surg 1968;34(11):768–74.

132. Figueroa JE, Maxfield WS, Batson HM, Birchall R. Radioisotope renal function studies in human renal allografts: value in the differential diagnosis of oliguria in the presence of obstructive disease with and without urinary extravasation. J Urol 1968;100(2):104–8.

133. Lubin E, Lewitus Z, Rosenfield J, Levi N. Kidney scanning with hippuran, a necessary complement for correct interpretation of renography in the transplanted kidney. In: Medical radioisotope scintigraphy Proceedings of a symposium held by the International Atomic Energy Agency in Salzburg, August 6–15, 1968, and 1969. Vienna: International Atomic Energy Agency, 1969.

134. Magnusson G, Collste L, Franksson C, Lundgren G. Radiorenography in Clinical Transplantation. Scand J Urol Nephrol 1967;1: 132–51.

135. Treves ST, Lebowitz R, Kuruc A, Heyman S, Rose P. Kidneys. In: Treves S, ed. Pediatric Nuclear Medicine. New York: Springer-Verlag, 1985:63–103.

136. Zum Winkel K, Harbst H, Schenck P, et al. Sequential scintigraphy in renal transplantation. In: Medical Radioisotope Scintigraphy: Proceedings of a Symposium Held by the International Atomic Energy Agency in Salzburg, August 6–15, 1968 and 1969. Vienna: International Atomic Energy Agency, 1969.

137. Harmon WE, Stablein D, Alexander SR, Tejani A. Graft thrombosis in pediatric renal transplant recipients. A report of the North American Pediatric Renal Transplant Cooperative Study. Transplantation 1991;51(2):406–12.

138. Spigos DG, Tan W, Pavel DG, Mozes M, Jonasson O, Capek V. Diagnosis of urine extravasation after renal transplantation. AJR 1977;129(3):409–13.

139. Kenny RW, Ackery DM, Fleming JS, Goddard BA, Grant RW. Deconvolution analysis of the scintillation camera renogram. Br J Radiol 1975;48(570):481–6.

140. Short MD, Glass HI, Chisholm GD, Vernon P, Silvester DJ. Gamma-camera renography using 123I-hippuran. Br J Radiol 1973;46(544): 289–94.

141. Gates GF. Glomerular filtration rate: estimation from fractional renal accumulation of 99mTc-DTPA (stannous). AJR 1982;138(3): 565–70.

142. Decostre PL, Salmon Y. Temporal behavior of peripheral organ distribution volume in mammillary systems. II. Application to background correction in separate glomerular filtration rate estimation in man. J Nucl Med 1990;31(10): 1710–6.

143. Takaki Y, Kojima A, Tsuji A, Nakashima R, Tomiguchi S, Takahashi M. Quantification of renal uptake of technetium-99m-DTPA using planar scintigraphy: a technique that considers organ volume. J Nucl Med 1993;34(7):1184–9.

144. Schlegel JU, Hamway SA. Individual renal plasma flow determination in 2 minutes. J Urol 1976;116(3):282–5.

145. Moser E, Jocham D, Beer M, Bull U. Effects of obstruction on single-kidney function: clinical and experimental results with 131I-hippurate and 99mTc-DMSA. Nuklearmedizin 1980;19(6):257–62.

146. Diffey BL, Hall FM, Corfield JR. The 99mTc-DTPA dynamic renal scan with deconvolution analysis. J Nucl Med 1976;17(5):352–5.

147. Oppenheim AV, Willsky AS, Young IT. Signals and Systems. Englewood Cliffs, NJ: Prentice-Hall, 1983.

148. Piepsz A, Ham HR, Erbsmann F, et al. A cooperative study on the clinical value of dynamic renal scanning with deconvolution analysis. Br J Radiol 1982;55(654):419–33.

149. Erbsmann F, Strugven J, Ham H, Piepsz A. Analysis of errors and systemic biases in the calculation of the renal retention function. In: Information Processing in Medical Imaging (Proceedings of the Vth International Conference), 1978. Nashville: ORNL/BCTIC, 1978.

150. Fleming JS, Goddard BA. A technique for the deconvolution of the renogram. Phys Med Biol 1974;19(4):546–9.

151. Gamel J, Rousseau WF, Katholi CR, Mesel E. Pitfalls in digital computation of the impulse response of vascular beds from indicator-dilution curves. Circ Res 1973;32(4):516–23.

152. Kuruc A, Caldicott WJ, Treves S. An improved deconvolution technique for the calculation of renal retention functions. Comput Biomed Res 1982;15(1):46–56.

153. Kainer G, McIlveen B, Hoschl R, Rosenberg AR. Assessment of individual renal function in children using 99mTc-DTPA. Arch Dis Child 1979;54(12):931–6.

154. Huttunen K, Huttunen NP, Koivula A, Ahonen A, Puukka R. 99mTc-DTPA—a useful clinical tool for the measurement of glomerular filtration rate. Scand J Urol Nephrol 1982;16(3):237–41.

155. Powers TA, Stone WJ, Grove RB, et al. Radionuclide measurement of differential glomerular filtration rate. Invest Radiol 1981;16(1):59–64.

156. Kuruc A, Treves ST, Rosen PR, Greenberg D. Estimating the plasma time-activity curve during radionuclide renography. J Nucl Med 1987;28(8):1338–40.

157. Owen JE, Walker RG, Willems D, Guignard PA, d'Apice AJ. Cadmium telluride detectors in the external measurement of glomerular filtration rate using 99mTc-DTPA (Sn): comparison with 51Cr-EDTA and 99mTc-DTPA (Sn) plasma sample methods. Clin Nephrol 1982;18(4):200–3.

158. Rossing N, Bojsen J, Frederiksen PL. The glomerular filtration rate determined with 99mTc-DTPA and a portable cadmium telluride detector. Scand J Clin Lab Invest 1978;38(1):23–8.

159. Blaufox MD, Potchen EJ, Merrill JP. Measurement of effective renal plasma flow in man by external counting methods. J Nucl Med 1967;8(2):77–85.

160. Sapirstein LA, Vidt DG, Mandel MJ, Hanusek G. Volumes of distribution and clearances of intravenously injected creatinine in the dog. Am J Physiol 1955;181(2):330–6.

161. Rootwelt K, Falch D, Sjokvist R. Determination of glomerular filtration rate (GFR) by analysis of capillary blood after single shot injection of 99mTc-DTPA. A comparison with simultaneous 125I-iothalamate GFR estimation showing equal GFR but difference in distribution volume. Eur J Nucl Med 1980;5(2):97–102.

162. Hall JE, Guyton AC, Farr BM. A single-injection method for measuring glomerular filtration rate. Am J Physiol 1977;232(1):F72–6.

163. Ham HR, Piepsz A. Estimation of glomerular filtration rate in infants and in children using a single-plasma sample method. J Nucl Med 1991;32(6):1294–7.

164. Piepsz A, Dobbeleir A, Erbsmann F. Measurement of separate kidney clearance by means of 99mTc-DTPA complex and a scintillation camera. Eur J Nucl Med 1977;2(3):173–7.

165. Piepsz A, Denis R, Ham HR, Dobbeleir A, Schulman C, Erbsmann F. A simple method for measuring separate glomerular filtration rate using a single injection of 99mTc-DTPA and the scintillation camera. J Pediatr 1978;93(5):769–74.

166. Gordon I, Anderson PJ, Orton M, Evans K. Estimation of technetium-99m-MAG3 renal clearance in children: two gamma camera techniques compared with multiple plasma samples. J Nucl Med 1991;32(9):1704–8.

167. Bailey SM, Evans DW, Fleming HA. Intravenous urography in investigation of hypertension. Lancet 1975;2(7924):57–8.

168. Chervu LR, Blaufox MD. Renal radiopharmaceuticals—an update. Semin Nucl Med 1982;12(3):224–45.

169. Ram MD, Evans K, Chisholm GD. A single injection method for measurement of effective renal plasma flow. Br J Urol 1968;40(4):425–8.

170. Razzak MA, Botti RE, MacIntyre WJ, Pritchard WH. External monitoring of I131–hippuran disappearance as a measure for renal blood flow. Int J Appl Radiat Isot 1967;18(12):825–8.

171. Mackay A, Eadie AS, Cumming AM, Graham AG, Adams FG, Horton PW. Assessment of total and divided renal plasma flow by 123I-hippuran renography. Kidney Int 1981;19(1):49–57.

172. Heidenreich P, Lauer O, Fendel H, Oberdorfer M, Pabst HW. Determination of total and individual kidney function in children by means of 123–I-hippuran whole body clearance and scintillation camera. Pediatr Radiol 1981;11(1):17–27.

173. Thompson IM Jr, Boineau FG, Evans BB, Schlegel JU. The renal quantitative scintillation camera study for determination of renal function. J Urol 1983;129(3):461–5.

174. Tauxe WN, Tobin M, Dubovsky EV, Bueschen AJ, Kontzen F. A macrofunction for computer processing of comprehensive renal function studies. Eur J Nucl Med 1980;5(2):103–8.

11
Vesicoureteral Reflux

S.T. Treves and Ulrich V. Willi

Vesicoureteric reflux (VUR) is caused by a failure of the ureterovesical valve mechanism. This failure may be due to a congenital variation, a pathologic process, an infection, or immaturity that distorts the anatomy or function (or both) of the ureterovesical junction. Passive and active factors characterize the normal valve mechanism of the ureterovesical junction. Passive factors include the obliquity of entry of the ureter into the bladder; the length of the intramural ureter, particularly of its submucosal segment; and the ratio of the length of the submucosal tunnel to the diameter of the ureter. The active factors include the contraction of the ureterotrigonal muscles, which close the ureteral meatus and the submucosal tunnel, and active ureteral peristalsis, as seen during diuresis.[1] The intravesical ureter becomes longer with age, often producing sufficient length to convert a refluxing ureterovesical junction into a nonrefluxing one. The principal long-term consequence of VUR, particularly when associated with infection, is the development of pyelonephritis, which in turn may lead to scarring, hypertension, and chronic renal failure.

Incidence

The exact incidence of VUR in the general population is not known. Approximately 1% (7 of 535) of apparently normal neonates, infants, and children were found to have VUR.[1] The incidence of VUR in siblings of children with reflux is much greater than in the general population. At Children's Hospital Boston, we evaluated 60 asymptomatic siblings of refluxing children using radionuclide cystography and found VUR in 45%.[2,3] Others' findings are similar.[4-6] A study at Children's Hospital Boston revealed that six of 16 refluxing-symptom-free siblings of children with VUR had evidence of cortical renal damage as assessed by technetium-99m–dimercaptosuccinic acid (^{99m}Tc)-DMSA scintigraphy.[7-10] DMSA cortical scintigraphy provides an early indicator of renal drainage, and it should be considered in the assessment of symptomatic and asymptomatic siblings of refluxing children. Using radionuclide cystography, we have also found asymptomatic reflux in parents of index children with VUR.

Spontaneous Cessation of Reflux

The concept that VUR tends to disappear spontaneously with growth and maturation is well accepted. Spontaneous cessation of reflux was reported in approximately 71% of children and 79% of ureters studied by Normand and Smellie[11] in 1979. The most important factor in the resolution of VUR seemed to be the apparent diameter of the ureter. Resolution of VUR took place in 85% of ureters of normal caliber but in only 41% of dilated ureters. In addition, these authors reported that 65% of ureters associated with scarred kidneys also ceased to reflux spontaneously.

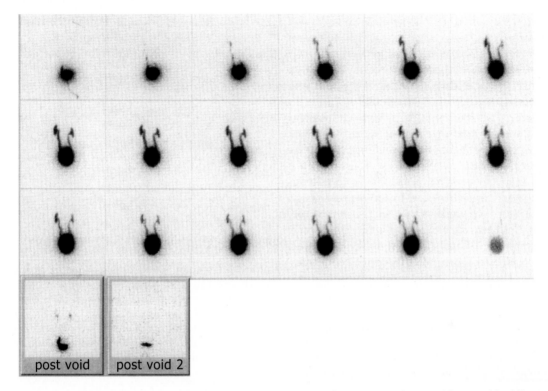

post void   post void 2

FIGURE 11.1. Bilateral vesicoureteric reflux, as shown by radionuclide cystography. Initial left reflux followed by right reflux reaching the renal pelves. Reflux appears early and persists during the entire voiding phase. The patient could not void while on the examination table. Postvoid images reveal complete drainage of tracer from the ureteropelvicaliceal systems.

Diagnosis

During the past several years, the method most frequently used for the detection of VUR has been radiographic voiding cystourethrography (VCUG). This well-established method has been an invaluable tool that has improved the understanding and treatment of VUR. It provides fine anatomic detail of the bladder and the urethra. In patients with reflux, it clearly outlines the anatomy of the pelvicaliceal systems, the ureters, and their insertion into the bladder. It has some limitations, however, including relatively high gonadal radiation exposure and low temporal resolution, which prevents diagnosis of intermittent VUR. During the past several years, radionuclide cystography (RNC) has gained increasing acceptance for the initial diagnosis and follow-up of VUR (Fig. 11.1). Advantages of RNC include low gonadal radiation exposure, high temporal resolution, and high sensitivity for the detection of VUR. Also RNC may be less expensive to perform than VCUG.[12] However, RNC cannot delineate the anatomy of the bladder and urethra. Some investigators have found that RNC is more sensitive than VCUG; both studies should be considered complementary in some cases.[13–15]

Grading the Severity of Vesicoureteric Reflux

The severity of VUR has been classified by its morphologic appearance on VCUG. A report by an international group studying VUR adopted a classification of reflux illustrated in

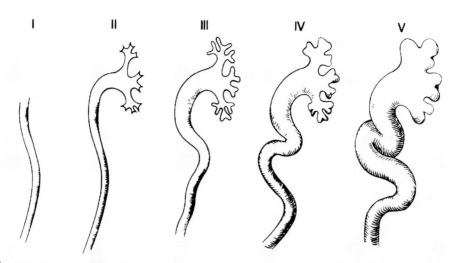

FIGURE 11.2. Grading of vesicoureteral reflux by voiding cystourethrography, international study classification. Grade I: ureter only. Grade II: ureter, pelvis, and calyces; no dilatation, normal caliceal fornices. Grade III: mild or moderate dilatation or tortuosity of ureter (or both) and mild or moderate dilatation of renal pelvis but no or slight blunting of fornices. Grade IV: moderate dilatation or tortuosity of ureter (or both) and moderate dilatation of renal pelvis and calyces. Complete obliteration of sharp angles of fornices but maintenance of papillary impressions in majority of calyces. Grade V: gross dilatation and tortuosity of ureter; gross dilatation of renal pelvis and calyces; papillary impressions are no longer visible in most calyces.

Figure 11.2.[16] This grading system is convenient for communication but need not be applied rigidly in an individual case.[1] Moreover, this classification is not exact, as VUR appearances vary over a continuum and often some VURs do not fall precisely within one of the five grades. In fact, the same patient may be classified with a grade II reflux during one examination and a grade I or III at another.

A practical problem is presented when one is asked to compare the VCUG and RNC findings for the same patient to determine if reflux has changed over time. Comparing the five VCUG grades of reflux with reflux severity on RNC is difficult; because of inherent technical differences between these two methods, a direct comparison may not be entirely appropriate. With RNC it is possible to recognize at least three degrees of reflux severity (Fig. 11.3).[17] The least severe degree shows reflux limited to the distal ureter without reaching the renal pelvis (Fig. 11.4). This picture corresponds to grade I reflux and can be called RNC grade 1. Another appearance is that of a small volume of VUR reaching the renal pelvis with minimal or no visualization of the ureter (Fig. 11.5). This picture corresponds to radiographic grades II or III, as it is not possible by the radionuclide technique to assess finely the diameter of the ureter and the anatomy of the pelvicaliceal system (RNC grade 2). Finally, the radionuclide cystogram could reveal a large volume of reflux reaching a dilated pelvicaliceal system with definite or marked dilatation and even elongation and tortuosity of the ureter corresponding in appearance to radiographic grades IV and V (RNC grade 3) (Figs. 11.6 and 11.7).

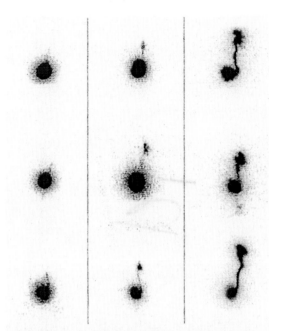

RNC Grade 1   RNC Grade 2   RNC Grade 3

FIGURE 11.3. Reflux severity in radionuclide cystography (RNC).

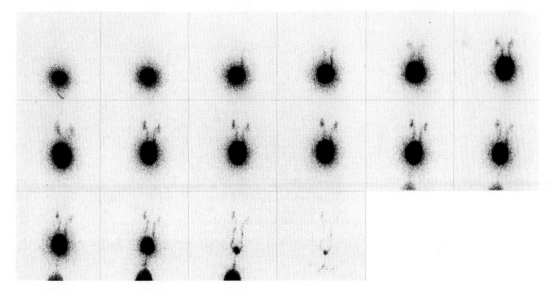

FIGURE 11.4. Distal left vesicoureteric reflux, RNC severity grade 1. Reflux is limited to the left distal ureter without reaching the renal pelvis.

FIGURE 11.5. Bilateral vesicoureteric reflux, RNC severity grade 2. Reflux reaches both renal pelves and persists during the filling and voiding phases of the RNC. At the end of voiding, a significant amount of tracer has drained out of the renal pelves, ureters, and bladder.

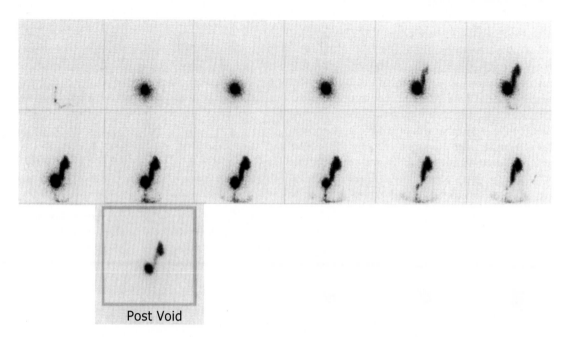

FIGURE 11.6. Severe unilateral vesicoureteric reflux, RNC severity grade 3. Reflux is visualized in a dilated right ureter and renal pelvis. A postvoid image reveals significant retention of tracer in the renal pelvicaliceal system and ureter with secondary bladder filling.

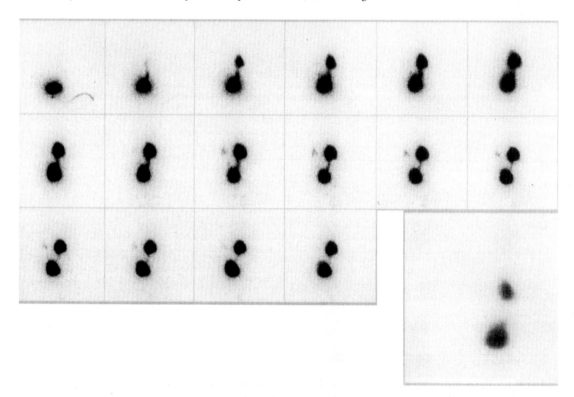

FIGURE 11.7. Severe right vesicoureteric reflux (RNC severity grade 3) and mild to moderate left vesicoureteric reflux (RNC grade 2). Right reflux appears early at low bladder volume and persists during the entire examination. A postvoid image (bottom right) reveals secondary bladder filling and significant retention of tracer in the right renal pelvis. In addition there is mild to moderate left vesicoureteric reflux reaching the renal pelvis. Left reflux occurs at higher bladder volumes, is intermittent, and drains rather rapidly even during bladder filling.

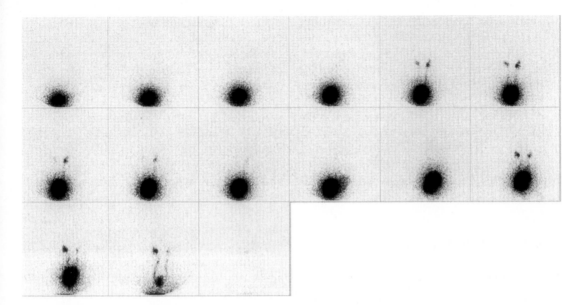

FIGURE 11.8. Intermittent bilateral vesicoureteric reflux. Mild to moderate reflux appears almost simultaneously during the mid-filling phase in both ureters and renal pelves. During the mid- to late filling phase, reflux subsides temporarily in both sides and reappears during the late filling and voiding phases.

Variability of Low-Grade Vesicoureteric Reflux

Vesicoureteric reflux is not a constant phenomenon. As mentioned earlier, approximately two thirds of VUR disappears spontaneously as a result of the patient's growth and maturation. In addition, low-grade VUR varies from moment to moment and from examination to examination. In our observation, using RNC, VUR varies also with bladder volume, voiding or filling, patient position, and level of anxiety. Reflux may be present during most of the filling and voiding phases of the radionuclide cystogram, or it may be intermittent (Fig. 11.8).[17,18] Therefore, it is clear that one normal examination is not sufficient to ensure that VUR has disappeared. Serial cystograms over several (6 to 12) months are needed to ensure complete cessation of reflux.[19] We have evaluated 480 ureters from 240 patients on two separate occasions when patients underwent RNC. The period between observations averaged 13 months (3 months to 3.7 years). None of the patients had prior surgery, neurogenic bladder, or other anatomic abnormality. This study revealed that 85% of the ureters showed either no change (55%) or decrease (30%) in reflux severity. However, 15% revealed an apparent worsening in reflux severity (9%), or reflux was detected only on the second RNC (6%). Two-stage RNC has also shown the variable nature of VUR.[20,21] Treatment programs for VUR, therefore, should take into account the variability of low grade reflux.

Treatment

Typically, patients with low-grade reflux are treated with a regimen of long-term antibiotic prophylaxis. With severe reflux, spontaneous resolution of reflux can occur but is less likely. Therefore, surgical treatment is more common in these patients. Continuous antibiotic therapy may be given to these patients provided their urine remains sterile, frequent urine cultures are performed, and that serial evaluation for reflux is carried out. This routine requires careful compliance by the patient and parents.

Surgical treatment of VUR has a high degree of success in experienced hands ($\approx 95\%$), offers an immediate correction of the anatomic problem, and reduces the risk of pyelonephritis. Neither medical nor surgical treatment, however, seems to offer a clear advantage related to subsequent development of hypertension or impairment of renal growth. Whichever form of therapy is chosen, long-term follow-up and observation are essential to assess the patient's progress and the presence of complicating factors, such as residual VUR, pyelonephritis, new scarring, hypertension, or renal dysfunction.

Radionuclide Cystography

Indications

Radionuclide cystography is indicated in four principal settings (Table 11.1). Because of its safety, high sensitivity, and minimal radiation exposure, RNC is an ideal method for the initial diagnosis of VUR in children. The clinical acceptance and effectiveness of this method is evidenced by the steady growth in the number of RNC studies performed in our institution. Radionuclide cystography is indicated for the follow-up of patients who have been diagnosed previously with VUR and are receiving long-term prophylactic antibiotic therapy. Patients undergoing this type of treatment are usually monitored for reflux every 6 to 12 months. Radionuclide cystography is an effective technique for evaluating the results of surgical repair of VUR. In addition, and because of the reasons mentioned above (low radiation dose, high sensitivity), RNC is a highly useful method for the diagnosis of familial reflux.

Methods

There are two principal nuclear medicine methods to diagnose VUR: direct RNC and

TABLE 11.1. Indications for radionuclide cystography

Initial diagnosis of vesicoureteric reflux (VUR)
Follow-up of previously diagnosed VUR to assess for spontaneous resolution
Assessment of antireflux surgery
Diagnosis of familial VUR

indirect radionuclide cystography (IRC). The direct method requires bladder catheterization to introduce the radionuclide into the bladder in a retrograde fashion. Indirect radionuclide cystography does not require catheterization. Studies comparing RNC with IRC have suggested that RNC is more sensitive than IRC.[22–24] However, RNC is an invasive technique, so IRC may still have a role in the diagnosis of VUR in cooperative patients and in those who refuse catheterization.[25] Indirect radionuclide cystography requires that the patient refrain from voiding until the time of examination. Increased urinary output caused by recent administration of a diuretic (e.g., furosemide) or an intravenous contrast agent for urography or overhydration can interfere with the detection of VUR. Therefore, cystography should be performed first, or one should wait 1 day after administration of these agents.

Patient Preparation

The same patient preparation applies for both direct RNC and IRC. A complete explanation of the procedure should be given to the patient and parents. When done with patience and understanding, such a conversation can reduce anxiety before the examination. In addition, we find it helpful to hand out or mail a brochure with information and instructions for the RNC.[17,26] If a patient is unusually apprehensive about the procedure, we schedule it for another day. We do not use sedation for RNC. The patient is instructed to void in the bathroom before the examination if possible, and then to lie supine on the examination table for the study (see below).

Direct Radionuclide Cystography

Radionuclide cystography can detect small volumes of reflux, as little as 0.2mL at 2cm from the projected edge of the bladder.[18] In most cases RNC is a stress test of the ureterovesical junction. It is a rather invasive procedure and requires bladder catheterization, the bladder being filled in a retrograde fashion with a fluid at a higher rate than is natural. The radiation exposure to the patient with RNC is low, with a gonadal absorbed radiation dose of less than 3 mrad (0.03 mGy). Radionuclide cystography is highly sensitive, and the operator has greater control of the procedure than with IRC. Patients of all ages can be examined. As part of the procedure, a urine sample under aseptic conditions is obtained for culture.

Radiopharmaceutical

Technetium-99m (^{99m}Tc) as pertechnetate is used. The usual administered dose is 1 to 2 mCi (37 to 74 MBq).

Equipment and Recording

The examination table is covered with plastic-lined absorbent paper to contain any spilled tracer and to reduce contamination of the table. A gamma scintillation camera system equipped with a high-resolution collimator is used. In our practice, the RNC is recorded as a series of 10-second frames in a 128×128 matrix format for the duration of the filling and voiding phases of the study. Postvoid images are routinely obtained if the patient is not able to empty the bladder while on the imaging table.

Catheterization

Sterile urethral catheterization trays prepared for each study contain the following items: three small containers, cotton, and a sterile towel with a central opening. Other materials needed include antiseptic solution (Hibiclens, Stuart Pharmaceuticals, Wilmington, DE), sterile water, anesthetic jelly (Xylocaine, AstraZeneca, Wilmington, DE), a 10-mL syringe with a blunt, tapered adapter ("fistula tip"). Catheters of two sizes are used: a 2.6-mm-diameter catheter (French 8) for most patients and a 1.5-mm-diameter catheter (French 5) for infants.

The success of the examination depends to a great extent on careful catheterization technique. Inexperience is the most frequent cause of iatrogenic damage to the male urethra. If necessary, a parent or aide assists in immobilizing the patient, who lies supine and is encouraged to relax. The so-called frog position is useful in catheterizing females. The periurethral area in females and the glans penis in males is carefully cleansed with antiseptic solution and sterile water warmed to body temperature before use. The catheter is lubricated with the anesthetic jelly to facilitate a smooth insertion. Using a directed bright spotlight, the female urethral orifice must be clearly identified before attempting catheterization.

In females the catheter should be introduced easily in one motion, without hesitation. Any additional contact with the area surrounding the urethral orifice should be avoided because it causes discomfort. This point cannot be emphasized enough, because a child who has had a bad first experience with this procedure is not likely to cooperate in the future.

In boys the urethra is anesthetized. The penis is held with one hand, while lidocaine (5 to 10 mL) is slowly injected into the urethra using the blunt adapter. Slow and deep breathing helps to relax the sphincter and allows anesthesia of the entire urethra. Slightly squeezing the anterior portion of the penis for a minute prevents the lidocaine from draining out. The catheter is then gently and continuously introduced into the bladder. Encourage the patient to breathe deeply and attempt to void, which may relax the sphincter. If the sphincter remains closed, the catheter should be kept under continuous and mild pressure against it. In most cases, the catheter eventually glides through the sphincter.

Do not try to overcome a closed or spastic sphincter by repeated back-and-forth motions of the catheter as it may result in urethral injury. In the rare instance when it is necessary to repeat the urethral anesthesia, a second attempt at catheterization is almost always successful.

Once the catheter has been advanced beyond the sphincter, most children cooperate. The residual bladder volume is then measured. The catheter is fixed with adhesive surgical tape to the inner thigh in girls and to the dorsal shaft

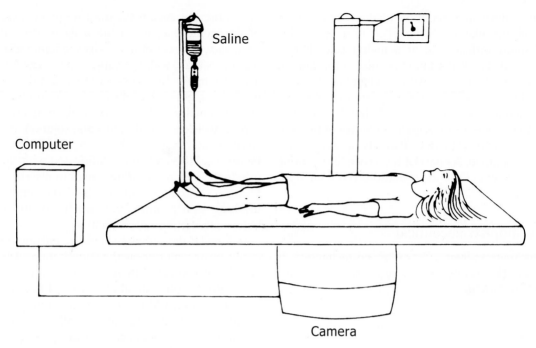

FIGURE 11.9. Method of direct radionuclide cystography.

of the penis in boys. Leaving the catheter in place until the end of the study allows for a repeat examination in case of failure, as well as for additional filling of the bladder. In most cases, however, the catheter is removed gently before the patient voids. Some investigators have suggested direct RNC by direct percutaneous administration rather than bladder catheterization.[27]

Filling and Voiding

The child is encouraged to lie quietly on the table. A calm environment and dim room lighting during the procedure often have a quieting effect. Many patients (and parents) find that watching a small ceiling-mounted TV while the study is in progress greatly helps reduce anxiety and makes the time pass more quickly.

The tracer is administered directly into the patient's bladder via the catheter.* The bottle

*For computerized radionuclide cystography (CRVC), the radiopharmaceutical is mixed with the saline in the bottle and infused into the bladder (see Appendix).

of 500 mL of normal saline (or irrigating solution) is suspended 70 to 90 cm above the bladder and connected to the catheter (Fig. 11.9). The saline solution is allowed to drain freely into the bladder. In our practice, we examine most patients in the supine position to more easily control the examination. However, the RNC can be performed in the sitting or semirecumbent position if so desired.

While the bladder is filling, the operator monitors the entire examination on the computer monitor. The end of the filling phase is usually indicated by a bladder volume appropriate for the patient's age (see below) or a reduction or cessation of the infusate's rate of flow. When the bladder is filled to its capacity, voiding is usually initiated without delay. Careful and complete collection of the voided fluid is necessary for quantitation (see Appendix). We use a plastic urinal for both girls and boys. In girls its lower border is gently pressed against the perineum and inner thighs. If patients cannot void in the supine position, they are asked to try voiding in the sitting position.

The technologist or physician conducting the study should record the following: residual bladder volume, the fact that a urine sample was obtained under aseptic conditions for culture, any problems during the catheterization or the procedure, and voided volume. A technologist's RNC data sheet is reproduced in (Fig. 11.10). The data can be entered directly on computer.

Functional Bladder Capacity

Knowledge of the expected functional bladder capacity is useful for evaluation of VUR in children. However, a priori prediction of bladder capacity in children is difficult. Subjective criteria of complete bladder filling produced by the patient (toes curling upward, jiggling leg movements, complaints of urgency) should be noted, but their value may be unreliable.

Although bladder capacity generally increases with age and maturation, its variability at a given age or in a given patient may correspond to 100% or more of the mean volume. Influences operating at the time of examination may cause the functional bladder capacity to be different from the actual capacity. Mechanical factors, such as rapid filling of the bladder, irritation from the catheter, or low temperature of the instilled fluid, can induce high bladder tonus and thus lower bladder capacity. Apprehension may provoke the same response. Uninhibited bladder contractions related to irritability from severe inflammation characteristically cause intermittent pain and urgency and tend to keep bladder capacity low. In most of the children with urinary tract infection (UTI) in our series, however, bladder capacity did not seem to be affected.[17] Most of our patients were studied after antibiotic treatment of their UTI.

Information about bladder capacity on previous studies, mean values, and observation of the infusion flow rate should aid the operator in filling the patient's bladder to its approximate functional capacity. Several studies have addressed bladder capacity as a function of age in children, but published studies have included fewer than 250 observations.[18,28–31] Those reports have indicated a linear relationship between age and functional bladder capacity. The following formula has been suggested[28]: bladder capacity (ounces) = age (years) plus 2.

In addition, for children up to 1 year of age a linear regression has been suggested[29]: capacity (mL) = [7.0 × weight (kg)] − 1.2. A study in our laboratory using direct RNC suggested that this relationship was not linear.[18]

More recently we have reviewed the functional bladder capacities for more than 4000 RNC examinations in children under 13 years of age. The relationship of functional bladder capacity and age seems to be nonlinear, and it can be described by a power model: $Y = \beta_o X^{\beta_1}$, where Y is the estimated bladder capacity; β_o is the volume (constant); X is the age; and β_1 is the slope power (Fig. 11.11).[32]

Analysis of Radionuclide Cystography

In routine practice, analysis of RNC is visual. The RNC should be viewed whenever possible on cinematic display, and the interpreter should be able to vary the playback speed and the contrast of the dynamic image set. With most low-grade reflux, the volume and amount of activity of refluxed tracer is much smaller than the activity within the bladder, so reflux could be missed if no contrast enhancement is used. No single approach covers all cases. Generally, it is useful to vary the upper threshold in the range between 5% and 15% of the maximum level of activity in the image. Evaluation of the RNC with a series of static images is generally effective; however, evaluation on cinematic display is unquestionably superior and is strongly recommended to achieve a higher diagnostic yield. Even with patient motion, dynamic evaluation enables the operator to distinguish scatter from minimal reflux better than on serial static images. Motion correction helps in the assessment of RNC where the patient has moved during the examination.

Time-activity curves from regions of interest over the renal, ureteral, and vesical regions can be utilized for quantitative evaluation of reflux, bladder volumes, and voiding flow rates with RNC. (See the Appendix for discussion of computerized voiding cystography.) Meticulous attention to technique and complete avoidance of patient motion are mandatory for this approach.[17]

DIVISION OF NUCLEAR MEDICINE
CHILDREN'S HOSPITAL, BOSTON
Radionuclide Cystogram

FIGURE 11.10. Direct radionuclide cystography data sheet.

Indications:

Findings:

The child urinated prior to catheterization? Yes ☐

No ☐   Explain:

Were there problems with catheterization? No ☐

Yes ☐   Explain:

Residual urine volume _____ ml.

Urine sent for culture?   Yes ☐

No ☐   Explain:

Bladder capacity _____ ml.

Patient voided _____ ml on the table.

☐   Patient did not void on the table.

☐   Post void image obtained.

Impression:

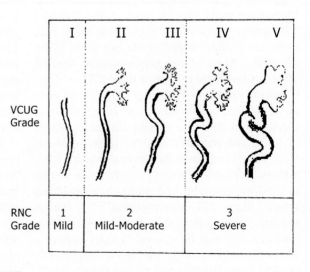

_____ M.D.

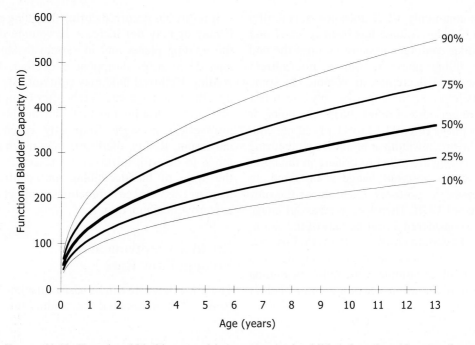

FIGURE 11.11. Functional bladder capacities versus ages in children less than 13 years of age.

Reporting Results

The RNC report should address at least the following information: voiding prior to the examination, residual bladder volume, the fact that a urine sample obtained under aseptic conditions was collected and sent to the laboratory for culture, problems with catheterization or the procedure, volume infused in the bladder, volume voided, presence and severity of reflux, and comparison with previous examinations (same, better, or worse). Most of our patients see a urologist after completion of RNC study; in our practice, the RNC report and images are immediately transmitted to the referring urologist.

Vesicoureteric Reflux in Radionuclide Cystography

An analysis of 135 consecutive radionuclide studies in our hospital revealed a 32% incidence of VUR, usually RNC grades 1 or 2. Reflux was present in 47% of the nonsurgical patients and in 11% of the patients evaluated after surgery. It was unilateral in 60% and bilateral in 40%. Unilateral reflux occurred in the right and left ureters with equal frequency. In the 59 refluxing renal units, reflux occurred during filling and voiding in 80%, whereas reflux present during voiding only was seen in 17% of the ureters. These findings underscore the importance of examining the patient during voiding as well as during filling. The remaining 3% of ureters refluxed during bladder filling only. Almost 80% of those patients with reflux during filling and voiding refluxed 2 to 34 mL (average 7 mL).[17]

Patterns of Reflux

The ability to continuously monitor during RNC permits observation of several dynamic patterns of reflux. Continuously increasing reflux characteristically occurs during the early or mid-filling phase, supposedly through a patulous ureteral orifice that allows the bladder and ureter(s) to behave as a single chamber. This is the most severe reflux. Occurrence of reflux in this condition appears to be independent of intravesical pressure, which is usually low during the beginning of bladder filling.[33]

Most commonly, VUR does not start until a certain bladder volume has been reached and then either continues to increase until the end of the filling phase or shows intermittent increases and decreases in volume. In some patients, however, there may be only one or few transient episodes of reflux during the filling or voiding phase (Figs. 11.12 to 11.14). Some children who are unwilling or unable to void during the cystogram are asked to urinate in the bathroom, and a postvoid image is obtained. In some cases, the postvoid image shows the only evidence of VUR. Therefore, a postvoid image must be considered a routine part of the examination. In certain cases of bilateral reflux, one ureter can be seen to begin refluxing at a certain bladder volume, with reflux beginning in the contralateral ureter at a greater bladder volume.

If reflux has occurred during the filling phase, it may or may not increase in volume during the voiding phase, and in certain instances it may decrease or disappear altogether during voiding. Refluxed fluid may continuously drain into the bladder immediately after completion of voiding, despite the fact that at this time intravesical pressure frequently reaches its maximum. Reflux, therefore, may not have as much to do with intravesical pressure as with the state of bladder filling and contraction insofar as these functions affect the ureterovesical junction.

Bladder Emptying and Voiding Flow Rate

The urine flow rate can be easily calculated with RNC.[34,35] We calculated the voiding flow rates

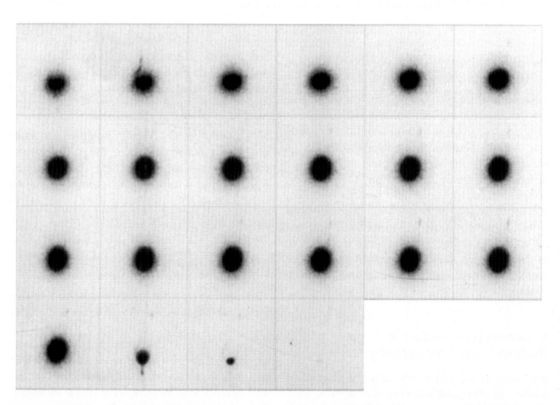

FIGURE 11.12. Intermittent mild bilateral vesicoureteric reflux. Early (low bladder volume) left vesicoureteric reflux (VUR) subsides rapidly. As the RNC progresses toward the end of filling, there is mild bilateral VUR. An image obtained following the completion voiding reveals complete drainage of both ureteropelvicaliceal systems and the bladder.

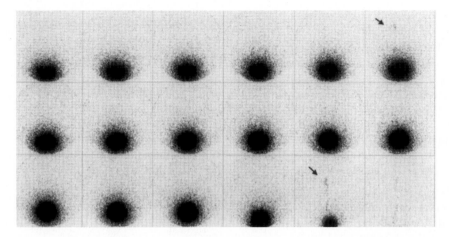

FIGURE 11.13. Mild intermittent left vesicoureteric reflux. Left VUR is visualized briefly during the mid-filling phase; it then disappears completely and returns during the voiding phase (arrows).

in 75 patients.[17] The average rate in 26 normal children was 10.2 mL/sec [range 2.0 to 21.0 mL/sec ± 4.5 standard deviation (SD)]. In 49 abnormal patients (reflux with or without infection or previous surgery), the voiding flow rates averaged 10.5 mL/sec (range 1.4 to 31.0 mL/sec ± 5.7 SD). In all 75 patients, the average voiding flow rate was 10.4 mL/sec (range 1.4 to 31.0 mL/sec ± 5.3 SD). The average voiding flow rate seemed to relate to the initial bladder volume and thus to age. The greater the initial bladder volume, the higher was the voiding flow rate. The presence of an indwelling catheter did not seem to reduce the voiding

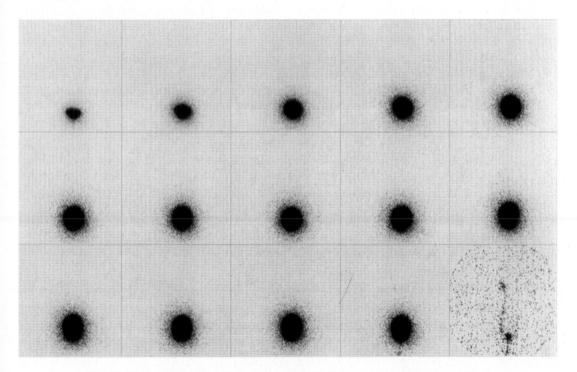

FIGURE 11.14. Mild left vesicoureteric reflux. Reflux is seen only during voiding.

flow rate significantly. In patients with an indwelling catheter, it averaged 10.7 mL/sec (range 2.0 to 31.0 mL/sec), whereas in those without a catheter the average flow rate was 9.8 mL/sec (range 1.4 to 25.0 mL/sec). The voiding time was 10 to 116 seconds (average 35 seconds). With the exception of a few extreme values, the voiding time in normal patients is comparable to that in patients with reflux.

Children usually do not use abdominal straining during voiding.[36] When they do, the urinary flow either increases or decreases, probably reflecting whether the external sphincter is contracted along with the abdominal muscles.[37] Thus urging the child to strain in order to void may be counterproductive.

Residual Bladder Volume

Residual volumes measured by catheterization and RNC may or may not be the same, and in many instances there is gross discrepancy between these two measurements for any number of reasons (Fig. 11.15). For example, the patient may not adequately empty the bladder because of some underlying abnormality such as aberrant micturition, as in some cases of reflux or dysuria.[38] The bladder may not be properly drained because the tip of the catheter abuts the bladder wall, or the patient may simply be unwilling or unable to void because of the unnatural situation.[39]

We have observed more complete emptying of the bladder in patients whose bladders were filled to a maximum or optimal volume during cystography. Apparently, high tonicity of the bladder wall induced adequate contraction and more complete emptying. A large residual volume in children at the beginning or end of the study does not necessarily mean that the patient has a significant abnormality. On the other hand, demonstration of an empty bladder is useful.

Urine Culture

We reviewed the results of urine culture in 113 consecutive children referred for radionuclide cystography. Urinary infection with *Escherichia coli* or *Streptococcus faecalis* was found in 11%

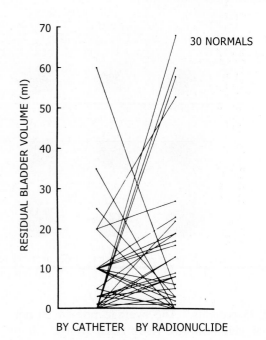

FIGURE 11.15. Residual bladder volumes measured in the same patients by catheterization and by radionuclide cystography in 30 normal children.

despite their history of continuous antibiotic treatment and careful follow-up by their physicians. Patients on antibiotic treatment and those who had undergone surgery showed a nearly equal incidence of urinary infection. Our experience agrees with that of other workers, suggesting that reflux and infection are independent of one another.[40-44]

Dosimetry

For children undergoing RNC between ages 1 and 10, the absorbed radiation dose estimates for the bladder wall are 18 to 27 mrad (0.18 to 0.27 mGy) and for ovaries 1 to 2 mrad (10 to 20 mGy). The testicular dose is less than the dose to the ovaries. The dose to the kidneys is estimated to be 0.02 to 0.04 mrad/mL of reflux per minute of residence in the collecting system. The estimated dose to the ureter in reflux is 1.3 mrad (13 mGy)/minute, which is the same as the dose to a sphere of 1 mL filled with ^{99m}Tc at a concentration of 2 mCi (74 MBq)/L.[17,45-47] The dose to the ovaries is 100 to 200 times less with RNC than with conventional VCUG and 20 to 40 times less than pulsed fluoroscopy.[17,48,49] In our dose calculations, the residence time for the activity in the bladder was determined from the duration of the study in patients of various age groups. The empty bladder mass was estimated by extrapolation from data in adults, using growth curves.[50]

Indirect Radionuclide Cystography

The principal advantages of IRC are that it can demonstrate reflux under physiologic conditions. It uses radiopharmaceuticals that, after intravenous injection, are rapidly eliminated in the urine and not retained in the renal parenchyma. Vesicoureteric reflux can be detected during voiding only. This technique has the advantage that it permits evaluation of renal function and urine drainage as well as detection of VUR. Indirect radionuclide cystography is less traumatic for the patient than RNC, physically and emotionally. It does not

require catheterization, and allows the bladder to be filled and emptied physiologically (Fig. 11.16). The minimal risk of induced infection is eliminated with IRC. But IRC cannot detect VUR that occurs during the filling period only.

The patient can void in the usual position, so the competence of the vesicoureteral mechanism is tested under normal voiding pressures.[25] A relative disadvantage of IRC is that it requires complete patient cooperation. Clearly, IRC is not meant for newborns, infants, and those patients who cannot or will not cooperate. Another disadvantage of IRC is that it requires that the imaging room be available when the patient is ready to void.

Radiopharmaceuticals

The radiopharmaceuticals technetium-99m-disodium [N-[N-N-(mercaptoacetyl)glycyl]-glycinato(2-)-N,N',N'',S]oxotechnetate(2-) (^{99m}Tc-MAG$_3$) or ^{99m}Tc–diethylenetriamine pentaacetic acid (^{99m}Tc-DTPA) are suitable

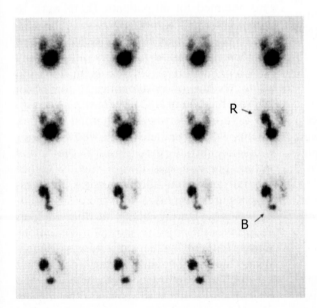
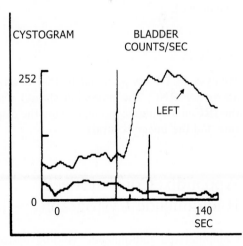

FIGURE 11.16. Indirect radionuclide cystography (^{99m}Tc-MAG$_3$). Left: The bladder is filled with radiotracer; as the patient voids, there is left vesicoureteric reflux (R) and secondary bladder (B) filling. Right: The time-activity curve from a region of interest over the left kidney reveals a sharp increase coinciding with the reflux seen on the images. (*Source:* Courtesy of Dr. Isky Gordon, Hospital for Sick Children, London, England.)

agents for IRC. ^{99m}Tc-MAG$_3$ is a better choice, as it results in less body background. The intravenous administered dose should be the same used for dynamic renal scintigraphy.

Recording

Indirect radionuclide cystography should be preceded by a conventional dynamic renal scan in order to evaluate renal function and assess complete drainage of tracer from the kidneys. Ideally, no significant amount of tracer should be present in the renal regions prior to the start of the IRC, as VUR may be difficult to detect in the presence of residual tracer in the pelvicaliceal system. For the voiding phase, the patient is positioned in the sitting position with the gamma camera centered over the region of the bladder and kidneys. The patient voids into a urinal, a bedpan, or a specially made console. Precautions to reduce contamination of the equipment and the room must be taken. Recording is begun when the patient is ready to void and continues until the end of voiding. Additional images may have to be obtained following voiding. The IRC is recorded using the same camera and computer acquisition parameters described under RNC (see above).

Analysis

Analysis of IRC is identical to that described above for RNC. The physician should review the IRC in a dynamic mode, varying the display rate and the image contrast.

Appendix: Computerized Radionuclide Cystography

Computerized radionuclide voiding cystography (CRVC) is a refinement of RNC. It is a quantitative method and enables simultaneous measurement of bladder volumes and pressures. When using CRVC, the following parameters are obtained:

1. Volume of the bladder at the first occurrence of reflux and at the time of maximum reflux during filling and/or voiding
2. Maximum bladder volume (end of filling)
3. Volumes of reflux (initial, maximum, residual)
4. Residual bladder volume
5. Average voiding flow rate
6. Bladder pressures

Intravesical Pressure

With CRVC, it is possible to simultaneously record the radionuclide cystogram and the intravesical pressures. Using a double-lumen catheter, one channel is used for infusion and the other is connected to a pressure transducer. We use a 3-mm-diameter double-lumen catheter (French 9). The pressure transducer output is connected through an analog-to-digital converter to the computer. Time-activity and time-pressure curves can then be displayed simultaneously.[17,51,52]

In a study in our institution aimed at establishing normal and abnormal ranges of intravesical pressure, measurements during RNC were obtained for 40 patients. There were 16 normal children, 15 with reflux, and nine who had previous surgery. In the normal children maximum intravesical pressures during filling were 15 to 80 cm H$_2$O (average 42 cm H$_2$O) and during voiding or postvoiding 24 to 136 cm H$_2$O (average 78 cm H$_2$O). There was no significant difference between the normal children, patients with reflux, and those who had prior reimplants. In all these groups, the initial voiding pressure was always slightly higher than the maximum filling pressure. Intravesical pressures decreased with increasing bladder volume. During filling of the bladder, the intravesical pressure showed a continuous increase until full bladder capacity was reached. Toward the end of voiding, a pressure peak that occurred after contraction characterized the pressure curve. In most instances, the highest recorded intravesical pressure was reached during this moment after contraction.

There is no satisfactory proof of the concept that intravesical pressure causes VUR.[53] A relationship between intravesical pressure and cortical renal damage in the absence of infection remains widely debated,[54] although in patients with VUR there are alterations in renal blood flow during voiding.[55] Renal damage from pyelotubular backflow has also been considered.[56] It has been clearly demonstrated in children under 6 years of age, but mainly in infants, that massive reflux in the presence of urinary tract infection leads to renal damage.[40,53,57–60]

Studies in rabbits reveal that renal blood flow decreases with acute increase of pressures in the pelvicaliceal system. This is reversible.[61] Intrarenal reflux seems to play an important role in the etiology of renal damage.[62] Because intravesical pressure is higher in younger than older children, it follows that intravesical pressure decreases with increasing bladder capacity. With renal damage occurring mainly in younger children, perhaps there is some relationship between intravesical pressure and reflux nephropathy. In the absence of a barrier at the ureterovesical junction, the upper urinary system and the bladder act as a single chamber. Studies in our laboratory seem to indicate that intravesical pressure is probably least important in terms of etiology, management, and prognosis of reflux provided that distal obstruction or neurogenic dysfunction is not present. Most of our patients exhibited reflux during filling at a relatively large bladder volume. The increasing bladder volume during the cystogram probably influences the anatomy and competence of the ureterovesical junction more than the increase in pressure.

In the growing child, maturation of the ureterovesical junction probably implies not only lengthening of the intravesical ureter, but also strengthening of the specific musculature related to the ureterovesical junction. Therefore decreasing occurrence of reflux with age is to be expected.[63–65] Controversy still exists about maturation of the ureterovesical junction.[44,66] Reflux only during voiding may be related to the changing anatomic condition of the ureterovesical junction during bladder contraction. The intravesical pressure at the initiation of voiding is not significantly higher than at the end of filling. Reflux that occurs at low bladder volume is more damaging.[67]

Analysis

With CRVC, the sequential images of the cystogram are displayed on the computer monitor and evaluated visually (see above). If reflux is present, regions of interest (ROIs) are drawn over the kidneys and bladder. In addition, another region near the bladder is selected to correct for background scatter.

It is important to determine if patient motion occurred during the study because it invalidates any attempts at quantitation. Motion correction should be applied. Time-activity curves are calculated for each ROI.

To obtain and estimate the volumes of reflux, bladder capacity, and residual capacity, a relation between activity and volume is obtained. Assuming that attenuation of the gamma rays is constant, that the radioisotope is well mixed with the solution of saline, and that a negligible amount of urine is produced by the kidneys during the study, the counts recorded are proportional to the volume(s):

$$V = RC \qquad (1)$$

where V is volume, R is a constant, and C is counts. Note that 0 counts represents zero volume. The constant R is calculated by relating the voided volume to the drop in total vesical counts during the voiding phase of the study. At the beginning of the voiding phase, the volume is V_0 and the counts are C_0. At the end of the voiding phase, the volume is V_e and the counts C_e. Substituting these values into Eq. 1 yields:

$$V_0 = RC_0 \qquad (2)$$

$$V_e = RC_e \qquad (3)$$

Subtracting Eq. 3 from Eq. 2 yields:

$$R = \frac{V_0 - V_e}{C_0 - C_e} = \frac{V}{C} = \frac{\text{change in volume}}{\text{change in counts}} \qquad (4)$$

Once the ratios are calculated, it is easy to obtain any volume of interest for any particular time of the study (e.g., maximum volume of reflux). One simply has to multiply the ratio R by the number of counts over a particular region at a given frame. After the counts in each region are converted to volumes, it is possible to calculate rates of flow. To obtain the average voiding flow rate, the count loss during voiding must be divided by the time of voiding and multiplied by the constant R.

$$\text{Average flow rate} = R = \frac{\Delta V}{AT} \quad (5)$$

References

1. Ransley PG. Vesicoureteric reflux. In: Williams DI, Johnston JH, eds. Pediatric Urology. London: Butterworth, 1982.
2. Noe HN. The long-term results of prospective sibling reflux screening. J Urol 1992;148(5 pt 2): 1739–42.
3. Van den Abbeele AD, Treves ST, Lebowitz RL, et al. Vesicoureteral reflux in asymptomatic siblings of patients with known reflux: radionuclide cystography. Pediatrics 1987;79(1):147–53.
4. Kenda RB, Fettich JJ. Vesicoureteric reflux and renal scars in asymptomatic siblings of children with reflux. Arch Dis Child 1992;67(4):506–8.
5. Ataei N, Madani A, Esfahani ST, et al. Screening for vesicoureteral reflux and renal scars in siblings of children with known reflux. Pediatr Nephrol 2004;19(10):1127–31.
6. Houle AM, Cheikhelard A, Barrieras D, Rivest MC, Gaudreault V. Impact of early screening for reflux in siblings on the detection of renal damage. BJU Int 2004;94(1):123–5.
7. Buonomo C, Treves ST, Jones B, Summerville D, Bauer S, Retik A. Silent renal damage in symptom-free siblings of children with vesicoureteral reflux: assessment with technetium Tc 99m dimercaptosuccinic acid scintigraphy. J Pediatr 1993;122(5 Pt 1):721–3.
8. Sukan A, Bayazit AK, Kibar M, et al. Comparison of direct radionuclide cystography and voiding direct cystography in the detection of vesicoureteral reflux. Ann Nucl Med 2003;17(7): 549–53.
9. Gordon I, Barkovics M, Pindoria S, Cole TJ, Woolf AS. Primary vesicoureteric reflux as a predictor of renal damage in children hospitalized with urinary tract infection: a systematic review and meta-analysis. J Am Soc Nephrol 2003;14(3): 739–44.
10. McLaren CJ, Simpson ET. Vesico-ureteric reflux in the young infant with follow-up direct radionuclide cystograms: the medical and surgical outcome at 5 years old. BJU Int 2002;90(7): 721–4.
11. Normand LCS, Smellie J. Vesicoureteric reflux: the case for conservative management. In: Hodson J, Kincaid-Smith P, eds. Reflux Nephropathy. New York: Masson, 1979.
12. Medina LS, Aguirre E, Altman NR. Vesicoureteral reflux imaging in children: comparative cost analysis. Acad Radiol 2003;10(2): 139–44.
13. Polito C, Rambaldi PF, La Manna A, Mansi L, Di Toro R. Enhanced detection of vesicoureteric reflux with isotopic cystography. Pediatr Nephrol 2000;14(8–9):827–30.
14. Poli-Merol ML, Francois S, Pfliger F, et al. Interest of direct radionuclide cystography in repeated urinary tract infection exploration in childhood. Eur J Pediatr Surg 1998;8(6): 339–42.
15. Saraga M, Stanicic A, Markovic V. The role of direct radionuclide cystography in evaluation of vesicoureteral reflux. Scand J Urol Nephrol 1996;30(5):367–71.
16. Medical versus surgical treatment of primary vesicoureteral reflux: report of the International Reflux Study Committee. Pediatrics 1981; 67(3):392–400.
17. Willi U, Treves ST. Radionuclide voiding cystography. In: Treves ST, ed. Pediatric Nuclear Medicine. New York: Springer-Verlag, 1985: 105–20.
18. Willi U, Treves S. Radionuclide voiding cystography. Urol Radiol 1983;5(3):161–73, 175.
19. Grmek M, Fettich J. The importance of follow-up of children with vesicoureteral reflux grade 1. Acta Paediatr 2003;92(4):435–8.
20. Pozderac RV, Becker CJ, Reitelman C, Kuhns LR. Comparison of single and two stage radionuclide cystography (RNC) for evaluation of reflux. J Nucl Med 1990;31:893(abstr).
21. Neel KF, Shillinger JF. The prevalence of persistent vesicoureteral reflux after 1 negative nuclear medicine cystogram. J Urol 2000;164(3 pt 2):1067–9.
22. Bower G, Lovegrove FT, Geijsel H, Van der Schaff A, Guelfi G. Comparison of "direct" and "indirect" radionuclide cystography. J Nucl Med 1985;26(5):465–8.
23. Conway JJ, Belman AB, King LR. Direct and indirect radionuclide cystography. Semin Nucl Med 1974;4(2):197–211.

24. Majd M, Kass EJ, Belman AB. Radionuclide cystography in children: comparison of direct (retrograde) and indirect (intravenous) techniques. Ann Radiol (Paris) 1985;28(3–4):322–8.

25. Gordon I, Peters AM, Morony S. Indirect radionuclide cystography: a sensitive technique for the detection of vesicoureteral reflux. Pediatr Nephrol 1990;4(6):604–6.

26. Hass EA, Solomon DJ. Telling children about diagnostic radiology procedures. Radiology 1977;124(2):521.

27. Wilkinson AG. Percutaneous direct radionuclide cystography in children: description of technique and early experience. Pediatr Radiol 2002;32(7):511–7.

28. Berger RM, Maizels M, Moran GC, Conway JJ, Firlit CF. Bladder capacity (ounces) equals age (years) plus 2 predicts normal bladder capacity and aids in diagnosis of abnormal voiding patterns. J Urol 1983;129(2):347–9.

29. Fairhurst JJ, Rubin CM, Hyde I, Freeman NV, Williams JD. Bladder capacity in infants. J Pediatr Surg 1991;26(1):55–7.

30. Koff SA. Estimating bladder capacity in children. Urology 1983;21(3):248.

31. Starfield B. Functional bladder capacity in enuretic and nonenuretic children. J Pediatr 1974;111:167–72.

32. Treves ST, Zurakowski D, Bauer SB, Mitchell KD, Nichols DP. Functional bladder capacity measured during radionuclide cystography in children. Radiology 1996;198(1):269–72.

33. Lattimer JK, Apperson JW, Gleason DM, Baker D, Flemming SS. The pressure at which reflux occurs, an important indicator of prognosis and treatment. J Urol 1963;89:395–404.

34. Spencer RP, Treves S. Bladder emptying flow rate as a function of bladder volume. Yale J Biol Med 1971;44(2):199–205.

35. Strauss BS, Blaufox MD. Estimation of residual urine and urine flow rates without urethral catheterization. J Nucl Med 1970;11(2):81–4.

36. Gierup J. Micturition studies in infants and children. Normal urinary flow. Scand J Urol Nephrol 1970;4(3):191–7.

37. Whitaker J, Johnston GS. Urinary flow rate with two techniques of bladder pressure measurement. Invest Urol 1966;4(3):235–8.

38. Hutch JA. Aberrant micturition. J Urol 1966;96(5):743–5.

39. Poznanski E, Poznanski AK. Psychogenic influences on voiding: observations from voiding cystourethrography. Psychosomatics 1969;10(6):339–42.

40. Cremin BJ. Observations on vesico-ureteric reflux and intrarenal reflux: a review and survey of material. Clin Radiol 1979;30(6):607–21.

41. Faure C. Le reflux vesico-ureteral. In: Lefebvre J, ed. Traite de Radiodiagnostic. Paris: Masson et Cie, 1973.

42. Friedland GW. Recurrent urinary tract infections in infants and children. Radiol Clin North Am 1977;15(1):19–35.

43. Stephens FD. Urologic aspects of recurrent urinary tract infection in children. J Pediatr 1972;80(5):725–37.

44. Stephens FD, Lenaghan D. The anatomical basis and dynamics of vesicoureteral reflux. J Urol 1962;87:669–80.

45. Dilman LD, Van der Lage FC. Radionuclide decay schemes and nuclear parameters for use in radiation dose estimation. In: Society of Nuclear Medicine, ed. NM/Medical Internal Radiation Dose Committee Pamphlet No. 10. New York: Society of Nuclear Medicine, 1975.

46. Loevinger R, Berman M. A revised schema for calculating the absorbed dose from biologically distributed radionuclides. In: Society of Nuclear Medicine, ed. NM/Medical Internal Radiation Dose Committee Pamphlet No. 1. New York: Society of Nuclear Medicine, 1975.

47. Snyder WS, Ford MR, Warner GG. Estimates of specific absorbed fractions for photon sources uniformly distributed in various organs of heterogenous phantom. In: Society of Nuclear Medicine, ed. NM/Medical Internal Radiation Dose Committee Pamphlet No. 5. New York: Society of Nuclear Medicine, 1978.

48. Fendel H. Radiation exposure due to urinary tract disease. In: Kaufmann HJ, ed. Progress in Pediatric Radiology. Basel, New York: S. Karger, 1970:116–35.

49. Leibovic SJ, Lebowitz RL. Reducing patient dose in voiding cystourethrography. Urol Radiol 1980;2:103–7.

50. Snyder WS, Cook MJ, Nasset ES. Report of the Task Group on Reference Man: a report. In: International Commission on Radiological Protection. Oxford; New York: Pergamon Press, 1975.

51. Papachristou F, Printza N, Doumas A, Koliakos G. Urinary bladder volume and pressure at reflux as prognostic factors of vesicoureteral reflux outcome. Pediatr Radiol 2004;34(7):556–9.

52. Cooper CS, Madsen MT, Austin JC, Hawtrey CE, Gerard LL, Graham MM. Bladder pressure at the onset of vesicoureteral reflux determined by

nuclear cystometrogram. J Urol 2003;170(4 pt 2):1537–40; discussion 1540.

53. Smith JC. Urethral resistance to micturition. Br J Urol 1968;40(2):125–56.

54. Bailey RR. Sterile reflux: is it harmless? In: Hodson J, Kincaid-Smith P, eds. Reflux Nephropathy. New York: Masson, 1979.

55. Orr WA, Kimbrough H, Gillenwater JY. Alterations in renal blood flow with voiding in the presence of vesicoureteral reflux. J Urol 1971;106(2):214–9.

56. King LR. Vesicoureteral reflux: history, etiology, and conservative management. In: Kelalis PP, King LR, Belman AB, eds. Clinical Pediatric Urology, vol 2. Philadelphia: Saunders, 1976.

57. Hodson CJ, Edwards D. Chronic pyelonephritis and vesico-ureteric reflex. Clin Radiol 1960;11:219–31.

58. Rolleston GL, Shannon FT, Utley WL. Follow-up of vesico-ureteric reflux in the newborn. Kidney Int Suppl 1975;4:S59–64.

59. Rolleston GL, Shannon FT, Utley WL. Relationship of infantile vesicoureteric reflux to renal damage. Br Med J 1970;1(694):460–3.

60. Smellie J, Edwards D, Hunter N, Normand IC, Prescod N. Vesico-ureteric reflux and renal scarring. Kidney Int Suppl 1975;4:S65–72.

61. Treves ST, Packard AB, Fung LC. Assessment of rapid changes in renal blood flow with (191m)Ir, an ultra-short-lived radionuclide. J Nucl Med 2004;45(3):508–11.

62. Rolleston GL, Maling TM, Hodson CJ. Intrarenal reflux and the scarred kidney. Arch Dis Child 1974;49(7):531–9.

63. Hutch JA. Theory of maturation of the intravesical ureter. J Urol 1961;86:534–8.

64. Tanagho EA, Meyers FH, Smith DR. Urethral resistance: its components and implications. I. Smooth muscle component. Invest Urol 1969; 7(2):136–49.

65. Tanagho EA, Meyers FH, Smith DR. Urethral resistance: its components and implications. II. Striated muscle component. Invest Urol 1969; 7(3):195–205.

66. Lyon RP, Marshall S, Tanagho EA. Theory of maturation: a critique. J Urol 1970;103(6):795–800.

67. Tepmongkol S, Chotipanich C, Sirisalipoch S, Chaiwatanarat T, Vilaichon AO, Wattana D. Relationship between vesicoureteral reflux and renal cortical scar development in Thai children: the significance of renal cortical scintigraphy and direct radionuclide cystography. J Med Assoc Thai 2002;85(suppl 1):S203–9.

12
Calculation of Glomerular Filtration Rate

Robert E. Zimmerman, Karl Mitchell, and Royal T. Davis

Serial measurement of the glomerular filtration rate (GFR) is recognized as an important assessment of the status of kidney function for individuals in certain disease states and especially for those undergoing chemotherapy. To be clinically useful the method used to measure GFR must compare favorably to the GFR gold standard, which is the urinary clearance of inulin, and the variance between successive serial measurements must be kept small.

Methods that have been used in the clinical laboratory to measure GFR include urinary and plasma clearance of inulin, urinary and plasma clearance of creatinine, plasma clearance of chromium-51–ethylenediaminetetraacetic acid (^{51}Cr-EDTA), plasma clearance of iodine-125 (^{125}I)–sodium-iothalamate, plasma clearance of sodium iothalamate using fluorescent activation analysis of stable iodine, and plasma clearance of ^{99m}Tc–diethylenetriamine pentaacetic acid (^{99m}Tc-DTPA).[1] Each of these methods has some systematic differences when compared to the gold standard method, clearance of inulin, because the agents used may bind to plasma proteins, renal tubular effects will affect clearance, and details of the analysis may vary.[1,2] Clearance of these agents is best described by a two-compartment exponential curve with a fast component of about 20 minutes and a slower component of several hundred minutes. Often the fast compartment is ignored so that the number of blood samples is minimized. The slower component can be analyzed using one to four plasma samples with increasing accuracy as more samples are used. Ignoring the fast com-ponent in this way systematically overestimates the GFR measurement. Correction factors among the different techniques have been derived, and they are sometimes used. Fortuitously, the factors tend to cancel each other, resulting in less difference than might otherwise be expected.[1,2]

To be used serially in children, the method employed must be relatively noninvasive, well tolerated, and easily implemented. Perhaps the method that comes closest to meeting these requirements for measurement of GFR in children is that using ^{99m}Tc-DTPA with serial blood samples. In vivo imaging of ^{99m}Tc-DTPA has been used to determine GFR, but its reproducibility is not good enough for many of the indications for GFR measurements. Therefore, measurement of the serum clearance of ^{99m}Tc-DTPA is preferred. While measuring the serum clearance of ^{99m}Tc-DTPA is conceptually simple, it is necessary to emphasize the importance of the use of good laboratory techniques and attention to detail in order to attain GFR estimates of acceptable clinical accuracy. Such a technique was published in 1993 by Rodman et al.[2] They also determined a reduced blood sampling schedule that results in an accurate and precise measurement of GFR.

Based on this work, the Nuclear Medicine Division at Children's Hospital Boston implemented a protocol to perform GFR measurements in children using three blood samples at 2, 3, and 4 hours. The protocol is shown in Figure 12.1. Both unfiltered and ultrafiltered samples are processed. The ultrafiltered

Indications: Estimation of GFR

Radiopharmaceutical: Commercial Name: ^{99m}Tc-DTPA
                                  Generic Name: diethylenetriaminepentaacetic acid
                                  Vendor: Several

Dose: 1.85 MBq/kg (50 µCi/kg)
           Minimum 11.1 MBq (300 µCi)
           Maximum 111 MBq (3 mCi)

Patient Preparation: The patient should be hydrated either orally or intravenously (10 ml/kg) over a 30-min period prior to the radiopharmaceutical administration. Height and weight must be recorded prior to the exam.

> (1) Preferably, it will be arranged that patient will have a venous line in place that can be accessed for 2, 3, and 4 hr blood drawings
> (2) Oncology patients with high flow lines (CVL, central venous line) in place after a peripheral injection of the radiopharmaceutical will have their CVL accessed for the 2, 3, and 4 hr blood drawings. The CVL will only be used by those technologists trained to do so.
> (3) When a CVL or intracath is not placed, the patient will receive 1 venopuncture for the radiopharmaceutical injection followed by 3 separate venopunctures for blood drawings at 2, 3, and 4 hr for GFR calculations.

Route of administration: Intravenously, followed by a 5-10 ml flush: The injection is critical. Any indication of infiltration will invalidate the study.

Procedure: Calculate the patient dose according to weight. Assay the prepared dose in the dose calibrator noting the time and activity on the worksheet. Secure an IV and inject the patient followed by a 5-10 ml saline flush. Note the time on the worksheet. Take a 1-min image over the injection site to ensure proper administration of the radiopharmaceutical. Assay the syringe, noting the time and activity on the worksheet. The patient is instructed to return at 2, 3, and 4 hrs post-injection to have blood samples drawn (use red-top tubes for blood samples (3-4 ml). Record time that samples are drawn on the worksheet.

Note: When accessing "high flow lines" or intracaths, flush lines with 5 ml of saline and withdraw 2 ml of blood and discard. Then proceed with 3-4 ml blood sample drawing for GFR calculation.

Standard Preparation: Draw up approximately 18 MBq (500 µCi) of 99mTc-DTPA in a syringe. Assay and record activity and time on the worksheet. Inject 50% into a volumetric flask containing 250 ml of water. The injected standard activity should be approximately 9 MBq (250 µCi). Re-assay the standard syringe, noting the time and remaining activity on the worksheet.

FIGURE 12.1. Protocol for glomerular filtration rate (GFR) determination in use at Children's Hospital Boston. Good laboratory technique and attention to detail is required in preparing the samples for counting.

Pipette Standards: label 4 tubes as described below:

```
S100a - 100 µl
S100b - 100 µl
S200a - 200 µl
S200b - 200 µl
```

Blood Samples: Allow blood to clot at room temperature, then centrifuge blood tubes at 3500 rpm for 5 min to separate serum. Prepare and label three serum tubes as follows:

```
S2 - 2 hour sample
S3 - 3 hour sample
S4 - 4 hour sample
```

Serum Method: Pipette two 200-µl serum samples from each blood sample (2, 3, 4 hr), label tubes as follows:

```
S2a S3a S4a
S2b S3b S4b
```

Ultrafiltration (UF) Method: Pipette two 500 µl serum samples from each blood sample into labeled ultra-filtration units (Centrifree, Amicon #4104 Millipore Corporation, Billerica, MA). Label as follows:

```
U2a U3a U4a
U2b U3b U4b
```

Centrifuge UF units at 500 rpm for 30 min. Pipette 200 µl from each UF unit into tubes labeled as follows and dilute samples up to 1 ml and cap tubes:

```
F2a F3a F4a
F2b F3b F4b
```

Sample Counting: Perform the routine quality control on the well counter/spectrometer prior to counting. Count all samples in the well counter/spectrometer. Sample for 1 min each. Record 1 min background reading. Fill in the worksheet with results.

Analysis: Run the CH GFR program on the ICON computer to fit curve and calculated GFR in ml/min, ml/min/m^2 and ml/min/1.73m^2.

FIGURE 12.1. *Continued*

samples have had the protein components of plasma removed that may have bound some ^{99m}Tc-DTPA. The analysis is performed as described by Rodman and colleagues[2] by fitting the percentage dose per liter at each time point for the processed samples to a single exponential function of the form:

$$C(t) = C_0 e^{-\frac{\ln(2)t}{T}}$$

where C is the concentration expressed as percentage dose per liter (% dose/L) for the ultra-filtered samples, C_0 is the theoretical initial concentration, and T is the clearance half-time for the slow compartment. Results are presented only for the ultrafiltered samples as gross clearance in milliliters per minute and milliliters per minute normalized to square meters of body surface area (BSA) and the commonly used units of milliliters per minute normalized to 1.73 times BSA. Body surface area is calculated from the patient's height and weight using the formula of DuBois and DuBois[3]:

$$BSA(m^2) = 0.007184 \times Height\ (cm)^{0.725}$$
$$\times Weight\ (kg)^{0.425}$$

Other parameters reported in Figure 12.2A include the clearance half-time in minutes, initial concentration C_0, and volume of distribution VD, which is the injected activity divided by the initial concentration C_0, in units of %

dose/L. The half-time, VD, and the graph can serve as checks on the quality of the data that were used in the GFR calculation and can aid in the interpretation of the results. The abbreviated report is shown in Figure 12.2B, along with the most meaningful of the results.

Normal values for GFR in children have been given in various places over the years. However, normal values for ^{99m}Tc-DTPA have not been widely published for children. Table 12.1 gives the values reported by Chantler and Barratt[4] for normal GFR for different age groups. Note the wide range for normals. Often it is the reproducibility of the measurement and not the absolute value that is most important, as changes in GFR can be more important in monitoring the status of kidney function.

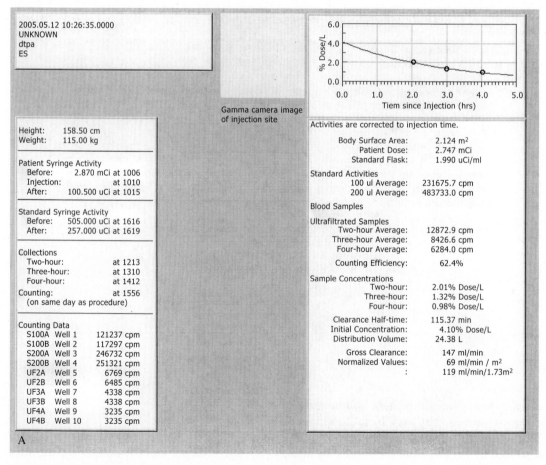

FIGURE 12.2. A: Comprehensive results page summarizing the raw and intermediate data as well as the results of the calculation of GFR. Presenting the raw data and intermediate data aids in the interpretation of the reliability of the final GFR calculation. B: Final results page for the GFR calculation. This page contains only the most relevant results of the GFR calculation.

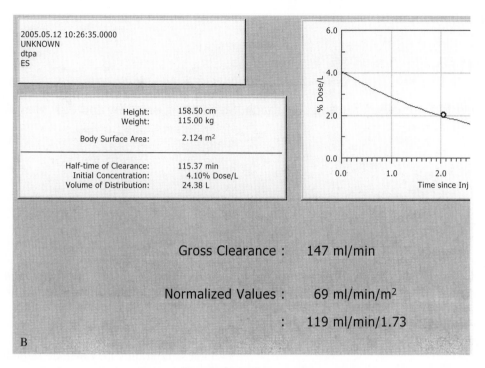

FIGURE 12.2. *Continued*

TABLE 12.1. Normal glomerular filtration rate (GFR) for different ages

Age	GFR (mL/min/1.73 m²)	
	Mean	Range (±2 SD)
Premature	47	29–65
2–8 days	38	26–60
4–28 days	48	28–68
35–95 days	58	30–86
1–5.9 mo	77	41–103
6–11.9 mo	103	49–157
12–19 mo	127	63–191
2–12 years	127	89–165
Adult males	131	88–174
Adult females	117	87–147

References

1. Chantler C, Barratt TM. Laboratory evaluation. In: Holliday MA, Vernier RL, Barratt TM, et al., eds. Pediatric Nephrology, 2nd ed. Baltimore: Williams & Wilkins, 1987:282–98.

2. Rodman JH, Maneval DC, Magill HL, et al. Measurement of Tc-99m DTPA serum clearance for estimating glomerular filtration rate in children with cancer. Pharmacotherapy 1993; 13(1):10–6.

3. DuBois D, DuBois EF. A formula to estimate the approximate surface area if height and weight be known. Arch Intern Med 1916;17:863–71.

4. Chantler C, Barratt TM. Laboratory evaluation. In: Holliday MA, Vernier RL, Barratt TM, et al., eds. Pediatric Nephrology, 2nd ed. Baltimore: Williams & Wilkins, 1987:288.

13
Bone

Leonard P. Connolly, Laura A. Drubach, Susan A. Connolly, and S.T. Treves

Skeletal scintigraphy is a highly sensitive technique for diagnosis of bone disorders. This chapter reviews the performance and interpretation of skeletal scintigraphy in children and concentrates on pathologic conditions that occur predominantly or exclusively in children.

General Considerations

Radiopharmaceuticals

Technetium-99m (^{99m}Tc)-labeled diphosphonates are the most widely used radiopharmaceuticals for skeletal scintigraphy. Diphosphonates are analogues of pyrophosphate, a normal constituent of bone. The ^{99m}Tc-labeled diphosphonates concentrate in amorphous calcium phosphate and crystalline hydroxyapatite. The distribution of these tracers reflects blood flow and bone formation. Tracer that does not localize to bone is cleared by the kidneys.

We use 0.2 mCi (7.4 MBq)/kg of ^{99m}Tc–methylene diphosphonate for skeletal scintigraphy. The minimum dose administered is 1.0 mCi (37 MBq) when only static images are obtained and 2.0 mCi (74 MBq) for three-phase imaging. The maximum administered dose is 20 mCi (740 MBq).

Fluorine-18 is an alternative radiopharmaceutical that distributes according to regional blood flow and osteoblastic activity. Positron emission tomography using ^{18}F offers the advantage of higher spatial resolution than standard skeletal scintigraphy. An administered dose of 0.06 mCi (2.2 MBq)/kg to a maximum of 4 mCi (148 MBq) has been used in children.[1]

Imaging Techniques

Skeletal scintigraphy may include radionuclide angiography, tissue phase imaging, and skeletal phase imaging (Fig. 13.1). The need to include all three phases depends on the clinical question and the patient's condition. Three-phase imaging is particularly helpful for assessing children with suspected musculoskeletal infection. A four-phase study, which is rarely needed in children, includes an additional set of skeletal phase images between 6 and 24 hours following tracer administration.

For radionuclide angiography, a gamma camera equipped with a high sensitivity collimator is used. Recording begins immediately after bolus administration. We record images at one frame per second for 60 seconds on a 128×128 matrix. Tracer distribution reflects regional blood flow during this phase.

Immediately following the radionuclide angiogram, a tissue phase image is obtained for 300,000 to 500,000 counts on a 256×256 matrix. Tissue phase images can be obtained in various projections or of different areas but generally should be completed within 5 minutes of administration.[3] Tissue phase images depict tracer in the blood pool, soft tissue, and sites of highly active bone formation, such as the physes.

We perform skeletal phase imaging 2 to 4 hours after radiopharmaceutical administra-

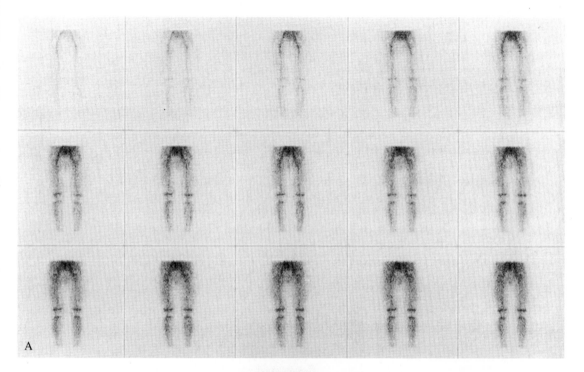

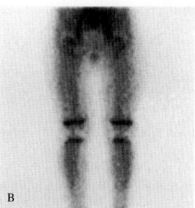

FIGURE 13.1. Three-phase skeletal scintigraphy. A: Radionuclide angiography (anterior projection) shows symmetric blood flow to the hips and knees. B: Tissue phase imaging shows tracer within the soft tissues and bone. C: Skeletal phase imaging reveals normal symmetric tracer distribution. Note that the patellae and naviculars are not visualized because they have not begun ossification in this 2-year-old girl. D: Pinhole magnification images confirm the symmetric uptake at the hips and knees. Note the clarity with which the capital femoral epiphyses are depicted and the absence of uptake in the unossified ischiopubic synchondroses, trochanters, and patellae. (*Source:* Connolly and Treves,[2] with permission.)

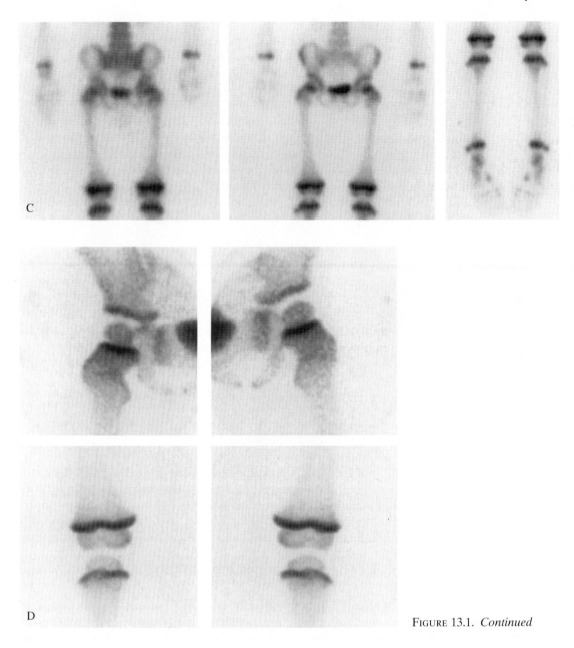

FIGURE 13.1. *Continued*

tion. By this time, tracer has localized to the skeleton and almost completely cleared from the soft tissues. Skeletal phase imaging is obtained in either a multiple-spot (Fig. 13.2) or whole-body (Fig. 13.3) format and may include magnification or tomographic imaging. The format is chosen considering a patient's condition, available instrumentation, and the preference of the interpreting physician. Multiple-spot technique provides images with slightly better resolution than does the whole-body method. The whole-body technique is faster to complete than multiple-spot scintigraphy, especially when a dual-detector system is used to simultaneously obtain anterior and posterior images. Imaging in the whole-body format requires the patient to remain still for a longer continuous time period than does imaging with individual spot images. A high-resolution collimator is used.

FIGURE 13.2. Multiple-spot technique. Note the intense uptake at growth centers. Images of the thorax, abdomen, pelvis, and hips were obtained in anterior and posterior projections. A: The skull was imaged in both lateral projections as well as in the anterior and posterior projections. B: The upper extremities were imaged in a posterior projection and the lower extremities in an anterior projection. (*Source:* Connolly and Treves,[2] with permission.)

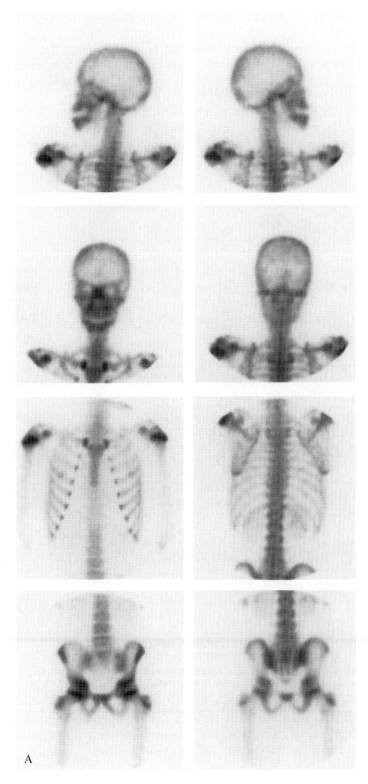

A

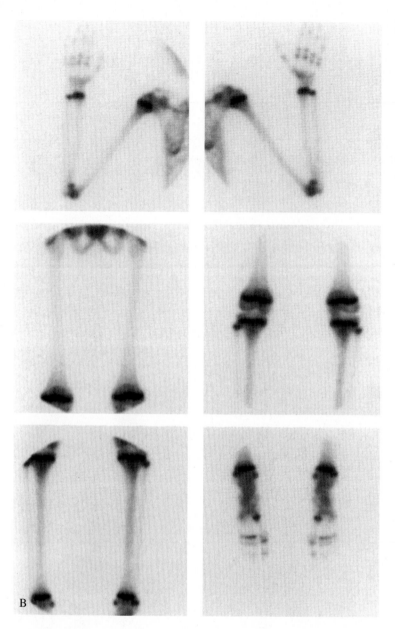

FIGURE 13.2. *Continued*

Magnification scintigraphy is most useful for assessing small structures such as the femoral capital epiphysis (Fig. 13.1) and the small bones of the hands and feet. It can also help assess bone along growth centers when high-resolution collimation is not sufficient. Spatial resolution of the gamma camera system is optimized with a small-aperture (2 to 3 mm) pinhole collimator. Other methods of magnification, including the use of a converging collimator and electronic magnifi-

cation (zoom), are less satisfactory. To take advantage of its high resolution and magnification capabilities, a pinhole collimator is brought as close as possible to the structure of interest, which is centered in the field of view. Count densities of 100,000 to 150,000 should be obtained.[2,4]

Single photon emission computed tomography (SPECT) provides better three-dimensional lesion localization and greater contrast than does planar imaging. Skeletal

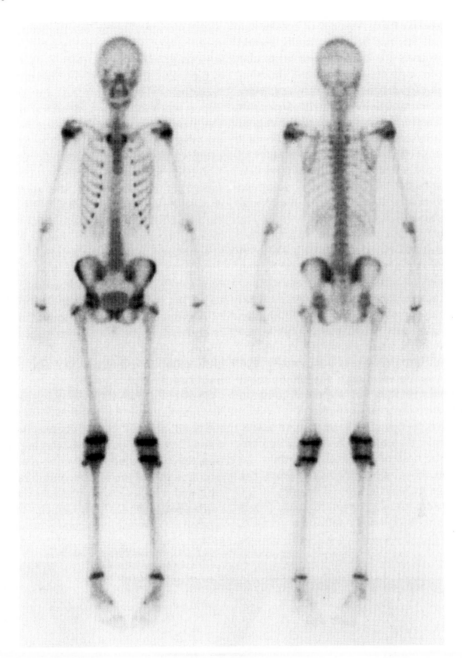

FIGURE 13.3. Whole-body skeletal scintigraphy. These anterior (left) and posterior (right) images of a 13-year-old girl were obtained with a moving detector system. (*Source:* Connolly and Treves,[2] with permission.)

SPECT is particularly useful in the diagnosis of focal abnormalities of the spine.

Potential Pitfalls for Interpretation

Interpretation of pediatric skeletal scintigraphy requires familiarity with differences between the appearance of pediatric and adult skeletal scintigrams as well as age- and gender-related variations within the children. Some patterns are worth noting due to their frequency or potential to be mistaken for pathology.

In order to be demonstrated with skeletal scintigraphy, structures must be ossified or undergoing ossification. Absence of uptake in a structure that has not begun to ossify should not be mistaken for evidence of avascular necrosis. From a practical standpoint, this consideration is of greatest importance regarding the capital femoral epiphysis, patella, and tarsal navicular (Fig. 13.1). Ossification of the capital femoral epiphysis occurs between the ages of 2 and 7 months. The patella ossifies between 18 months and 6 years of age. The tarsal navicular is the last tarsal bone to ossify, doing so between the ages of 1 and $3\frac{1}{2}$ years in girls and 3 and $5\frac{1}{2}$ years in boys.

A striking difference in the scintigraphic appearance of the immature pediatric skeleton compared to the mature adult skeleton is high uptake at the physeal growth centers of long bones and apophyseal growth centers of flat and irregular bones (Figs. 13.2 and 13.3). This high uptake reflects a rich blood supply and active enchondral ossification.[5,6] The appearance of ossification centers is occasionally misinterpreted as representing a pathologic state. A brief review of some of the more common sources of such error is warranted.

The skull is particularly challenging to assess. Physiologically high uptake is variably demonstrated at the base of the skull, the orbits, the nasal region, the temporomandibular joints, the mastoid regions, and the cranial sutures.

The sternum usually develops from single manubrial and xiphoid ossification centers and three separate mesosternal centers.[7] These centers may be depicted scintigraphically as regions of high uptake (Fig. 13.4). Commonly, two or three linear bands of high uptake corresponding to synchondroses are shown. The upper synchondrosis is identified in adults as the manubriosternal joint. Other patterns that are observed in children include paired ossification centers, which create an appearance that has been termed a "double sternum," and failure of ossification of the sternal bodies exclusive of the manubrium.[8] The latter two variants are somewhat more common in children with congenital heart disease but are also encountered in healthy children.[9]

High uptake at the ossification centers adjacent to the costochondral junctions and at the apophysis of the inferior scapular tip (Fig. 13.5) often projects over the posterior and posterolateral aspects of the ribs on posterior scintigrams. Oblique projections and images with the arms raised and lowered can help exclude rib pathology.

The ischiopubic synchondrosis, a cartilaginous junction between the inferior pubic ramus and the ischium, usually ossifies between the ages of 4 and 12 years. Prior to the beginning of ossification, the ischiopubic synchondrosis appears as a discontinuity of the inferior pubic ramus (Figs. 13.1 and 13.6). Uptake becomes high during ossification (Figs. 13.7 to 13.9). This high uptake is often asymmetric, particularly around the age

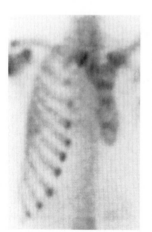
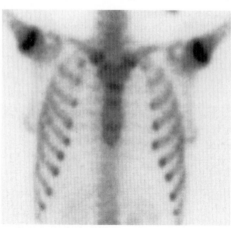
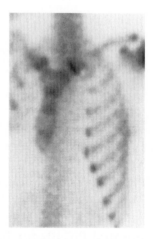

FIGURE 13.4. Sternal ossification centers. Three bands of high uptake corresponding to sternal growth centers are identified in an 18-year-old man. (*Source:* Connolly and Treves,[2] with permission.)

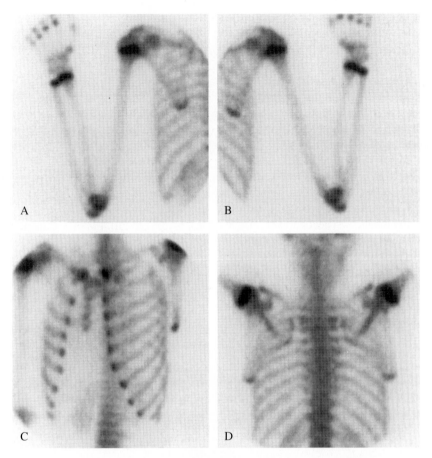

FIGURE 13.5. Scapular apophyses. Uptake is higher at the apophyses of the inferior scapular tips than in adjacent bone. These apophyses overlie ribs on the posterior projections (A,B). Oblique imaging (C) and posterior imaging with the arms raised (D) depict the apophyses separate from the ribs. (*Source:* Connolly and Treves,[2] with permission.)

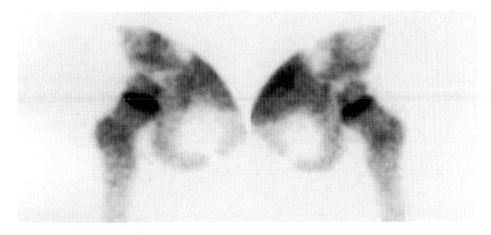

FIGURE 13.6. Ischiopubic synchondroses. Pinhole imaging shows no uptake at the right and left synchondroses of a 5-year-old girl. (*Source:* Connolly and Treves,[2] with permission.)

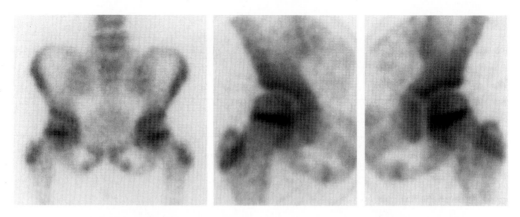

FIGURE 13.7. Ischiopubic synchondroses. High-resolution planar and pinhole images show symmetrically high uptake at the ischiopubic synchondroses of a 9-year-old girl. (*Source:* Connolly and Treves,[2] with permission.)

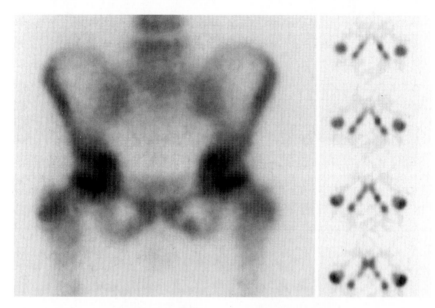

FIGURE 13.8. Ischiopubic synchondroses. High-resolution planar scintigraphy images (left image) and axial single photon emission computed tomography (SPECT) show asymmetric higher uptake at the left ischiopubic synchondrosis of an 8-year-old girl. (*Source:* Connolly and Treves,[2] with permission.)

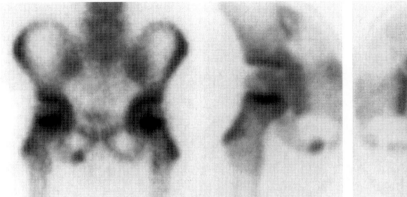
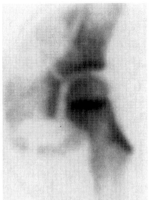

FIGURE 13.9. Ischiopubic synchondroses. There is intense uptake at the right and no uptake at the left ischiopubic synchondrosis. Note that the greater trochanters have not begun ossification. (*Source:* Connolly and Treves,[2] with permission.)

of 8 years (Figs. 13.8 and 13.9). An asymmetric anatomic appearance to the ischiopubic synchondroses is also common radiographically.[10] Some imaging specialists experience difficulty in confidently excluding osteomyelitis when symptoms are referable to the ischiopubic region. With awareness of the normal pattern of uptake, this should rarely pose a significant problem, however. High uptake in adjacent bone and poor definition of the synchondrosis's margins are signs of pathology.[11,12]

The tibial tubercle, which originates as an inferior extension of the proximal tibial chondroepiphysis, develops a secondary ossification center by 7 to 9 years of age. The epiphyseal tubercle center fuses with the main proximal tibial center at approximately 15 years of age. Closure of the tubercle physis occurs between the ages of 13 and 15 years in females and 15 and 19 years in males. From the time the secondary ossification center develops until its complete closure, high uptake is present (Fig. 13.10).

In the feet, high uptake is very commonly seen from early in life through the teenage years at a growth center at the first metatarsal base (Fig. 13.11) and the apophysis along the posterior calcaneal border (Fig. 13.12).

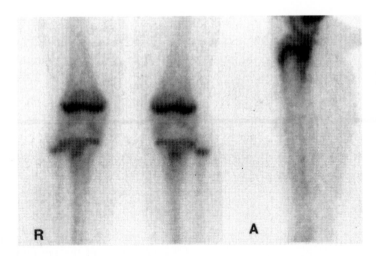

FIGURE 13.10. Tibial tubercle. Prominent uptake is frequently identified at the tibial tubercles (R, right; A, anterior). (*Source:* Connolly and Treves,[2] with permission.)

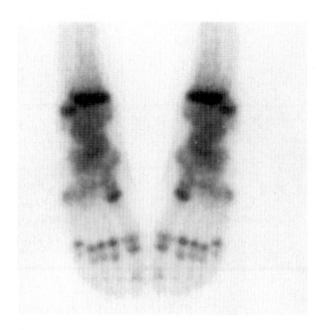

FIGURE 13.11. Metatarsal growth centers. High uptake is shown at metatarsal and phalangeal growth centers. (*Source:* Connolly and Treves,[2] with permission.)

Clinical Applications

Infection, Inflammation, and Avascular Necrosis

Acute Osteomyelitis

Acute osteomyelitis is a common pediatric problem that occurs at any age. Acute osteomyelitis of the immature skeleton is usually the result of hematogenous spread of bacteria. Nearly one third of patients have a history of upper respiratory infection, otitis media, or other infection that may be the source of bacteremia.[13] A history of recent trauma to the affected bone is elicited in one third of cases, suggesting that traumatized bone is at increased risk of osteomyelitis.[14] Direct puncture wounds and spread of infection from

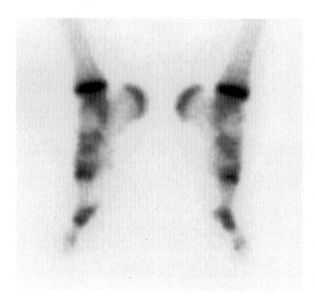

FIGURE 13.12. Calcaneal apophysis. High uptake along the posterior calcaneus corresponds to the calcaneal apophysis. (*Source:* Connolly and Treves,[2] with permission.)

contiguous structures such as the skin or paranasal sinuses account for a small percentage of cases. *Staphylococcus aureus* is the infective organism in approximately three fourths of cases.[15,16] One third of neonatal cases are caused by group B β-hemolytic streptococcus.[17] Less common causative organisms include salmonella species, mycobacterium, fungi, and viral agents. *Pseudomonas aeruginosa* is associated with acute osteomyelitis secondary to penetrating foot wounds.

The long bones are involved in approximately three fourths of cases. Acute osteomyelitis of the long bones predominantly affects the metaphysis (Figs. 13.13 to 13.15). Blood-borne organisms become lodged in the metaphyses due to high vascularity but slow flow in looping sinusoidal vessels. The most rapidly growing and largest metaphyses are affected most often. In decreasing order of frequency, the distal femur, proximal femur, proximal tibia, distal tibia, proximal humerus, distal humerus, fibula, and other long bones are involved.[18] The epiphysis is commonly involved in infants and children less than 18 months of age because transphyseal vessels allow infection to spread. After these vessels are obliterated, the physis serves as a natural barrier to spread of infection. Occasionally the epiphysis is involved primarily or as a result of septic arthritis in children of all ages (Fig. 13.16). Primary diaphyseal involvement with acute hematogenous osteomyelitis is unusual, but loose attachment of the periosteum to the cortex permits subperiosteal spread of metaphyseal infection into and along the diaphysis.

The flat and irregular bones are involved in approximately 25% of cases (Figs. 13.17 to 13.19). Acute osteomyelitis of the flat and irregular bones characteristically develops in bone adjacent to cartilage. These regions, termed metaphyseal equivalents, have a similar vascular anatomy to that of the long bone metaphyses. The most common sites of involvement, in decreasing order of frequency, are the ilium, vertebrae, calcaneus, ischium, scapula, talus, pubis, patella, tarsal navicular, and sternum.[18]

Early diagnosis of acute osteomyelitis helps lessen the risk of complications such as sepsis, chronic infection, and growth arrest. Unfortunately, diagnosis can be quite difficult clinically. Limping or refusal to bear weight is often the only symptom. Pain, when present, is often poorly localized or referred. Swelling and tenderness are often absent. Fever may accompany other signs, may be the only sign, or may be absent. Hematologic analysis may be within normal parameters. The erythrocyte sedimentation rate (ESR) is elevated in 90% of cases but is a very nonspecific indicator.[19] Only about one third of affected children have leukocytosis and less than one half have positive blood cultures. A diagnosis of acute osteomyelitis is established most accurately by a positive culture from a bony aspirate, but such aspirations are culture-positive in only about 70% of cases.[13] The diagnosis is often based on imaging findings.

The imaging evaluation of children with suspected acute osteomyelitis usually begins with radiographs. Acute osteomyelitis is rarely diagnosed with radiographs in the early stages. Deep soft tissue swelling, obliteration of soft tissue planes, and subcutaneous edema can be evident within 48 hours of infection but are neither consistently observed nor specific. Osseous manifestations of focal or confluent radiolucencies and periosteal new bone are not visualized until 7 to 10 days after the onset of infection because radiographs are insensitive to loss of less than 30% of bone matrix.[14,16] Further imaging is generally required to assist in evaluating cases of suspected acute osteomyelitis. The modalities most frequently employed for this purpose are skeletal scintigraphy and magnetic resonance imaging (MRI).

Skeletal scintigraphy is highly reliable in the early diagnosis of acute osteomyelitis. The sensitivity of three-phase skeletal scintigraphy has been estimated as 94% and the specificity as 95%.[20] It is worth noting that diagnostic aspiration and antibiotic therapy do not need to be delayed until scintigraphy is completed because fine-needle aspiration does not alter the scintigraphic findings[21-23] and antibiotic therapy does not lead to rapid normalization of scintigraphy. Early reports of poor results in the diagnosis of neonatal osteomyelitis[24-27] have been contradicted by a later study that

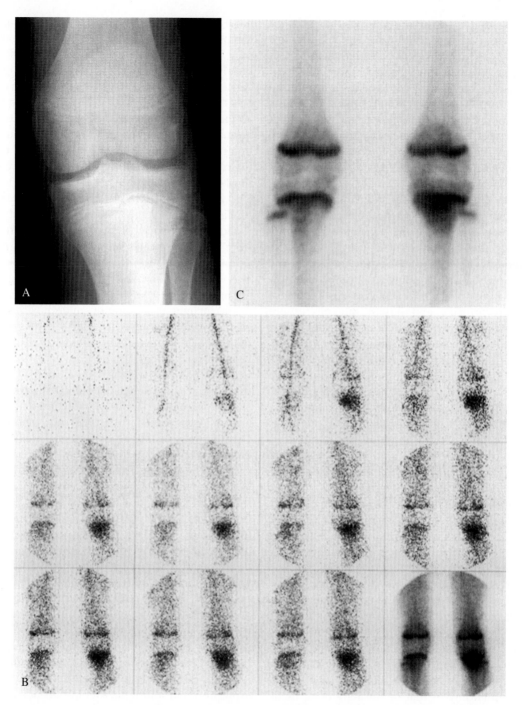

FIGURE 13.13. Acute osteomyelitis. The left knee appears normal radiographically (A). Anterior angiographic (B), tissue (B, lower right panel), and skeletal phase (C) images show high localization and uptake in the left proximal tibial metaphysis. (*Source:* Connolly and Treves,[2] with permission.)

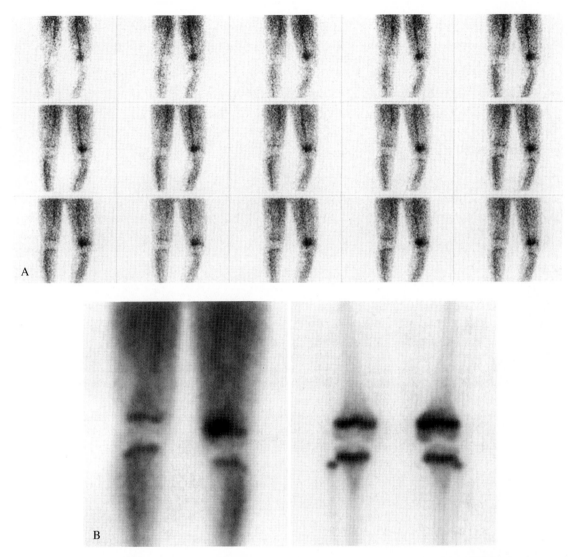

FIGURE 13.14. Acute osteomyelitis. A: Radionuclide angiography (anterior projection) demonstrates asymmetrically high tracer delivery to the left distal femoral metaphysis. B: Tissue and skeletal phase imaging (left and right panels respectively) show high localization and uptake in the medial aspect of the left distal femoral metaphysis. (*Source:* Connolly and Treves,[2] with permission.)

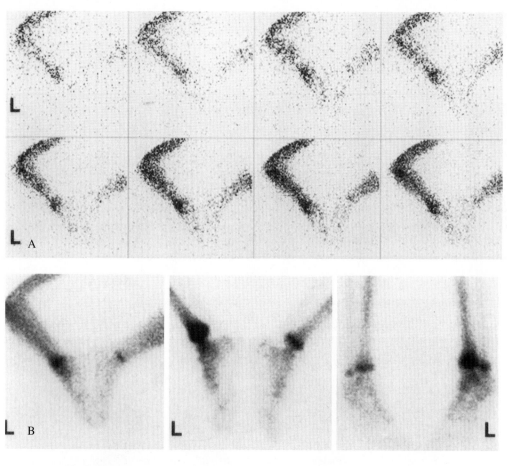

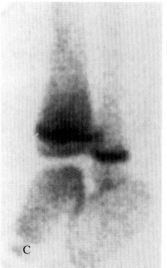

FIGURE 13.15. Acute osteomyelitis. A: Radionuclide angiography reveals asymmetrically high tracer delivery to the left ankle and lower leg (L, left). B: Tissue phase imaging (left panel) shows high localization diffusely in the left lower leg with focal prominence at the ankle. Skeletal phase images (middle and right panels) demonstrate focally intense uptake in the distal left tibial metaphysis. C: The abnormality is quite evident by pinhole imaging. (*Source:* Connolly and Treves,[2] with permission.)

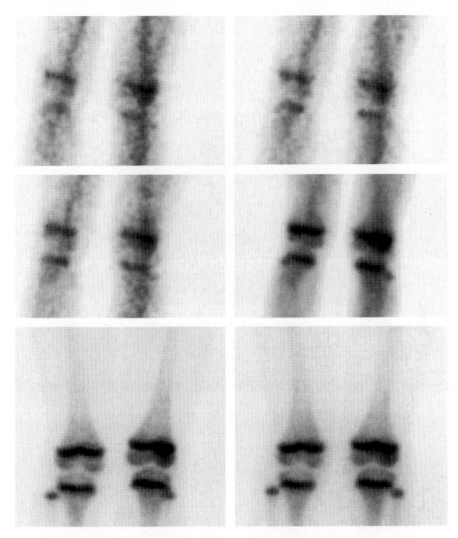

FIGURE 13.16. Epiphyseal osteomyelitis. Angiographic and tissue phase imaging (anterior projection) show high localization at the distal left femoral epiphysis laterally. Skeletal phase imaging in the anterior (lower left panel) and posterior (lower right panel) projections show focally high uptake at that site. (*Source:* Connolly and Treves,[2] with permission.)

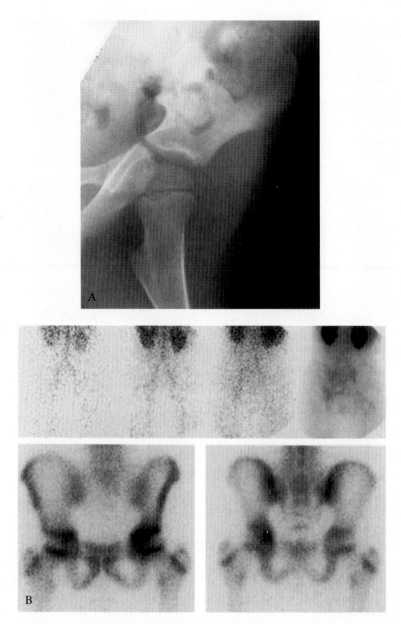

FIGURE 13.17. Acute osteomyelitis. A: A radiograph of an 11-year-old with left hip pain reveals no osseous abnormality. B: Only slight asymmetrically high localization is evident at the left hip on three selected posterior images from radionuclide angiography (upper row left). Tissue phase (upper right, posterior projection) and skeletal phase images (lower left, anterior projection; lower right, posterior projection) show high localization and uptake in the left acetabulum. C: The uptake abnormality is confirmed with coronal (upper row) and axial (lower row) SPECT. (*Source:* Connolly and Treves,[2] with permission.)

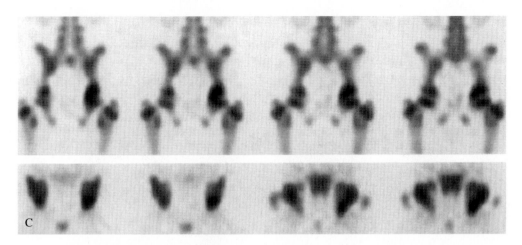

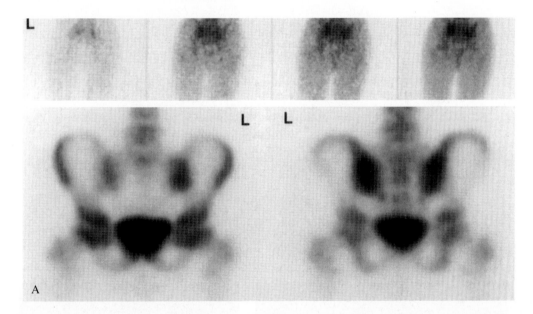

FIGURE 13.17. *Continued*

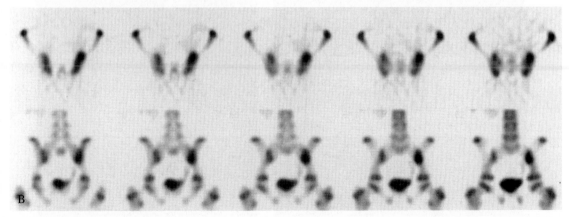

FIGURE 13.18. Acute osteomyelitis. Posterior angiographic and tissue phase images (A, upper row) reveal high localization in the region of the left sacroiliac joint. Skeletal phase images (A, lower row) and SPECT (B) show high uptake in the left ilium. (*Source:* Connolly and Treves,[2] with permission.)

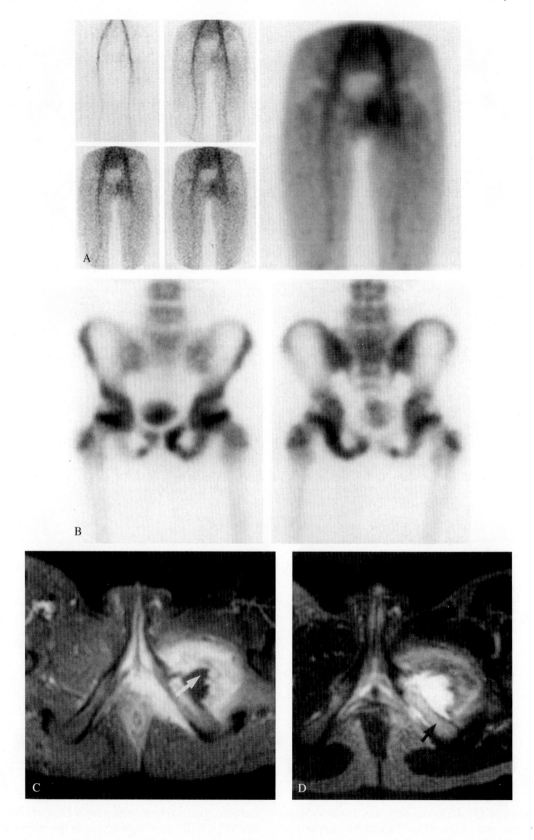

◀

FIGURE 13.19. Acute osteomyelitis. A: Selected anterior images from a radionuclide angiogram (left and middle panels) and a tissue phase image (right panel) show high localization in the left inguinal region. B: Anterior (left) and posterior skeletal phase images show high uptake in the left ischium and pubis. C,D: Magnetic resonance imaging (MRI) shows an abscess centered about the left ischiopubic synchondrosis. The postgadolinium image (C) shows moderate to marked enhancement and an area of central liquefaction (arrow). The left ischium has increased T2 signal (D, arrow). (*Source:* Connolly and Treves,[2] with permission.)

indicated skeletal scintigraphy was a reliable tool for detecting sites of acute osteomyelitis during the first 6 weeks of life.[28] Nevertheless, it is prudent to be particularly cautious in excluding acute osteomyelitis in neonates on the basis of skeletal scintigraphy.

With the ^{99m}Tc-labeled diphosphonates, three-phase scintigraphy centered over the region of highest clinical suspicion should be performed. Skeletal phase images should include a survey of the whole body because osteomyelitis, particularly in neonates[17,24–26,28] but also in older children,[19,29] can present with referred pain or be multifocal and because conditions such as Ewing sarcoma, leukemia, and neuroblastoma[30] may clinically mimic acute osteomyelitis. Pinhole imaging is useful in some cases (Fig. 13.15). When pelvic osteomyelitis is suspected, SPECT may be helpful (Figs. 13.17 and 13.18).

Skeletal scintigraphy is usually positive by 24 to 72 hours after symptom onset. Typically, high localization is shown on angiographic and tissue phase images, and high uptake is shown on the skeletal phase images. Focally low localization and uptake, with or without adjacent high localization and uptake, have been observed in acute osteomyelitis of long and flat bones (Fig. 13.20).[26,28,31,32] This pattern, often referred to as "cold" osteomyelitis, most likely reflects regional ischemia in the early thrombotic phase or regional vascular tamponade later in the course of the disease. Causes of tamponade include intraosseous pressure from inflammation, edema, or abscess, subperiosteal extension of infection or fluid, and joint effusion. The prognosis may be poorer in those with "cold osteomyelitis."[33] The incidence of "cold osteomyelitis" is higher in the neonate than in older children.[26,28]

The emergence of MRI has raised questions regarding how suspected acute osteomyelitis is best approached from an imaging standpoint. Changes in signal intensity resulting from increased fluid in the bone marrow allow the detection of acute osteomyelitis by MRI within 24 to 48 hours following symptom onset. Marrow edema appears as low signal intensity on T1-weighted and high signal intensity on T2-weighted MRI. Abnormal perfusion, indicative of ischemia, necrosis, or intraosseous abscess, can be demonstrated with gadolinium-enhanced MRI.[14] Magnetic resonance imaging is also useful in identifying extension of infection into the physis, in which case MRI assists with surgical treatment aimed at decreasing the risk of growth arrest.

The sensitivity of MRI relative to that of scintigraphy has not been established.[34] Experience at our institution suggests that it is reasonable to consider skeletal scintigraphy and MRI as equally sensitive for the early diagnosis of acute osteomyelitis.[35] The main advantages of scintigraphy are that whole-body

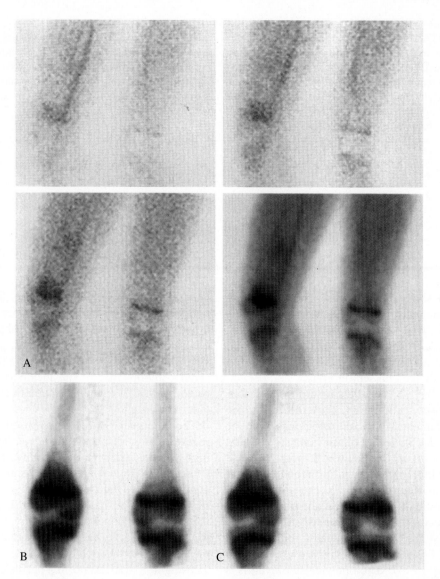

FIGURE 13.20. Acute osteomyelitis: cold osteo-myelitis. Selected anterior images from the radionu-clide angiogram and the tissue phase image of a 13-year-old boy show high localization in the distal right femoral metaphysis and less prominently in the midthigh or femur (A). Skeletal phase images in the anterior (B) and posterior (C) projections show high right femoral metaphyseal uptake, with a region of low uptake in the adjacent diaphysis. A large amount of subperiosteal pus was drained surgically. (*Source:* Connolly and Treves,[2] with permission.)

imaging is relatively easy and that sedation is rarely needed even in children under 6 years of age. The main advantage of MRI is its ability to show intraosseous, subperiosteal, and soft tissue abscesses.[36] This consideration is most important with pelvic osteomyelitis, which is accompanied by soft-tissue abscesses that require drainage in about 20% of cases (Fig. 13.19),[35] and with vertebral infection.

Subacute and Chronic Osteomyelitis

Subacute osteomyelitis may result from unsuccessful or no treatment of acute osteomyelitis.[33,37] The long bones are predominantly affected. Subacute osteomyelitis may persist for months or years and then is considered chronic.[38] Hematologic analysis is even less revealing than in acute osteomyelitis. The ESR is usually elevated but to a lesser degree than with acute osteomyelitis. The white blood cell count is usually normal, and blood cultures typically do not yield growth of organisms. *Staphylococcus aureus* is often cultured from the involved bone.[39]

Subacute or chronic osteomyelitis is usually identified radiographically. The lesions are most commonly metaphyseal but may extend into or primarily involve the epiphysis or diaphysis. The most common radiographic manifestation is a well-defined radiolucency that corresponds to a localized (Brodie) abscess, often surrounded by a sclerotic rim. The other common radiographic manifestation is irregular cortical resorption accompanied by periosteal reaction. The former appearance may be difficult to distinguish from that of osteoid osteoma, and the latter may be difficult to distinguish from that of Ewing sarcoma.[14,40,41] Skeletal scintigraphy typically shows high uptake at sites of subacute or chronic osteomyelitis.

Chronic Recurrent Multifocal Osteomyelitis

Chronic recurrent multifocal osteomyelitis (CRMO) is a rare and poorly understood disease. It occurs most frequently between the ages of 7 and 14 years. Females are affected approximately twice as often as males. Chronic recurrent multifocal osteomyelitis is insidious in onset. Localized pain and soft tissue swelling are the usual presenting complaints. Chronic recurrent multifocal osteomyelitis follows an unpredictable and episodic but self-limited course over a period of months to years until spontaneous resolution occurs. Bone aspirates or biopsy specimens reveal chronic inflammatory changes. Organisms do not grow from culture and antibiotics do not alter the clinical course.[42,43]

Radiographically, lytic destruction is usually the first manifestation (Figs. 13.21 and 13.22). Sclerosis becomes apparent later. The most common sites of involvement are the long bone metaphyses. Other sites include the spine, pelvis, and clavicles. Distribution is typically asymmetric.[42] The appearance and presentation often suggests a skeletal malignancy. Biopsy is frequently required for this differentiation. Skeletal scintigraphy may be abnormal, typically showing high uptake, before radiographic manifestations develop and is particularly useful in demonstrating multifocality.[44]

Vertebral Infection

Diskitis, vertebral osteomyelitis, and epidural abscess constitute a spectrum of inflammatory disorders of the pediatric spine.

Diskitis is an inflammation of the intervertebral disk space that is probably due to a low-grade bacterial or viral infection. Organisms reach the intervertebral disk through vessels that originate in the marrow space of a contiguous vertebra, traverse the vertebral end plate, and enter the nucleus pulposus and annulus fibrosus. This vascular network is prominent through the age of 8 years but may persist through 30 years of age.[45–47]

Diskitis most commonly affects children between the ages of 6 months and 4 years and involves the lumbar spine, particularly L1-2, L2-3, and L3-4. A second, lower epidemiologic peak occurs between 10 and 14 years of age. The thoracic spine is more commonly involved in these older children.

The clinical presentation of children with diskitis is notoriously nonspecific. Fever is usually absent or low grade. Younger children

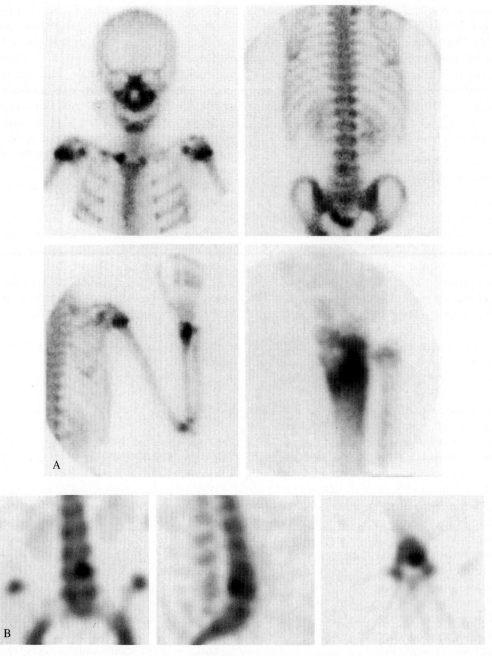

FIGURE 13.21. Chronic recurrent multifocal osteomyelitis. A: High uptake is shown at sites of involvement in the right clavicle, L4, the sacrum, and the distal right radius. A region of lower uptake adjacent to the focal concentration in the radius is better demonstrated with the pinhole image (lower right) than the high-resolution planar image of the right radius. B: With SPECT, the L4 abnormality is shown to involve the posteromedial vertebral body. (*Source:* Connolly and Treves,[2] with permission.)

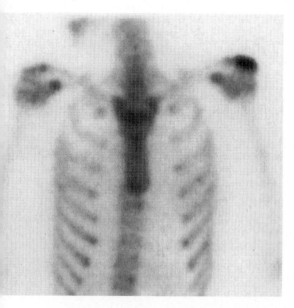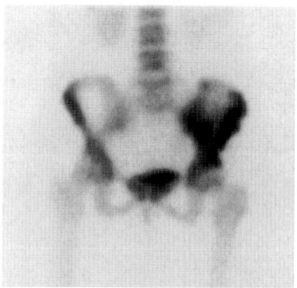

FIGURE 13.22. Chronic recurrent multifocal osteomyelitis. High uptake is present in the left acromion process and the left ilium. (*Source:* Connolly and Treves,[2] with permission.)

frequently present with reluctance or refusal to walk and bear weight. Back or abdominal pain may be present, especially in older children. Hematologic evaluation often reveals only an elevated ESR and mild leukocytosis. Blood and biopsy cultures are positive in one third to one half of all patients with diskitis. The cultured organism is usually *S. aureus.* A course of antibiotics is generally employed even when blood or biopsy cultures are negative for growth.[48]

Radiographs are often normal at the time of presentation. Disk space narrowing, with or without erosion of the adjacent endplates, usually becomes evident only after inflammation has been present for at least 2 weeks. Skeletal scintigraphy is expected to be abnormal in patients with symptoms for more than 7 days.[48,49] The typical scintigraphic appearance is high uptake involving the vertebral end plates and bodies on each side of the inflamed disk (Fig. 13.23). High uptake may reflect microtrauma due to loss of the cushioning effect of the disk and extrusion of disk material through the vertebral ring apophysis into the vertebral body and does not require infection of the vertebrae themselves.

Vertebral osteomyelitis differs from diskitis in that there is involvement and often eventual loss of height of a vertebral body. In children, vertebral osteomyelitis predominantly occurs before the age of 10 years. The clinical presentation is often identical to that described for diskitis, although systemic signs are more common. Skeletal scintigraphy typically reveals high uptake in a single vertebra (Fig. 13.24).[50,51] The scintigraphic appearance may resemble that of diskitis, however. Without loss of vertebral body height or direct bacterial culture from bone, it is often not possible to differentiate vertebral osteomyelitis from diskitis.

Single photon emission computed tomography increases the sensitivity of scintigraphy for the diagnosis of diskitis and vertebral osteomyelitis.[52] It is most useful when planar images are normal or equivocal.[51]

Paraspinal or epidural abscess can occur in association with diskitis or vertebral osteomyelitis but also can occur in their absence.[51] Significant neurologic deficits may result from epidural abscess, necessitating a prompt diagnosis to prevent permanent damage. Because neurologic symptoms may be absent or minimal, MRI is useful in excluding

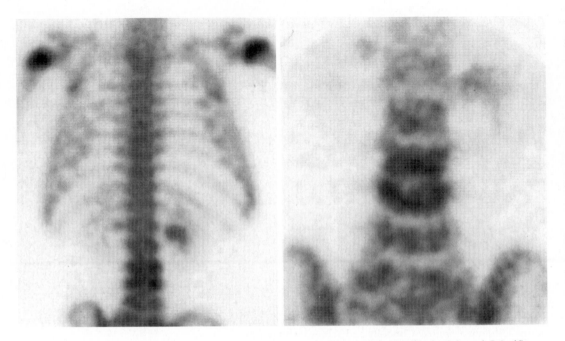

FIGURE 13.23. Diskitis. Posterior planar and pinhole images show high uptake in L3 and L4. (*Source:* Connolly and Treves,[2] with permission.)

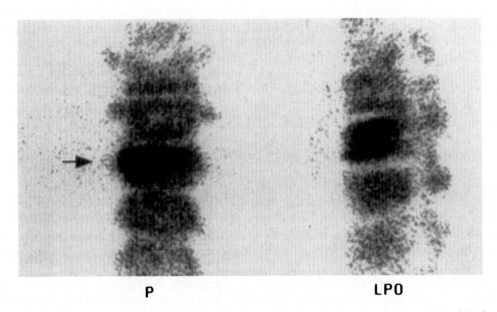

P   LPO

FIGURE 13.24. Vertebral osteomyelitis. Pinhole images show marked uptake in the L1 vertebral body.

an associated soft tissue or epidural abscess or, in cases of diskitis, in determining the effect of extruded disk material on the spinal canal.[53]

Septic Arthritis and Transient Synovitis

Septic arthritis and transient synovitis are the most frequently encountered joint-related conditions in children suspected of having acute osteomyelitis. These conditions usually affect the hip and knee.[54]

Septic arthritis typically occurs before 3 years of age. Organisms enter the joint by hematogenous seeding of the synovium, by spread from acute osteomyelitis of intraarticular bone, or by direct puncture wounds. Within a joint, pathogenic organisms find an environment consisting of transudative joint fluid and avascular cartilage that is hospitable for their proliferation. Defense mechanisms are overwhelmed with pathogenic bacteria, such as *S. aureus*. Lytic enzymes, including proteases, collagenases, and peptidases in purulent articular fluid destroy articular and epiphyseal cartilages.

Epiphyseal ischemia secondary to intracapsular pressure from an effusion may progress to infarction. Ischemia is a particular concern at the hip because perfusion of the capital femoral epiphysis is largely reliant on the lateral ascending cervical artery, which courses within the hip joint.[55] The vascular supply of the femoral capital epiphysis in young children warrants review in this context.[56] The proximal femur receives its blood supply via an extracapsular vascular ring formed by two primary branches of the deep femoral artery, the medial circumflex and lateral circumflex arteries, and the artery of the ligamentum teres. Ascending cervical vessels that arise from the vascular ring are the most important source of blood to the epiphysis. The posterior and lateral aspects of the ring are formed by the medial circumflex artery. The terminal branch of the medial circumflex artery, the lateral ascending cervical artery, provides the largest volume of blood to the epiphysis. This vessel enters the capsule posterolaterally and gives off a rete of branching arterioles that extend medially and anteriorly to supply the entire epiphysis. The anastomotic network of the anterior portion of the ring, which is formed by the lateral circumflex artery, is much less extensive than that of the posterior portion of the ring.

Transient synovitis (toxic synovitis, observation hip, irritable hip) is an idiopathic condition. Affected children are typically 5 to 10 years of age, but there is considerable overlap in the age distribution of children with this condition and septic arthritis. There is a slight male predominance. Transient synovitis is largely a diagnosis of exclusion.[57] Symptoms usually subside following a short period of rest.

As with osteomyelitis, the imaging evaluation of children with suspected septic arthritis and transient synovitis typically begins with radiographs. A joint effusion is manifested radiographically by obliteration of fat pads, joint space widening, or even partial subluxation. Radiographs may appear normal despite an effusion particularly at the hip.[58] Ultrasonography is invaluable for detection of hip effusion.[59] A hip effusion appears ultrasonographically as an anechoic or hypoechoic area separating the proximal femoral metaphysis from the joint capsule. Echogenic material within an effusion suggests septic arthritis,[60] but this finding is neither specific nor sensitive. Examination of aspirated joint fluid is needed to distinguish septic arthritis from transient synovitis or other effusion-causing conditions.

Once a diagnosis is established by joint aspiration, further imaging may not be needed. However, some children with undiagnosed septic arthritis or transient synovitis are referred for skeletal scintigraphy. Others require better exclusion of periarticular osseous pathology. Skeletal scintigraphy of joints affected by either condition may show high periarticular localization during the angiographic and tissue phases and high uptake in periarticular bone during the skeletal phase (Figs. 13.25 and 13.26). The study may be normal, particularly in transient synovitis.[33,61–63] A focal area of high uptake indicates osseous pathology, usually osteomyelitis associated with septic arthritis (Fig. 13.27).

Ischemia is manifested scintigraphically as low or absent uptake in the capital femoral

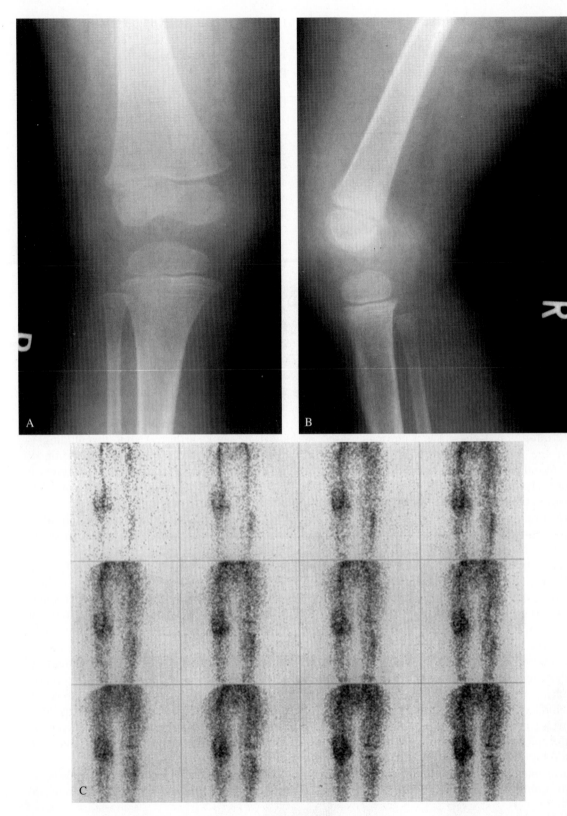

FIGURE 13.25.

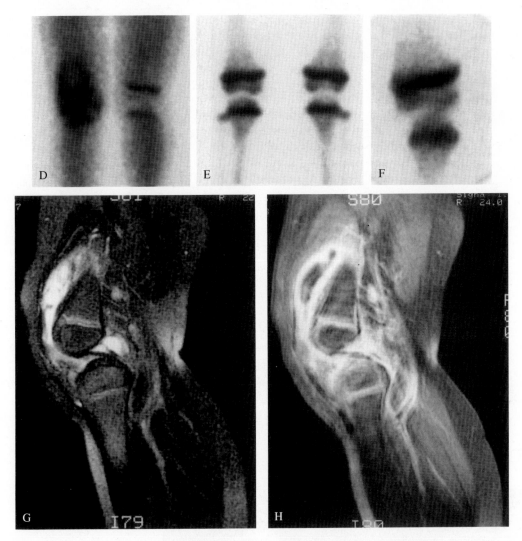

FIGURE 13.25. Transient synovitis. Anteroposterior (A) and lateral (B) radiographs of a 3-year-old girl with painful swelling of the right knee reveal a joint effusion but no osseous abnormality. Radionuclide angiography shows high tracer delivery to the right knee (C). High localization on the tissue phase image (D) outlines the suprapatellar bursa. Skeletal phase images (E: planar; F: pinhole, right knee) reveal mildly high uptake affecting the articulating surfaces of the distal femur and proximal tibia. Sagittal T2-weighted MRI of the right knee reveals a joint effusion (G). Enhancement of thickened synovium is seen on T1-weighted image following gadolinium (H). (*Source:* Connolly and Treves,[2] with permission.)

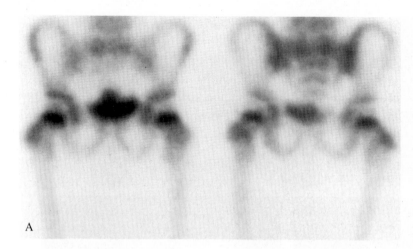

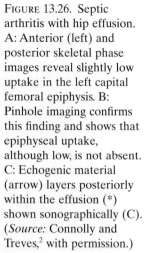

FIGURE 13.26. Septic arthritis with hip effusion. A: Anterior (left) and posterior skeletal phase images reveal slightly low uptake in the left capital femoral epiphysis. B: Pinhole imaging confirms this finding and shows that epiphyseal uptake, although low, is not absent. C: Echogenic material (arrow) layers posteriorly within the effusion (*) shown sonographically (C). (*Source:* Connolly and Treves,[2] with permission.)

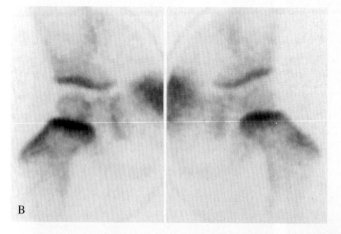

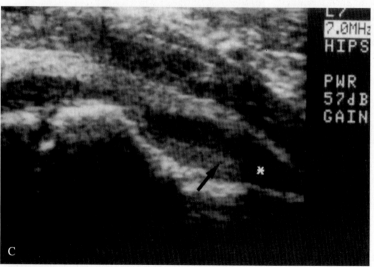

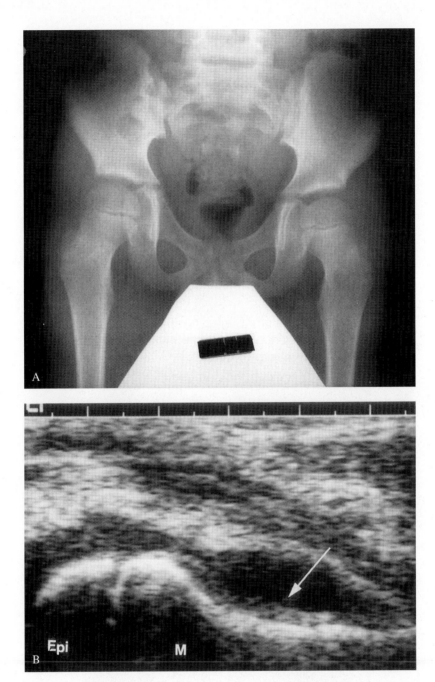

FIGURE 13.27. Acute osteomyelitis and septic arthritis. A: The bones of the left hip appear normal radiographically. Asymmetry to the acetabular "teardrop" distance suggests a left hip effusion. B: Ultrasonography reveals a moderate left hip effusion (arrow, epi: capital femoral epiphysis, m: metaphysis). C: Radionuclide angiography (anterior projection) indicates high perfusion to the left hip region. D: Diffusely high localization persists on tissue phase imaging (left panel). A skeletal phase image (right panel) shows high uptake in the left proximal femoral metaphysis. E: The abnormality is better depicted with pinhole magnification. (Source: Connolly and Treves,[2] with permission.)

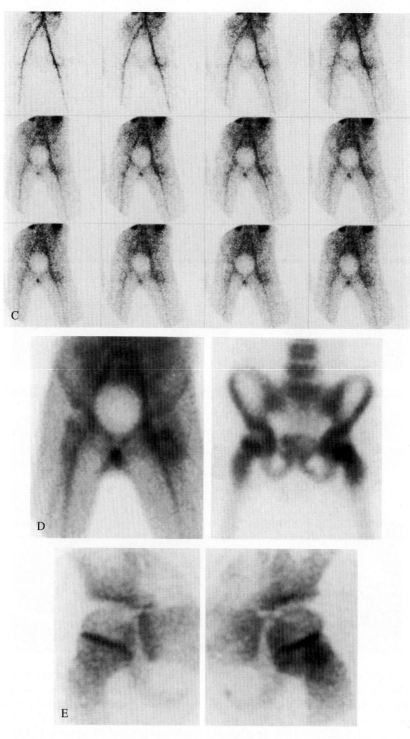

FIGURE 13.27. *Continued*

epiphysis and subcapital physis during the angiographic and tissue phases. Depending on the degree of vascular impairment, skeletal phase images may show similarly impaired uptake or may be normal.

The differential diagnosis of joint conditions is wide and includes Legg-Calvé-Perthes disease, juvenile rheumatoid arthritis, rheumatic fever, Kawasaki disease, and Lyme disease.

Legg-Calvé-Perthes Disease

Legg-Calvé-Perthes disease is idiopathic avascular necrosis (AVN) of the immature capital femoral epiphysis. Most patients are Caucasian boys between the ages of 5 and 8 years. Almost 90% of Legg-Calvé-Perthes disease is unilateral. Limping is the most common symptom. Hip, thigh, or knee pain may be present. Clinical presentation is typically insidious and the diagnosis is usually made with radiographs. The earliest finding is a subchondral lucency. Small size, sclerosis, and fragmentation of the affected epiphysis are shown later. Skeletal scintigraphy is most useful when radiographs are negative and symptoms are not well localized. Scintigraphic abnormalities predate radiographic manifestations by up to 6 weeks.[64] The sensitivity of skeletal scintigraphy exceeds 90%.[64-67] Absence of uptake in the capital femoral epiphysis is the earliest scintigraphic finding (Fig. 13.28). Pinhole magnification may be needed to show this abnormality. Uptake by the subcapital physis is often higher on the involved side.[33]

When the diagnosis is established by radiographs or scintigraphy, some advocate using sequential skeletal scintigraphy to depict the way in which uptake returns to the epiphysis. A column of uptake in the lateral epiphysis is believed to reflect recanalization of vessels (Fig. 13.29). This appearance is considered to have a more favorable prognosis than when uptake returns across the base of the epiphysis, which is believed to result from development of new vessels.[68,69]

It is reasonable to consider MRI as being as sensitive as skeletal scintigraphy for Legg-Calvé-Perthes disease. There is evidence favoring each modality, and either can be falsely negative.[70] Signal changes indicating marrow edema are early signs of Legg-Calvé-Perthes disease.[71,72] Absence of marrow enhancement following gadolinium helps to confirm avascularity.[73,74] Magnetic resonance imaging is very useful for showing abnormalities of the synovium and the growth cartilage of the epiphysis and physis.[75-77] Because nourishment of the synovium and epiphyseal cartilage is by synovial fluid, there may be overgrowth of these structures relative to the avascular epiphysis. Resultant loss of containment of the femoral head within the acetabulum may require surgery to reduce stress on the developing femoral head and promote its normal development and shaping.[78] Transphyseal bone bridging is a strong predictor of growth disturbance.[76] Like skeletal scintigraphy, MRI shows findings suggesting the two patterns of revascularization.[79]

The differential diagnosis of Legg-Calvé-Perthes disease includes AVN, which can occur with sickle cell disease and other hemoglobinopathies, Gaucher disease, corticosteroid use, hypothyroidism, and irradiation. Bilaterality in particular raises concern for an underlying condition.[14]

Sickle Cell Anemia

Sickle cell anemia is a hemoglobinopathy in which valine replaces glutamic acid at the sixth position of the β-globulin chain (hemoglobin S). Changes in deoxygenated hemoglobin S result in erythrocyte rigidity and fragility. Children with sickle cell anemia are at risk for avascular necrosis of bone caused by vascular occlusion, osteomyelitis, and septic arthritis (Figs. 13.30 and 13.31). Skeletal pain in these children is more frequently related to a sickle cell crisis with bone infarction than it is to infection. Differentiation between bone infarction and osteomyelitis presents a clinical challenge in some cases. The degree of fever and leukocytosis may be similar. The ESR may be low, normal, or elevated, and radiographs may be normal, reveal only soft tissue swelling, or show bone destruction and periosteal reaction with either bone infarction or osteomyelitis in children with sickle cell anemia.

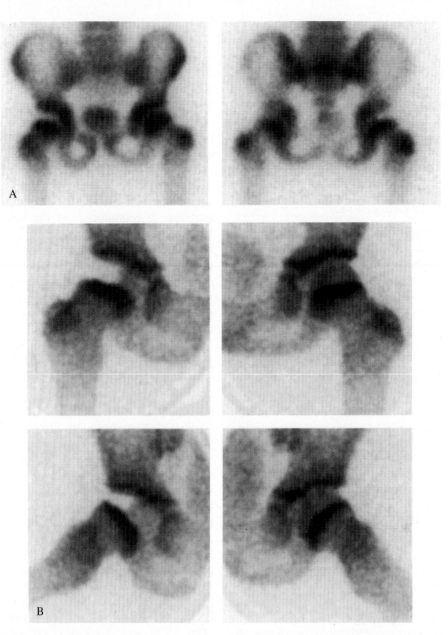

FIGURE 13.28. Legg-Calvé-Perthes disease. High resolution planar (A, anterior projection and posterior projection) and pinhole (B, anterior and frog lateral projections) scintigraphy shows no uptake in the right capital femoral epiphysis. Note that uptake in the acetabulum should not be misinterpreted as being within the medial portions of the epiphysis. The affected epiphysis appeared normal radiographically. (*Source:* Connolly and Treves,[2] with permission.)

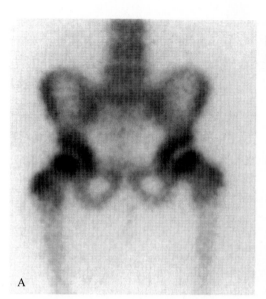

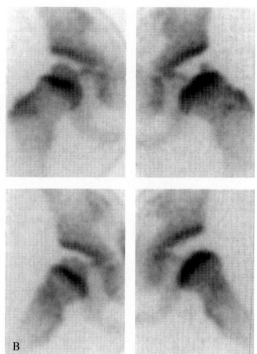

A

B

FIGURE 13.29. Legg-Calvé-Perthes disease. A: High-resolution planar imaging suggests low or absent uptake in the left capital femoral epiphysis. B: Pinhole imaging in the anterior projection shows a lateral column of intact uptake (upper row). This column is not visualized in the frog lateral position (lower row) due to rotation of the epiphysis. (*Source:* Connolly and Treves,[2] with permission.)

Skeletal scintigraphy does not reliably distinguish bone infarction from osteomyelitis in sickle cell patients. High or low tracer localization and uptake are observed with either. Early in the course of symptoms, high localization on the angiographic and tissue phase images and high uptake on the skeletal phase images are more suggestive of osteomyelitis. Skeletal scintigraphy of children with sickle cell disease and bone pain usually demonstrates multiple sites of abnormal localization due to prior bone infarctions. Skeletal scintigraphy also reveals extraosseous abnormalities in some children with sickle cell anemia. Abnormal localization in the spleen is observed secondary to splenic infarction (Figs. 13.30, 13.31).[80] Localization in other infarcted tissue, including cerebral tissue, has also been reported.[81] Prominent renal tracer localization occurs, usually due to altered iron distribution and repeated transfusions.[82]

Trauma

Skeletal scintigraphy is a highly sensitive tool that can be abnormal within a few hours of skeletal injury.[83,84] In pediatrics, skeletal scintigraphy is particularly useful for detecting injuries associated with child abuse, learning to walk, and sports.

Child Abuse

Identification of abused infants and children is essential if they are to be protected from further and perhaps fatal injury. Since Caffey's[85] early radiographic description of skeletal injuries in abused children, imaging has come to play a primary role in the evaluation of suspected pediatric victims of physical abuse. The most frequent sites of skeletal injury are the long bones, ribs, and skull.

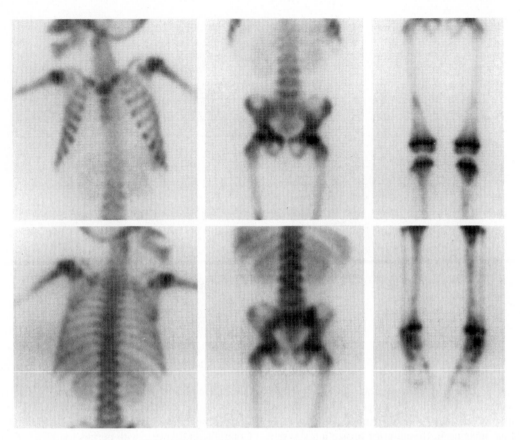

FIGURE 13.30. Sickle cell anemia. Multiple sites of abnormal uptake are demonstrated in the long bones and pelvis. The most intense focus in the right pubis corresponded to a fracture through infarcted bone. Tracer accumulation within the spleen is best identified on the posterior images (lower row). (*Source:* Connolly and Treves,[2] with permission.)

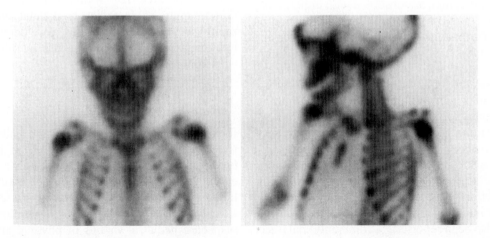

FIGURE 13.31. Sickle cell anemia. Absence of uptake in the upper sternum was due to an acute infarction. (*Source:* Connolly and Treves,[2] with permission.)

Infants and young children who have been victims of abuse are often too young to verbally localize the sites of trauma or pain. Subsequently, evaluation of the entire skeleton is an essential component of their evaluation. Radiographic skeletal surveys performed for this purpose include anteroposterior and lateral views of the skull and thorax, lateral views of the spine, an anteroposterior view of the abdomen and pelvis, and anteroposterior views of the three segments of each extremity.[86] Additional films may be obtained of sites considered suspicious for injury. Skeletal scintigraphy is performed with multiple-spot imaging of the entire skeleton. With both radiography and scintigraphy, careful patient positioning, use of high-quality imaging systems, and strict attention to detail are essential.

The types of injury associated with child abuse can be understood by considering the primary mechanisms of injury. With infants, assault frequently entails the victim being grasped about the thorax, facing the assailant, and violently shaken. Metaphyseal and rib fractures are characteristic (Figs. 13.32 to 13.34). Metaphyseal fractures result from shearing forces on the immature primary spongiosa. The metaphyseal predilection reflects the weakness of newly formed bone adjacent to the physis. These fractures most frequently involve the tibia, distal femur, and proximal humerus. They are often bilateral. A planar series of microfractures through the immature primary spongiosa is present.[87] Rib fractures occur at sites of compression, posteriorly near the costovertebral junction where the rib is compressed against the transverse process, laterally, and anteriorly.[88] Abused older children are often grasped by an extremity and shaken. With this type of abuse, torsional forces can cause a metaphyseal

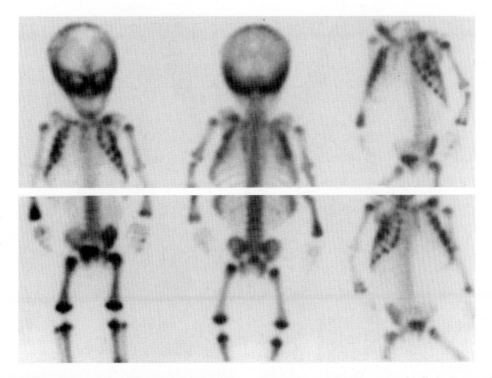

FIGURE 13.32. Child abuse. Skeletal scintigraphy (anterior, posterior, and anterior oblique projections) reveals high uptake in the left clavicle, multiple right and left ribs laterally, multiple left ribs at the costovertebral junctions, the left ilium and the femoral, tibial and humeral diaphyses bilaterally. The appearance of the physes and adjacent metaphyses indicates definite injuries to the distal right radius, both proximal femora and the left proximal tibia and possible injuries of the distal femoral and right proximal tibial metaphyses. (*Source:* Connolly and Treves,[2] with permission.)

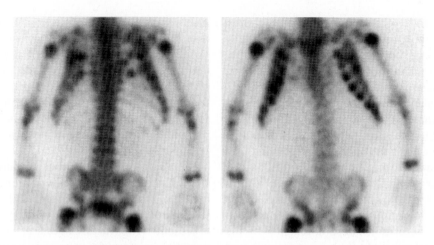

FIGURE 13.33. Child abuse. Skeletal scintigraphy reveals evidence of multiple posterior and lateral rib fractures. (*Source:* Connolly and Treves,[2] with permission.)

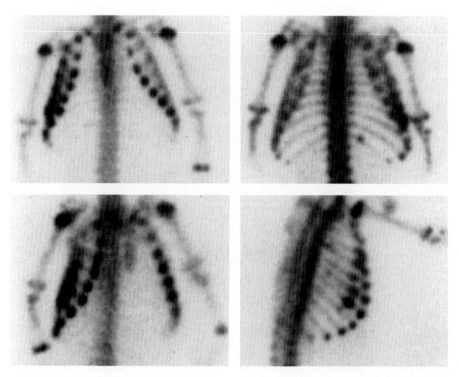

FIGURE 13.34. Child abuse. Skeletal scintigraphy shows sites of high uptake in multiple ribs anterolaterally and the right 11th rib posteriorly. The right anterior oblique projection (lower left panel) and right lateral projection (lower right panel) assist in delineating the extent of injury to the anterolateral right 3rd to 8th ribs. (*Source:* Connolly and Treves,[2] with permission.)

fracture, whereas direct pressure can result in a diaphyseal fracture or a periosteal injury.[89] Abused infants and children are also subject to blunt trauma to any bone. Often, more than one mechanism of injury is active.

Protocols for evaluating suspected victims of child abuse vary based on individual preferences and expertise. A radiographic skeletal survey is usually the initial step. Radiographs are useful for showing fractures, estimating fracture age and stage of healing, demonstrating displacement, and checking for underlying pathology (e.g., osteogenesis imperfecta). Skeletal scintigraphy is most useful when radiographs are negative or detection of additional fractures to those shown radiographically would be useful in establishing the diagnosis. Use of both modalities can maximize the detection of both individual victims and individual fractures. The importance of identifying individual victims is self-apparent. The significance of detecting individual fractures is that the social and legal outcomes of child abuse are related to the number, extent, and severity of lesions that are defined.[89–92] Even with a combined modality approach, many abused children will not have evidence of skeletal trauma.[88,93] Further evaluation should not be deferred solely on the basis of negative radiographic and scintigraphic surveys.

Of the most common fractures, scintigraphy has proven to be especially useful for showing high uptake associated with rib fractures.[88,94,95] Due to superimposed soft tissue and osseous structures, rib fractures are often not apparent radiographically until a callus forms. Scintigraphy is also highly reliable in detecting diaphyseal injuries, which are also well demonstrated radiographically; a focal abnormality is occasionally shown, but it is more common to see diffusely high uptake. Metaphyseal injuries are typically detected radiographically. The radiographic appearance of these fractures depends on the orientation of the x-ray beam to the metaphyseal fragment. A metaphyseal fracture appears as a crescent ("bucket-handle" fracture) when imaged obliquely and as two peripheral triangles ("corner" fracture) when imaged tangentially.[14,86,87] Metaphyseal fractures may be manifested scintigraphically by alterations in the normal shape of the physis or as heightened intensity of physeal uptake that may extend to affect the metaphysis.[95] Although some have found scintigraphy very sensitive for detecting metaphyseal injuries,[89,95] metaphyseal foci of high uptake may be obscured by the intensely tracer-avid physis, and isolated physeal abnormalities are very subjective observations. Skull fractures are typically linear, nondepressed, and often hairline. These fractures incite minimal osteoblastic response, so they are often not identified with skeletal scintigraphy even when evident radiographically. When scintigraphy is positive for skull fracture, the appearance is typically diffusely high uptake at the fracture site (Fig. 13.35).

Toddler Injuries

Fractures of the lower extremity occur due to falls, unaccustomed stress, or both as children develop walking skills between the ages of 9 months and 3 years.

The best known is the spiral or oblique fracture of the tibia, commonly referred to as a toddler's fracture (Figs. 13.36 and 13.37).[96] Radiographic findings, if present, are often subtle. The fracture may not be visualized by standard anteroposterior and lateral radiographs because of its orientation. Oblique radiographs are useful but are seldom obtained unless the diagnosis is specifically questioned. Other relatively common sites of fracture in toddlers include the upper tibia, the calcaneus (Fig. 13.38), and the cuboid (Fig. 13.39).[97–100] Radiographic findings are often subtle or absent with these fractures too.

High sensitivity, a wide field of view, and the ability to perform the study without sedation makes skeletal scintigraphy highly valuable for diagnosis of fractures in toddlers whose radiographs are negative.[97–102] Tibial fractures usually cause diffusely high diaphyseal uptake (Fig. 13.36). A spiral orientation is sometimes evident (Fig. 13.37). Focal, linear, or diffusely high uptake is seen with upper tibial, calcaneal, and cuboidal fracture. Fractures often cause high localization during the angiographic and tissue phases as well as high uptake during the skeletal phases (Fig. 13.36).

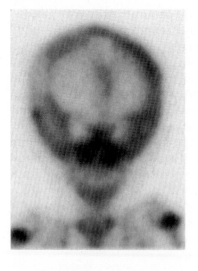
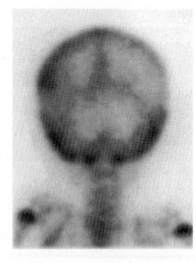

FIGURE 13.35. Child abuse. Asymmetrically high uptake is shown in the left temporal, parietal, and occipital bones (anterior, posterior, left and right lateral images) of a child whose radiographic survey revealed a linear left parietal fracture. (*Source:* Connolly and Treves,[2] with permission.)

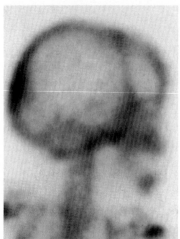
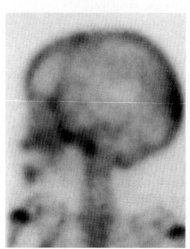

Stress Injuries

The number of children and adolescents involved in organized sports has increased dramatically over recent decades. More participation has led to more sports-related injuries, particularly overuse injuries.

Overuse injuries result from repetitive submaximal musculoskeletal loading during efforts to build and sustain strength and endurance. Stress on bone triggers a coordinated response that involves resorption mediated by osteoclasts and repair and hypertrophy mediated by osteoblasts.[103–105] Optimally, the resultant changes are functional and adaptive. For

example, tibial bone density, cortical thickness, and diaphyseal diameter increase in runners. A partial or complete disruption of bone, a stress fracture, may occur when there is a disproportion in favor of osteoclastic activity.

Stress fractures are considered fatigue fractures when the injured bone is otherwise normal. The vast majority of stress fractures in athletes are fatigue fractures. Stress fractures are considered insufficiency fractures when there is an underlying abnormality in the injured bone. The most common underlying condition is osteoporosis. Although osteoporosis is predominantly a condition of postmenopausal women, it occurs in girls and young

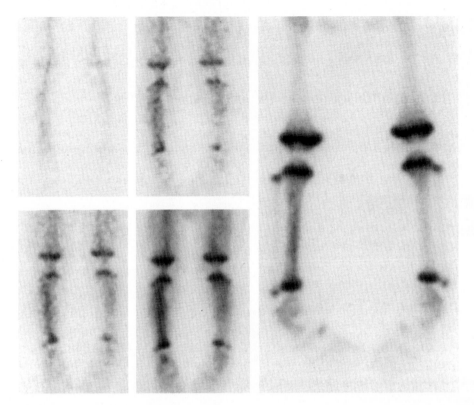

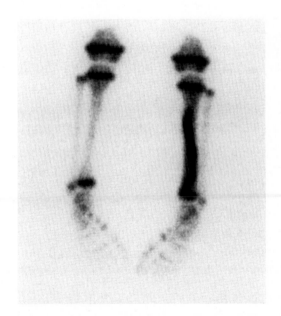

FIGURE 13.36. Toddler's fracture. Selected images from radionuclide angiography and a tissue phase image indicate high tracer delivery to the right calf of a 22-month-old girl. The skeletal phase image shows diffusely high uptake in the right tibial diaphysis. (*Source:* Connolly and Treves,[2] with permission.)

FIGURE 13.37. Toddler's fracture. A well-defined region of markedly high uptake delineates a spiral fracture in a 2-year-old boy.

women as part of the female athlete triad. The other two components of this triad are disordered eating and amenorrhea.

Skeletal scintigraphy is generally considered the gold standard for diagnosis of stress injuries to bone.[106] Stress injuries related to sports are often the same in children as those that occur in adults. Injuries of the back, hip, and pelvis that are either more commonly or exclusively encountered in children are emphasized in this section.

Low Back Pain in Young Athletes

Low back pain is more often of skeletal origin in children and teenagers than in adults. Spondylolysis is a particularly common etiology.[107]

Spondylolysis is stress fracture of the pars interarticularis. Ethnic and familial variations in its incidence suggest that heredity plays a predisposing role in some cases.[108–110] This is due to either the angulation of the spinal lamina

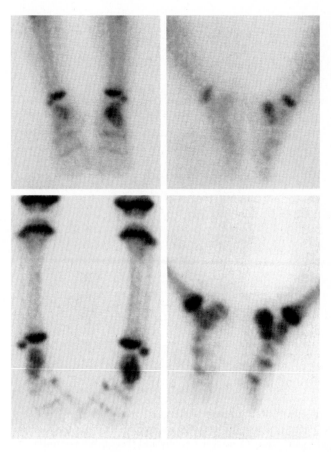

FIGURE 13.38. Calcaneal injury in a toddler. Tissue phase (upper panels) and skeletal phase (lower panels) images demonstrate diffusely high localization and uptake in the left calcaneus of a 25-month-old girl who was favoring her left lower extremity. (*Source:* Connolly and Treves,[2] with permission.)

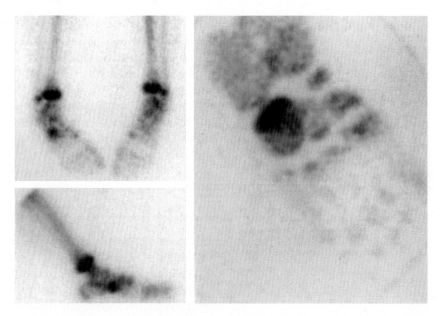

FIGURE 13.39. Cuboid injury in a toddler. Diffusely high uptake is identified with planar imaging (left panels). Pinhole imaging (right panel) shows focally high uptake at the base of the right cuboid. (*Source:* Connolly and Treves,[2] with permission.)

and facets or a congenital weakness in the pars interarticularis.[111] Spondylolysis occurs in association with many athletic activities, particularly gymnastics, diving, and contact sports.[51] Hyperextension is the mechanism of injury. The lower lumbar levels are most commonly affected. Bilateral spondylolysis may result in spondylolisthesis, which is anterior subluxation of the involved vertebra.

Lateral radiographs including a coned-down view of the lumbosacral junction are often useful for showing spondylolysis and always useful for assessing spondylolisthesis. The typical radiographic appearance of spondylolysis is a radiolucency crossing a pars interarticularis. Sclerosis may also be evident due to healing at the fracture site or remodeling and enlargement of the contralateral pedicle.[112] Several methods for quantitating the degree of spondylolisthesis have been described. A simple, reproducible one is to divide the distance slipped by the anteroposterior dimension of the vertebral body below. Radiographs in flexion and extension may be useful to assess mobility of the affected vertebra.

Scintigraphy is used for demonstrating evidence of stress associated with radiographically occult injuries to the partes interaticulares and as a means of assessing metabolic activity when spondylolysis is evident radiographically. The typical appearance is focally high uptake in a pars interarticularis (Figs. 13.40 to 13.42). This high uptake may be due to fracture or to stress remodeling without frank fracture. Planar skeletal scintigraphy is more sensitive than plain film radiography, and SPECT is more sensitive than planar scintigraphy for demonstrating stress changes in a pars interarticularis. An increase of about 50% in diagnostic yield with SPECT relative to planar scintigraphy warrants the use of SPECT in children with suspected spondylolysis.[113]

The primary considerations for differential diagnosis of high uptake in the region of a lumbar pars interarticularis are osteoid osteoma and facet joint arthropathy. The degree of uptake is usually greater with osteoid osteoma than with pars interarticularis stress, but the appearance of the two processes overlaps and the opposite can be the case. High uptake in the facet joint regions is a sensitive but nonspecific finding with facet joint arthropathy.[114] Because of the proximity of the facet joints and partes interarticulares, facet joint arthropathy and pars interarticularis stress can appear identical on skeletal scintigraphy. Patient age is often the leading factor used for their differentiation; facet joint arthropathy is a common cause of low back pain in adults but not in adolescents.

Although skeletal scintigraphy is most often obtained to detect evidence of pars interarticularis stress in young athletes with low back pain, abnormalities supportive of other diagnoses are also shown. These abnormalities are typically stress-related.[115,116] A particularly common diagnosis is stress associated with a lumbosacral transitional vertebra. This anatomic variant is characterized by an enlarged transverse process that follows the contour of the sacral ala. The large transverse process usually articulates with the sacrum through a joint space. Repetitive flexion and extension stress the transverse-sacral articulation, which is part of the weight-bearing platform.[117,118] High uptake at the transverse-sacral articulation of young patients with lumbosacral transitional vertebrae can support a diagnosis of stress at this site as the cause of pain (Fig. 13.43). Sclerosis and other changes are usually not radiographically evident, but there are trends for MRI and computed tomography (CT) to show findings that imply stress or motion at the articulation.[116]

Other stress-related causes of low back pain that may be associated with scintigraphic abnormalities include injuries to the vertebral bodies, transverse processes, and spinous processes.[115,116]

Growth centers surrounding the vertebral body's end plate (vertebral ring apophyses) and at the tips of the spinous and transverse processes can be injured prior to ossification. Disk material may penetrate an injured vertebral ring apophysis.[119–122] Anterior and less commonly posterior or lateral displacement of disk material can separate a segment of the vertebral body (Fig. 13.44). When this segment is ossified, the radiographic appearance is referred to as a limbus vertebra. Penetration of disk material anteriorly, centrally, or posteriorly

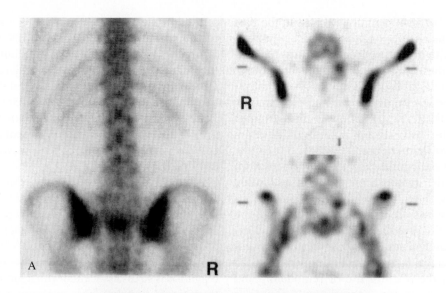

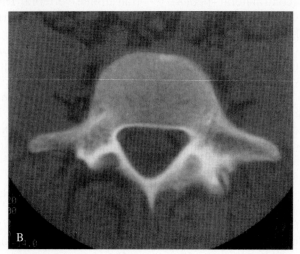

FIGURE 13.40. Pars interarticularis stress. A: High uptake in the left L5 pars interarticularis is suggested by a posterior planar image (left panel) and convincingly indicated by SPECT (right panels, axial and coronal images shown). B: Computed tomography demonstrates corresponding sclerosis involving the left pars interarticularis. (*Source:* Connolly and Treves,[2] with permission.)

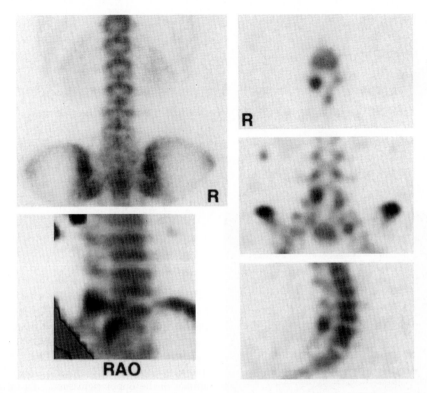

FIGURE 13.41. Pars interarticularis stress. A posterior planar image shows no uptake abnormality. High uptake involving the right L5 pars interarticularis is seen with axial, coronal, sagittal and volume ren- dered (displayed in the right anterior oblique pro- jection) SPECT. (*Source:* Connolly and Treves,[2] with permission.)

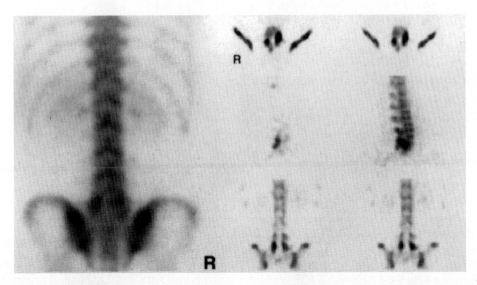

FIGURE 13.42. Pars interarticularis stress. A posterior planar image reveals high uptake on the right and less prominently on the left at L5. Axial, sagittal, and coronal SPECT indicate stress of the bilateral L5 partes interarticulares. (*Source:* Connolly and Treves,[2] with permission.)

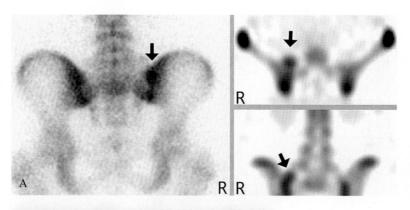

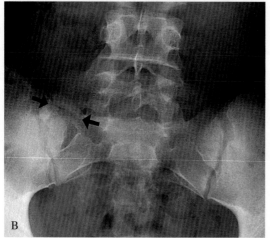

FIGURE 13.43. Lumbosacral transitional vertebra. A: Planar imaging (left panel, posterior projection) shows asymmetrically higher uptake along the upper right sacroiliac joint (arrow). SPECT (right panels, transverse and coronal images) shows focally high uptake in the upper right sacral ala (arrows). B: A radiograph indicates that the high uptake correlates with the articulation between a lumbosacral transitional vertebra and the sacrum (arrows). (*Source:* Connolly et al.,[115] with permission.)

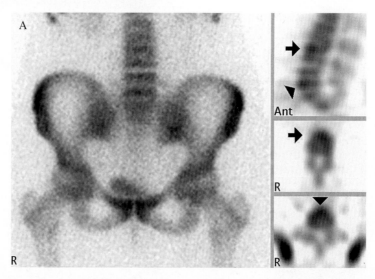

FIGURE 13.44. Vertebral ring apophyseal injuries. A: Skeletal scintigraphy was performed in a 15-year-old female gymnast with low back pain. Anterior planar imaging shows prominent uptake along the anterior and inferior margins of the L4 and L5 vertebral bodies, an appearance that can be within the physiologic range. SPECT delineates foci of high uptake at the anterosuperior margin of the L4 body (arrow) and the anteroinferior margin of the L5 body (arrowhead).

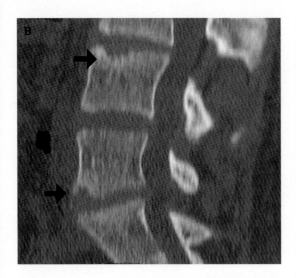

FIGURE 13.44. B: Computed tomography (CT) shows corresponding depressions of the vertebral bodies (arrows) where the ring apophysis has been penetrated. (*Source:* Connolly et al.,[115] with permission.)

without an associated ossified fragment creates a cartilaginous (Schmorl's) node. Extrusions at multiple levels with associated kyphosis create the appearance of Scheuermann's disease, which typically affects the thoracic spine but can affect the lumbar spine. Limbus vertebra, cartilaginous node, and Scheuermann's disease are radiographic diagnoses that are occasionally suggested by skeletal scintigraphy when uptake is focally higher in a region along vertebral body end plates. Skeletal scintigraphy should not be used to exclude these diagnoses because it is often negative or only very subtly abnormal.[123] Growth centers at the tips of the spinous and transverse processes are ossifying during the years in which spondylolysis is characteristically encountered. Injuries can result from repetitive traction such as that exerted by the dorsolumbar fascia on the spinous processes. The value of skeletal scintigraphy for diagnosis of injuries to these structures is limited by uptake being physiologically high at growth centers. Nevertheless, focally higher uptake at a particular level can help direct clinical examination or support clinical findings (Fig. 13.45).

Pelvic Apophyseal Avulsions

During the teenage years, apophyses appear in the iliac crest, anterior superior iliac spine, anterior inferior iliac spine, the ischium, the lesser trochanter, and the greater trochanter. Until these apophyses ossify, they are the weakest point in the musculotendinous unit and are prone to being avulsed in response to sudden forceful or repetitive muscular traction.[124] Muscles attaching on these apophyses include the abdominal wall musculature (iliac crest), the sartorius and tensor fascia lata (anterosuperior iliac spine), the rectus femoris (anteroinferior iliac spine), the hamstrings and adductors (ischium), the iliopsoas (lesser trochanter), and the external rotators (greater trochanter). Pelvic and proximal femoral apophyseal avulsions are most common in sprinters, football players, ballet dancers, and jumpers. Acute onset of pain during strenuous activity is typically described. Displacement of an avulsed apophysis is usually apparent radiographically. Avulsions of the anterior inferior iliac spine and the iliac crest apophyses may show relatively little displacement and escape detection, however. Displacement is sometimes minimal with avulsions at other sites as well. An avulsion fracture should be suspected in adolescents with hip, pelvic, or low back pain and asymmetrically high uptake corresponding to a pelvic or hip apophysis (Figs. 13.46 and 13.47).

Slipped Capital Femoral Epiphysis

Slipped capital femoral epiphysis (SCFE) is an epiphyseal separation. Muscular traction displaces the femoral neck anterolaterally relative to the separated epiphysis. The epiphysis, which is held in the acetabulum, rotates medially and posteriorly. The peak incidence of SCFE is during the pubertal growth spurt. Children with SCFE usually are overweight, slightly tall for their ages, and tend to have some delay in skeletal maturation. Children of African ancestry are particularly susceptible. A combination of mechanical shearing forces and a predisposing hormonal influence have been implicated. Slipped capital femoral epiphysis is bilateral in as many as 30% of cases. Other settings in

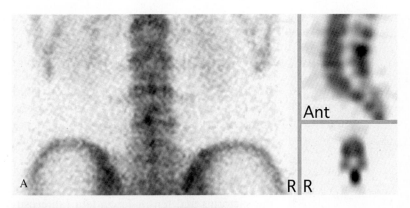

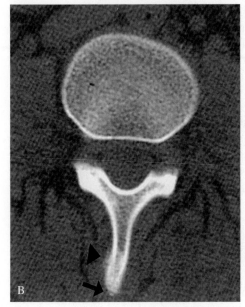

FIGURE 13.45. A: Skeletal scintigraphy (left, planar imaging; right, sagittal and axial SPECT) shows marked uptake at the L4 spinous process tip of a 13-year-old female gymnast. Note that uptake is also high at other spinous process tips but to a lesser degree; physiologic uptake at spinous process apophyses makes their evaluation difficult and very subjective. B: CT shows reactive sclerosis along the spinous process (arrowhead) and a small bony fragment (arrow) at the tip. (*Source:* Connolly et al.,[115] with permission.)

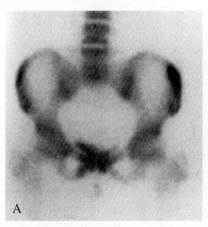

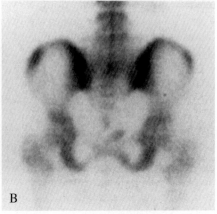

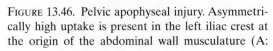

FIGURE 13.46. Pelvic apophyseal injury. Asymmetrically high uptake is present in the left iliac crest at the origin of the abdominal wall musculature (A: anterior projection; B: posterior projection). (*Source:* Connolly and Treves,[2] with permission.)

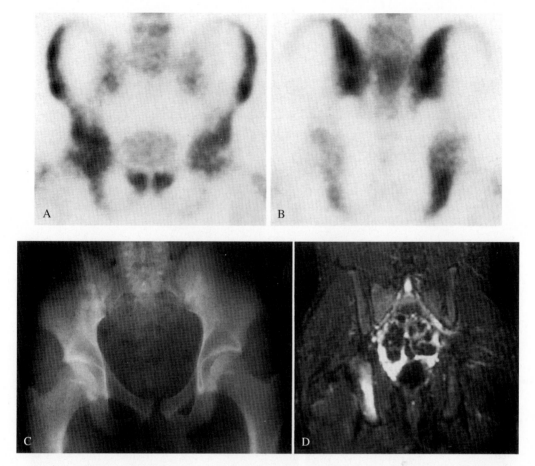

FIGURE 13.47. Apophyseal injury. High uptake is seen in the right ischium on the anterior (A) and posterior (B) planar skeletal scintigrams. C: A radiograph does not show an avulsed fragment. D: A coronal T2-weighted fat suppressed image reveals increased signal corresponding to the uptake abnormality in the right ischium. (*Source:* Connolly and Treves,[2] with permission.)

which SCFE occurs include renal osteodystrophy, hypothyroidism, hypopituitarism with growth hormone deficiency, and following pelvic and femoral irradiation. These associations are particularly common when SCFE occurs before 10 years of age.[14,33] Children with SCFE typically present with hip or groin pain. A change in gait or range of motion at the involved hip may occur. Treatment of SCFE is aimed primarily at preventing further slippage. Operative pin fixation generally provides good long-term functional outcome for mild slips. Techniques to reduce the degree of slippage that are employed in cases where the slip is severe carry a significant risk of complications including AVN, chondrolysis, and degenerative changes.[125]

The diagnosis is usually made with radiographs. Radiographic signs may be subtle on the anteroposterior projection so a true lateral or frog-leg lateral projection is important. Skeletal scintigraphy may show accentuated high uptake in, or apparent widening of, the physis (Fig. 13.48). These findings, when present, may be subtle and are quite subjective. Magnetic resonance imaging, which can delineate widening and irregularity of the growth plate on T1-weighted images before a SCFE is shown radiographically, is therefore preferred for assessment of suspected radiographically

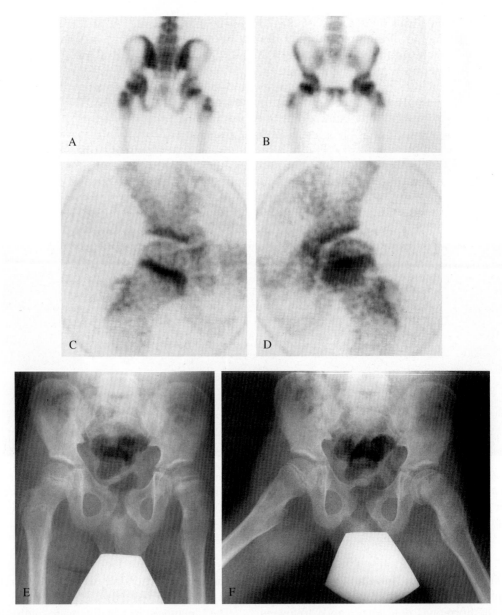

FIGURE 13.48. Slipped capital femoral epiphysis. Posterior (A) and anterior (B) skeletal phase planar images reveal high uptake in the left femoral metaphysis. This finding, which was detected incidentally on a study performed for long-term neuroblastoma follow-up, is better demonstrated with pinhole magnification (C,D). An anteroposterior radiograph (E) reveals widening of the left proximal femoral physis and joint space. A suggestion of medial displacement of the femoral capital epiphysis relative to the metaphysis is confirmed by a frog leg lateral radiograph (F). (*Source:* Connolly and Treves,[2] with permission.)

occult SCFE.[126] Skeletal scintigraphy can be useful for assessing the vascularity of the femoral head. Ischemia complicating SCFE, with or without therapeutic pinning, results in absent uptake by the femoral head (Fig. 13.49).[127] In patients with continued pain during treatment, scintigraphy has been used to assess the physiologic status of the subcapital physis

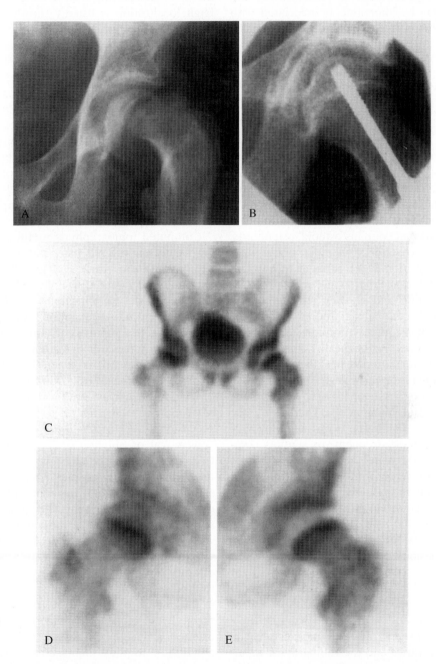

FIGURE 13.49. Slipped capital femoral epiphysis. An anteroposterior radiograph (A) reveals marked displacement of the left femoral capital epiphysis relative to the metaphysis. Following open reduction and internal fixation (B), anterior planar (C) and pinhole magnification images (D: right hip; E: left hip) show no uptake in the left epiphysis. (*Source:* Connolly and Treves,[2] with permission.)

when a recurrent slip is suspected. No uptake at the physis provides evidence of growth plate closure and indicates that recurrence is unlikely (Fig. 13.50). Chondrolysis, which may result from penetration of pins into the hip joint or may be idiopathic, is associated with high acetabular uptake, but this is a nonspecific finding.[128]

Benign Tumors and Tumor-Like Lesions

Osteoid Osteoma

Osteoid osteoma is a relatively common osseous lesion that is best classified as a benign neoplasm, although inflammatory, traumatic, and vascular etiologies have been suggested.[129] Microscopically, osteoid osteoma consists of a central nidus that contains osteoid, osteoblasts, and vascular channels. The nidus is less than 1.5 cm in size. It may be situated in cortical, medullary, or cancellous bone or in a subperiosteal location and is often surrounded by dense reactive trabecular bone. A related lesion, osteoblastoma, is virtually identical to osteoid osteoma histologically. The primary point of differentiation is size; the nidus of an osteoblastoma is larger than 1.5 cm.

Most osteoid osteomas are detected in adolescents and young adults. There is a male predominance. The lesion is rare in nonwhites. Pain is the most frequent presenting complaint. Often the pain is relieved by salicylates and is most intense at night. Intralesional pressure due to vasodilatation mediated by prostaglandins within the nidus may be the cause of pain.[130,131]

Appendicular lesions are more common than vertebral lesions. In the long bones, osteoid osteomas are almost always diaphyseal or metaphyseal. Vertebral osteoid osteomas occur most often in the posterior elements and are often near the apex of a scoliotic curve.[129]

Radiographs are often diagnostic, but the appearance varies and the radiographic manifestations of diseases such as osteomyelitis, stress fracture, and osteosarcoma overlap with those of osteoid osteoma.[132] The typical radiographic appearance of a cortical osteoid osteoma is a radiolucency, corresponding to the nidus, with surrounding sclerosis and cortical thickening.[133]

Skeletal scintigraphy is essentially 100% sensitive for the detection of osteoid osteoma.[134] High localization is usually shown on angiographic and tissue phase imaging. Skeletal phase images show well-localized, focal, marked uptake in osteoid osteomas (Figs. 13.51 to 13.53). A characteristic appearance is intense uptake in the nidus surrounded by less marked but still high uptake in reactive bone (Fig. 13.51).[135,136] This pattern is most commonly observed with lesions of the appendicular skeleton and is best demonstrated by pinhole magnification imaging.[137] Single photon emission computed tomography can help localize an osteoid osteoma in anatomically complex areas such as the spine.

Computed tomography is useful in evaluating suspected osteoid osteomas that do not demonstrate the classic radiographic appearance and in delineating the nidus. The nidus of an osteoid osteoma appears as a well-defined, oval or round, low-attenuation lesion that contains variable amounts of mineralization.[129] Magnetic resonance imaging may also demonstrate the nidus but is generally less reliable than CT for this purpose. Due to the presence of extensive marrow and soft tissue edema, MRI may be suggestive of a more aggressive process.[138,139]

Removal or ablation of the nidus is curative. Intraoperative scintigraphy helps localize the nidus for surgical excision and guide its complete removal.[140-143] Intraoperative pinhole magnification scintigraphy (Fig. 13.53) allows the surgeon to minimize the amount of bone removed, an important consideration in the weight-bearing bones and vertebrae where osteoid osteomas typically occur.[143] Nonoperative techniques designed to limit bone resection in patients with osteoid osteoma have gained favor. These include CT-guided percutaneous excision[144-146] and CT-guided radiofrequency ablation.[147] Medical management with long-term use of nonsteroidal antiinflammatory agents is an alternative in cases where excision or ablation carries a significant risk of disability or would be highly complex.[148] This

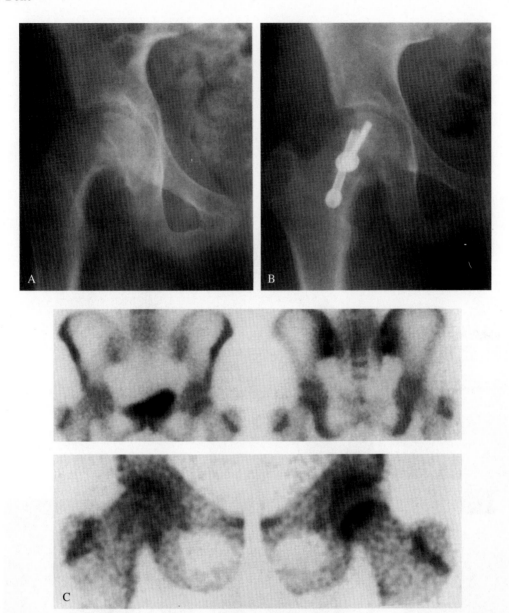

FIGURE 13.50. Slipped capital femoral epiphysis. A: A radiograph reveals a slipped right capital femoral epiphysis. B: The patient returned 14 months following open reduction and internal fixation with right thigh pain. C: Scintigraphy confirmed closure of the right subcapital physis (upper row, anterior and posterior planar images; lower row, right and left hip pinhole images). The left subcapital physis remained open. (*Source:* Connolly and Treves,[2] with permission.)

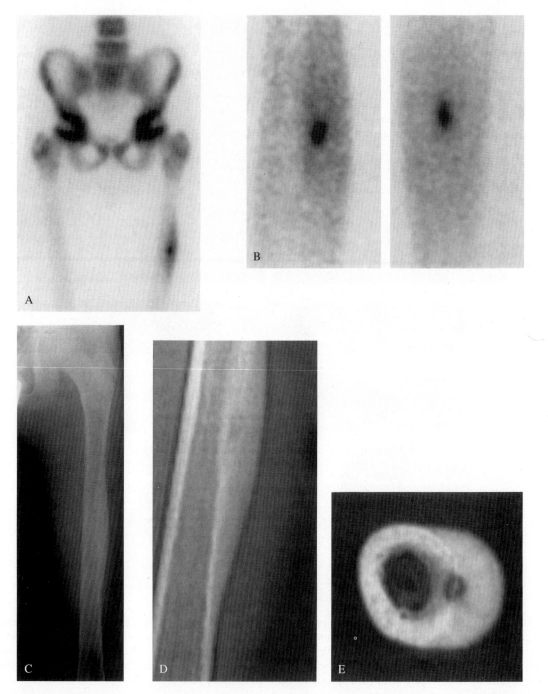

FIGURE 13.51. Osteoid osteoma. High resolution planar (A) and pinhole scintigraphy (B, anterior projection and lateral projections) show marked focal uptake in the nidus of an osteoid osteoma surrounded by less prominent uptake in reactive bone. Extensive cortical thickening surrounding the radiolucent nidus is shown with a radiograph (C) and with a scout image obtained for computed tomography (D). The nidus is shown by CT (E). (*Source:* Connolly and Treves,[2] with permission.)

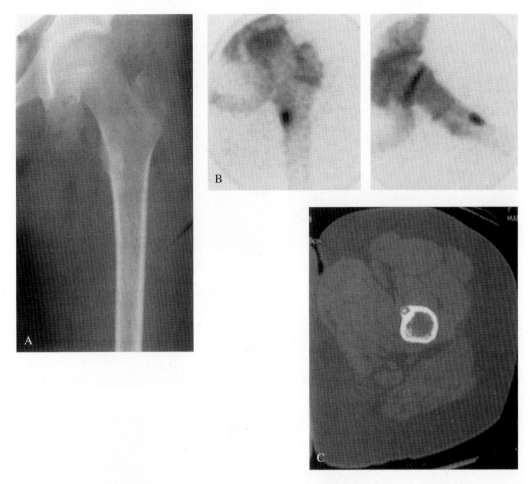

FIGURE 13.52. Osteoid osteoma. A: A radiograph reveals a subtle area of sclerosis just inferior to the left lesser trochanter. B: Skeletal scintigraphy (anterior and frog leg lateral pinhole images) demonstrates intense uptake in the nidus with mildly high uptake in adjacent bone. C: The nidus appears as a radiolucent lesion with central calcification on CT. (*Source:* Connolly and Treves,[2] with permission.)

observational approach is supported by the concept that osteoid osteoma is a self-limited lesion that eventually heals. The 6 to 15 years that this healing process may require[149–151] is unacceptable for most patients, however.

Benign Cortical Lesions

Benign cortical lesions include fibrous cortical defect, nonossifying fibroma, and the avulsive cortical irregularity of the distal medial femoral metaphysis. Fibrous cortical defect and nonossifying fibroma are histologically similar cortical rests of fibrous tissue found in metaphyses. Fibrous metaphyseal defects are present in about 40% of boys and 30% of girls during development. A lesion that is larger than 5 mm and extends into the medullary canal is referred to as a nonossifying fibroma (NOF). Smaller lesions that are confined to the cortex are

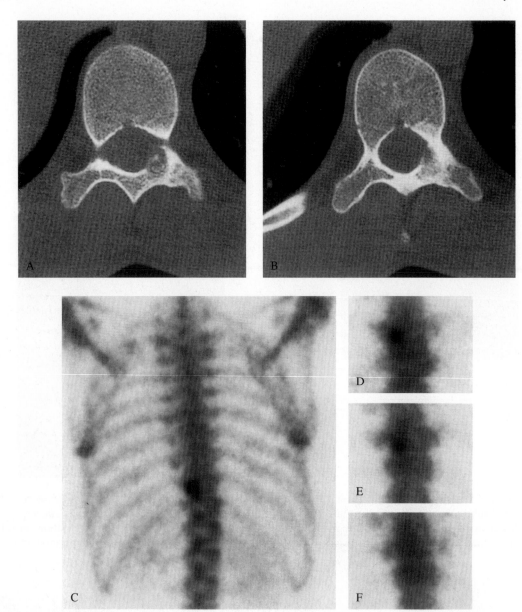

FIGURE 13.53. Osteoid osteoma. Computed tomography depicts calcification within the radiolucent nidus in the left pedicle of T10 (A) and adjacent sclerosis (B). Skeletal scintigraphy (posterior projection) shows intense uptake in the nidus (C). Intraoperative pinhole scintigraphy also demonstrates focal intense uptake prior to attempted excision (D). Focal uptake persisted (E) following an initial attempt at removal but was no longer present after further curettage (F). (*Source:* Connolly and Treves,[2] with permission.)

referred to as fibrous cortical defects. Benign cortical lesions fill with bone and regress before adulthood. Fibrous cortical defects appear radiographically as intracortical lucent lesions, often with sclerotic rims. Nonossifying fibromas appear as eccentric multiloculated metaphyseal or metadiaphyseal lucencies. Pathologic fracture is rare unless a NOF exceeds half the diameter of the involved bone.[152] Avulsive cortical irregularity is characterized by radiolucency, cortical roughening, or both. This radiographic appearance to the medial distal femoral metaphysis is common between 3 and 17 years of age, particularly in males, and is likely due to stress at the insertion of the gastrocnemius muscle.[14] Skeletal scintigraphy of benign cortical lesions reveals either normal or mildly high uptake.[33,153–155] Pathologic fracture should be considered when marked uptake is present, especially if there are related symptoms.[156,157]

Simple Bone Cyst

Simple bone cysts are serosanguinous or serous fluid-filled cavities with thin fibrous linings. The proposed etiology is interstitial fluid stasis secondary to trauma or venous obstruction. Almost all are solitary lesions. The great majority arise in the metaphysis of the long bones, mainly the humerus and femur. As the bone grows, the physis grows away from the lesion, which comes to lie in a diaphyseal or metadiaphyseal location. This lesion is often detected as an incidental radiographic finding. The primary significance is a risk for fracture.

The characteristic radiographic appearance is an expansile, thin-walled, intramedullary lucent lesion.[33] Depending on the size and location of the cyst, skeletal scintigraphy may be normal, reveal minimally high uptake around the periphery of the cyst, or show focally low uptake without such a surrounding rim (Fig. 13.54). Pathologic fracture typically results in focal or diffusely high uptake.[33]

Aneurysmal Bone Cyst

An aneurysmal bone cyst is an expansile lytic lesion that consists of vascular stroma, fibrous tissue, and blood or other fluid. Aneurysmal bone cysts are found slightly more frequently in females than males. As many as 30% may develop as a result of a vascular anomaly in other benign and malignant lesions, including osteosarcoma.[33]

Aneurysmal bone cysts usually appear as eccentric, lytic, expansile, occasionally trabeculated lesions (Fig. 13.55). Most long bone lesions are metaphyseal. Involvement of the posterior elements, often extending into the vertebral body, is characteristic of spinal lesions (Fig. 13.56).[158]

Angiographic and tissue phase images usually show high localization. Skeletal phase images typically demonstrate peripherally high and centrally low uptake (Fig. 13.55).[33,159] Abnormalities due to aneurysmal bone cysts may be best shown during the angiographic and tissue phases when the lesion is located deeply, such as in the pelvis (Fig. 13.57).[160] Skeletal scintigraphy does not differentiate an aneurysmal bone cyst that is associated with another lesion from one that is not, except in cases where metastatic lesions are detected.[33,159] Multiple fluid-fluid levels as shown by MRI or CT are characteristic of,[161] but not specific for,[162] an aneurysmal bone cyst.

Fibrous Dysplasia

Fibrous dysplasia is a mesodermal developmental abnormality in which the medullary space is replaced by a mixture of fibrous stroma and trabeculae of woven bone. There are monostotic and polyostotic forms. Patients with fibrous dysplasia typically present in the first two decades of life. Symptoms are often nonspecific and include pain, tenderness, and limp. Monostotic fibrous dysplasia may be detected as an incidental radiographic finding. Pathologic fracture, bowing deformity, leg length discrepancy, and facial asymmetry occur, particularly with polyostotic involvement. Pigmented cutaneous macules (café-au-lait spots) are present in one third to one half of patients with polyostotic fibrous dysplasia. The clinical significance of fibrous dysplasia stems from the skeletal complications and from the

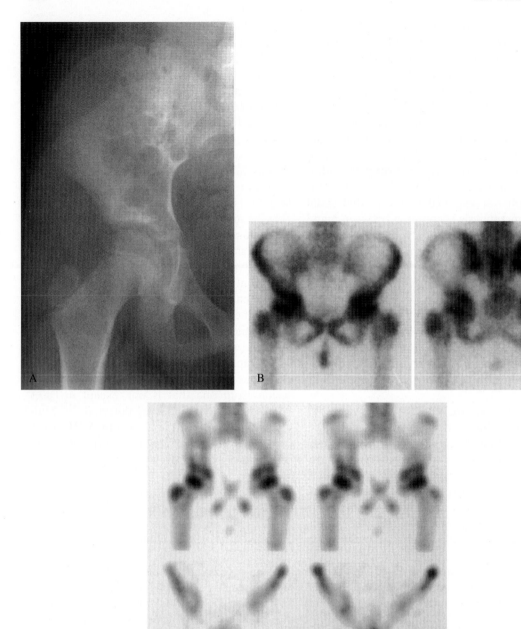

FIGURE 13.54. Simple bone cyst. A: A pelvic radiograph shows a multiloculated radiolucency in the right ilium. B: Anterior (left panel) and posterior (right panel) images demonstrate only slightly high uptake in the right ilium adjacent to the sacroiliac joint. C: An area of low uptake corresponding to the cyst is shown with SPECT. (*Source:* Connolly and Treves,[2] with permission.)

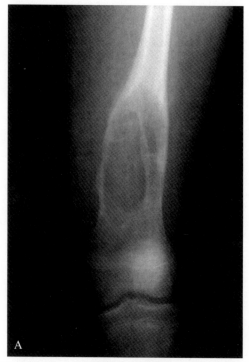

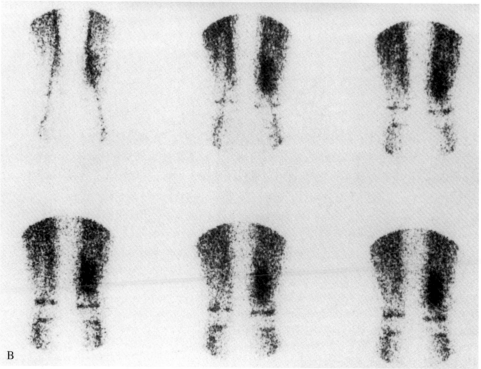

FIGURE 13.55. Aneurysmal bone cyst. A radiograph (A) shows eccentric radiolucent expansion of the distal left femoral diaphysis. Radionuclide angiography (B) and tissue phase imaging (C) shows high localization in the entire lesion. Skeletal phase imaging (D) shows high uptake along the lesion's periphery and centrally low uptake. (*Source:* Courtesy of Drs. J. Sty and R.G. Wells, Children's Hospital of Wisconsin.)

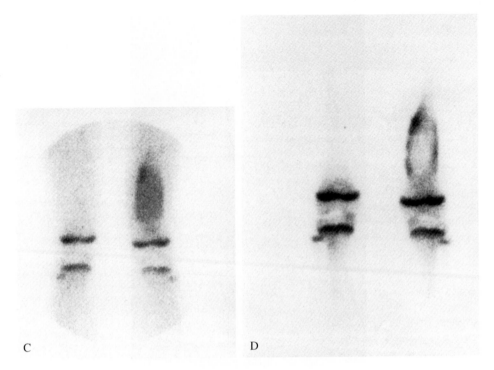

C   D

FIGURE 13.55. *Continued*

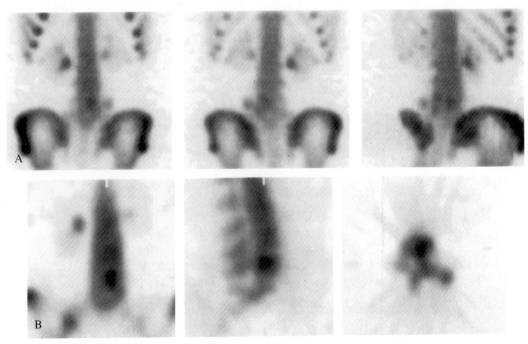

FIGURE 13.56. Aneurysmal bone cyst. A: Volume rendered anterior, posterior, and right posterior oblique SPECT images show high uptake in the left lateral aspect of L5 extending into the adjacent soft tissues. B: Coronal, sagittal, and transverse SPECT show high uptake and a region of low uptake in the vertebral body. C: A lytic lesion involving the left L5 pedicle and vertebral body is depicted radiographically). D,E: Computed tomography (D) and MRI (E) show an expansile lytic mass that is centered in the left pedicle of L5 and extends into the L5 vertebral body. Multiple fluid-fluid levels are present within the mass. (*Source:* Connolly and Treves,[2] with permission.)

FIGURE 13.56. *Continued*

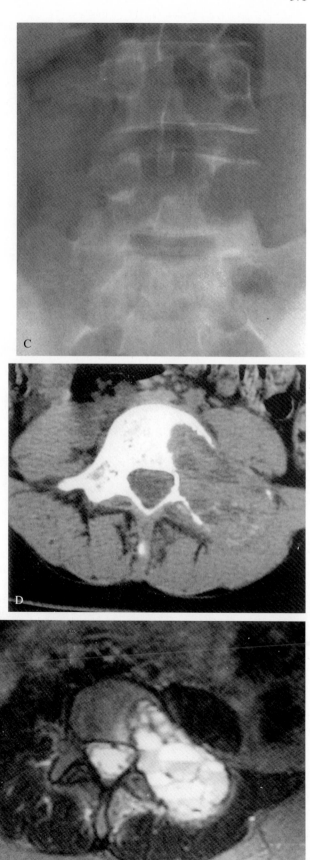

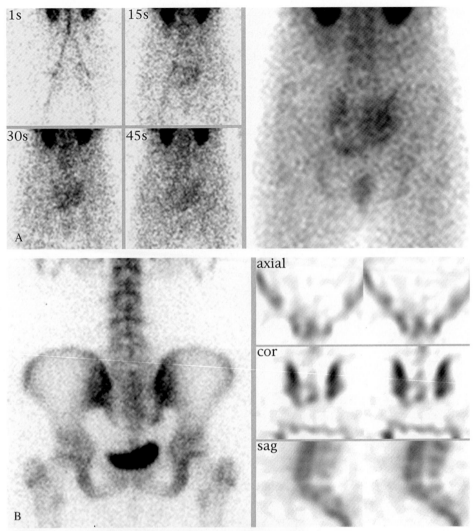

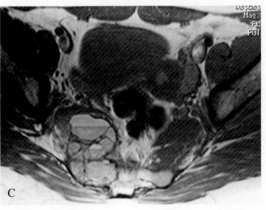

FIGURE 13.57. Aneurysmal bone cyst. A: Skeletal scintigraphy was performed to assess a 13-year-old girl who had experienced 6 weeks of pain in the right buttock and posterior thigh. Selected frames from angiographic and tissue phase imaging (posterior projection) show high localization related to the right middle to lower sacrum and sacroiliac joint. B: Skeletal phase imaging demonstrates only subtle findings. Posterior planar imaging and SPECT show mildly high uptake along the inferolateral margin of the middle to lower right sacrum. SPECT also reveals a region of low uptake. C: Magnetic resonance imaging (fast spin echo) shows multiple fluid-fluid levels in the lesion. (*Source:* Rajadhyaksha et al.[160] with permission.)

association between endocrine dysfunctions, particularly precocious sexual development in girls, with the polyostotic form (McCune-Albright syndrome).[163,164]

Any bone can be affected. Monostotic disease most frequently involves the ribs, femur, tibia, and craniofacial bones. Polyostotic disease is typically unilateral or, when bilateral, markedly asymmetric. The femur, tibia, pelvis, and foot are most commonly affected. Rib, craniofacial, and upper extremity lesions are also relatively common. In both forms, craniofacial involvement characteristically affects the skull base and the sinuses.[163]

The radiographic appearance of fibrous dysplasia varies. The most characteristic finding is mild expansion of a bone by an ill-defined homogeneous radiolucency with poorly structured trabeculations. The lesions are often described as flame-shaped and of a ground-glass appearance. A thick sclerotic margin is sometimes present.[163] The lesions of fibrous dysplasia typically show high uptake (Fig. 13.58) due to the presence of immature woven bone and associated abnormal ossification.

Osteochondroma and Enchondroma

Osteochondroma (exostosis), the most common benign tumor of bone, appears radiologically as a sessile or pedunculated osseous excrescence whose cortex and medullary cavity are continuous with those of adjacent normal bone (Fig. 13.59). Osteochondromas typically arise in a metaphysis, most commonly about the knee. Most occur sporadically, but small osteochondromas may result from radiation therapy during childhood.[165] Computed tomography or MRI can demonstrate a thick cartilaginous cap during childhood. Multiple osteochondromas occur in patients with hereditary multiple exostoses. This skeletal dysplasia predominantly affects males and is typically diagnosed by age 2 years. Marked modeling abnormalities, including shortening, broadening, and metaphyseal flaring, are present.[33,166]

An enchondroma is a benign tumor of mature hyaline cartilage (Fig. 13.60). The vast majority of enchondromas occur as solitary lesions and appear radiographically as expansile lucent lesions. Punctate calcifications are present in enchondromas of older children and adults. The most common locations are the metacarpals and phalanges, but any bone preformed in cartilage can be affected.[166] Multiple enchondromas occur sporadically and in enchondromatosis (Ollier's disease). Bowing and shortening deformities and pathologic fractures are common with enchondromatosis.

Benign cartilaginous tumors are at risk for malignant transformation, mainly to chondrosarcoma and predominantly in the conditions with multiple lesions.[166]

The degree of uptake in osteochondromas and enchondromas varies. High uptake in these lesions results from hyperemia, enchondral ossification, and reactive bone formation. High uptake is typically depicted in the cartilaginous cap of osteochondromas in the immature skeleton. Skeletal scintigraphy does not distinguish lesions that have undergone malignant transformation from those that have not. Proposed criteria for this distinction, including uptake that increases over time, high uptake after skeletal maturity, and high uptake relative to an internal standard such as bone along the sacroiliac joint, have not been validated. Normal or low uptake relative to adjacent bone does not exclude malignant transformation.[167-170]

Infantile Cortical Hyperostosis

Infantile cortical hyperostosis, also known as Caffey disease, is a disease of unknown etiology characterized by hyperplasia of subperiosteal bone and soft tissue swelling. It occurs during infancy. The mandible is the most common site. Lesions have also been observed in the skull, clavicles, ribs, scapulae, long bones, and metatarsals. Recovery is the rule and usually occurs within weeks to a year. Radiographs show cortical thickening and periosteal new bone formation. During healing there may be laminated periosteal reaction, cortical thinning, and increase in bone size.[171,172] During the active

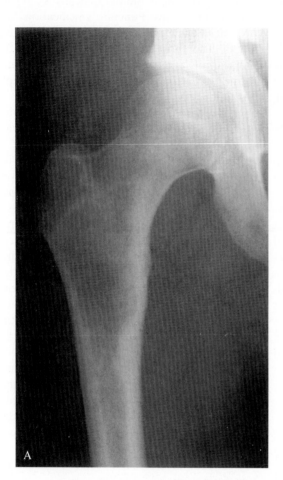

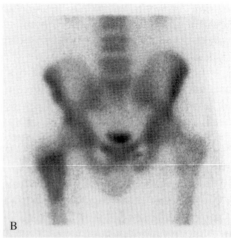

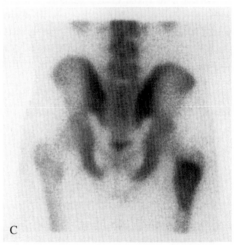

FIGURE 13.58. Fibrous dysplasia. A radiograph reveals a ground-glass radiolucency of the right femur with thinning of the endosteal cortex (A). Skeletal scintigraphy in the anterior (B) and poste- rior (C) projections demonstrates high uptake along the lesion's periphery. (*Source:* Connolly and Treves,[2] with permission.)

phase of the disease, skeletal scintigraphy reveals intense uptake in the involved bone.

Langerhans Cell Histiocytosis

Langerhans cell histiocytosis (LCH), formerly referred to as histiocytosis X, is a disease char- acterized by nonneoplastic proliferation of Langerhans cells.[173] These cells arise in the bone marrow or from cells that originate in the bone marrow and mature in the epidermis, dermal lymphatics, and lymph nodes. Langerhans cells present antigens to T lymphocytes. Birbeck granules, which are centrally striated rod- shaped organelles, are their distinctive feature.[174] Langerhans cell histiocytosis has been postulated to result from abnormal immune regulation[173] and clonal cellular proliferation.[175]

Although histologically benign, LCH may follow an aggressive clinical course. It

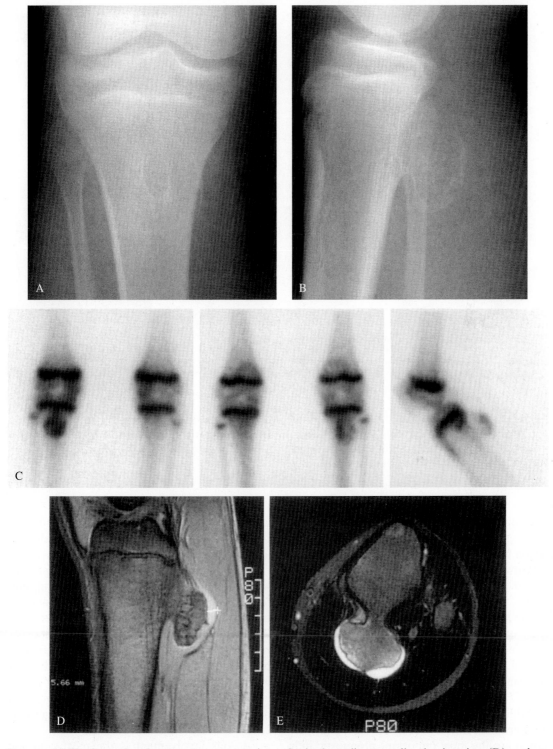

FIGURE 13.59. Osteochondroma. Anteroposterior (A) and lateral (B) radiographs of the right tibia show an osteochondroma. High uptake overlying the right metadiaphyseal tibia on anterior and posterior images is shown to correspond to the periphery of the osteochondroma in a lateral projection (C). Sagittal gradient recall echo imaging (D) and an axial T2-weighted image (E) show an approximately 5.7-mm-thick cartilaginous cap that corresponds to the site of high uptake. (*Source:* Connolly and Treves,[2] with permission.)

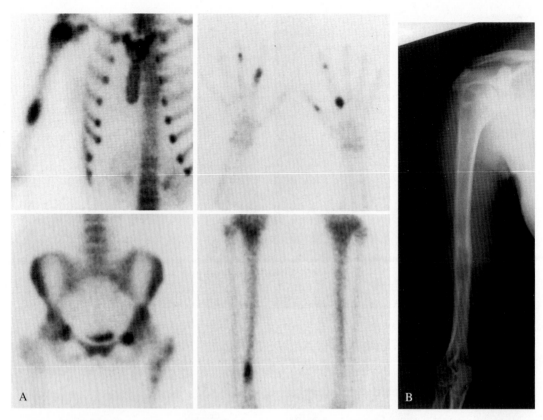

FIGURE 13.60. Enchondromas. A: Areas of high uptake are present in the right humerus, sternal manubrium, multiple phalanges of the hands, the left acetabulum, the left femur, and the right tibia. B: A correlative radiograph demonstrate a radiolucent lesions in the right humerus. (*Source:* Connolly and Treves,[2] with permission.)

encompasses a wide spectrum of disease ranging from a single, self-limited skeletal lesion to disseminated, often fatal, visceral and marrow infiltration. The classic clinical groupings of disease patterns as eosinophilic granuloma, Hand-Schüller-Christian disease, and Letterer-Siwe disease were differentiated on the basis of their clinical course and the extent to which bone and the reticuloendothelial system are involved. Because significant overlap exists between these syndromes, cases of LCH are more accurately classified on an individual basis without reference to these eponyms. Extent of disease and age at presentation are the most important prognostic indicators.[14] Children less than 2 years of age with disseminated disease have a high likelihood of disease progression and the poorest prognosis.

Children who present with disease limited to bone are unlikely to develop systemic disease and have a favorable prognosis.[173,176]

Children with osseous LCH often present with localized pain, soft tissue swelling, and tenderness. Clinical presentation occasionally mimics that of osteomyelitis.[173] Children with disseminated disease may present with nonspecific systemic signs or with complaints referable to sites of involvement, such as the liver or lungs. Diabetes insipidus can result from extension of skull or orbital lesions or from neurohypophyseal infiltration of Langerhans cells.[177]

Osseous involvement is the most common manifestation of LCH. Lesions in the skull, mandible, spine, pelvis, and ribs account for about two thirds of lesions.[178] Long bones, where the lesions are usually diaphyseal, occasionally metaphyseal, and rarely epiphyseal,[173] are involved in about one third of cases.[178] The radiographic appearance of osseous LCH varies. The most common appearance is a lytic lesion with little or no reactive bone formation. A characteristic finding is a lytic skull lesion with beveled edges due to uneven destruction of the inner and outer tables. In the spine, the vertebral body is usually involved; vertebra plana results in some cases.[33]

On skeletal scintigraphy (Figs. 13.61 and 13.62), LCH lesions often demonstrate low uptake with or without surrounding high uptake. In some cases, only high uptake, which may be intense, is apparent. High uptake is due to osseous repair rather than the lesion itself. Lesions that incite little or no reparative response are quite subtle and difficult to identify.

Whether skeletal scintigraphy or the radiographic skeletal survey is more sensitive for detecting osseous lesions of LCH has been the subject of controversy. The conventional teaching that radiographs are more sensitive is largely based on comparisons using

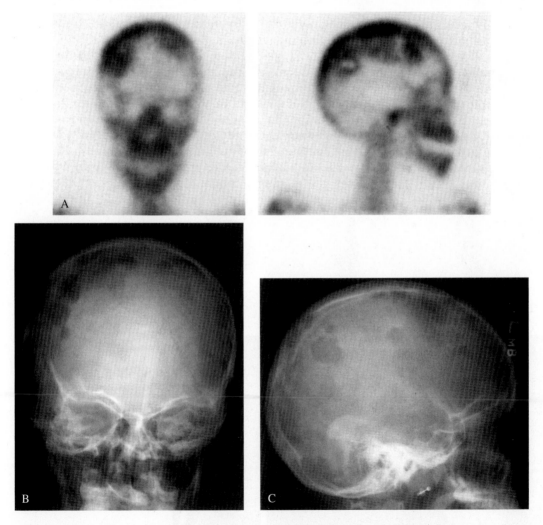

FIGURE 13.61. Langerhans cell histiocytosis. A: Anterior and lateral images depict extensive areas of low and high uptake within the skull. B,C: Correlative radiographs show multiple radiolucencies. (*Source:* Connolly and Treves,[2] with permission.)

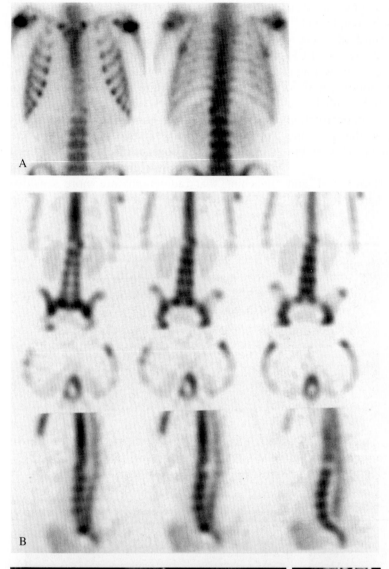

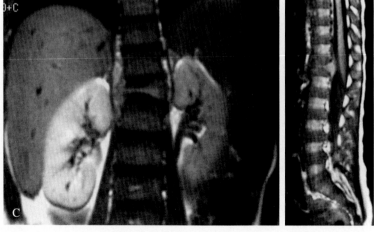

FIGURE 13.62. Langerhans cell histiocytosis. A: An anterior planar image reveals low uptake in the right aspect of T12 and high uptake in the left aspect of that vertebrae on anterior and posterior images. B: The distribution of radiotracer is better depicted with SPECT. C: MRI shows collapse of the central and right portions of the T12 vertebral body. Posterior displacement of the conus is depicted on the sagittal MRI. (*Source:* Connolly and Treves,[2] with permission.)

early-generation gamma cameras, studies comparing scintigrams performed following therapy with plain films obtained prior to therapy, studies in which plain films were interpreted with knowledge of scintigraphic findings, and studies that did not separate lesions according to anatomic regions.[179] More recent work indicates that scintigraphy is more sensitive for detecting lesions at some locations, mainly the ribs, spine, and pelvis, and plain films are more sensitive for detecting lesions at other sites, particularly the skull.[180] Lesion detection is therefore optimized by combined radiographic and scintigraphic imaging.

Treatments of osseous LCH include observation without intervention, surgical excision, radiation therapy, and intralesional steroid administration. Multiagent chemotherapy is used in cases with systemic involvement.[173] Bone marrow transplantation is used in some children with disseminated involvement.[181]

Oncology

Osteosarcoma

Osteosarcoma is the most common primary bone malignancy of childhood. This tumor usually originates within the medullary space. It occasionally arises from the surface of a bone in periosteal and parosteal forms. Histologically, the diagnosis of osteosarcoma requires neoplastic osteoid and osseous tissue. Chondroid or fibrous tissue is frequently present. Osteosarcoma is classified as osteoblastic, chondroblastic, fibroblastic, or of mixed cellularity based on the relative distribution of tissue types or as telangiectatic when there are large cystic spaces containing blood, scant osteoid, and massive cellular necrosis. The tumor is graded as high or low based on aggressiveness and degree of cellular differentiation.[182]

The incidence of osteosarcoma peaks between the ages of 15 and 25 years. Children younger than 6 years of age are very rarely affected. Patients typically present with localized pain, swelling, or both.[166] Pathologic fracture occurs in about 5% of cases. Fracture disrupts barriers to tumor spread and worsens prognosis.[14,183] Osteosarcoma is predominantly a lesion of the long bones, where it is typically metaphyseal in location. The distal femur, proximal tibia, and proximal humerus are most commonly affected.[166,182] Flat bones are involved in 10% of cases.[14]

The etiology is unknown. In a minority of cases, osteosarcoma develops as a late complication of radiation therapy or chemotherapy. Children with the genetic or hereditary type of retinoblastoma are predisposed to osteosarcoma; this risk is increased by radiation or chemotherapy.[184,185] Very rarely, osteosarcoma develops in benign lesions including fibrous dysplasia, infarction, chronic osteomyelitis, osteoblastoma, and aneurysmal bone cyst.[182,184,186,187]

The most common locations of osteosarcoma metastases are lung and bone. Pulmonary metastases usually precede skeletal metastases. Skeletal metastases involve sites distant from the primary tumor or the same bone in which the primary tumor is located (skip metastasis). A small percentage of patients have multiple skeletal lesions at diagnosis (osteosarcomatosis). Osteosarcomatosis is likely due to skeletal metastases rather than multiple primary lesions in most cases.[188]

The treatment of choice for osteosarcoma is wide resection. Reconstruction with a cadaveric allograft, bone prosthesis, or both is often performed.[183] Chemotherapy is used pre- and postoperatively. Other treatments include tibiofemoral rotationplasty for distal femoral osteosarcoma and amputation. The choice of procedure depends on multiple factors that include the overall prospects for survival, psychological effects, estimated likelihood of recurrence, and probability of restoring function.[183] The 10-year survival rate of osteosarcoma patients exceeds 70%.[189] Death is frequently due to pulmonary metastatic disease and rarely to local recurrence. The highest survival rates are realized in patients without metastatic disease at presentation and greater than 90% to 95% tumoral necrosis following preoperative chemotherapy.[190,191]

The radiographic appearance of osteosarcoma reflects bone production and destruction. Radiographs typically reveal a large bone-forming lesion. Radiolucent areas of lysis are frequently intermixed with radiodense areas of sclerosis. In some tumors, particularly aggressive and telangiectatic lesions, the lytic component predominates. The cortex is destroyed and an aggressive-appearing periosteal reaction, such as a Codman's triangle or a spiculated "sunburst" pattern, is often present. There is usually an associated soft tissue mass that may contain areas of malignant bone.[14]

The primary tumor typically demonstrates marked uptake on skeletal scintigraphy (Figs. 13.63 and 13.64).[192] Regions of low uptake within viable nonossified tumor and necrotic tumor are also frequently present (Fig. 13.64). High uptake often extends beyond the pathologic confines of the tumor, so skeletal scintigraphy does not effectively define tumoral margins.[193–195] This extended pattern usually involves bone in continuity with, or immedi-

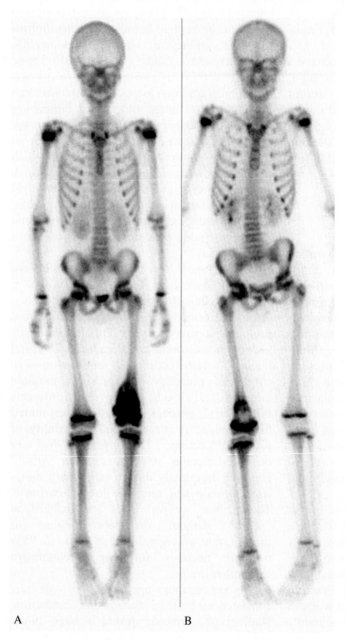

A   B

FIGURE 13.63. A: Marked uptake is shown in a left distal femoral osteosarcoma. B: In another patient, a mixed pattern of high and low uptake is associated with a right distal femoral osteosarcoma that extended from the distal diaphysis to the physis. The asymmetrically higher uptake in uninvolved femur and tibia is due to hyperemia. (*Source:* Connolly et al.,[192] with permission.)

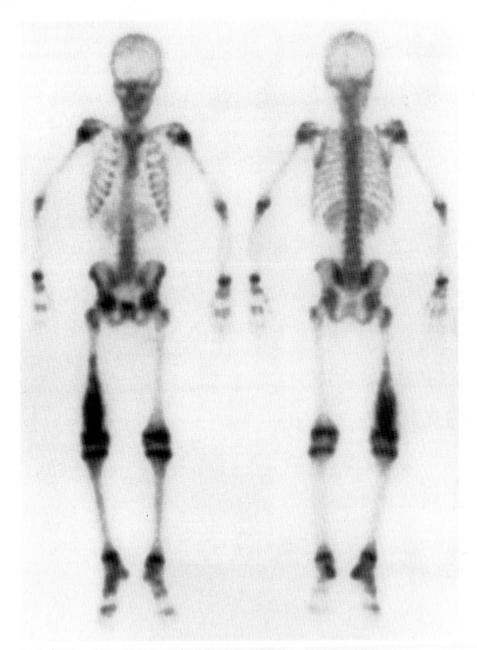

FIGURE 13.64. Metastatic osteosarcoma. Anterior and posterior whole-body images show intense uptake in a right femoral osteosarcoma. Separate foci of high uptake in the mid-diaphysis and at the level of the lesser trochanter indicate skip metastases. (*Source:* Connolly and Treves,[2] with permission.)

ately across the joint adjacent to, the tumor, but can involve an entire ipsilateral extremity. Marrow hyperemia, medullary reactive bone, and periosteal new bone have been demonstrated in some cases that exhibited this pattern.[193]

Skeletal scintigraphy is used for the detection of metastases at diagnosis and during follow-up. Skeletal metastases appear as areas of high uptake (Figs. 13.64 and 13.65) and are often radiographically occult or asymptomatic.[196,197] Skeletal metastases may demonstrate the

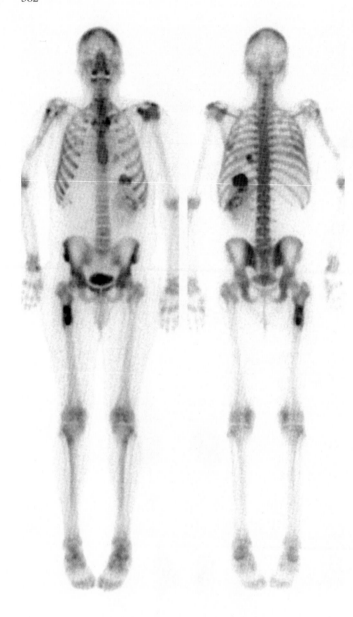

FIGURE 13.65. Metastatic osteosarcoma. A skeletal metastasis in the right proximal femur and nonskeletal metastases involving the left lung, left adrenal gland, and left kidney are shown in a patient who underwent resection of a right humeral osteosarcoma and allograft reconstruction 7 years previously. High uptake along the right humeral allograft is due to an old allograft fracture. (*Source:* Connolly et al.,[192] with permission.)

scintigraphic flare phenomenon during therapy.[198] This pattern is characterized by increasing intensity of uptake at sites of known metastases or by the appearance of new foci of high uptake on a study obtained within months of a therapeutic intervention despite clinical improvement.[199] It is likely due to bone repair. The flare phenomenon should be considered in patients who appear to be responding well clinically. Excluding disease progression remains the primary concern, particularly when new abnormalities are detected. Unfortunately, a patient's subsequent clinical and imaging course are the only reliable arbiters in some cases. Skeletal scintigraphy typically shows regression of a flare phenomenon over 4 to 6 months.[199] Skeletal scintigraphy may show extraosseous metastases due to osteoid production (Fig. 13.65).[196,200–202]

When interpreting follow-up studies, imaging specialists must be familiar with the normal appearance of allografts and amputation stumps.

Transplantation of a cadaveric bone allograft is frequently performed as part of a limb-sparing procedure. The goal is to preserve function. Intercalary allografts reestablish a segment of a long bone exclusive of the epiphysis and articulating surfaces. Osteoarticular allografts include the epiphysis and articulating surfaces. Allografts are incorporated into the skeleton by a process referred to as creeping substitution. After capillaries invade the allograft, osteocytes deposit new bone on the allograft matrix and resorb the allogeneic bone.[203–205] A study on retrieved cadaveric bone allografts shows that this process is limited to the allograft ends and superficial layers and involves no more than 20% of the allogeneic bone by 5 years.[206]

Allografts have a characteristic scintigraphic appearance that reflects their incorporation process (Figs. 13.66 to 13.68). A cadaveric bone allograft usually appears as an area of low to absent uptake. A peripheral rim of uptake that slightly exceeds uptake in soft tissue is often present.[207] The rim likely represents a thin seam of new bone that develops on allograft surfaces.[206] The scintigraphic appearance has been described as being tramline.[208] With long-term follow-up, uptake may become more diffuse in the allograft.[209] High uptake is typically present at the junction between native and allograft bone and at sites of plate and screw fixation. High uptake is often identified along joint surfaces articulating with an allograft. This is attributable to stress-induced changes in host joints secondary to degeneration of allograft cartilage.[206] Complications, the most common of which is fracture,[209] alter the scintigraphic appearance of allografts. Allograft fractures usually occur 2 years or longer postoperatively and result from mechanical stress (Fig. 13.69). Fractures that occur within 18 months of surgery are usually due to rejection and associated with allograft dissolution.[210] Most allograft infections occur in the first months postoperatively.[211] Local recurrence usually occurs in host bone or adjacent soft tissue but may extend to involve the allograft (Fig. 13.70).[208]

Skeletal scintigraphy typically reveals evidence of bone stress after lower extremity allograft reconstruction or amputation. Typical locations of skeletal stress are the lower extremity contralateral to an allograft or ampu-

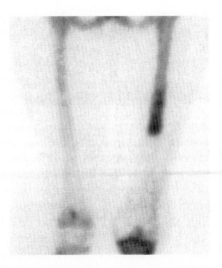
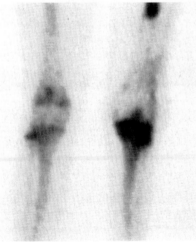

FIGURE 13.66. Allograft. Osteoarticular allograft. A distal left femoral osteoarticular allograft appears as an area of low to absent uptake. Its periphery is outlined by a rim of uptake slightly greater than that in adjacent soft tissues. High uptake in the left mid-femoral diaphysis is due to a plate and screw fixation device. High uptake is demonstrated in the articulating surfaces of the tibia. (*Source:* Connolly and Treves,[2] with permission.)

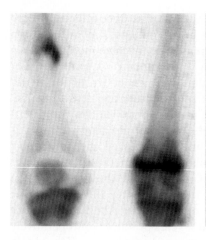 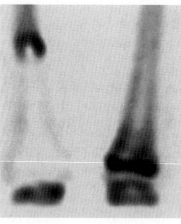

FIGURE 13.67. Osteoarticular allograft. High uptake is present at the junction with native bone and in the articulating tibial plateaus. Planar imaging (left panel) and SPECT (right panel) show uptake faintly outlining the allograft. (*Source:* Connolly and Treves,[2] with permission.)

tation, the lower extremity ipsilateral to an allograft, and the pelvis. On a single study, the distinction between skeletal stress and metastatic disease can be difficult, leaving individual practitioners to rely heavily on their previous experience. In general, stress changes tend to appear as more diffuse abnormalities. Focal abnormalities due to osteosarcoma metastases tend to show more intense uptake than do those

related to bone stress. There is considerable overlap, however, and some uncertainties are resolved only by clinical follow-up and additional imaging with radiography, CT, or MRI. Following amputation and the fitting of a prosthesis, high uptake is commonly seen at the tip of the bone through which amputation has been performed.[212] With tibiofemoral rotationplasty, stress changes are also apparent, particularly in the foot and ankle that act on the prosthesis (Fig. 13.71).

Ewing Sarcoma

Ewing sarcoma is the second most common primary bone malignancy of childhood. Ewing sarcoma has several different genotypes that share a common neuroectodermal origin and, with primitive neuroectodermal tumor (PNET), constitute what is considered a group of related tumors.[213] Ewing sarcoma is composed of small round cells. Absence of lobular rosettes, neuron specific enolase, and neurosecretory granules helps differentiate Ewing sarcoma from PNET.[214] The histologic features of Ewing sarcoma resemble those of other small round cell tumors of childhood, such as neuroblastoma, leukemia, and lymphoma.[215,216] The incidence of Ewing sarcoma is highest in the second decade of life. Almost all cases occur between the ages of 5 and 30 years. Caucasians are predominantly affected.[14,33,166,182]

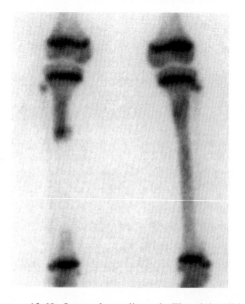

FIGURE 13.68. Intercalary allograft. The right tibial allograft appears as a region of absent uptake. High up-take is present at the proximal junction with the native bone. (*Source:* Connolly and Treves,[2] with permission.)

Pain and swelling are the most common symptoms. A palpable mass is often present. The patient may be febrile. Hematologic analysis

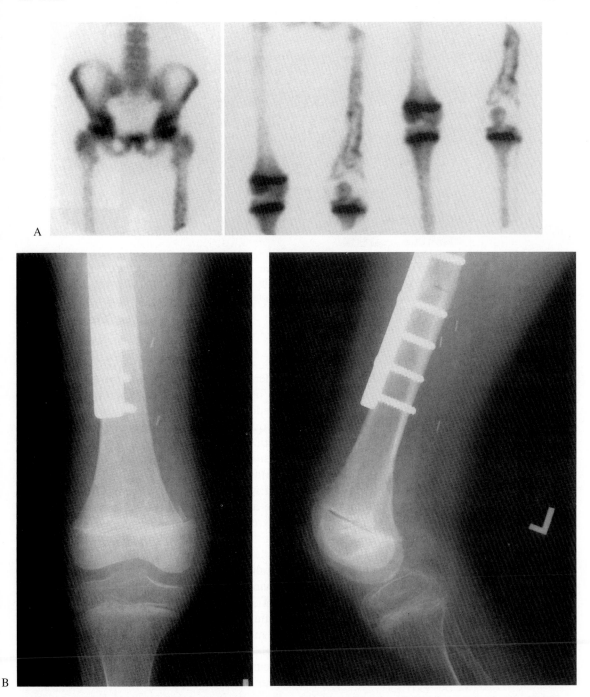

FIGURE 13.69. Allograft fracture. A 9-year-old girl had an osteosarcoma of her left distal femur, which was resected. A skeletally immature allograft was used for limb salvage. A: Skeletal scintigraphy shows uptake within the allograft that is variably of lesser and greater intensity to that in native bone. B: Anteroposterior and lateral radiographs reveal separation of the allograft epiphysis and a small metaphyseal fracture fragment medial to the distal femur. (*Source:* Connolly and Treves,[2] with permission.)

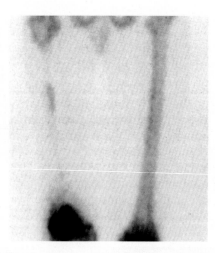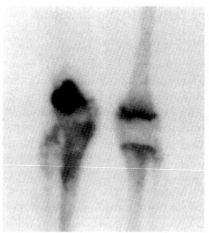

FIGURE 13.70. Local recurrence and metastases following allograft. High uptake in the right distal femur and proximal tibia is secondary to recurrent and metastatic disease in this child who had undergone allograft reconstruction following excision of a right femoral osteosarcoma. (*Source:* Connolly and Treves,[2] with permission.)

reveals elevation of the ESR, leukocytosis, and anemia in some cases. The constellation of clinical and hematologic findings occasionally suggests a diagnosis of osteomyelitis.[14,33,166,182]

In patients up to the age of 20 years, Ewing sarcoma most often affects the appendicular skeleton, particularly the femur, tibia, and humerus. Ewing sarcoma of the long bones is centered in the metaphysis slightly more often than the diaphysis. Metaphyseal lesions are typically eccentrically positioned and tend to extend into the diaphysis. Pelvic, rib, and vertebral lesions predominate in patients older than 20 years of age.[14] Skeletal metastases often precede pulmonary metastases and are present in 10% to 20% of patients at diagnosis.[33] Therapy entails multiagent chemotherapy for eradication of microscopic or overt metastatic disease and irradiation and/or surgery for control of the primary lesion. Because late recurrence is not uncommon, resection of the primary tumor has gained favor.[217]

Ewing sarcoma is usually revealed with radiographs. Permeative, poorly marginated osteolysis and a thin, laminated or spiculated periosteal reaction are relatively common findings. Reactive bone is common in flat bones and in cancellous bone of the metaphysis and ribs.

Sclerosis is occasionally intermixed with areas of osteolysis. Ewing sarcoma rarely appears predominantly sclerotic. A soft tissue mass is frequently present. Ewing sarcoma may be entirely or predominantly within the soft tissues and can erode a bone's cortical surface.[14,33]

Ewing sarcoma usually causes high uptake in the affected bone (Figs. 13.72 to 13.74). Some aggressive lesions appear as areas of predominantly or entirely low uptake.[218] An extended pattern occurs in some cases.[166] Skeletal tracer localization in the soft tissue component of a Ewing sarcoma is occasionally observed.

The primary role of skeletal scintigraphy in patients with Ewing sarcoma is to detect skeletal metastases, which typically appear as focally high uptake (Fig. 13.74). A flare response may occur in skeletal metastases of patients treated with chemotherapy. Increasing localization in the soft tissue component of Ewing sarcoma has been reported as a manifestation of the flare phenomenon.[190]

Nonskeletal Malignancies

Skeletal scintigraphy is used in staging and during follow-up of a number of nonskeletal

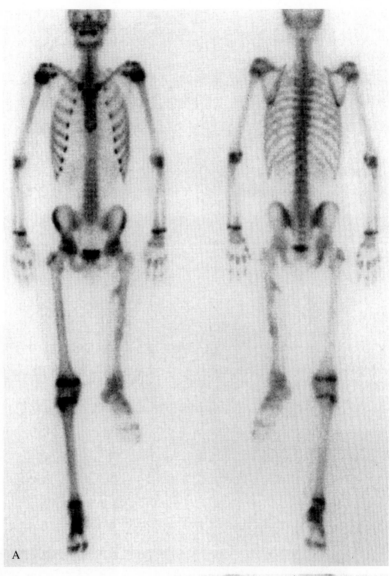

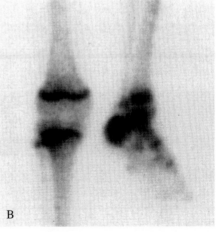

FIGURE 13.71. Femorotibial rotationplasty. A: Whole-body images of a 15-year-old following left femorotibial rotationplasty. B: One year later, there is diffusely high uptake in the left calcaneus secondary to fracture. (*Source:* Connolly and Treves,[2] with permission.)

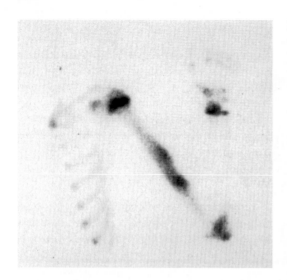

FIGURE 13.72. Ewing sarcoma. Skeletal scintigraphy demonstrates high uptake surrounding an area of cortical excavation in the left midhumeral diaphysis. (*Source:* Connolly and Treves,[2] with permission.)

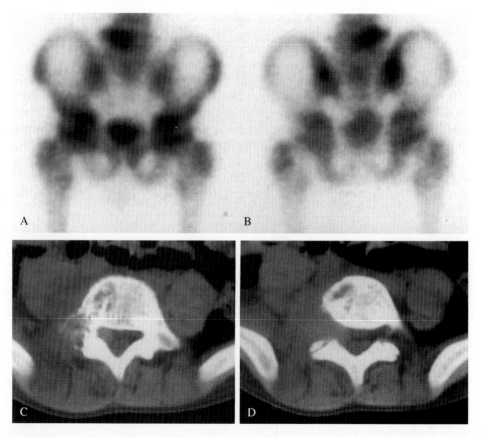

FIGURE 13.73. Ewing sarcoma. Skeletal scintigraphy (A: anterior; B: posterior) shows marked uptake at L5. Computed tomography (C,D) shows permeative osteolysis of the right L5 pedicle and the right side of the vertebral body. A soft tissue component extends into the L5-S1 neural foramen (D). (*Source:* Connolly and Treves,[2] with permission.)

FIGURE 13.74. Metastatic Ewing sarcoma. Metastases from a lesion in the right proximal femur are shown in the left femur, the right proximal humerus, and the left mid-humerus.

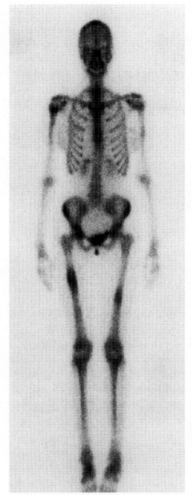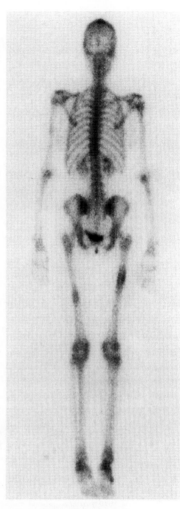

malignancies in children, most importantly neuroblastoma, some lymphomas, medulloblastoma, rhabdomyosarcoma, retinoblastoma, and renal tumors other than Wilms' tumor. Nonskeletal malignancies, particularly neuroblastoma and leukemia, are occasionally first indicated by skeletal scintigraphy when the presenting symptoms are caused by skeletal metastases.[3,30] A characteristic appearance of neuroblastoma results from localization of tracer in the primary tumor (Figs. 13.75 and 13.76), which occurs in 40% to 85% of cases, along with multiple skeletal sites of abnormal uptake.[219-223] Although as many as 80% of children with leukemia may have skeletal abnormalities that are associated with abnormal uptake,[224] skeletal scintigraphy is not routinely

performed because osseous disease does not affect treatment or prognosis.

Skeletal metastases most often appear as sites of high uptake (Fig. 13.77). Low uptake may occur with aggressive lesions or ischemia. Skeletal metastases that exhibit low uptake are most closely associated with neuroblastoma and leukemia, although metastases of these tumors more often show high uptake. Some skeletal metastases cause relatively little or no alteration in uptake. Metaphyseal lesions are especially notorious for escaping detection in children with neuroblastoma and are partly responsible for the higher diagnostic yield of metaiodobenzylguanidine (MIBG) scintigraphy (Figs. 13.76 and 13.77) for detecting skeletal disease in that malignancy. Skeletal scintigraphy

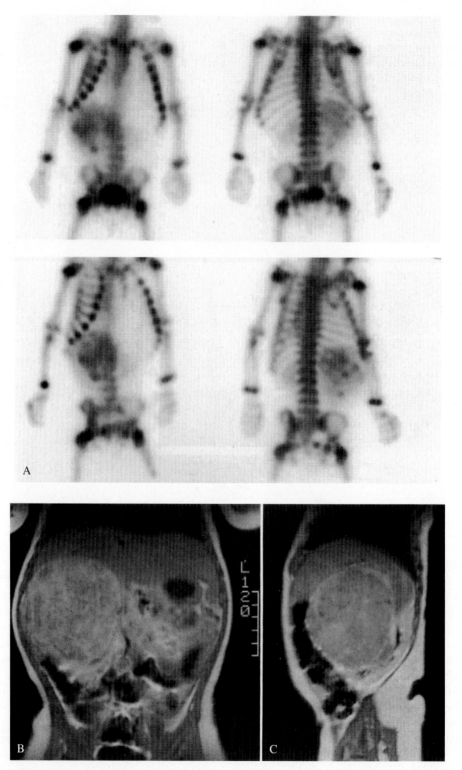

FIGURE 13.75. Neuroblastoma. Skeletal scintigraphy (A) shows abnormal tracer localization within the right upper quadrant (anterior, posterior, right anterior oblique, and right posterior oblique projections). Gadolinium-enhanced T1-weighted coronal (B) and sagittal (C) images demonstrate a large heterogenously enhancing right adrenal mass. (*Source:* Connolly and Treves,[2] with permission.)

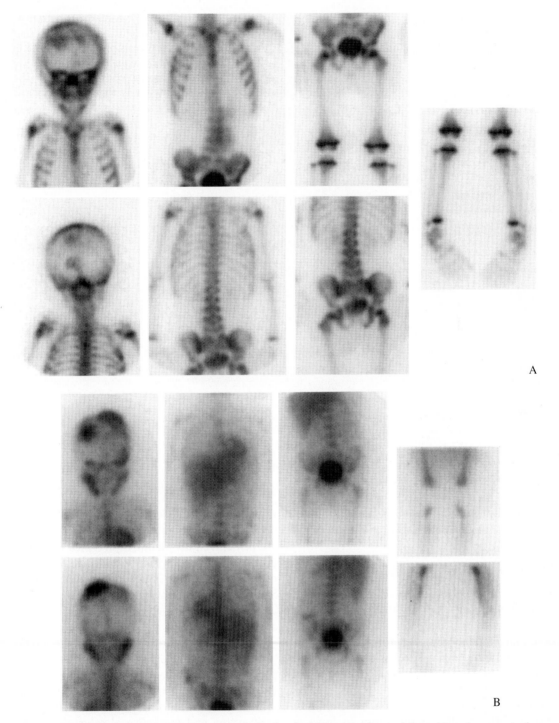

FIGURE 13.76. Metastatic neuroblastoma. A: Skeletal scintigraphy reveals tracer localization in the soft tissues to the left of the lumbar spine (upper row: anterior projection; lower row: posterior projection; tibiae: anterior projection). Multiple foci of high uptake are depicted in the calvarium, periorbital facial bones, spine, pelvis, and long bone metaphyses. B: The abnormal foci shown by skeletal scintigraphy correspond to sites of abnormal ^{123}I-MIBG uptake in this child with a paraortic neuroblastoma and widespread metastases. (*Source:* Connolly and Treves,[2] with permission.)

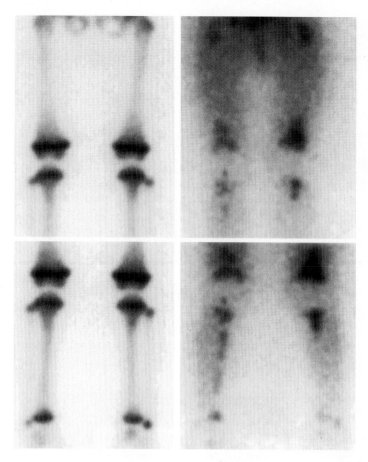

FIGURE 13.77. Metastatic neuroblastoma. Skeletal scintigraphy (left panels) reveals prominent uptake in the proximal and distal femoral and tibial metaphyses bilaterally. The distribution is slightly asymmetric, being greater in the left than right distal femoral and proximal metaphyses. Metastatic disease is confirmed with ^{123}I-MIBG imaging (right panels). (*Source:* Connolly and Treves,[2] with permission.)

occasionally shows tracer accumulation in nonskeletal metastases of neuroblastoma.[225,226]

Skeletal Effects of Antineoplastic Therapy

The risk of radiation injury is greater in the growing skeleton than in the mature adult skeleton. This risk increases with the growth potential of bone and therefore is highest in young children and at sites of active growth. Growth may be disturbed in bone exposed to a radiation dose of 400 cGy and can be arrested with exposure to 1200 to 2000 cGy (Fig. 13.78).[227–229] Radiation injury to bone is most closely associated with regional high-dose therapy, in which case the changes are confined to the radiation port. Total body irradiation, as is used prior to bone marrow transplantation, places the entire immature skeleton at risk for

radiation injury.[230] Radiation exerts its effect primarily on osteoblasts and leads to immediate or delayed cell death, injury with recovery, arrested cellular division, abnormal repair, or neoplasia. Vascular injury also plays a role.[229] Skeletal abnormalities due to radiation therapy include growth disturbance, avascular necrosis, and neoplasia.

Radiation injury of the long bones is manifested radiographically as abnormal tubulation, premature epiphyseal fusion, physeal widening due to arrested physeal ossification, metaphyseal fraying due to impaired endochondral ossification, and metaphyseal sclerosis due to increased mineral deposition and deficient chondroclasis and osteoclasis.[14] Radiation injury of the femoral capital epiphysis radiographically simulates Legg-Calvé-Perthes disease, and radiation injury to the proximal

FIGURE 13.78. Radiation effect. Skeletal scintigraphy was performed in a 15-year-old girl who had undergone pelvic radiation for treatment of bladder rhabdomyosarcoma at the age of 18 months and had a right slipped femoral capital epiphysis. Whole-body images show a disproportionately small pelvis as well as high physeal uptake associated with the known injury. (*Source:* Stauss et al.,[227] with permission.)

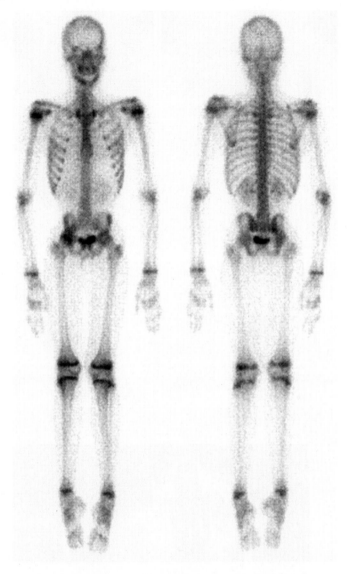

femoral physis may lead to a SCFE.[231] Impaired endochondral ossification in vertebral bodies produces end-plate irregularity, an altered trabecular pattern, and loss of vertebral height. Kyphosis and scoliosis may result.[228,229] Early following radiation therapy, there is high uptake due to hyperemia and inflammation. Later, there is low uptake due to decreased vascularity (Fig. 13.79).

Benign or malignant bone lesions occasionally develop secondary to radiation therapy. The most common lesion is osteochondroma,

which may arise in any bone subjected to radiation in the range of 1200 cGy or greater. This lesion typically arises within 5 years of treatment.[165] Osteosarcoma may develop years after radiation therapy. Children with hereditary retinoblastoma are especially prone to this complication (Fig. 13.80). To be considered a radiation-induced sarcoma, a tumor must develop along the path of a radiation beam at least 3 years after radiation therapy. The mean latent period is 11 years. A radiation dose of 3000 cGy is usually required.[229]

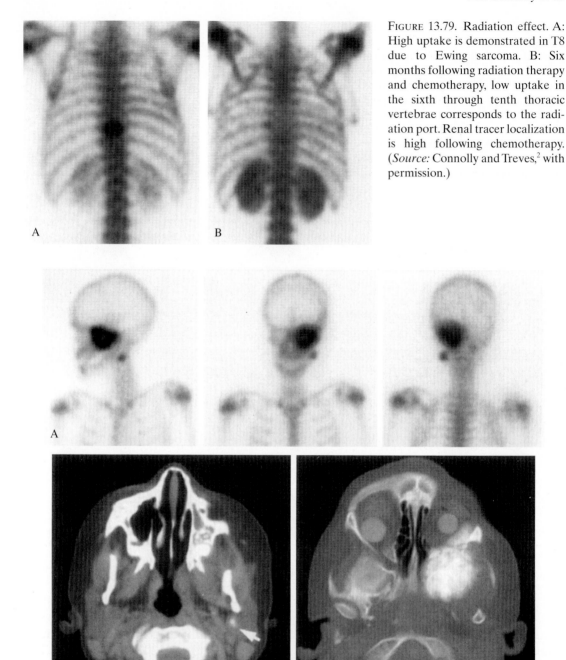

FIGURE 13.79. Radiation effect. A: High uptake is demonstrated in T8 due to Ewing sarcoma. B: Six months following radiation therapy and chemotherapy, low uptake in the sixth through tenth thoracic vertebrae corresponds to the radiation port. Renal tracer localization is high following chemotherapy. (*Source:* Connolly and Treves,[2] with permission.)

FIGURE 13.80. Osteosarcoma following radiation. This 6-year-old boy was diagnosed with bilateral familial retinoblastoma at 2 years of age. Treatment had included radiation, chemotherapy, and bilateral enucleation. A: Left lateral, anterior, and posterior skeletal scintigraphy images depict intense uptake in the left orbit and a focus of high localization related to the left mandible. B: Computed tomography shows the latter finding to be due to a calcified metastasis within the parotid nodal tissue (white arrow). C: The primary mass, which demonstrates whorl-like osseous matrix on CT, arose from the greater wing of the sphenoid bone and the lateral orbital wall. Note the bilateral ophthalmic prostheses. (*Source:* Connolly and Treves,[2] with permission.)

Chemotherapy is associated with induction of second malignancies, including osteosarcoma in children who have received alkylating agents, and disturbed bone formation. Methotrexate osteopathy is a particularly important bone formation disturbance associated with chemotherapy in children. It most often affects children receiving low-dose, long-term, oral-maintenance methotrexate for acute leukemia but may also occur with high-dose, short-term, intravenous methotrexate therapy.[232] Methotrexate osteopathy is a possible etiology for metaphyseal foci of high uptake in children receiving, or who have recently received, this agent. Correlation with radiographs permits the diagnosis to be reached. Severe osteopenia, dense zones of provisional calcification, transverse metaphyseal bands, and metaphyseal fractures are typically evident radiographically.[232] Other skeletal abnormalities related to chemotherapeutic regimens include ifosfamide-induced hypophosphatemic rickets[233] and steroid osteopathy. Inclusion of colony-stimulating factors in pediatric chemotherapeutic regimens may be associated with prominent axial and juxtaarticular uptake similar to what has been described in adults.[234]

References

1. Lim R, Fahey FH, Laffin S, et al. Early experience with fluorine-18 bone PET in young athletes (abstract). J Nucl Med 2005; in press.
2. Connolly LP, Treves ST. Pediatric Skeletal Scintigraphy: With Multimodality Imaging Correlation. New York: Springer-Verlag, 1998.
3. Shalaby-Rana E, Majd M. (99m)Tc-MDP scintigraphic findings in children with leukemia: value of early and delayed whole-body imaging. J Nucl Med 2001;42(6):878–83.
4. Connolly LP, Treves ST, Connolly SA, et al. Pediatric skeletal scintigraphy: applications of pinhole magnification. Radiographics 1998; 18(2):341–51.
5. Christensen SB, Krogsgaard OW. Localization of Tc-99m MDP in epiphyseal growth plates of rats. J Nucl Med 1981;22(3):237–45.
6. Comar CL, Lotz WE, Boyd GA. Autoradiographic studies of calcium, phosphorus and strontium distribution in the bones of the growing pig. Am J Anat 1952;90(1):113–29.
7. Ogden JA, Conlogue GJ, Bronson ML, et al. Radiology of postnatal skeletal development. II. The manubrium and sternum. Skeletal Radiol 1979;4(4):189–95.
8. Mandell GA, Heyman S. Absent sternum on bone scan. Clin Nucl Med 1983;8(7):327.
9. Steiner RM, Kricun M, Shapiro J. Absent mesosternum in congenital heart disease. AJR 1976;127(6):923–5.
10. Caffey J, Ross SE. The ischiopubic synchondrosis in healthy children: some normal roentgenologic findings. AJR Radium Ther Nucl Med 1956;76(3):488–94.
11. Cawley KA, Dvorak AD, Wilmot MD. Normal anatomic variant: scintigraphy of the ischiopubic synchondrosis. J Nucl Med 1983;24(1): 14–6.
12. Kloiber R, Udjus K, McIntyre W, et al. The scintigraphic and radiographic appearance of the ischiopubic synchondroses in normal children and in osteomyelitis. Pediatr Radiol 1988;18(1):57–61.
13. Scott RJ, Christofersen MR, Robertson WW Jr, et al. Acute osteomyelitis in children: a review of 116 cases. J Pediatr Orthop 1990;10(5): 649–52.
14. Laor T, Jaramillo D, Oestrich A. Skeletal system. In: Kirks DR, Griscom NT, eds. Practical Pediatric Imaging: Diagnostic Radiology of Infants and Children, 3rd ed. Philadelphia: Lippincott-Raven, 1998:327–510.
15. Capitanio MA, Kirkpatrick JA. Early roentgen observations in acute osteomyelitis. AJR Radium Ther Nucl Med 1970;108(3):488–96.
16. Faden H, Grossi M. Acute osteomyelitis in children. Reassessment of etiologic agents and their clinical characteristics. Am J Dis Child 1991;145(1):65–9.
17. Asmar BI. Osteomyelitis in the neonate. Infect Dis Clin North Am 1992;6(1):117–32.
18. Nixon GW. Acute hematogenous osteomyelitis. Pediatr Ann 1976;5(1):64–81.
19. Nelson JD. Acute osteomyelitis in children. Infect Dis Clin North Am 1990;4(3):513–22.
20. Schauwecker DS. The scintigraphic diagnosis of osteomyelitis. AJR 1992;158(1):9–18.
21. Canale ST, Harkness RM, Thomas PA, et al. Does aspiration of bones and joints affect results of later bone scanning? J Pediatr Orthop 1985;5(1):23–6.
22. McCoy JR, Morrissy RT, Seibert J. Clinical experience with the technetium-99 scan in children. Clin Orthop Rel Res 1981(154): 175–80.

23. Traughber PD, Manaster BJ, Murphy K, et al. Negative bone scans of joints after aspiration or arthrography: experimental studies. AJR 1986;146(1):87–91.

24. Ash JM, Gilday DL. The futility of bone scanning in neonatal osteomyelitis: concise communication. J Nucl Med 1980;21(5):417–20.

25. Majd M, Frankel RS. Radionuclide imaging in skeletal inflammatory and ischemic disease in children. AJR 1976;126(4):832–41.

26. Mok PM, Reilly BJ, Ash JM. Osteomyelitis in the neonate. Clinical aspects and the role of radiography and scintigraphy in diagnosis and management. Radiology 1982;145(3):677–82.

27. Sullivan DC, Rosenfield NS, Ogden J, et al. Problems in the scintigraphic detection of osteomyelitis in children. Radiology 1980; 135(3):731–6.

28. Bressler EL, Conway JJ, Weiss SC. Neonatal osteomyelitis examined by bone scintigraphy. Radiology 1984;152(3):685–8.

29. Howman-Giles R, Uren R. Multifocal osteomyelitis in childhood. Review by radionuclide bone scan. Clin Nucl Med 1992;17(4): 274–8.

30. Applegate K, Connolly LP, Treves ST. Neuroblastoma presenting clinically as hip osteomyelitis: a "signature" diagnosis on skeletal scintigraphy. Pediatr Radiol 1995;25 Suppl 1:S93–6.

31. Jones DC, Cady RB. "Cold" bone scans in acute osteomyelitis. J Bone Joint Surg Br 1981; 63–B(3):376–8.

32. Teates CD, Williamson BR. "Hot and cold" bone lesion in acute osteomyelitis. AJR 1977;129(3):517–8.

33. Sty JR, Wells RG, Starshak RJ, et al. The musculoskeletal system. In: Sty JR, ed. Diagnostic imaging of infants and children. Gaithersburg, MD: Aspen, 1992:233–405.

34. Harcke HT. Role of imaging in musculoskeletal infections in children. J Pediatr Orthop 1995;15(2):141–3.

35. Connolly LP, Connolly SA, Drubach LA, et al. Acute hematogenous osteomyelitis of children: assessment of skeletal scintigraphy-based diagnosis in the era of MRI. J Nucl Med 2002;43(10):1310–6.

36. Dangman BC, Hoffer FA, Rand FF, et al. Osteomyelitis in children: gadolinium-enhanced MR imaging. Radiology 1992;182(3): 743–7.

37. King DM, Mayo KM. Subacute haematogenous osteomyelitis. J Bone Joint Surg Br 1969;51(3): 458–63.

38. David R, Barron BJ, Madewell JE. Osteomyelitis, acute and chronic. Radiol Clin North Am 1987;25(6):1171–201.

39. Morrissy RT. Bone and joint sepsis. In: Morrissy RT, Weinstein SLV, eds. Lovel and Winter's Pediatric Orthopedics. Philadelphia: Lippincott-Raven, 2001:459–505.

40. Roberts JM, Drummond DS, Breed AL, et al. Subacute hematogenous osteomyelitis in children: a retrospective study. J Pediatr Orthop 1982;2(3):249–54.

41. Bogoch E, Thompson G, Salter RB. Foci of chronic circumscribed osteomyelitis (Brodie's abscess) that traverse the epiphyseal plate. J Pediatr Orthop 1984;4(2):162–9.

42. Brown T, Wilkinson RH. Chronic recurrent multifocal osteomyelitis. Radiology 1988;166 (2):493–6.

43. Giedion A, Holthusen W, Masel LF, et al. Subacute and chronic "symmetrical" osteomyelitis. Ann Radiol (Paris) 1972;15(3):329–42.

44. Mandell GA, Contreras SJ, Conard K, et al. Bone scintigraphy in the detection of chronic recurrent multifocal osteomyelitis. J Nucl Med 1998;39(10):1778–83.

45. Ratcliffe JF. An evaluation of the intra-osseous arterial anastomoses in the human vertebral body at different ages. A microarteriographic study. J Anat 1982;134(pt 2):373–82.

46. Ratcliffe JF. Anatomic basis for the pathogenesis and radiologic features of vertebral osteomyelitis and its differentiation from childhood discitis. A microarteriographic investigation. Acta Radiol Diagn (Stockh) 1985;26(2): 137–43.

47. Wiley AM, Trueta J. The vascular anatomy of the spine and its relationship to pyogenic vertebral osteomyelitis. J Bone Joint Surg Br 1959;41–B:796–809.

48. Wenger DR, Bobechko WP, Gilday DL. The spectrum of intervertebral disc-space infection in children. J Bone Joint Surg Am 1978; 60(1):100–8.

49. Fischer GW, Popich GA, Sullivan DE, et al. Diskitis: a prospective diagnostic analysis. Pediatrics 1978;62(4):543–8.

50. Treves ST, Connolly LP, Kirkpatrick JA, et al. Bone. In: Treves ST, ed. Pediatric Nuclear Medicine, 2nd ed. New York: Springer-Verlag, 1995:233–301.

51. Sty JR, Wells RG, Conway JJ. Spine pain in children. Semin Nucl Med 1993;23(4):296–320.

52. Swanson D, Blecker I, Gahbauer H, et al. Diagnosis of discitis by SPECT technetium-99m

MDP scintigram. A case report. Clin Nucl Med 1987;12(3):210–1.

53. Jaramillo D, Treves ST, Kasser JR, et al. Osteomyelitis and septic arthritis in children: appropriate use of imaging to guide treatment. AJR 1995;165(2):399–403.

54. Ozonoff MB. Generalized orthopedic diseases of childhood. In: Ozonoff MB, ed. Pediatric Orthopedic Radiology, 2nd ed. Philadelphia: Saunders, 1992:461–568.

55. Conway JJ. A scintigraphic classification of Legg-Calve-Perthes disease. Semin Nucl Med 1993;23(4):274–95.

56. Chung SM. The arterial supply of the developing proximal end of the human femur. J Bone Joint Surg Am 1976;58(7):961–70.

57. Kocher MS, Zurakowski D, Kasser JR. Differentiating between septic arthritis and transient synovitis of the hip in children: an evidence-based clinical prediction algorithm. J Bone Joint Surg Am 1999;81(12):1662–70.

58. Volberg FM, Sumner TE, Abramson JS, et al. Unreliability of radiographic diagnosis of septic hip in children. Pediatrics 1984;74(1):118–20.

59. Zawin JK, Hoffer FA, Rand FF, et al. Joint effusion in children with an irritable hip: US diagnosis and aspiration. Radiology 1993; 187(2):459–63.

60. Zieger MM, Dorr U, Schulz RD. Ultrasonography of hip joint effusions. Skeletal Radiol 1987;16(8):607–11.

61. Kloiber R, Pavlosky W, Portner O, et al. Bone scintigraphy of hip joint effusions in children. AJR 1983;140(5):995–9.

62. Minikel J, Sty J, Simons G. Sequential radionuclide bone imaging in avascular pediatric hip conditions. Clin Orthop Rel Res 1983(175): 202–8.

63. Sty JR, Wells RG, Smith WB. The child with acute leg pain. Semin Nucl Med 1988;18(2): 137–58.

64. Bensahel H, Bok B, Cavailloles F, et al. Bone scintigraphy in Perthes disease. J Pediatr Orthop 1983;3(3):302–5.

65. Calver R, Venugopal V, Dorgan J, et al. Radionuclide scanning in the early diagnosis of Perthes' disease. J Bone Joint Surg Br 1981;63–B(3):379–82.

66. Cavailloles F, Bok B, Bensahel H. Bone scintigraphy in the diagnosis and follow up of Perthes' disease. Eur J Nucl Med 1982;7(7):327–30.

67. Sutherland AD, Savage JP, Paterson DC, et al. The nuclide bone-scan in the diagnosis and management of Perthes' disease. J Bone Joint Surg Br 1980;62(3):300–6.

68. Comte F, De Rosa V, Zekri H, et al. Confirmation of the early prognostic value of bone scanning and pinhole imaging of the hip in Legg-Calve-Perthes disease. J Nucl Med 2003;44(11):1761–6.

69. Tsao AK, Dias LS, Conway JJ, et al. The prognostic value and significance of serial bone scintigraphy in Legg-Calve-Perthes disease. J Pediatr Orthop 1997;17(2):230–9.

70. Sebag GH. Disorders of the Hip. Magn Reson Imaging Clin North Am 1998;6(3):627–41.

71. Bos CF, Bloem JL, Bloem RM. Sequential magnetic resonance imaging in Perthes' disease. J Bone Joint Surg Br 1991;73(2):219–24.

72. Pinto MR, Peterson HA, Berquist TH. Magnetic resonance imaging in early diagnosis of Legg-Calve-Perthes disease. J Pediatr Orthop 1989;9(1):19–22.

73. Vande Berg B, Malghem J, Labaisse MA, et al. Avascular necrosis of the hip: comparison of contrast-enhanced and nonenhanced MR imaging with histologic correlation. Work in progress. Radiology 1992;182(2):445–50.

74. Ducou le Pointe H, Haddad S, Silberman B, et al. Legg-Perthes-Calve disease: staging by MRI using gadolinium. Pediatr Radiol 1994; 24(2):88–91.

75. Kumasaka Y, Harada K, Watanabe H, et al. Modified epiphyseal index for MRI in Legg-Calve-Perthes disease (LCPD). Pediatr Radiol 1991;21(3):208–10.

76. Jaramillo D, Kasser JR, Villegas-Medina OL, et al. Cartilaginous abnormalities and growth disturbances in Legg-Calve-Perthes disease: evaluation with MR imaging. Radiology 1995; 197(3):767–73.

77. Egund N, Wingstrand H. Legg-Calve-Perthes disease: imaging with MR. Radiology 1991; 179(1):89–92.

78. Weinstein SLV. Legg-Calvé-Perthes disease. In: Lovell WW, Winter RB, Morrissy RT, et al., eds. Lovell and Winter's Pediatric Orthopaedics, 4th ed. Philadelphia: Lippincott-Raven, 1996:951–92.

79. Lamer S, Dorgeret S, Khairouni A, et al. Femoral head vascularisation in Legg-Calve-Perthes disease: comparison of dynamic gadolinium-enhanced subtraction MRI with bone scintigraphy. Pediatr Radiol 2002;32(8): 580–5.

80. Fischer KC, Shapiro S, Treves S. Visualization of the spleen with a bone-seeking radionuclide in a child with sickle-cell anemia. Radiology 1977;122(2):398.

81. Hung GL, Stewart CA, Yeo E, et al. Incidental demonstration of cerebral infarction on bone scintigraphy in sickle cell disease. Clin Nucl Med 1990;15(10):671–2.

82. Sty JR, Babbitt DP, Sheth K. Abnormal Tc-99m-methylene diphosphonate accumulation in the kidneys of children with sickle cell disease. Clin Nucl Med 1980;5(10):445–7.

83. Fordham EW, Ramachandran PC. Radionuclide imaging of osseous trauma. Semin Nucl Med 1974;4(4):411–29.

84. Harcke HT Jr. Bone imaging in infants and children: a review. J Nucl Med 1978;19(3): 324–9.

85. Caffey J. Multiple fractures in the long bones of infants suffering from chronic subdural hematoma. AJR 1946;56:163–73.

86. Kleinman PK. Imaging of child abuse: an update. In: Kirks DR, ed. Emergency Pediatric Radiology. Reston, VA: American Roentgen Ray Society, 1995:189–95.

87. Kleinman PK, Marks SC, Blackbourne B. The metaphyseal lesion in abused infants: a radiologic-histopathologic study. AJR 1986;146(5): 895–905.

88. Kleinman PK. Diagnostic imaging in infant abuse. AJR 1990;155(4):703–12.

89. Conway JJ, Collins M, Tanz RR, et al. The role of bone scintigraphy in detecting child abuse. Semin Nucl Med 1993;23(4):321–33.

90. Conway JJ. Further comments on the role of the radionuclide skeletal survey in the diagnosis of the suspected abused child. Radiology 1983;148:574–5.

91. Jaudes PK. Comparison of radiography and radionuclide bone scanning in the detection of child abuse. Pediatrics 1984;73(2):166–8.

92. Kleinman PK, Blackbourne BD, Marks SC, et al. Radiologic contributions to the investigation and prosecution of cases of fatal infant abuse. N Engl J Med 1989;320(8):507–11.

93. Merten DF, Radkowski MA, Leonidas JC. The abused child: a radiological reappraisal. Radiology 1983;146(2):377–81.

94. Smith FW, Gilday DL, Ash JM, et al. Unsuspected costo-vertebral fractures demonstrated by bone scanning in the child abuse syndrome. Pediatr Radiol 1980;10(2):103–6.

95. Sty JR, Starshak RJ. The role of bone scintigraphy in the evaluation of the suspected abused child. Radiology 1983;146(2):369–75.

96. Dunbar JS, Owen HF, Nogrady MB, et al. Obscure tibial fracture of infants—the toddler's fracture. J Can Assoc Radiol 1964;15:136–44.

97. Swischuk LE, John SD, Tschoepe EJ. Upper tibial hyperextension fractures in infants: another occult toddler's fracture. Pediatr Radiol 1999;29(1):6–9.

98. Starshak RJ, Simons GW, Sty JR. Occult fracture of the calcaneus—another toddler's fracture. Pediatr Radiol 1984;14(1):37–40.

99. Blumberg K, Patterson RJ. The toddler's cuboid fracture. Radiology 1991;179(1):93–4.

100. Englaro EE, Gelfand MJ, Paltiel HJ. Bone scintigraphy in preschool children with lower extremity pain of unknown origin. J Nucl Med 1992;33(3):351–4.

101. John SD, Moorthy CS, Swischuk LE. Expanding the concept of the toddler's fracture. Radiographics 1997;17(2):367–76.

102. Miller JH, Sanderson RA. Scintigraphy of toddler's fracture. J Nucl Med 1988;29(12): 2001–3.

103. Lanyon LE. Functional strain in bone tissue as an objective, and controlling stimulus for adaptive bone remodelling. J Biomech 1987; 20(11–12):1083–93.

104. Lanyon LE. Functional strain as a determinant for bone remodeling. Calcif Tissue Int 1984; 36(suppl 1):S56–61.

105. Maffulli N, King JB. Effects of physical activity on some components of the skeletal system. Sports Med 1992;13(6):393–407.

106. Anderson MW, Greenspan A. Stress fractures. Radiology 1996;199(1):1–12.

107. Micheli LJ. Low back pain in the adolescent: differential diagnosis. Am J Sports Med 1979; 7(6):362–4.

108. Albanese M, Pizzutillo PD. Family study of spondylolysis and spondylolisthesis. J Pediatr Orthop 1982;2(5):496–9.

109. Fredrickson BE, Baker D, McHolick WJ, et al. The natural history of spondylolysis and spondylolisthesis. J Bone Joint Surg Am 1984;66(5):699–707.

110. Wynne-Davies R, Scott JH. Inheritance and spondylolisthesis: a radiographic family survey. J Bone Joint Surg Br 1979;61–B(3): 301–5.

111. Wiltse LL. The etiology of spondylolisthesis. Am J Orthop 1962;44–A:539–60.

112. Wilkinson RH, Hall JE. The sclerotic pedicle: tumor or pseudotumor? Radiology 1974; 111(3):683–8.

113. Bellah RD, Summerville DA, Treves ST, et al. Low-back pain in adolescent athletes: detection of stress injury to the pars interarticularis with SPECT. Radiology 1991;180(2):509–12.

114. Holder LE, Machin JL, Asdourian PL, et al. Planar and high-resolution SPECT bone imaging in the diagnosis of facet syndrome. J Nucl Med 1995;36(1):37–44.

115. Connolly LP, Drubach LA, Connolly SA, et al. Young athletes with low back pain: skeletal scintigraphy of conditions other than pars interarticularis stress. Clin Nucl Med 2004; 29(11):689–93.

116. Connolly LP, d'Hemecourt PA, Connolly SA, et al. Skeletal scintigraphy of young patients with low-back pain and a lumbosacral transitional vertebra. J Nucl Med 2003;44(6):909–14.

117. Wigh RE. The thoracolumbar and lumbosacral transitional junctions. Spine 1980;5(3):215–22.

118. Wigh RE. The transitional lumbosacral osseous complex. Skeletal Radiol 1982;8(2):127–31.

119. Ghelman B, Freiberger RH. The limbus vertebra: an anterior disc herniation demonstrated by discography. AJR 1976;127(5):854–5.

120. Goldman AB, Ghelman B, Doherty J. Posterior limbus vertebrae: a cause of radiating back pain in adolescents and young adults. Skeletal Radiol 1990;19(7):501–7.

121. Henales V, Hervas JA, Lopez P, et al. Intervertebral disc herniations (limbus vertebrae) in pediatric patients: report of 15 cases. Pediatr Radiol 1993;23(8):608–10.

122. Swischuk LE, John SD, Allbery S. Disk degenerative disease in childhood: Scheuermann's disease, Schmorl's nodes, and the limbus vertebra: MRI findings in 12 patients. Pediatr Radiol 1998;28(5):334–8.

123. Mandell GA, Morales RW, Harcke HT, et al. Bone scintigraphy in patients with atypical lumbar Scheuermann disease. J Pediatr Orthop 1993;13(5):622–7.

124. Fernbach SK, Wilkinson RH. Avulsion injuries of the pelvis and proximal femur. AJR 1981;137(3):581–4.

125. Kehl DK. Slipped capital femoral epiphysis. In: Lovell WW, Winter RB, Morrissy RT, et al., eds. Lovell and Winter's Pediatric Orthopaedics, 4th ed. Philadelphia: Lippincott-Raven, 1996: 993–1022.

126. Umans H, Liebling MS, Moy L, et al. Slipped capital femoral epiphysis: a physeal lesion diagnosed by MRI, with radiographic and CT correlation. Skeletal Radiol 1998;27(3):139–44.

127. Gelfand MJ, Strife JL, Graham EJ, et al. Bone scintigraphy in slipped capital femoral epiphysis. Clin Nucl Med 1983;8(12):613–15.

128. Smergel EM, Harcke HT, Pizzutillo PD, et al. Use of bone scintigraphy in the management of slipped capital femoral epiphysis. Clin Nucl Med 1987;12(5):349–53.

129. Kransdorf MJ, Stull MA, Gilkey FW, et al. Osteoid osteoma. Radiographics 1991;11(4): 671–96.

130. Makley JT. Prostaglandins—a mechanism for pain mediation in osteoid osteoma. Orthop Trans 1982;6:72.

131. Schulman L, Dorfman HD. Nerve fibers in osteoid osteoma. J Bone Joint Surg Am 1970;52(7):1351–6.

132. Freiberger RH, Loitman BS, Helpern M, et al. Osteoid osteoma; a report on 80 cases. AJR Radium Ther Nucl Med 1959;82(2):194–205.

133. Swee RG, McLeod RA, Beabout JW. Osteoid osteoma. Detection, diagnosis, and localization. Radiology 1979;130(1):117–23.

134. Lisbona R, Rosenthall L. Role of radionuclide imaging in osteoid osteoma. AJR 1979;132(1): 77–80.

135. Helms CA. Osteoid osteoma. The double density sign. Clin Orthop Relat Res 1987(222): 167–73.

136. Helms CA, Hattner RS, Vogler JB 3rd. Osteoid osteoma: radionuclide diagnosis. Radiology 1984;151(3):779–84.

137. Roach PJ, Connolly LP, Zurakowski D, et al. Osteoid osteoma: comparative utility of high-resolution planar and pinhole magnification scintigraphy. Pediatr Radiol 1996;26(3):222–5.

138. Hayes CW, Conway WF, Sundaram M. Misleading aggressive MR imaging appearance of some benign musculoskeletal lesions. Radiographics 1992;12(6):1119–34; discussion 35–6.

139. Assoun J, Richardi G, Railhac JJ, et al. Osteoid osteoma: MR imaging versus CT. Radiology 1994;191(1):217–23.

140. Rinsky LA, Goris M, Bleck EE, et al. Intraoperative skeletal scintigraphy for localization of osteoid-osteoma in the spine. Case report. J Bone Joint Surg Am 1980;62(1):143–4.

141. Simons GW, Sty J. Intraoperative bone imaging in the treatment of osteoid osteoma of the femoral neck. J Pediatr Orthop 1983;3(3): 399–402.

142. Sty J, Simons G. Intraoperative 99m technetium bone imaging in the treatment of benign osteoblastic tumors. Clin Orthop Rel Res 1982(165):223–7.

143. Taylor GA, Shea N, O'Brien T, et al. Osteoid osteoma: localization by intraoperative magnification scintigraphy. Pediatr Radiol 1986; 16(4):313–16.

144. Towbin R, Kaye R, Meza MP, et al. Osteoid osteoma: percutaneous excision using a CT-guided coaxial technique. AJR 1995;164(4): 945–9.

145. Mazoyer JF, Kohler R, Bossard D. Osteoid osteoma: CT-guided percutaneous treatment. Radiology 1991;181(1):269–71.

146. Baunin C, Puget C, Assoun J, et al. Percutaneous resection of osteoid osteoma under CT guidance in eight children. Pediatr Radiol 1994;24(3):185–8.

147. Rosenthal DI, Alexander A, Rosenberg AE, et al. Ablation of osteoid osteomas with a percutaneously placed electrode: a new procedure. Radiology 1992;183(1):29–33.

148. Kneisl JS, Simon MA. Medical management compared with operative treatment for osteoid-osteoma. J Bone Joint Surg Am 1992;74(2): 179–85.

149. Golding JS. The natural history of osteoid osteoma; with a report of twenty cases. J Bone Joint Surg Br 1954;36–B(2):218–29.

150. Moberg E. The natural course of osteoid osteoma. J Bone Joint Surg Am 1951;33(A:1): 166–70.

151. Vickers CW, Pugh DC, Ivins JC. Osteoid osteoma; a fifteen-year follow-up of an untreated patient. J Bone Joint Surg Am 1959;41–A(2):357–8.

152. Arata MA, Peterson HA, Dahlin DC. Pathological fractures through non-ossifying fibromas. Review of the Mayo Clinic experience. J Bone Joint Surg Am 1981;63(6): 980–8.

153. Burrows PE, Greenberg ID, Reed MH. The distal femoral defect: technetium-99m pyrophosphate bone scan results. J Can Assoc Radiol 1982;33(2):91–3.

154. Dunham WK, Marcus NW, Enneking WF, et al. Developmental defects of the distal femoral metaphysis. J Bone Joint Surg Am 1980;62(5): 801–6.

155. Kumar R, Madewell JE, Lindell MM, et al. Fibrous lesions of bones. Radiographics 1990;10(2):237–56.

156. Brenner RJ, Hattner RS, Lillien DL. Scintigraphic features of nonosteogenic fibroma. Radiology 1979;131(3):727–30.

157. Drubach LA, Connolly SA, Treves ST, et al. Stress-induced fracture involving a nonossifying fibroma. Clin Nucl Med 2004;29(1):41–2.

158. Kransdorf MJ, Sweet DE. Aneurysmal bone cyst: concept, controversy, clinical presentation, and imaging. AJR 1995;164(3):573–80.

159. Hudson TM. Scintigraphy of aneurysmal bone cysts. AJR 1984;142(4):761–5.

160. Rajadhyaksha C, Connolly LP, Connolly SA, et al. Aneurysmal bone cyst of the sacrum: value of three-phase imaging. Clin Nucl Med 2003;28(11):933–5.

161. Hudson TM, Hamlin DJ, Fitzsimmons JR. Magnetic resonance imaging of fluid levels in an aneurysmal bone cyst and in anticoagulated human blood. Skeletal Radiol 1985;13(4): 267–70.

162. Tsai JC, Dalinka MK, Fallon MD, et al. Fluid-fluid level: a nonspecific finding in tumors of bone and soft tissue. Radiology 1990;175(3): 779–82.

163. Kransdorf MJ, Moser RP Jr, Gilkey FW. Fibrous dysplasia. Radiographics 1990;10(3): 519–37.

164. Mirra JM, Gold RH. Fibrous dysplasia. In: Mirra JM, Picci P, Gold RH, eds. Bone Tumors: Clinical, Radiologic, and Pathologic Correlations. Philadelphia: Lea & Febiger, 1989: 191–226.

165. Libshitz HI, Cohen MA. Radiation-induced osteochondromas. Radiology 1982;142(3): 643–7.

166. Hudson TM. Radiologic-Pathologic Correlation of Musculoskeletal Lesions, 1st ed. Baltimore: Williams & Wilkins, 1987.

167. Epstein DA, Levin EJ. Bone scintigraphy in hereditary multiple exostoses. AJR 1978; 130(2):331–3.

168. Hudson TM, Springfield DS, Spanier SS, et al. Benign exostoses and exostotic chondrosarcomas: evaluation of cartilage thickness by CT. Radiology 1984;152(3):595–9.

169. Hendel HW, Daugaard S, Kjaer A. Utility of planar bone scintigraphy to distinguish benign osteochondromas from malignant chondrosarcomas. Clin Nucl Med 2002;27(9): 622–4.

170. Lange RH, Lange TA, Rao BK. Correlative radiographic, scintigraphic, and histological evaluation of exostoses. J Bone Joint Surg Am 1984;66(9):1454–9.

171. Caffey J, Silverman FA. Infantile cortical hyperostoses: preliminary report on a new syndrome. AJR 1945;54:1–3.

172. Padfield E, Hicken P. Cortical hyperostosis in infants: a radiological study of sixteen patients. Br J Radiol 1970;43(508):231–7.

173. Stull MA, Kransdorf MJ, Devaney KO. Langerhans cell histiocytosis of bone. Radiographics 1992;12(4):801–23.

174. Cline MJ. Histiocytes and histiocytosis. Blood 1994;84(9):2840–53.

175. Willman CL. Detection of clonal histiocytes in Langerhans cell histiocytosis: biology and clinical significance. Br J Cancer Suppl 1994;23: S29–33.

176. Dimentberg RA, Brown KL. Diagnostic evaluation of patients with histiocytosis X. J Pediatr Orthop 1990;10(6):733–41.

177. Broadbent V, Dunger DB, Yeomans E, et al. Anterior pituitary function and computed tomography/magnetic resonance imaging in patients with Langerhans cell histiocytosis and diabetes insipidus. Med Pediatr Oncol 1993;21(9):649–54.

178. Kirks DR, Taybi H, Histiocytosis X. In: Parker BR, Castellino RA, eds. Pediatric Oncologic Radiology. St. Louis: Mosby, 1977:209–34.

179. Schaub T, Ash JM, Gilday DL. Radionuclide imaging in histiocytosis X. Pediatr Radiol 1987;17(5):397–404.

180. Dogan AS, Conway JJ, Miller JH, et al. Detection of bone lesions in Langerhans cell histiocytosis: complementary roles of scintigraphy and conventional radiography. J Pediatr Hematol Oncol 1996;18(1):51–8.

181. Stoll M, Freund M, Schmid H, et al. Allogeneic bone marrow transplantation for Langerhans' cell histiocytosis. Cancer 1990;66(2):284–8.

182. Resnick D. Tumors and tumor-like lesions of bone: radiographic principles. In: Resnick D, ed. Diagnosis of Bone and Joint Disorders, 3rd ed. Philadelphia: Saunders, 1995:3613–27.

183. Aboulafia AJ, Malawer MM. Surgical management of pelvic and extremity osteosarcoma. Cancer 1993;71(10 suppl):3358–66.

184. Meadows AT, Baum E, Fossati-Bellani F, et al. Second malignant neoplasms in children: an update from the Late Effects Study Group. J Clin Oncol 1985;3(4):532–8.

185. Link MP, Eilber F. Osteosarcoma. In: Pizzo PA, Poplack DG, eds. Principles and Practice of Pediatric Oncology, 2nd ed. Philadelphia: JB Lippincott, 1993:841–66.

186. Resnick D, Kyriakos K, Greenway GD. Tumors and tumor-like lesions of bone: imaging and pathology of specific tumors. In: Resnick D, ed. Diagnosis of Bone and Joint Disorders, 3rd ed. Philadelphia: Saunders, 1995:3662–97.

187. Newton WA Jr, Meadows AT, Shimada H, et al. Bone sarcomas as second malignant neoplasms following childhood cancer. Cancer 1991;67(1): 193–201.

188. Hopper KD, Moser RP Jr, Haseman DB, et al. Osteosarcomatosis. Radiology 1990;175(1): 233–9.

189. Glasser DB, Lane JM, Huvos AG, et al. Survival, prognosis, and therapeutic response in osteogenic sarcoma. The Memorial Hospital experience. Cancer 1992;69(3):698–708.

190. Meyers PA, Heller G, Healey J, et al. Chemotherapy for nonmetastatic osteogenic sarcoma: the Memorial Sloan-Kettering experience. J Clin Oncol 1992;10(1):5–15.

191. Bacci G, Picci P, Ruggieri P, et al. Primary chemotherapy and delayed surgery (neoadjuvant chemotherapy) for osteosarcoma of the extremities. The Istituto Rizzoli Experience in 127 patients treated preoperatively with intravenous methotrexate (high versus moderate doses) and intraarterial cisplatin. Cancer 1990;65(11):2539–53.

192. Connolly LP, Drubach LA, Ted Treves S. Applications of nuclear medicine in pediatric oncology. Clin Nucl Med 2002;27(2):117–25.

193. Chew FS, Hudson TM. Radionuclide bone scanning of osteosarcoma: falsely extended uptake patterns. AJR 1982;139(1):49–54.

194. Goldman AB, Braunstein P. Augmented radioactivity on bone scans of limbs bearing osteosarcomas. J Nucl Med 1975;16(5):423–4.

195. Thrall JH, Geslien GE, Corcoron RJ, et al. Abnormal radionuclide deposition patterns adjacent to focal skeletal lesions. Radiology 1975;115(3):659–63.

196. Rees CR, Siddiqui AR, duCret R. The role of bone scintigraphy in osteogenic sarcoma. Skeletal Radiol 1986;15(5):365–7.

197. McKillop JH, Etcubanas E, Goris ML. The indications for and limitations of bone scintigraphy in osteogenic sarcoma: a review of 55 patients. Cancer 1981;48(5):1133–8.

198. Herrlin K, Willen H, Wiebe T. Flare phenomenon in osteosarcoma after complete remission. J Nucl Med 1995;36(8):1429–31.

199. Podoloff DA. Malignant bone disease. In: Henkin RE, Boles MA, Dillehay GL, et al., eds. Nuclear Medicine, 2nd ed. Philadelphia: Mosby Year Book, 1996:1208–22.

200. Vanel D, Henry-Amar M, Lumbroso J, et al. Pulmonary evaluation of patients with osteosarcoma: roles of standard radiography, tomography, CT, scintigraphy, and tomoscintigraphy. AJR 1984;143(3):519–23.

201. Kirks DR, McCook TA, Merten DF, et al. The value of radionuclide bone imaging in selected

patients with osteogenic sarcoma metastatic to lung. Pediatr Radiol 1980;9(3):139–43.

202. Hoefnagel CA, Bruning PF, Cohen P, et al. Detection of lung metastases from osteosarcoma by scintigraphy using 99mTc-methylene diphosphonate. Diagn Imaging 1981;50(5): 277–84.

203. Aro HT, Aho AJ. Clinical use of bone allografts. Ann Med 1993;25(4):403–12.

204. Friedlaender GE. Bone grafts. The basic science rationale for clinical applications. J Bone Joint Surg Am 1987;69(5):786–90.

205. Mankin HJ, Springfield DS, Gebhardt MC, et al. Current status of allografting for bone tumors. Orthopedics 1992;15(10):1147–54.

206. Enneking WF, Mindell ER. Observations on massive retrieved human allografts. J Bone Joint Surg Am 1991;73(8):1123–42.

207. Bar-Sever Z, Connolly LP, Gebhardt MC, et al. Scintigraphy of lower extremity cadaveric bone allografts in osteosarcoma patients. Clin Nucl Med 1997;22(8):532–5.

208. Roebuck DJ, Griffith JF, Kumta SM, et al. Imaging following allograft reconstruction in children with malignant bone tumours. Pediatr Radiol 1999;29(10):785–93.

209. Alman BA, De Bari A, Krajbich JI. Massive allografts in the treatment of osteosarcoma and Ewing sarcoma in children and adolescents. J Bone Joint Surg Am 1995;77(1):54–64.

210. Berrey BH Jr, Lord CF, Gebhardt MC, et al. Fractures of allografts. Frequency, treatment, and end-results. J Bone Joint Surg Am 1990; 72(6):825–33.

211. Dick HM, Strauch RJ. Infection of massive bone allografts. Clin Orthop Relat Res 1994(306):46–53.

212. Ben Ami T, Treves ST, Tumeh S, et al. Stress fractures after surgery for osteosarcoma: scintigraphic assessment. Radiology 1987;163(1): 157–62.

213. Triche TJ. Pathology of pediatric malignancies. In: Pizzo PA, Poplack DG, eds. Principles and Practice of Pediatric Oncology, 2nd ed. Philadelphia: JB Lippincott, 1993.

214. Marina NM, Etcubanas E, Parham DM, et al. Peripheral primitive neuroectodermal tumor (peripheral neuroepithelioma) in children. A review of the St. Jude experience and controversies in diagnosis and management. Cancer 1989;64(9):1952–60.

215. Horowitz ME, DeLaney TE, Malawer MM, et al. Ewing's sarcoma family of tumors: Ewing's sarcoma of bone and soft tissue and the peripheral primitive neuroectodermal tumors. In: Pizzo PA, Poplack DG, eds. Principles and Practice of Pediatric Oncology, 2nd ed. Philadelphia: JB Lippincott, 1993:795–821.

216. Crist WM, Kun LE. Common solid tumors of childhood. N Engl J Med 1991;324(7):461–71.

217. O'Connor MI, Pritchard DJ. Ewing's sarcoma. Prognostic factors, disease control, and the reemerging role of surgical treatment. Clin Orthop Rel Res 1991(262):78–87.

218. Bushnell D, Shirazi P, Khedkar N, et al. Ewing's sarcoma seen as a "cold" lesion on bone scans. Clin Nucl Med 1983;8(4):173–4.

219. Smith FW, Gilday DL, Ash JM, et al. Primary neuroblastoma uptake of 99m-technetium methylene diphosphonate. Radiology 1980; 137(2):501–4.

220. Young G, L'Heureux P. Extraosseous tumor uptake of 99m technetium phosphate compounds in children with abdominal neuroblastoma. Pediatr Radiol 1978;7(3):159–63.

221. Podrasky AE, Stark DD, Hattner RS, et al. Radionuclide bone scanning in neuroblastoma: skeletal metastases and primary tumor localization of 99mTc-MDP. AJR 1983;141(3): 469–72.

222. Martin-Simmerman P, Cohen MD, Siddiqui A, et al. Calcification and uptake of Tc-99m diphosphonates in neuroblastomas: concise communication. J Nucl Med 1984;25(6):656–60.

223. Howman-Giles RB, Gilday DL, Ash JM. Radionuclide skeletal survey in neuroblastoma. Radiology 1979;131(2):497–502.

224. Clausen N, Gotze H, Pedersen A, et al. Skeletal scintigraphy and radiography at onset of acute lymphocytic leukemia in children. Med Pediatr Oncol 1983;11(4):291–6.

225. Mandell GA, Heyman S. Extraosseous uptake of technetium-99m MDP in secondary deposits of neuroblastoma. Clin Nucl Med 1986;11(5): 337–40.

226. Connolly LP, Bloom DA, Kozakewich H, et al. Localization of Tc-99m MDP in neuroblastoma metastases to the liver and lung. Clin Nucl Med 1996;21(8):629–33.

227. Stauss J, Connolly LP, Drubach LA, et al. Pelvic hypoplasia after radiation therapy. Clin Nucl Med 2003;28(10):847–8.

228. Warner WW. Kyphosis. In: Lovell WW, Winter RB, Morrissy RT, et al., eds. Lovell and Winter's Pediatric Orthopaedics, 4th ed. Philadelphia: Lippincott-Raven, 1996:687–716.

229. Dalinka MK, Haygood TM. Radiation changes. In: Resnick D, ed. Diagnosis of Bone and Joint

Disorders, 3rd ed. Philadelphia: Saunders, 1995:3276–308.

230. Fletcher BD, Crom DB, Krance RA, et al. Radiation-induced bone abnormalities after bone marrow transplantation for childhood leukemia. Radiology 1994;191(1):231–5.

231. Wolf EL, Berdon WE, Cassady JR, et al. Slipped femoral capital epiphysis as a sequela to childhood irradiation for malignant tumors. Radiology 1977;125(3):781–4.

232. Ecklund K, Laor T, Goorin AM, et al. Methotrexate osteopathy in patients with osteosarcoma. Radiology 1997;202(2):543–7.

233. Silberzweig JE, Haller JO, Miller S. Ifosfamide: a new cause of rickets. AJR 1992;158(4):823–4.

234. Stokkel MP, Valdes Olmos RA, Hoefnagel CA, et al. Tumor and therapy associated abnormal changes on bone scintigraphy. Old and new phenomena. Clin Nucl Med 1993;18(10): 821–8.

14
Pediatric Oncology

Hossein Jadvar and Barry L. Shulkin

The incidence of cancer is estimated to be 133.3 per million children in the United States.[1] Although cancer is much less common in children than in adults (only about 2% of all cancers occur before 15 years of age), it is still an important cause of mortality in pediatrics. Approximately 10% of deaths during childhood are attributable to cancer, making it the leading cause of childhood death from disease.[2] Nuclear imaging has played an increasingly important role in diagnosis, staging, treatment monitoring, surveillance, and prognostication in children with cancer.

Common radiotracers used in imaging cancer have included gallium-67 citrate (^{67}Ga), thallium-201 chloride (^{201}Tl), technetium-99m sestamibi (^{99m}Tc-MIBI), and more recently fluorine-18-fluorodeoxyglucose (^{18}F-FDG). The mechanism of ^{67}Ga uptake in tumor is uncertain but appears to be related to blood flow, increased capillary permeability, and transferrin. [201]Tl uptake in tumor is primarily dependent on blood flow, tumor viability, tumor type, and the adenosine triphosphatase (ATPase)-dependent Na-K pump. The mechanism of ^{99m}Tc-MIBI uptake in tumors is associated with regional blood flow, tissue viability, cell membrane potential, and mitochondrial content. The uptake level is also inversely related to the degree of P transporter glycoprotein, an energy-dependent efflux pump responsible for multidrug resistance. The enhanced glucose metabolism of tumors is reflected by high FDG uptake mediated by increased expression of glucose transporters and increased activity of hexokinase.

Traditional planar and single photon emission computed tomography (SPECT) imaging systems have been complemented by the rapid emergence of positron emission tomography (PET), and more recently the hybrid positron emission tomography–computed tomography (PET-CT) imaging systems. Technical issues specific to performing PET and PET-CT in children such as radiation dosimetry, physical location of the PET-CT unit, the roles of CT and nuclear medicine technologists, the methodology for study interpretation, use of intravenous and sugar-free oral contrasts for the CT portion of the examination, and the management of hyperglycemia have been reviewed elsewhere.[3–10] This chapter reviews the clinical role of nuclear imaging in pediatric oncology and particularly emphasizes the promising clinical applications of PET and PET-CT.

Brain Tumors

Brain tumors are the most common nonhematologic tumors of childhood. They account for about 20% of all pediatric malignancies. The majority of pediatric brain tumors arise from neuroepithelial tissue. Tumors are subclassified histopathologically by cell type and are graded for degree of malignancy using criteria that include mitotic activity, infiltration, and anaplasia.[11,12] In the posterior fossa, medulloblastoma, cerebellar astrocytoma, ependymoma, and brainstem gliomas are most common. Tumors about the third ventricle include tumors that arise from suprasellar, pineal, and ventricular tissue. The most common neoplasms about the third ventricle are optic and hypothalamic gliomas, craniopharyngiomas, and germ cell tumors. Supratentorial tumors are most often astrocytomas, many of which are low grade.[12]

Magnetic resonance imaging (MRI) and CT are the principal imaging modalities used in staging and following children with brain tumors. Their main limitation is the inability to distinguish viable recurrent or residual tumor from abnormalities resulting from surgery or radiation. Single photon emission computed tomography with either ^{201}Tl or ^{99m}Tc-MIBI has proven valuable for this determination in a number of pediatric brain tumors.[13–16] Neither [201]Tl-201 nor ^{99m}Tc-MIBI localizes in the brain by blood–brain barrier breakdown. ^{99m}Tc-MIBI, however, normally accumulates in the choroids plexus.[15] Both ^{201}Tl and ^{99m}Tc-MIBI display low accumulation in necrosis while tumor frequently shows high uptake levels. Combined ^{201}Tl and ^{99m}Tc–hexamethylpropyleneamine oxime (^{99m}Tc-HMPAO) imaging increases the specificity for discriminating post-therapy changes from recurrent tumor. Low ^{201}Tl uptake combined with low perfusion on HMPAO imaging suggests necrosis.[17]

Use of FDG-PET in brain tumors has been widely reported in series that predominantly include adult patients for whom FDG-PET has helped distinguish viable tumor from posttherapeutic changes.[18–20] High FDG uptake relative to adjacent brain indicates residual or recurrent tumor, whereas low or absent FDG uptake is observed in areas of necrosis (Fig. 14.1). This distinction is most readily made with high-grade tumors that show high uptake of FDG at diagnosis. Even with high-grade tumors, the presence of microscopic tumor foci is not excluded by an FDG-PET study that does not show increased uptake. Furthermore, in the immediate posttherapy period, elevated FDG uptake may persist.[21,22] Fluorodeoxyglucose PET has been applied to tumor grading and prognostication. Higher-grade aggressive tumors typically have higher FDG uptake than do lower grade tumors.[23] Low-grade tumors typically appear isometabolic or hypometabolic relative to the metabolic activity of the normal

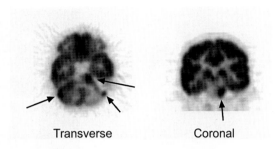

Transverse   Coronal

FIGURE 14.1. Fluorodeoxyglucose positron emission tomography (FDG-PET) scans from a 6-year-old with recurrent anaplastic ependymoma. Areas of increased uptake representing recurrent tumor are indicated by arrows.

brain gray matter. The development of hypermetabolism as evidenced by increased FDG uptake in a low-grade tumor that appeared hypometabolic at diagnosis indicates degeneration to a higher grade.[24] Shorter survival times have been reported for patients whose tumors show the highest degree of FDG uptake.[25–27] In a series of children affected by neurofibromatosis who had low-grade astrocytomas, high tumoral glucose metabolism shown by FDG-PET was a more accurate predictor of tumor behavior than was histologic analysis.[28] Combining FDG-PET and MRI in the planning of stereotactic brain biopsies has also been reported to improve the diagnostic yield in infiltrative, ill-defined lesions and to reduce sampling in high-risk functional areas.[29]

Lymphoma

Lymphomas of non-Hodgkin's and Hodgkin's types account for between 10% and 15% of pediatric malignancies. Non-Hodgkin's lymphoma occurs throughout childhood. Lymphoblastic and small-cell tumors, including Burkitt's lymphoma, are the most common histologic types. The disease is usually widespread at diagnosis. Mediastinal and hilar involvement are common with lymphoblastic lymphoma. Burkitt's lymphoma most often occurs in the abdomen. Hodgkin's disease has a peak incidence during adolescence. Nodular sclerosing and mixed cellularity are the most common his-

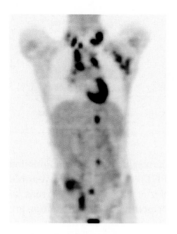
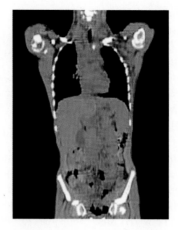
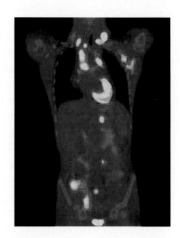

FIGURE 14.2. An 11-year-old boy with nodular scle-rosing Hodgkin's disease, status post–biopsy of the left axilla. FDG PET–computed tomography (CT) images demonstrate hypermetabolic nodal disease involving the left axilla, bilateral supraclavicular, mediastinal, gastrohepatic ligament, retroperitoneal, and right iliac nodal basins.

tologic types. The disease is rarely widespread at diagnosis, and the majority of cases have intrathoracic nodal involvement.[1,30] The prog-noses in these diseases are related to accurate initial staging, adequate primary treatment, accurate detection of recurrence, and early institution of secondary or salvage therapy.

Scintigraphy with ^{67}Ga has proven useful in staging and monitoring therapeutic response of children with non-Hodgkin's and Hodgkin's lymphomas[31-34] In low-grade lymphomas, ^{201}Tl uptake may be higher than that in intermediate and high-grade varieties.[35,36] Similar to ^{67}Ga, FDG uptake is generally greater in higher than in lower grade lymphomas.[37,38] Fluorodeoxyglu-cose PET has been shown to reveal sites of nodal and extranodal disease that are not detected by conventional staging methods, resulting in upstaging of disease[37-45] (Figs. 14.2 and 14.3). Fluorodeoxyglucose PET at the time

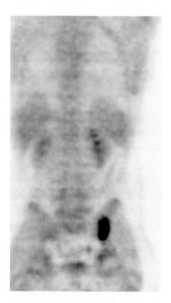
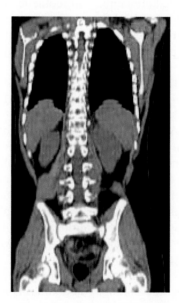
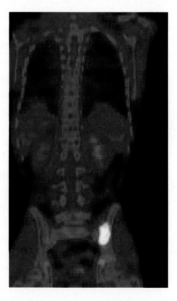

FIGURE 14.3. A 13-year-old boy with PET-CT demonstration of osseous lymphoma involving the left medial ilium with associated sclerotic changes on noncontrast CT and no associated soft tissue mass or involvement of the left sacroiliac (SI) joint space.

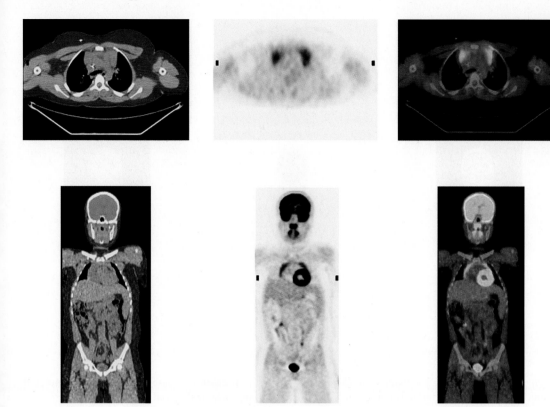

FIGURE 14.4. A 12-year-old boy with history of embryonal cell carcinoma of the liver. FDG-PET images (center panel) show increased uptake of FDG on both sides of the mediastinum representing thymic rebound. Previous FDG-PET scan 6 months earlier did not show uptake in this region.

of initial evaluation has also been recently shown to change disease stage and treatment in up to 10% to 23% of children with lymphoma.[46,47] Identification of areas of intense FDG uptake within the bone marrow can be particularly useful in directing the site of biopsy or even eliminating the need for biopsy at staging.[40,48] Fluorodeoxyglucose PET is also useful in assessing residual soft tissue masses shown by CT after therapy. Absence of FDG uptake in a residual mass is predictive of remission, whereas high uptake indicates residual or recurrent tumor.[44] A negative FDG-PET scan after completion of chemotherapy, however, does not exclude the presence of residual microscopic disease.[49] The potential role of FDG-PET in radiation treatment planning for pediatric oncology including lymphoma has also been recently described.[50–52]

There are several potential pitfalls with both ^{67}Ga scintigraphy and FDG-PET that must be noted. These include high tracer uptake in

thymus and in skeletal growth centers, particularly the long bone physes[53–57] (Fig. 14.4). With the introduction of PET-CT imaging systems, it has been recognized that elevated FDG uptake in the normal brown adipose tissue may also be a source of false-positive findings[58–60] (Fig. 14.5). The common anatomic areas involved include the neck and shoulder region, axillae, mediastinum, and the paravertebral and perinephric regions. Neck brown fat hypermetabolism is seen significantly more in the pediatric population than in the adult population (15% vs. 2%, $p < .01$) and appears to be stimulated by cold temperatures.[58,59] Other potential pitfalls, which also apply to imaging adults, include variable FDG uptake in working skeletal muscles, the myocardium, the thyroid gland, and the gastrointestinal tract, as well as accumulation of FDG excreted into the renal pelvis and bladder and possible tracer accumulation in draining lymph nodes from extravasated tracer at the time of injection.[61] Diffuse high bone marrow

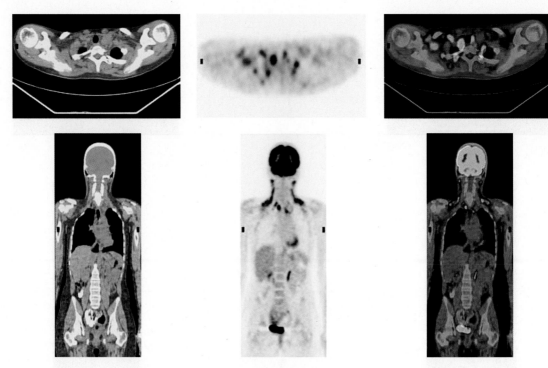

FIGURE 14.5. FDG-PET-CT images of a 15-year-old girl with Hodgkin's disease who recently completed chemotherapy. There is abundant uptake of FDG in cervical, supraclavicular, and mediastinal fat.

and splenic ^{67}Ga and FDG uptake following administration of hematopoietic stimulating factors may also resemble disseminated metastatic disease.[53,62,63] Elevated bone marrow FDG uptake has been observed in patients as late as 4 weeks following completion of treatment with granulocyte colony-stimulating factor (GCSF)[62] (Fig. 14.6). This observation probably reflects increased bone marrow glycolytic metabolism in response to hematopoietic growth factors.

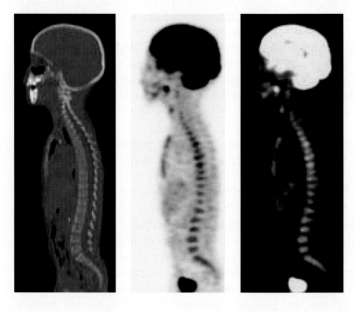

FIGURE 14.6. FDG-PET images of a 4-year-old boy undergoing chemotherapy for recurrent Wilms' tumor. Sagittal images show markedly increased uptake within the vertebral and sternal bone marrow. Patient was receiving granulocyte colony-stimulating factor at the time of the study.

Neuroblastoma

Neuroblastoma is the most common extracranial solid malignant tumor in children. The mean age of patients at presentation is 20 to 30 months; neuroblastoma is rare after the age of 5 years.[30,64] The most common location of neuroblastoma is the adrenal gland. Other sites of origin include the paravertebral and presacral sympathetic chain, the organ of Zuckerkandl, posterior mediastinal sympathetic ganglia, and cervical sympathetic plexuses. Gross or microscopic calcification is often present in the tumor. Two related neural crest tumors, ganglioneuroma and ganglioneuroblastoma, have been described. Some neuroblastomas spontaneously regress or mature into ganglioneuroma, which is benign. In fact, as Kushner[64] points out, screening programs of infants show that many cases escape detection because of spontaneous regression and maturation into benign lesions. However, the unpredictability and apparent infrequency of spontaneous regression and maturation, and the consequences of delaying therapy, require that treatment be initiated at diagnosis in most cases. It is therefore clinically critical to distinguish low-risk (90% survival) from high-risk (30% survival) patient subsets.[64]

Ganglioneuroblastoma is a malignant tumor that contains both undifferentiated neuroblasts and mature ganglion cells. Disseminated disease is present in up to 70% of neuroblastoma cases at diagnosis and most commonly involves cortical bone and bone marrow. Less frequently, there is involvement of liver, skin, or lung. A primary tumor is not detected in up to 10% of children with disseminated neuroblastoma.[65] The primary tumor may also go undetected in patients who present with paraneoplastic syndromes such as infantile myoclonic encephalopathy. Surgical excision is the preferred treatment of localized neuroblastoma. When local disease is extensive, intensive preoperative chemotherapy may be utilized. When distant metastases are present, surgical removal is not likely to improve survival. The prognosis in these cases is poor, but high-dose chemotherapy, total-body irradiation, and bone marrow reinfusion is beneficial for some children with this presentation.

Delineation of local disease extent is achieved with MRI, CT, and scintigraphic studies. These tests are also utilized in localizing the primary site in children who present with disseminated disease or with a paraneoplastic syndrome. Iodine-123-metaiodobenzylguanidine (^{123}I-MIBG) and indium-111 (^{111}In)–pentetreotide scintigraphy have been employed in these settings with a sensitivity of greater than 85% for detecting neuroblastoma. Uptake of ^{123}I-MIBG, which is an analogue of guanethidine and norepinephrine, into neuroblastoma is by a neuronal sodium- and energy-dependent transport mechanism[66] (Fig. 14.7). The localization of ^{111}In-pentetreotide in neuroblastoma reflects the presence of somatostatin type 2 receptors on some neuroblastoma cells.[67]

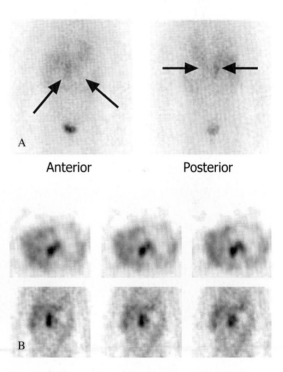

Anterior   Posterior

FIGURE 14.7. A: Planar images obtained 24 hours after ^{123}I-MIBG administration in a 3-year-old with residual abdominal neuroblastoma following bone marrow transplantation. Mildly increased uptake is seen in the right adrenal bed and possibly the left adrenal bed. B: Single photon emission computed tomography (SPECT) images (top row, transverse; bottom row, coronal) demonstrate clearly the abnormal uptake of MIBG in the residual tumor with extension across the midline.

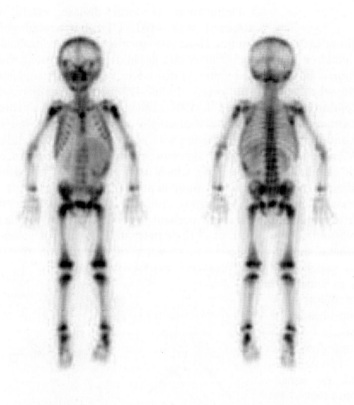

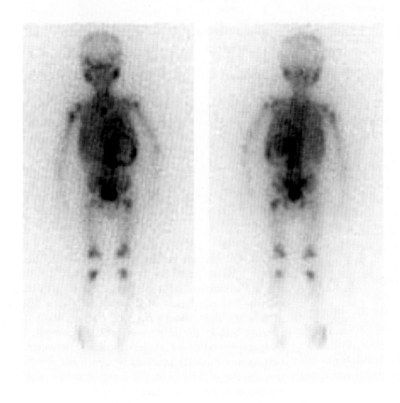

FIGURE 14.8. Bone scan (top) and ^{123}I-MIBG scan (bottom) of a 2-year-old with neuroblastoma studied at the time of presentation. Although the bone scan is abnormal, the extent of disease is much better portrayed with MIBG scintigraphy.

Bone scintigraphy has been most widely used for detection of skeletal involvement for staging (Fig. 14.8). ^{123}I-MIBG and, to a lesser extent, ^{111}In-pentetreotide imaging have also been increasingly used for detecting skeletal involvement.[68] Magnetic resonance imaging or CT cannot distinguish viable tumor from treatment-related scar or tumor that has matured into ganglioneuroma. Specificity in establishing residual viable tumor can be improved with ^{123}I-MIBG or ^{111}In-pentetreotide imaging when the primary tumor had been shown to accumulate one of these agents. These agents are also useful in assessing residual skeletal disease in patients with ^{123}I-MIBG or ^{111}In-pentetreotide avid skeletal metastases. Bone scintigraphy, however, is unable to distinguish active disease from bony repair on the basis of tracer uptake.

Neuroblastomas are metabolically active tumors. Neuroblastomas and their metastases avidly concentrated FDG prior to chemotherapy or radiation therapy in 16 of 17 patients studied with FDG-PET and MIBG imaging.[69] Uptake after therapy was variable but tended to be lower. Fluorodeoxyglucose and MIBG results were concordant in most instances. However, there were occasions when one agent accumulated at a site of disease and the other did not. Overall, MIBG imaging was considered superior to FDG-PET, particularly in delineation of residual disease. An advantage of FDG-PET is the initiation of imaging 60 minutes after FDG administration, whereas MIBG imaging is performed one or more days following tracer administration. Fluorodeoxyglucose PET may be of limited value for the evaluation of the bone marrow involvement of neuroblastoma due to mild FDG accumulation by the normal bone marrow.[69] A recent study has reported that once the primary tumor is resected, PET and bone marrow examination suffice for monitoring neuroblastoma patients at high risk for progressive disease in soft tissue, bone, and bone marrow.[70] Currently, the primary role of FDG-PET in neuroblastoma is in the evaluation of known or suspected neuroblastomas that do not demonstrate MIBG uptake.

Wilms' Tumor

Wilms' tumor is the most common renal malignancy of childhood. It is predominantly seen in younger children and uncommonly encountered after the age of 5 years.[1] Bilateral renal involvement occurs in about 5% of all cases and can be identified synchronously or metachronously.[71] An asymptomatic abdominal mass is the typical mode of presentation. Nephrectomy with adjuvant chemotherapy is the treatment of choice. Radiation therapy is used in selected cases when resection is incomplete. Scintigraphy has not played an important role in imaging of Wilms' tumor. Radiography, ultrasonography, CT, and MRI are commonly employed in anatomic staging and detection of metastases, which predominantly involve lung, occasionally liver, and only rarely other sites. Anatomic imaging is of limited value in the assessment for residual or recurrent tumor.[71] Mild ^{201}Tl uptake has been noted in Wilms' tumor.[72] Uptake of FDG by Wilms' tumor has been described,[73] but a role for FDG-PET in Wilms' tumor has not been established (Fig. 14.9). Normal excretion

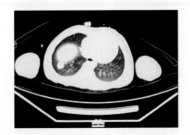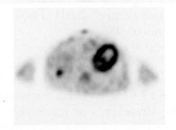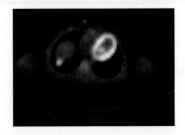

FIGURE 14.9. FDG-PET-CT scan of a 4-year-old with Wilms' tumor metastatic to the right lower lobe of the lung.

of FDG through the kidney is a limiting factor. However, careful correlation with anatomic cross-sectional imaging facilitates distinguishing tumor uptake from normal renal FDG excretion.

Bone Tumors

Osteosarcoma and Ewing's sarcoma are the two primary bone malignancies of childhood. Osteosarcoma is the more common and predominantly affects adolescents and young adults. A second peak affects older adults, predominantly individuals with a history of prior radiation to bone or Paget's disease. This tumor rarely affects children younger than 7 years of age. Osteosarcoma is typically a lesion of the long bones. The treatment of choice for osteosarcoma of an extremity is wide resection and limb-sparing surgery. Limb-sparing procedures entail the resection of tumor with a cuff of surrounding normal tissue at all margins, skeletal reconstruction, and muscle and soft tissue transfers. Employing current chemotherapeutic regimens pre- and postoperatively and imaging to define tumor extent and tumor viability preoperatively, limb-sparing procedures can be appropriately performed in 80% of patients with osteosarcoma.[74]

Most Ewing's sarcoma occurs between the ages of 5 and 30 with the highest incidence being in the second decade of life. Ewing's sarcoma most often affects the appendicular skeleton in patients younger than 20 years. Beyond that age, pelvic, rib, and vertebral lesion predominate. Therapy for Ewing's sarcoma involves irradiation and/or surgery for control of the primary lesion and multiagent chemotherapy for eradication of microscopic or overt metastatic disease. Because late recurrence is not uncommon, resection of the primary tumor is gaining favor for local disease control.[75]

Magnetic resonance imaging is used to define the local extent of osteosarcoma and Ewing's sarcoma in bone and soft tissue. However, signal abnormalities caused by peritumoral edema can result in an overestimation of tumor extension.[76] Scintigraphy has been used primarily to detect skeletal metastases of these tumors at diagnosis and during follow-up. With osteosarcoma, skeletal scintigraphy occasionally demonstrates extraosseous metastases, most often pulmonary, due to osteoid production by the metastatic deposits. Determination of preoperative chemotherapeutic response is important in planning limb-salvage surgery. Due to the nonspecific appearance of viable tumor on MRI, variable results have been reported for assessing chemotherapeutic response.[77–82] Gallium-67 scintigraphy has been employed for evaluation of osteosarcoma and Ewing's sarcoma, but it is not consistently accurate in defining the extent of bone lesion and in assessing treatment response because in the latter case the uptake may reflect healing and not necessarily residual tumor.[83,84] Scintigraphy with ^{201}Tl has been shown to be useful for assessing therapeutic response in osteosarcoma[85–90] and perhaps Ewing's sarcoma[86,87] Marked decrease in tumoral ^{201}Tl uptake indicates a favorable response to chemotherapy. ^{99m}Tc-MIBI may also be useful in osteosarcoma but seemingly not with Ewing's sarcoma.[91,92] The exact role of FDG-PET in osteosarcoma and Ewing's sarcoma has not yet been determined (Figs. 14.10 and 14.11). However, early experience suggests that in patients with Ewing's sarcoma, FDG-PET may play a role in monitoring response to therapy.[93–98] Fluorodeoxyglucose PET may be superior to bone scintigraphy for detecting osseous metastases from Ewing's sarcoma but may be less sensitive for those from osteosarcoma.[99] A second potential role is in assessing patients with suspected or known pulmonary metastases in osteosarcoma.

Soft Tissue Tumors

Rhabdomyosarcoma is the most common soft tissue malignancy of childhood. The peak incidence occurs between 3 and 6 years of age. Rhabdomyosarcomas can develop in any organ or tissue and do not usually arise in muscle. The most common anatomic locations are the head, particularly the orbit and paranasal sinuses, the neck, and the genitourinary tract.

FIGURE 14.10. A: Bone scan of an 11-year-old boy with metastatic osteosarcoma following left above-the-knee amputation. There is no abnormal uptake in the thorax. B: FDG-PET-CT scan shows metastatic disease in mediastinal and hilar lymph node regions.

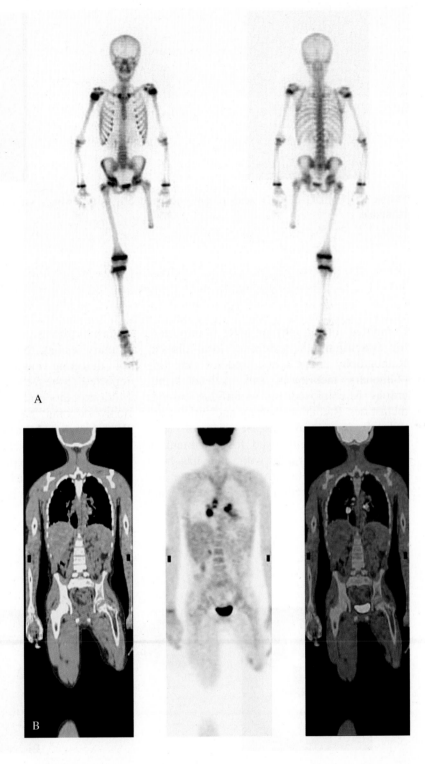

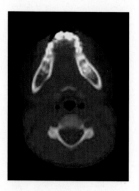
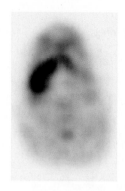
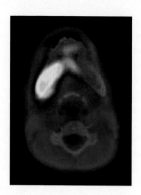

FIGURE 14.11. FDG-PET-CT scan of an 8-year-old boy with Ewing's sarcoma metastatic to the right mandible.

Computed tomography or MRI is important for establishing the extent of local disease. Radiography and CT are used for detecting pulmonary metastases, and skeletal scintigraphy is employed for identifying osseous metastases. Radiation therapy and surgery are utilized for local disease control, and chemotherapy is employed for treatment of metastases. Scintigraphy with ^{67}Ga has been shown to be valuable in the initial diagnosis, staging, and detection of recurrence and metastatic disease. In patients with gallium-avid primary lesions, the sensitivity and specificity for detecting metastatic disease has been reported to be 94% and 95%, respectively.[100] Mild to moderate ^{201}Tl uptake in rhabdomyosarcoma has also been described.[101] Rhabdomyosarcomas show variable degrees of FDG accumulation (Fig. 14.12). Cases showing the clinical utility of FDG-PET have been described, but the exact role of FDG-PET in rhabdomyosarcoma is yet to be determined.[93]

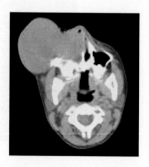
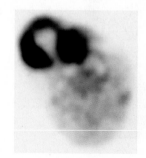
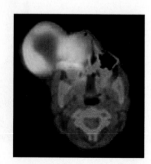

FIGURE 14.12. FDG-PET-CT scan of a 13-year-old girl with rhabdomyosarcoma of the right maxilla. There is considerable extracranial extension of the tumor. The center of the tumor is devoid of FDG activity following radiofrequency ablation.

References

1. Gurney JG, Severson RK, Davis S, Robinson LL. Incidence of cancer in children in the United States. Cancer 1995;75:2186–95.
2. Robinson L. General principles of the epidemiology of childhood cancer. In: Pizzo P, Poplack D, eds. Principles and Practice of Pediatric Oncology. Philadelphia: Lippincott-Raven, 1997:1–10.
3. Jones SC, Alavi A, Christman D, et al. The radiation dosimetry of 2-18F-fluoro-2-deoxy-D-glucose in man. J Nucl Med 1982;23:613–17.
4. Ruotsalainen U, Suhonen-Povli H, Eronen E, et al. Estimated radiation dose to the newborn in FDG-PET studies. J Nucl Med 1996;37:387–93.
5. Borgwardt L, Larsen HJ, Pedersen K, Hojgaard L. Practical use and implementation of PET in children in a hospital PET center. Eur J Nucl Med Mol Imaging 2003;30:1389–97.
6. Roberts EG, Shulkin BL. Technical issues in performing PET studies in pediatric patients. J Nucl Med Technol 2004;32:5–9.
7. Kaste SC. Issues specific to implementing PET-CT for pediatric oncology: what we have learned along the way. Pediatr Radiol 2004; 34:205–213.
8. Jadvar H, Connolly LP, Shulkin BL, et al. Positron emission tomography in pediatrics. In: Freeman LM, ed. Nuclear Medicine Annual. Philadelphia: Lippincott Williams & Wilkins, 2000:53–83.
9. Jadvar H, Connolly LP, Shulkin BL. PET imaging in pediatric disorders. In: Valk PE, Bailey DL, Townsend DW, Maisey MN, eds. Positron Emission Tomography: Basic Science and Clinical Practice. London: Springer-Verlag, 2003:755–74.
10. Shulkin BL. PET imaging in pediatric oncology. Pediatr Radiol 2004;34:199–204.
11. Kleihues P, Burger P, Scheithauer B. The new WHO classification of brain tumors. Brain Pathol 1993;3:255–68.
12. Robertson R, Ball WJ, Barnes P. Skull and brain. In: Kirks D, ed. Practical Pediatric Imaging. Diagnostic Radiology of Infants and Children. Philadelphia: Lippincott-Raven, 1997:65–200.
13. Maria B, Drane WB, Quisling RJ, Hoang KB. Correlation between gadolinium-diethylenetriaminepentaacetic acid contrast enhancement and thallium-201 chloride uptake in pediatric brainstem glioma. J Child Neurol 1997;12:341–8.
14. O'Tuama L, Janicek M, Barnes P, et al. Tl-201/Tc-99m HMPAO SPECT imaging of treated childhood brain tumors. Pediatr Neurol 1991;7:249–57.
15. O'Tuama L, Treves ST, Larar G, et al. Tl-201 versus Tc-99m MIBI SPECT in evaluation of childhood brain tumors: a within-subject comparison. J Nucl Med 1993;34:1045–51.
16. Rollins N, Lowry P, Shapiro K. Comparison of gadolinium-enhanced MR and thallium-201 single photon emission computed tomography in pediatric brain tumors. Pediatr Neurosurg 1995;22:8–14.
17. Zhang JJ, Park CH, Kim SM, et al. Dual isotope SPECT in the evaluation of recurrent brain tumor. Clin Nucl Med 1992;17:663–4.
18. Valk PE, Budinger TF, Levin VA, et al. PET of malignant cerebral tumors after interstitial brachytherapy. Demonstration of metabolic activity and correlation with clinical outcome. J Neurosurg 1988;69:830–8.
19. Di Chiro G, Oldfield E, Wright DC, et al. Cerebral necrosis after radiotherapy and/or intraarterial chemotherapy for brain tumors: PET and neuropathologic studies. AJR 1988; 150:189–97.
20. Glantz MJ, Hoffman JM, Coleman RE, et al. Identification of early recurrence of primary central nervous system tumors by 18F-fluorodeoxyglucose positron emission tomography. Ann Neurol 1991;29:347–55.
21. Janus T, Kim E, Tilbury R, et al. Use of 18F-fluorodeoxyglucose positron emission tomography in patients with primary malignant brain tumors. Ann Neurol 1993;33:540–8.
22. Rozental JM, Levine RL, Nickles RJ. Changes in glucose uptake by malignant gliomas: preliminary study of prognostic significance. J Neuron-Oncol 1991;10:75–83.
23. Schifter T, Hoffman JM, Hanson MW, et al. Serial FDG-PET studies in the prediction of survival in patients with primary brain tumors. J Comput Assist Tomogr 1993;17:509–61.
24. Francavilla TL, Miletich RS, Di Chiro G, et al. Positron emission tomography in the detection of malignant degeneration of low-grade gliomas. Neurosurgery 1989;24:1–5.
25. Patronas NJ, Di Chiro G, Kufta C, et al. Prediction of survival in glioma patients by means of positron emission tomography. J Neurosurg 1985;62:816–22.
26. Holthof VA, Herholz K, Berthold F, et al. In vivo metabolism of childhood posterior fossa tumors and primitive neuroectodermal tumors

before and after treatment. Cancer 1993: 1394–403.

27. Hoffman JM, Hanson MW, Friedman HS, et al. FDG-PET in pediatric posterior fossa brain tumors. J Comput Assist Tomogr 1992;16:62–8.

28. Molloy PT, Defeo R, Hunter J, et al. Excellent correlation of FDG PET imaging with clinical outcome in patients with neurofibromatosis type I and low-grade astrocytomas. J Nucl Med 1999;40:129P(abstr).

29. Pirotte B, Goldman S, Salzberg S, et al. Combined positron emission tomography and magnetic resonance imaging for the planning of stereotactic brain biopsies in children: experience in 9 cases. Pediatr Neurosurg 2003;38: 146–55.

30. Cohen MD. Imaging of Children with Cancer. St. Louis: Mosby Yearbook, 1992.

31. Rossleigh MA, Murray IPC, Mackey DWJ. Pediatric solid tumors: evaluation by gallium-67 SPECT studies. J Nucl Med 1990;31:161–72.

32. Howman-Giles R, Stevens M, Bergin M. Role of gallium-67 in management of paediatric solid tumors. Aust Paediatr J 1982;18:120–5.

33. Yang SL, Alderson PO, Kaizer HA, Wagner HA. Serial Ga-67 citrate imaging in children with neoplastic disease: concise communication. J Nucl Med 1979;20:210–14.

34. Sty JR, Kun LE, Starshak RJ. Pediatric applications in nuclear oncology. Semin Nucl Med 1985;15:17–200.

35. Waxman AD, Ramanna L, Said J. Thallium scintigraphy in lymphoma: relationship to gallium-67. J Nucl Med 1989;30:915(abstr).

36. Kaplan WD, Southee AE, Annese ML, et al. Evaluating low and intermediate grade non-Hodgkin's lymphoma with gallium-67 (Ga) and thallium-201 (Tl) imaging. J Nucl Med 1990; 31:793(abstr).

37. Okada J, Yoshikawa K, Imazeki K, et al. The use of FDG-PET in the detection and management of malignant lymphoma: correlation of uptake with prognosis. J Nucl Med 1991;32:686–91.

38. Rodriguez M, Rehn S, Ahlstrom H, et al. Predicting malignancy grade with PET in non-Hodgkin's lymphoma. J Nucl Med 1995;36: 1790–6.

39. Moog F, Bangerter M, Diederichs CG, et al. Lymphoma: role of whole-body 2-deoxy-2-F-18-fluoro-D-glucose (FDG) PET in nodal staging. Radiology 1997;203:795–800.

40. Moog F, Bangerter M, Diederichs CG, et al. Extranodal malignant lymphoma: detection with FDG PET versus CT. Radiology 1998; 206:475–81.

41. Okada J, Yoshikawa K, Itami M, et al. Positron emission tomography using fluorine-18-fluorodeoxyglucose in malignant lymphoma: a comparison with proliferative activity. J Nucl Med 1992;33:325–9.

42. Paul R. Comparison of fluorine-18-2-fluorodeoxyglucose and gallium-67 citrate imaging for detection of lymphoma. J Nucl Med 1987;28:288–92.

43. Newman JS, Francis IR, Kaminski MS, Wahl RL. Imaging of lymphoma with PET with 2-F-18–fluoro-2-deoxy-D-glucose: correlation with CT. Radiology 1994;190:111–16.

44. de Wit M, Bumann D, Beyer W, et al. Whole-body positron emission tomography (PET) for diagnosis of residual mass in patients with lymphoma. Ann Oncol 1997;8(suppl 1): 57–60.

45. Hudson MM, Krasin MJ, Kaste SC. PET imaging in pediatric Hodgkin's lymphoma. Pediatr Radiol 2004;34:190–8.

46. Montravers F, McNamara D, Landman-Parker J, et al. (18)F FDG in childhood lymphoma: clinical utility and impact on management. Eur J Nucl Med Mol Imaging 2002;29:1155–65.

47. Depas G, De Barsy C, Jerusalem G, et al. 18F-FDG PET in children with lymphomas. Eur J Nucl Med Mol Imaging 2005;32(1):31–8.

48. Carr R, Barrington SF, Madan B, et al. Detection of lymphoma in bone marrow by whole-body positron emission tomography. Blood 1998;91:3340–6.

49. Lavely WC, Delbeke D, Greer JP, et al. FDG PET in the follow-up of management of patients with newly diagnosed Hodgkin and non-Hodgkin lymphoma after first-line chemotherapy. Int J Radiat Oncol Biol Phys 2003;57:307–15.

50. Swift P. Novel techniques in the delivery of radiation in pediatric oncology. Pediatr Clin North Am 2002;49:1107–29.

51. Korholz D, Kluge R, Wickmann L, et al. Importance of F18-fluorodeoxy-D-2-glucose positron emission tomography (FDG-PET) for staging and therapy control of Hodgkin's lymphoma in childhood and adolescence—consequences for the GPOH-HD 2003 protocol. Onkologie 2003;26:489–93.

52. Krasin MJ, Hudson MM, Kaste SC. Positron emission tomography in pediatric radiation oncology: integration in the treatment-planning process. Pediatr Radiol 2004;34:214–21.

53. Kondoh H, Murayama S, Kozuka T, Nishimura T. Enhancement of hematopoietic uptake by granulocyte colony-stimulating factor in Ga-67 scintigraphy. Clin Nucl Med 1995;20:250–3.
54. Donahue DM, Leonard JC, Basmadjian GP, et al. Thymic gallium-67 localization in pediatric patients on chemotherapy: concise communication. J Nucl Med 1981;22(12):1043–8.
55. Patel PM, Alibazoglu H, Ali A, et al. Normal thymic uptake of FDG on PET imaging. Clin Nucl Med 1996;21:772–5.
56. Weinblatt ME, Zanzi I, Belakhlef A, et al. False positive FDG-PET imaging of the thymus of a child with Hodgkin's disease. J Nucl Med 1997;38:888–90.
57. Brink I, Reinhardt MJ, Hoegerle S, et al. Increased metabolic activity in the thymus gland studied with 18F-FDG PET: age dependency and frequency after chemotherapy. J Nucl Med 2001;42:591–5.
58. Yeung HW, Grewal RK, Gonen M, et al. Patterns of (18F)-FDG uptake in adipose tissue and muscles: a potential source of false-positives for PET. J Nucl Med 2003;44:1789–96.
59. Cohade C, Mourtzikos KA, Wahl RL. "USA-fat": prevalence is related to ambient outdoor temperature—evaluation with 18F-FDG PET/CT. J Nucl Med 2003;44:1267–70.
60. Weber WA. Brown adipose tissue and nuclear medicine imaging. J Nucl Med 2004;45:1101–3.
61. Delbeke D. Oncological applications of FDG PET imaging: colorectal cancer, lymphoma, and melanoma. J Nucl Med 1999;40:591–603.
62. Sugawara Y, Fisher SJ, Zasadny KR, et al. Preclinical and clinical studies of bone marrow uptake of fluorine-1-fluorodeoxyglucose with or without granulocyte colony-stimulating factor during chemotherapy. J Clin Oncol 1998; 16:173–80.
63. Hollinger EF, Alibazoglu H, Ali A, et al. Hematopoietic cytokine-mediated FDG uptake simulates the appearance of diffuse metastatic disease on whole-body PET imaging. Clin Nucl Med 1998;23:93–8.
64. Kushner BH. Neuroblastoma: a disease requiring a multitude of imaging studies. J Nucl Med 2004;45:1172–88.
65. Bousvaros A, Kirks DR, Grossman H. Imaging of neuroblastoma: an overview. Pediatr Radiol 1986;16:89–106.
66. Farahati J, Mueller SP, Coennen HH, et al. Scintigraphy of neuroblastoma with radiolabeled m-iodobenzylguanidine. In: Treves ST, ed. Pediatric Nuclear Medicine, 2nd ed. New York: Springer-Verlag, 1995:528–45.
67. Briganti V, Sestini R, Orlando C, et al. Imaging of somatostatin receptors by indium-111-pentetreotide correlates with quantitative determination of somatostatin receptor type 2 gene expression in neuroblastoma tumor. Clin Cancer Res 1997;3:2385–91.
68. Shulkin BL, Shapiro B, Hutchinson RJ. 131I-MIBG and bone scintigraphy for the detection of neuroblastoma. J Nucl Med 1992;33(10): 1735–40.
69. Shulkin BL, Hutchinson RJ, Castle VP, Yanik GA, Shapiro B, Sisson JC. Neuroblastoma: positron emission tomography with 2-fluorine-18-fluoro-2-deoxy-D-glucose compared with metaiodobenzylguanidine scintigraphy. Radiology 1996;199:743–50.
70. Kushner BH, Yeung HW, Larson SM, et al. Extending positron emission tomography scan utility to high-risk neuroblastoma: fluorine-18 fluorodeoxyglucose positron emission tomography as sole imaging modality in follow-up of patients. J Clin Oncol 2001;19:3397–405.
71. Barnewolt CE, Paltiel HJ, Lebowitz RL, Kirks DR. Genitourinary system. In: Kirks DR, ed. Practical Pediatric Imaging. Diagnostic Radiology of Infants and Children, 3rd ed. Philadelphia: Lippincott-Raven, 1997:1009–170.
72. Howman-Giles R, Uren R, White G, Shaw P. Tl-201 scintigraphy in pediatric solid tumors. J Nucl Med 1993;34:52(abstr).
73. Shulkin BL, Chang E, Strouse PJ, Bloom DA, Hutchinson RJ. PET FDG studies of Wilms tumors. J Pediatr Hematol Oncol 1997;19: 334–8(abstr).
74. McDonald DJ. Limb salvage surgery for sarcomas of the extremities. AJR 1994;163:509–13.
75. O'Connor MI, Pritchard DJ. Ewing's sarcoma. Prognostic factors, disease control, and the reemerging role of surgical treatment. Clin Orthop 1991;262:78–87.
76. Jaramillo D, Laor T, Gebhardt M. Pediatric musculoskeletal neoplasms. Evaluation with MR imaging. MRI Clin North Am 1996;4:1–22.
77. Frouge C, Vanel D, Coffre C, Couanet D, Contesso G, Sarrazin D. The role of magnetic resonance imaging in the evaluation of Ewing sarcoma—a report of 27 cases. Skeletal Radiol 1988;17:387–92.
78. MacVicar AD, Olliff JFC, Pringle J, et al. Ewing sarcoma: MR imaging of chemotherapy-induced changes with histologic correlation. Radiology 1992;184:859–64.

79. Lemmi MA, Fletcher BD, Marina NM, et al. Use of MR imaging to assess results of chemotherapy for Ewing sarcoma. AJR 1990;155: 343–6.

80. Erlemann R, Sciuk J, Bosse A, et al. Response of osteosarcoma and Ewing sarcoma to preoperative chemotherapy: assessment with dynamic and static MR imaging and skeletal scintigraphy. Radiology 1990;175:791–6.

81. Holscher HC, BLoem JL, Vanel D, et al. Osteosarcoma: chemotherapy-induced changes at MR imaging. Radiology 1992;182(3):839–44.

82. Lawrence JA, Babyn PS, Chan HS, et al. Extremity osteosarcoma in childhood: prognostic value of radiologic imaging. Radiology 1993;189:43–7.

83. Simon MA, Kirchner RT. Scintigraphic evaluation of primary bone tumors: comparison of technetium-99m phosphate and gallium citrate imaging. J Bone Joint Surg 1980;62:758–64.

84. Yeh SDJ, Rosen G, Caparros B, Benua RS. Semiquantitative gallium scintigraphy in patients with osteogenic sarcoma. Clin Nucl Med 1984;9:175–83.

85. Connolly LP, Laor T, Jaramillo D, et al. Prediction of chemotherapeutic response of osteosarcoma with quantitative thallium-201 scintigraphy and magnetic resonance imaging. Radiology 1996;201(P):349(abstr).

86. Lin J, Leung WT. Quantitative evaluation of thallium-201 uptake in predicting chemotherapeutic response of osteosarcoma. Eur J Nucl Med 1995;22:553–5.

87. Menendez LR, Fideler BM, Mirra J. Thallium-201 scanning for the evaluation of osteosarcoma and soft tissue sarcoma. J Bone Joint Surg 1993;75:526–31.

88. Ramanna L, Waxman A, Binney G, et al. Thallium-201 scintigraphy in bone sarcoma: comparison with gallium-67 and technetium-99m MDP in the evaluation of chemotherapeutic response. J Nucl Med 1990;31:567–72.

89. Rosen G, Loren GJ, Brien EW, et al. Serial thallium-201 scintigraphy in osteosarcoma. Correlation with tumor necrosis after preoperative chemotherapy. Clin Orthop 1993;293:302–6.

90. Ohtomo K, Terui S, Yokoyama R, et al. Thallium-201 scintigraphy to assess effect of chemotherapy to osteosarcoma. J Nucl Med 1996;37:1444–8.

91. Bar-Sever Z, Connolly LP, Treves ST, et al. Technetium-99m MIBI in the evaluation of children with Ewing's sarcoma. J Nucl Med 1997;38:13P(abstr).

92. Caner B, Kitapel M, Unlu M, et al. Technetium-99m-MIBI uptake in benign and malignant bone lesions: a comparative study with technetium-99m-MDP. J Nucl Med 1992;33:319–24.

93. Lenzo NP, Shulkin B, Castle VP, Hutchinson RJ. FDG PET in childhood soft tissue sarcoma. J Nucl Med 2000;41(5 suppl):96P(abstr).

94. Abdel-Dayem HM. The role of nuclear medicine in primary bone and soft tissue tumors. Semin Nucl Med 1997;27:355–63.

95. Shulkin BL, Mitchell DS, Ungar DR, et al. Neoplasms in a pediatric population: 2-F-18–fluoro-2-deoxy-D-glucose PET studies. Radiology 1995;194:495–500.

96. Franzius C, Sciuk J, Brinkschmidt C, et al. Evaluation of chemotherapy response in primary bone tumors with F-18 FDG positron emission tomography compared with histologically assessed tumor necrosis. Clin Nucl Med 2000; 25:874–81.

97. Hawkins DS, Rajendran JG, Conrad EU 3rd, et al. Evaluation of chemotherapy response in pediatric bone sarcomas by F-18-fluorodeoxy-D-glucose positron emission tomography. Cancer 2002;94:3277–84.

98. Brisse H, Ollivier L, Edeline V, et al. Imaging of malignant tumours of the long bones in children: monitoring response to neoadjuvant chemotherapy and preoperative assessment. Pediatr Radiol 2004;34:595–605.

99. Franzius C, Sciuk J, Daldrup-Link HE, et al. FDG-PET for detection of osseous metastases from malignant primary bone tumors: comparison with bone scintigraphy. Eur J Nucl Med 2000;27:1305–11.

100. Cogswell A, Howman-Giles R, Bergin M. Bone and gallium scintigraphy in children with rhabdomyosarcoma: a 10-year review. Med Pediatr Oncol 1994;22:15–21.

101. Nadel HR. Thallium-201 for oncological imaging in children. Semin Nucl Med 1993;23: 243–54.

15
Infection and Inflammation

Christopher J. Palestro, Charito Love, and Maria B. Tomas

Despite dramatic advances in its prevention and treatment, infection remains a major cause of morbidity in children, accounting for approximately 30% of childhood deaths worldwide.[1] The development of powerful antimicrobial agents has improved patient survival, but timely diagnosis is equally, if not more, important. In adults, most infections can be diagnosed with a thorough history, a complete physical examination, and appropriate laboratory tests. In the pediatric population, unfortunately, this is a difficult task. Children do not, or will not, verbalize their feelings, and the history is often little more than secondhand information obtained from a parent. The physical examination of an ailing child can be difficult, if not impossible. Further complicating matters is the fact that inflammatory conditions such as vasculitis and inflammatory disease may mimic infection. Consequently, empiric treatment with antibiotics, which may be neither appropriate nor effective, is often instituted. Imaging procedures are usually reserved for those patients in whom symptomatology or physical findings point to a specific region of the body. Because of concerns about radiation exposure, pediatricians tend to utilize nuclear imaging only as a last recourse, when all other resources have been exhausted. The nuclear physician is often faced with the formidable task of diagnosing and localizing infection and inflammation late in the course of an illness when an expeditious and correct diagnosis is even more critical.

Tracers

Methylene Diphosphonate (MDP)

The uptake of technetium-99m–methylene diphosphonate (^{99m}Tc-MDP) depends on blood flow and the rate of new bone formation. When performed for osteomyelitis, a three-phase study is usually done. Three–phase bone imaging consists of a dynamic imaging sequence, the perfusion phase, followed immediately by static images of the region of interest, the soft tissue phase. The third, or bone, phase is performed 2 to 4 hours later. Images should be acquired on a large field of view gamma camera equipped with a low-energy, high-resolution, parallel-hole collimator and a 15% to 20% window centered on 140 keV. The usual injected dose is 9 to 11 MBq (0.24–0.30 mCi)/kg of ^{99m}Tc-MDP.[2] The normal distribution of this tracer in children, by 2 hours after injection, includes the skeleton, genitourinary tract, and soft tissues. Intense, symmetric uptake in the physes of the long bones, which are centers of growth and hematopoietic production, is present. Intense uptake also can be appreciated in the marrow-rich flat facial bones.[3]

Gallium-67

For more than 30 years, gallium-67 (^{67}Ga)-citrate has been used for localizing foci of infection and inflammation. In spite of its disadvantages, including an inherent nonspecificity, the delay between injection and imaging, and a variable biodistribution that can confound image interpretation, gallium imaging remains both popular and useful, providing information that is complementary to, and at times not available from, other tests.

A group III transition metal with a half-life of 78 hours, ^{67}Ga emits a broad spectrum of gamma rays between 92 and 889 keV. The energies suitable for imaging include 92 keV (38%), 184 keV (23%), and 300 keV (16%). By 24 hours after injection about 10% to 25% of the administered dose is excreted via the kidneys. The large bowel is the principal excretory pathway beyond 24 hours. At 72 hours after injection about 75% of the administered dose remains in the body, equally distributed among soft tissues, bone/bone marrow, and liver.[4] The normal distribution is variable, however. Nasopharyngeal and lacrimal gland activity can

be quite prominent, even in the absence of disease. Breast uptake is usually faint and symmetric; intense uptake is associated with hyperprolactinemic conditions such as pregnancy, lactation, certain drugs, and hypothalamic lesions (Fig. 15.1).[5–8] In patients who have undergone multiple transfusions, increased renal, bladder, and bone activity, together with decreased hepatic and colonic activity, is often observed, presumably due to iron receptor saturation by exogenous iron from the transfused cells.[9] The magnetic resonance imaging (MRI) contrast agent gadolinium can cause a similar alteration in the biodistribution of gallium.[10]

Several factors govern the uptake of gallium in inflammation, and it is not necessary that they all be present for such uptake to occur. Following intravenous injection, more than 90% of circulating gallium is in the plasma, nearly all of it transferrin bound. Increased blood flow and increased vascular membrane

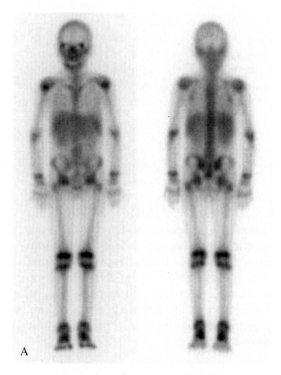

A

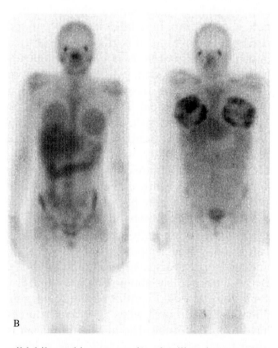

B

FIGURE 15.1. A: Normal anterior (left) and posterior (right) 72 hour images from a gallium scan performed on a 10-year-old patient. Note the uniformly intense activity in the ends of the long bones corresponding to active growth plates. B: Compare the mild, bilateral breast uptake of gallium in an asymptomatic 15-year-old girl (left) with the intense breast uptake in a 17-year-old girl (right) who had recently given birth.

permeability result in increased delivery to, and accumulation of, transferrin-bound gallium at inflammatory foci. Gallium also binds to lactoferrin, which is present in high concentrations in inflammatory foci. Direct uptake by certain bacteria, including *Staphylococcus aureus*, has been observed in vitro, and this too may account for gallium uptake in infection. Siderophores, small molecular weight chelates produced by bacteria for iron binding and transport, are gallium avid. It has been postulated that the siderophore-gallium complex is transported into the bacterium, where it remains until phagocytosed by macrophages. Although some gallium may be transported bound to leukocytes, it is important to note that, even in the absence of circulating leukocytes, gallium accumulates in infection.[4]

Imaging is usually performed 18 to 72 hours after injection of 1.5 to 2.6 MBq (0.04–0.07 mCi)/kg ^{67}Ga-citrate.[11,12] A gamma camera capable of imaging multiple energy peaks and equipped with a medium-energy collimator must be used. Gallium is excreted via the large bowel and colonic activity can make image interpretation difficult. The use of single photon emission computed tomography (SPECT) or delayed imaging facilitates image interpretation. Bowel preparation with laxatives prior to imaging is sometimes used, although its value is questionable.[4,12]

Labeled Leukocytes

In vitro labeling of leukocytes, a labor-intensive process that takes about 2 to 3 hours, is most often performed using the lipophilic compounds indium-111 (^{111}In)-oxyquinolone or technetium-99m–hexamethylpropyleneamine oxime (^{99m}Tc-HMPAO). The usual dose of ^{111}In-labeled leukocytes is 0.15 to 0.25 MBq (0.004–0.007 mCi)/kg; the usual dose of ^{99m}Tc-HMPAO–labeled leukocytes is 3.7 to 7.4 MBq (0.1–0.2 mCi)/kg.[13,14] A limiting factor to the use of labeled leukocyte imaging in children is the amount of blood that must be withdrawn in order to obtain a sufficiently large quantity of leukocytes to label and subsequently image. In adults and older children, 40 to 60 mL of whole blood can be confidently withdrawn without fear of precipitating a hemodynamic crisis. But this is not the case in younger children and infants, and unfortunately there are no data available on the smallest quantity of blood that must be withdrawn to satisfactorily perform the test. For safety reasons, not more than 5% of a child's total blood volume, or about 3.5 mL/kg, should be withdrawn. Using this guideline, we have successfully imaged infants as young as 6 weeks old, after labeling leukocytes separated from as little as 7 mL of blood.

Successful imaging with labeled white cells depends on intact chemotaxis, the number and types of cells labeled, and the cellular response to a particular inflammatory process. The conventional labeling process does not normally affect leukocyte chemotaxis. A circulating white count of at least 2 to 3×10^6/mL is probably needed to obtain satisfactory images. In most clinical settings, the majority of leukocytes labeled are neutrophils, and hence the procedure is most sensitive for identifying neutrophil-mediated inflammatory processes, such as bacterial infections. The procedure is not sensitive for detecting illnesses, such as sarcoidosis and tuberculosis, in which the predominant cellular response is not neutrophilic.[12,15]

Regardless of whether leukocytes are labeled with ^{111}In or ^{99m}Tc, intense diffuse, bilateral pulmonary activity is observed on images obtained shortly after injection. This activity decreases over time, reaching background levels within 4 hours (Fig. 15.2). This phenomenon is likely due to several factors. Neutrophils spend more time in contact with the pulmonary endothelium than they do in the systemic vascular bed. One reason for this is that the mean pressure across the pulmonary circulation is lower than that in the systemic circulation. Cell size is another factor. To pass through the pulmonary capillaries, which are about 5.5 μm in diameter, neutrophils, which are about 8 μm in diameter, must undergo cytoskeletal deformation. During the labeling procedure, neutrophils are activated. Activated cells are more rigid and less easily deformed and consequently pass more slowly through the pulmonary vessels. Activated leukocytes also adhere to the pulmonary capillaries for a longer period than do nonactivated cells. Finally, there is evidence that the in vitro

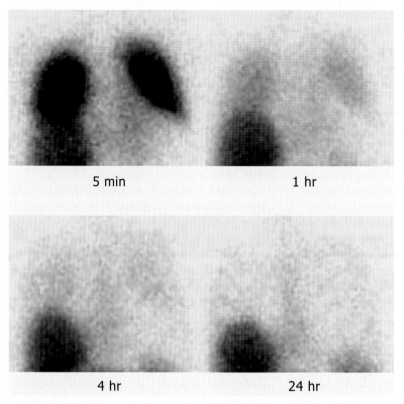

FIGURE 15.2. Labeled leukocyte images are characterized by intense pulmonary activity soon after injection. The intensity of this activity rapidly decreases, approaching background within about 4 hours after injection. This phenomenon is independent of the radiolabel used.

labeling procedure itself causes prolonged pulmonary transit of leukocytes, perhaps as a result of cell trauma during the labeling process.[16–18]

At 24 hours after injection, the usual imaging time for ^{111}In-labeled leukocytes, the normal distribution of activity is limited to the liver, spleen, and bone marrow (Fig. 15.3).[12,15] The normal biodistribution of ^{99m}Tc-HMPAO–labeled leukocytes is more variable. In addition to the reticuloendothelial system, activity is also normally present in the genitourinary tract, large bowel (within 4 hours after injection), blood pool, and occasionally the gallbladder.[12,15,19] The time interval between injection of ^{99m}Tc-HMPAO–labeled leukocytes and imaging varies with the indication; in general imaging is usually performed within a few hours after injection.

For ^{111}In-labeled leukocyte studies, images should be acquired on a large field of view gamma camera equipped with a medium-energy parallel-hole collimator. Energy dis-

crimination is accomplished by using a 15% window centered on the 174-keV photopeak and a 20% window centered on the 247-keV photopeak of [111]In. For ^{99m}Tc-labeled autologous leukocyte studies, a high-resolution, low-energy, parallel-hole collimator is used with a 15% to 20% window centered on the 140-keV photopeak of [99m]Tc.[12]

There are advantages and disadvantages to both [111]In- and ^{99m}Tc-labeled leukocytes. Advantages of ^{99m}Tc-labeled cells include a photon energy that is optimal for imaging using current instrumentation, a higher photon flux, and the ability to detect abnormalities within a few hours after injection. Disadvantages include genitourinary tract activity, which appears shortly after injection, and bowel activity, which appears by 4 hours after injection. The instability of the label and the short half-life of technetium-99m are disadvantages when delayed 24-hour imaging is needed. This occurs in those infections that tend to be indolent in nature and for which several hours may be necessary for

FIGURE 15.3. Normal anterior (left) and posterior (right) 24-hour whole-body images from an indium-111 (^{111}In)-labeled leukocyte study performed on a 9-year-old child. Activity is limited to the liver, spleen, and bone marrow. The distribution of hematopoietically active bone marrow varies with the age of the child, with decreasing appendicular activity, as the child grows older. Regardless of the radiolabel used, splenic uptake is normally more intense than hepatic uptake.

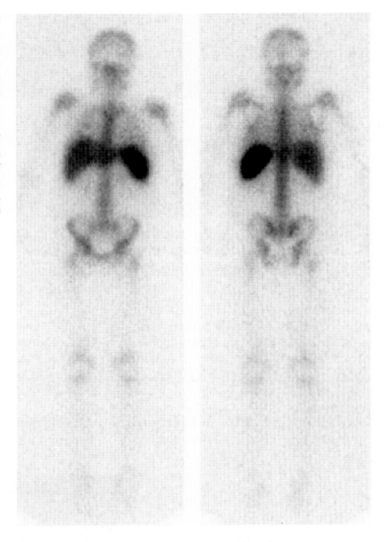

accumulation of a sufficient quantity of labeled leukocytes to be successfully imaged.[15]

The advantages of the ^{111}In label are the stability of the label, and a virtually constant normal distribution of activity limited to the liver, spleen, and bone marrow. The 67-hour physical half-life of ^{111}In allows for delayed imaging, which is valuable for musculoskeletal infection. There is another advantage to the use of indium-labeled leukocytes in musculoskeletal infection. Many of these patients require bone or marrow scintigraphy, which can be performed while the patient's cells are being labeled, as part of a simultaneous dual isotope acquisition, or immediately after completion of

the indium-labeled leukocyte study. When technetium-labeled leukocytes are used, an interval of least 48 hours is required between the white cell and bone or marrow scans.[15]

The disadvantages of the indium label include a low photon flux, less than ideal photon energies, and the fact that a 24-hour interval between injection and imaging are generally required.

^{99m}Tc-labeled leukocytes are best suited to imaging acute inflammatory conditions, such as inflammatory bowel disease, whereas ^{111}In-labeled white cells are preferred for more indolent conditions such as musculoskeletal infection.

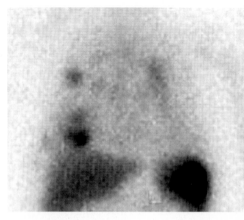
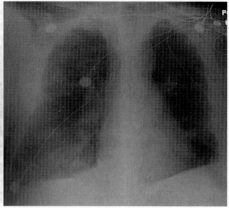

FIGURE 15.4. Bilateral, multifocal areas of pul-monary activity are present on the labeled leukocyte image of a patient with pneumonia (left). Bilateral infiltrates are present on the chest x-ray performed the same day (right).

To maximize the value of labeled leukocyte imaging, pitfalls of the technique must be recognized. Although pulmonary uptake of labeled leukocytes is a normal physiologic event during the first few hours after injection, by 24 hours such uptake is abnormal. Focal pul-monary uptake that is segmental or lobar in appearance is usually associated with bacterial pneumonia (Fig. 15.4). In addition to pneumo-nia, segmental/lobar pulmonary uptake of labeled leukocytes can be seen in patients with cystic fibrosis. This uptake is usually intense, multifocal, and bilateral, and is due to the accu-mulation of labeled leukocytes in pooled secre-tions in bronchiectatic regions of the lungs. In patients with cystic fibrosis, pulmonary uptake of labeled leukocytes cannot automatically be equated with infection (Fig. 15.5). Focal pul-

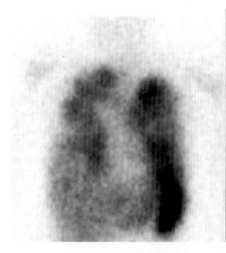
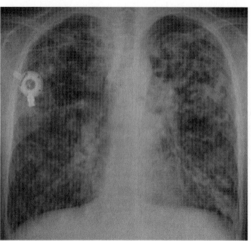

FIGURE 15.5. There is intense, multifocal, bilateral pulmonary uptake of labeled leukocytes (left) in a 15-year-old patient with cystic fibrosis. Chest radi-ograph (right), which demonstrates diffuse fibrotic changes with large bronchiectatic cavities and air-space infiltrates, was unchanged from prior studies, and the patient's respiratory status was stable. In the patient with cystic fibrosis, pulmonary uptake of labeled leukocytes cannot automatically be equated with infection. (Source: Love et al.,[17] with permission of the Radiological Society of North America.)

FIGURE 15.6. Anterior (left) and posterior (right) 24-hour whole-body images from labeled leukocyte study performed on a 9-year-old patient with septicemia but with no signs or symptoms referable to the respiratory tract. Note the diffuse bilateral pulmonary uptake of labeled leukocytes, which has been observed in the septic patient and is apparently of no clinical significance.

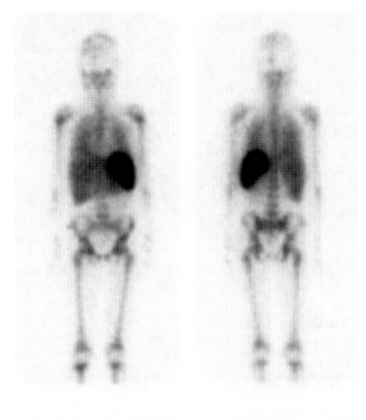

monary uptake that is not segmental or lobar is due to technical problems during labeling or reinfusion and is not usually associated with infection.[17,20,21]

Diffuse pulmonary uptake on images obtained more than 4 hours after reinjection of labeled cells is associated with a variety of pathologic conditions, including opportunistic infection, radiation pneumonitis, pulmonary drug toxicity, and adult respiratory distress syndrome. This pattern is almost never seen in bacterial pneumonia, however.[17,22–25]

Diffuse pulmonary uptake of labeled leukocytes can also be observed in septic patients whose chest x-rays are normal and who have no clinical evidence of respiratory tract inflammation or infection. It is believed that the circulating neutrophils are activated by cytokines, which are released peripherally in response to an infection. These activated neutrophils pool in the pulmonary circulation because it is more difficult for them to undergo the cytoskeletal deformation required to maneuver through the pulmonary circulation. The cytokines presumably also activate pulmonary vascular endothelial cells, causing increased adherence of leukocytes to the cell walls (Fig. 15.6).[17,25–28]

In-111–labeled leukocytes do not accumulate in normal bowel; such activity is abnormal. In hospitalized patients, a frequent cause of this activity is antibiotic-associated, or pseudomembranous, colitis. Other etiologies include inflammatory bowel disease, ischemic colitis, and gastrointestinal bleeding (Fig. 15.7).[12,15]

Labeled leukocytes do not accumulate in normally healing surgical wounds, so that the presence of such activity indicates infection. There are, however, certain exceptions. Granulating wounds, or wounds that heal by secondary intention, can appear as areas of intense

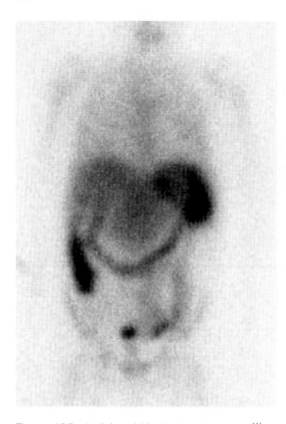

activity on leukocyte images even in the absence of infection. Examples include "ostomies" (tracheostomies, ileostomies, feeding gastrostomies, etc.) and skin grafts (Fig. 15.8).[29]

Focal uptake, especially when superficial in location, requires careful clinical correlation. Vascular access lines, dialysis catheters, and even lumbar punctures can all yield false-positive results in the absence of appropriate clinical history.[29]

^{99m}Tc-Fanolesomab

Considerable effort has been devoted to developing in vivo methods of labeling leukocytes, including use of peptides and antigranulocyte antibodies/antibody fragments. ^{99m}Tc-fanolesomab, approved for clinical use in the United States in 2004, is a monoclonal murine M class immunoglobulin that binds to CD15 receptors present on leukocytes. Originally raised against stage-specific embryonic antigen (SSEA)-1 in mice immunized with murine embryonal carcinoma F9 cells, this antibody has a molecular weight of approximately 900 kd. It exhibits a high affinity (association constant $K_d = 10^{-11}$ M) for the carbohydrate moiety 3-fucosyl-N-acetyl lactosamine contained in the CD15 antigen, which is expressed on human neutrophils, eosinophils, and lymphocytes. This agent pre-

FIGURE 15.7. Activity within the large bowel on ^{111}In-labeled leukocyte images is always abnormal. In patients receiving antibiotics, such uptake is often indicative of antibiotic associated colitis.

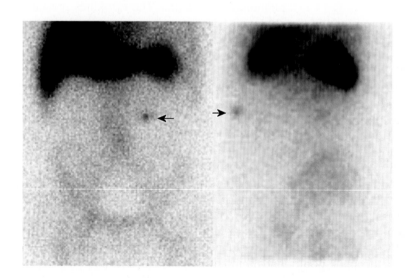

FIGURE 15.8. There is a superficial focus (arrows) of labeled leukocyte activity in the left upper abdomen of a patient with a feeding gastrostomy. Such uptake, which can be quite intense at times, is normally present around "ostomy" sites and does not indicate infection.

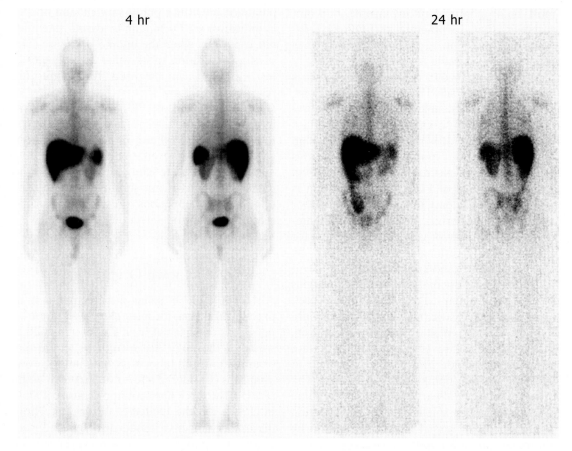

FIGURE 15.9. The normal distribution of ^{99m}Tc-fanolesomab, shortly after injection includes the liver, spleen, bone marrow, genitourinary tract, and blood pool (left). Colonic activity is often present at 24 hours (right).

sumably binds to circulating neutrophils that eventually migrate to the focus of infection, as well as to neutrophils and neutrophil debris containing CD15 receptors, already sequestered in the focus of infection.[30]

About 8 MBq (0.22 mCi)/kg of the radiolabeled compound, containing 75 to 125 μg antibody, is injected. Activity is initially distributed in the vasculature and eliminated from the blood with a mean linear half-life of 8 hours. Splenic and hepatic activity peak 25 to 35 minutes following injection (Fig. 15.9). In contrast to in vitro labeled leukocytes, there is no increased retention of activity in the lungs. The dose-limiting organ is the spleen, which receives an estimated 0.064 mGy/MBq (0.24 rad/mCi).[30]

Within 20 minutes after injection of fanolesomab, there is a transient drop in the number of circulating white cells. Return to baseline usually occurs within 45 minutes.[30] (Following reports of serious adverse events, this agent was withdrawn from the U.S. Market in December, 2005).

Fluorodeoxyglucose Positron Emission Tomography (FDG-PET)

Fluorine-18 fluorodeoxyglucose (^{18}F-FDG) is readily available, exquisitely sensitive, and relatively inexpensive. The procedure is rapidly completed, and the high-resolution tomographic positron emission tomography (PET) images are superior to those provided by most single photon emitting agents. It is not surprising that the potential of FDG-PET for detecting infection and inflammation has attracted considerable interest.

Fluorodeoxyglucose, a glucose analogue, is transported into cells via glucose transporters. Intracellular radiolabeled FDG is phosphorylated by hexokinase enzyme to ^{18}F-2'-FDG-6 phosphate, which does not easily pass through the cell membrane. Compared with glucose, this fluorinated deoxyglucose is not metabolized. Increased uptake of FDG in inflammation is related, at least in part, to an increased number of glucose transporters. In addition, in inflammation, the affinity of glucose transporters for deoxyglucose presumably is increased by various cytokines and growth factors.[31–37]

The normal distribution of FDG includes brain, myocardium, and genitourinary tract. Bone marrow, gastric, and bowel activity are variable. Thymic uptake, especially in children, can be prominent. Liver and spleen uptake are generally low-grade and diffuse, although in infection, splenic uptake may be intense. The spleen is an integral part of the body's immune system. Increased splenic activity in infection likely reflects increased glucose utilization by this organ, and it is important to recognize that this increased activity cannot automatically be attributed to infection or tumor of the organ itself.[31] The usual pediatric dose is 5 to 10 MBq (0.14–0.30 mCi)/kg.[38]

Indications

Opportunistic Infection

Nuclear medicine plays an important role in the detection of infections unique to the immunocompromised patient, and for most of them, gallium imaging is the radionuclide procedure of choice. Many opportunistic infections affect the lungs, and a normal gallium scan of the chest excludes infection with a high degree of certainty, especially in the setting of a negative chest radiograph. In the HIV-positive patient, lymph node uptake of gallium is most often due to mycobacterial disease or lymphoma. Focal, or localized, pulmonary parenchymal uptake of gallium is usually associated with bacterial

pneumonia. Diffuse pulmonary gallium uptake is indicative of *Pneumocystis carinii* pneumonia, especially when the uptake is intense (Fig. 15.10). In addition to its value as a diagnostic test, gallium can be used for monitoring response to therapy.[4,15,39]

Fluorodeoxyglucose PET is also a useful test in this population, especially in the central nervous system, where it accurately distinguishes lymphoma from toxoplasmosis.[31,40,41]

Labeled leukocyte scintigraphy, in contrast to gallium imaging, is not sensitive for detecting opportunistic infections presumably because most opportunistic infections do not incite a neutrophilic response.[4,15,22,39]

Fever of Unknown Origin

Although there is some disagreement on its precise definition, for most clinical situations, a persistent fever for at least 8 days in a child in whom a thorough history, complete physical examination, and laboratory data fail to reveal a cause, is considered a fever of unknown origin (FUO). The three most common causes of FUO in children in the United States are infectious diseases, connective tissue diseases, and neoplasms. In up to 20% of cases, however, a definitive diagnosis is never established. The most frequently diagnosed systemic infections in children with FUO include tuberculosis, brucellosis, tularemia, salmonellosis, and various viruses. Focal infections include urinary tract infection, osteomyelitis, and abdominal/pelvic abscesses. The connective tissue disorders most commonly presenting as FUO in children are juvenile rheumatoid arthritis, systemic lupus erythematosus, and undefined vasculitis. Leukemia and lymphoma are the malignancies most often presenting as FUO.[42]

The role of radionuclide studies in the evaluation of children with FUO has received only limited attention in the literature, and for the most part the results have been disappointing. Buonomo and Treves[43] reviewed gallium scintigraphy, and found that although the test was positive in three of five children with focal signs and symptoms, the test was positive in only one of 25 children with only systemic signs or symptoms. These investigators concluded

FIGURE 15.10. There is intense, diffuse bilateral pulmonary uptake of gallium 67 in a 20-year-old patient who had recently completed treatment for non-Hodgkin's lymphoma. Although diffuse lung uptake of gallium is not specific, the more intense the uptake, the more likely the patient is to have *Pneumocystis carinii* pneumonia.

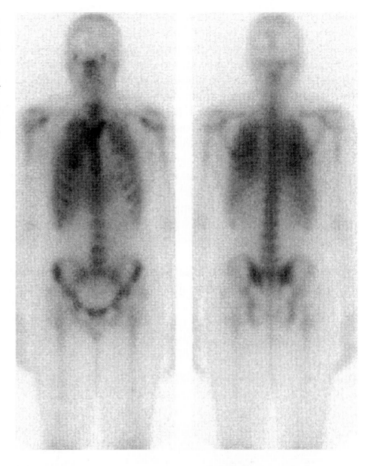

that gallium imaging is of little use in children with FUO who present with only systemic signs or symptoms.

Haentjens et al.[44] reviewed the results of labeled leukocyte imaging in 15 children and reported that false-negative results were found in five: pericarditis, osteomyelitis, hepatic abscess (two), and lung abscess. Williamson et al.[45] found that labeled leukocyte imaging was sensitive (94%) but not specific (57%). Steele et al.[46] found that imaging procedures, including radionuclide tests, rarely identified an unsuspected diagnosis.

Despite these disappointing results, clinicians do occasionally request radionuclide imaging for a child with FUO. The appropriate radionuclide study to perform, however, is open to debate. Labeled leukocyte imaging is more sensitive early in the course of an illness, whereas gallium is more sensitive later in the illness, and

the selection of the procedure could be determined by the duration of the illness. The etiologies of the FUO are numerous and it could be argued that the sensitive, but nonspecific, gallium should be the initial radionuclide study. Unfortunately, if one begins with gallium, it is necessary to wait a minimum of 7 to 10 days before performing a labeled leukocyte study. If labeled leukocyte imaging is performed first, however, one can immediately proceed to gallium imaging when necessary.[12,15] We generally begin with labeled leukocyte imaging and proceed to gallium imaging as needed. Regardless of which study is performed first, several days are required to complete both procedures.

Fluorodeoxyglucose PET is an intriguing and exciting alternative to the conventional radionuclide approach to the FUO. Fluorodeoxyglucose is similar to gallium; that is, though not specific, it is exquisitely sensitive, ideally suited to the evaluation of an entity with diverse etiologies. The short half-life of ^{18}F, moreover, does not delay the performance of any additional radionuclide studies that might be contemplated. Several studies support the use of FDG-PET in adults with FUO.[47–50] Blockmans et al.[47] reported that FDG-PET contributed helpful information in 41% of the patients studied. In a subgroup of patients who also underwent gallium imaging, FDG-PET was helpful in 35% of the cases, whereas gallium was helpful in 25%. These investigators concluded that FDG-PET compares favorably with gallium, and because of its rapid completion, could replace gallium scintigraphy as a radiopharmaceutical for the evaluation of patients with FUO (Fig. 15.11). Meller et al.[48] prospectively evaluated the utility of FDG-

PET in 20 patients with FUO. These investigators reported that FDG was 84% sensitive and 86% specific for identifying the source of the FUO. Among 18 patients who also underwent gallium imaging, FDG was more sensitive (81%) and more specific (86%) than gallium (67% sensitivity, 78% specificity). Bleeker-Rovers et al.[49] evaluated 35 patients with FUO and reported that FDG-PET studies were clinically helpful in 37% of the cases. The sensitivity and specificity of the test were 93% and 90%, respectively. The positive predictive value of the test was 87%, and the negative predictive value was 95%.

The potential value of this test has been further enhanced by preliminary data, which suggest that infective endocarditis and vasculitis, both of which can be the source of an FUO, and which were not previously amenable to detection with radionuclide studies, may be identified with FDG-PET.[51–54] Infective endocarditis is usually diagnosed by a combination of clinical and laboratory data together with the echocardiographic identification of valvular vegetations. Occasionally, however, vegetations are not infected. The intense echoes produced by the prosthesis may obscure small vegetations in patients with prosthetic heart valves. Yen et al.[51] found that, in spite of the normal myocardial FDG uptake, FDG-PET accurately identifies sites of infective endocarditis and may be a promising adjunct to echocardiography.

Vasculitis, an important cause of FUO in children, is characterized by inflammation and necrosis of blood vessel walls. The diagnosis is complicated by a lack of specific signs and symptoms, and imaging techniques are often used to confirm a suspected diagnosis in the absence of histologic proof, as well as to identify sites for biopsy.[31] Uptake of FDG in giant cell arteritis, Takayasu's arteritis, aortitis, and unspecified large vessel vasculitis have been described.[52–54] Blockmans et al.[53] observed abnormal vascular FDG uptake in 76% of 25 patients with proven temporal arteritis or polymyalgia rheumatica. Thoracic artery uptake had a positive predictive value of 93% and a negative predictive value of 80%. Meller et al.[54] found that FDG-PET identified more

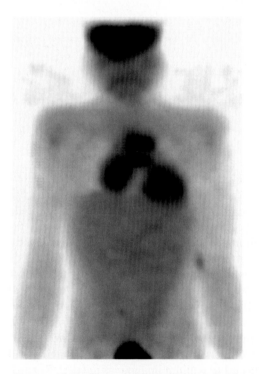

FIGURE 15.11. Fluorodeoxyglucose positron emission tomography (FDG-PET) imaging performed on a 14-year-old boy with a history of 3 weeks of intermittent fevers and a "widened mediastinum" on chest x-ray revealed hypermetabolic foci in the mediastinum. Lymph node biopsy was negative for tumor, but cultures subsequently grew Mycobacterium tuberculosis.

areas of involvement than MRI and was effective in the diagnosis and follow-up of patients with aortitis.

Other entities, including thromboembolic disease, childhood sarcoidosis, and chronic granulomatous disease, all of which can all present as an FUO, are associated with increased FDG uptake.[31]

Currently available data indicate that the negative predictive value of FDG-PET is very high; that is, a negative test makes it very unlikely that a morphologic origin of the fever will be identified. If borne out in larger series, FDG-PET, by reducing the number of imaging studies performed, may prove to be a very cost-effective method of investigating the FUO.

Appendicitis

Acute appendicitis presents as vague epigastric or periumbilical pain that increases in intensity, localizing in the right lower quadrant of the abdomen over the course of a few hours. Anorexia, nausea, and low-grade fever may also be present. There is localized right lower quadrant tenderness on deep palpation, coughing, or, on removal of the palpating hand, so-called rebound tenderness. Constipation and diarrhea are common in children. The erythrocyte sedimentation rate and C-reactive protein levels are increased, and leukocytosis may be present. This typical presentation of acute appendicitis, unfortunately, is found in only about 50% to 60% of patients, and is even less common in the very young, the very old, and women of childbearing age. Accurate and timely diagnosis can be clinically challenging; appendicitis is one of the most commonly misdiagnosed entities in emergency departments. Nearly 30% of pediatric patients ultimately diagnosed with acute appendicitis were originally misdiagnosed, and complications of a delayed, or missed, diagnosis, occur in up to 40% of these individuals.[55,56]

The conventional approach to the patient with an atypical or equivocal presentation for acute appendicitis includes a prolonged in-hospital stay for observation and frequent examination, as well as imaging studies, or discharge from the hospital with advice to return

if symptoms worsen. Ultrasonography has an accuracy of only about 30%. Computed tomography, with an accuracy of 93% to 94% with use of oral and intravenous (IV) contrast, requires some time for luminal contrast opacification to reach the area of the appendix, has decreased sensitivity in patients with low body fat content, and has the risk of allergic reaction to intravenous contrast.[12] In vitro labeled white cell imaging, using ^{99m}Tc-HMPAO–labeled leukocytes, accurately diagnoses early appendicitis. In a study of 100 pediatric patients with equivocal signs or symptoms, Rypins and Kipper[57] found that the test was 97% sensitive and 94% specific for diagnosing appendicitis. The negative predictive value of the test was 98%, and the negative laparotomy rate was only 4% compared to the current standard of about 12%. Disadvantages, however, include limited availability, lengthy preparation time (2 hours or more), the hazards associated with ex vivo leukocyte labeling, and in the case of small children, the amount of whole blood that must be withdrawn for the labeling process. Consequently, labeled leukocyte imaging has not gained widespread use for diagnosing appendicitis.

Recent studies have found that ^{99m}Tc-fanolesomab, which essentially labels leukocytes in vivo, is a valuable diagnostic adjunct in atypical appendicitis, and may, in fact, serve as a screening test for acute appendicitis.[58,59] In contrast to the conventional in vitro labeled leukocyte procedure, the agent requires no specially trained personnel, is supplied in kit form, and can be formulated in about 30 minutes.

A large multicenter trial, involving 200 patients between 5 and 86 years old, was conducted to assess the efficacy of fanolesomab for diagnosing acute appendicitis in patients with an equivocal presentation, to evaluate its safety, and to assess its potential impact on the clinical management of these patients.[59] There were 59 patients with histopathologically confirmed acute appendicitis. Sensitivity, specificity, and accuracy of fanolesomab were 91%, 86%, and 87%, respectively. The positive and negative predictive values of the test were 73% and 96%, respectively. The diagnosis of appendicitis was made in all cases within 90 minutes after

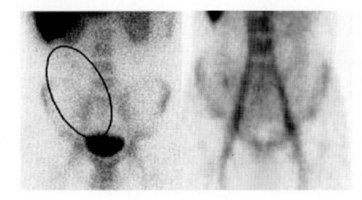

FIGURE 15.12. The so-called "appendicitis zone" in the right lower quadrant of the abdomen (left). Note the abnormal ^{99m}Tc-fanolesomab activity in this zone in a patient with appendicitis (right).

injection. Images became positive within 8 minutes in 50%, and within 50 minutes in 90%, of patients with acute appendicitis. In the subgroup of 48 pediatric patients, 5 to 17 years of age, the results were similar. The sensitivity, specificity, and accuracy of fanolesomab were 91%, 86%, and 88%, respectively. Positive and negative predictive values were 67% and 97%, respectively. The high negative predictive value is especially important, because a negative result means that acute appendicitis is very unlikely, thereby reducing unnecessary time in the hospital for observation, as well as unnecessary surgery. Finally, there was a significant improvement in making the appropriate management decision, both in patients with and in those without appendicitis, after the scan.

Imaging is carried out over a 90-minute period. Planar imaging is usually sufficient. Abnormal right lower quadrant activity in the "appendicitis zone" that persists over time is considered positive for appendicitis (Fig. 15.12).[59]

Inflammatory Bowel Disease

Inflammatory bowel disease (IBD) is a group of idiopathic, chronic disorders, of uncertain etiology, that include Crohn's disease and ulcerative colitis. The natural course of these disorders is one of unpredictable exacerbations and remissions. Although it can begin as early as the first year of life, IBD usually develops during adolescence and young adulthood and, in developed countries, is the major cause of chronic intestinal inflammation in children beyond the first few years of life.[60] Signs and symptoms of IBD in children are often nonspecific, and consequently this diagnosis is entertained in many children who ultimately are found to have other maladies. Definitive diagnosis is made with a combination of barium contrast radiography, upper gastrointestinal endoscopy, and colonoscopy with biopsy. Barium contrast radiography is associated with significant levels of ionizing radiation. Pediatric endoscopy requires special expertise and facilities, and sedation or general anesthesia may be necessary. Bowel evacuation regimens are a prerequisite for successful colonoscopy.[61] All of these tests are invasive, time consuming, and unpleasant for the patient. Thus, while radiologic studies and endoscopy are important for making the diagnosis of IBD, they are not appropriate screening tests, nor are they well suited for routine follow-up.

Though not a substitute for conventional diagnostic methods in pediatric IBD, labeled leukocyte imaging is very useful in a variety of situations. Several investigators have reported that the test is very sensitive for detecting IBD, with a high negative predictive value.[61–68] Because a negative study excludes, with a high degree of certainty, IBD as the cause of the patient's symptoms, labeled leukocyte imaging can be used a screening test to determine which children need to undergo more invasive investigation (Fig. 15.13). In the patient thought to

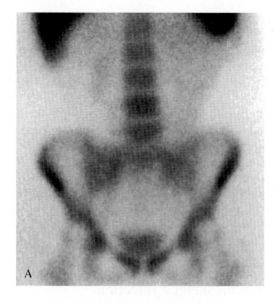

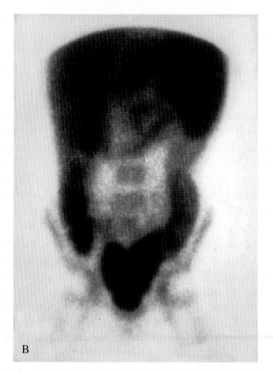

have ulcerative, or indeterminate, colitis, the presence of skip areas of activity in the colon, or the presence of small bowel activity, support the diagnosis of Crohn's disease (Fig. 15.14). The radionuclide study is also useful for patients who refuse endoscopy or contrast radiography and for those in whom these studies cannot be satisfactorily performed because of narrowing of the bowel lumen. The ability of the radionuclide study to differentiate active inflammation, which may respond to medical therapy, from scarring, which may require surgery, can have a significant impact on patient management.[63]

Radionuclide imaging can also be used to monitor patient response to therapy. Persistent bowel activity after a conventional course of therapy suggests that more intensive medical therapy, or even surgery, are in order. Similarly,

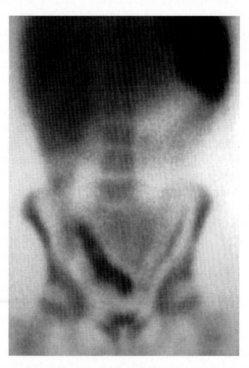

FIGURE 15.13. A: Normal ^{99m}Tc-labeled leukocyte image. Labeled leukocyte imaging is very sensitive for detecting inflammatory bowel disease (IBD). Consequently, in the symptomatic individual, a negative scan excludes IBD, with a high degree of certainty, as the cause of the patient's symptoms. B: There is intense labeled leukocyte activity throughout the colon in a patient with ulcerative colitis. (*Source:* Courtesy of Dr. Martin Charron.)

FIGURE 15.14. In addition to mild pancolonic activity, abnormal labeled leukocyte activity is also present in the distal jejunum/proximal ileum, and distal ileum. The presence of small bowel activity in the patient with colitis supports the diagnosis of Crohn's disease. (*Source:* Courtesy of Dr. Martin Charron.)

decreasing bowel uptake on serial studies confirms that the patient is responding to the therapeutic regimen, while persistent or recurrent uptake is indicative of residual disease or relapse. In the asymptomatic patient with elevated laboratory markers of inflammation, an abnormal labeled leukocyte study confirms the presence of active disease, and appropriate therapy can be instituted promptly. In the patient with a history of IBD and recurrent symptoms, but with a normal physical examination and normal laboratory tests, a negative leukocyte study effectively excludes active IBD as the cause of the symptoms.[63]

Although early studies were performed with ^{111}In-labeled autologous leukocytes, it is now agreed that ^{99m}Tc-HMPAO–labeled leukocytes should be used for the evaluation of IBD. Imaging at multiple time points maximizes the sensitivity of the test. In one series in which imaging was performed within 1 hour and again within 3 hours after injection, 12% of patients with disease were detected only on late images. Similarly, SPECT also increases the sensitivity of the test.[64] The caudal, or pelvic outlet, view facilitates detection of rectal disease that might otherwise be masked by urinary bladder activity. Physiologic bowel activity, probably due to hepatobiliary excretion of ^{99m}Tc-labeled hydrophilic complexes, appears on delayed images in up to 20% of children, and must be differentiated from activity secondary to inflammation. Physiologic activity appears in the distal small bowel no less than 3 hours after injection, is diffuse and mild in intensity, and migrates into the cecum by 4 hours. There must be no accumulation in other bowel segments.[64]

It is interesting to note that in a recent investigation in which labeled leukocyte imaging was found to be less accurate than previously reported, the presence of a stricture was considered diagnostic of active disease whether or not active inflammation was present, the pelvic outlet views apparently were not obtained, and the issue of physiologic bowel activity was not addressed.[69]

There are, however, some limitations to labeled leukocyte imaging. It cannot be the only imaging test used for IBD. It cannot define anatomic changes such as strictures, which are best delineated with endoscopy and contrast radiography. The test is less sensitive for upper, than for lower, gastrointestinal tract disease.[69,70] The sensitivity of the test also may be affected adversely by concomitant administration of corticosteroids.[63] Nevertheless, labeled leukocyte imaging is useful as an initial screening test to identify patients who need further investigation, for monitoring response to treatment, for detecting recurrent disease in patients who have completed treatment, and for determining the presence of active disease in patients whose physical presentation and laboratory test results are discordant.

Musculoskeletal Infection

Osteomyelitis

Infection of the bone, or osteomyelitis, is usually bacterial in origin, occurs most frequently in children less than 5 years of age, and most often is hematogenous in origin.[71–73] Osteomyelitis has a predilection for the highly vascular metaphyses of the long bones. Sluggish blood flow in the distal metaphyseal vessels makes them prone to necrosis and facilitates the deposition of blood–borne bacteria.[74] The distal femurs and the proximal tibiae and humeri are the most commonly involved bones.[71] Staphylococcus aureus is the most frequently encountered organism in pediatric osteomyelitis, except in neonates, where group A β-hemolytic streptococcus is the usual culprit.[75] Because the clinical manifestations may be subtle and may mimic other medical conditions, the diagnosis cannot be established solely on clinical grounds, especially in very young children and during the early stages of the disease, when appropriate treatment is more likely to eradicate the infection and prevent complications such as osteonecrosis and growth disturbance related to damage to the physes.[76] Consequently, imaging tests play an important role in the diagnosis of this entity.

In unviolated bone, focal hyperperfusion, focal hyperemia, and focally increased bony uptake on delayed images is the classic

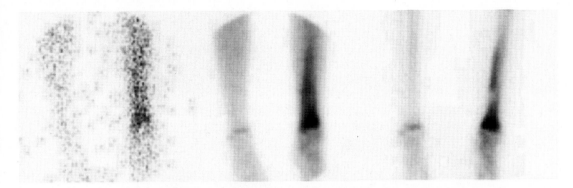

FIGURE 15.15. Focal hyperperfusion, focal hyperemia, and focally increased bone activity on a three-phase bone scan performed on a 10-year-old child with distal left tibial osteomyelitis.

appearance of osteomyelitis on the three-phase bone scan (Fig. 15.15).[77] There has been some controversy over the years about the value of bone scintigraphy in children, especially in neonates. Ash and Gilday[78] reported a sensitivity of only about 32% for bone scintigraphy in neonatal osteomyelitis, a marked contrast to the sensitivity of 100% in slightly older infants. These investigators concluded that neonatal osteomyelitis is a different disease from that in older infants and children. Berkowitz and Wenzel[79] reported similar findings in neonates. Sullivan et al.[80] reported that the appearance of childhood osteomyelitis on radionuclide bone imaging is very variable, and that a normal bone image does not exclude osteomyelitis. Subsequently, Bressler et al.[81] retrospectively reviewed the results of three-phase bone scintigraphy in neonates and found that all 15 sites of infection were identified on bone scintigraphy, although two (13%) of the 15 sites were photopenic.

The variable appearance of childhood osteomyelitis is probably related to the evolution of the disease itself. In children, especially neonates, subperiosteal edema, effusion, or vasospasm can cause occlusion of small vessels, reducing blood flow to the infected area. Early in the course of the disease, therefore, hyperperfusion and hyperemia may be absent, and on skeletal images the abnormality may appear as decreased, rather than increased, bony activity

(Fig. 15.16).[82] As blood flow is restored, bony uptake of the tracer gradually increases until it exceeds that in normal bone. At some point during the scintigraphic evolution of osteomyelitis, the intensity of tracer uptake in the infected bone will be indistinguishable from that in adjacent, normal, bone, and will go undetected. The focus of infection is typically located in the metaphysis, and the importance of meticulous technique to facilitate the discrimination of normally increased activity in the physis from abnormally increased uptake in the juxtaposed metaphysis cannot be overemphasized.[83]

Because prompt diagnosis of osteomyelitis in the child is critical, three-phase bone scintigraphy, even with its shortcomings, is usually the first radionuclide test performed. As osteomyelitis may be multifocal in children, the ability to image the whole body is an added benefit of this test.

For those studies that are normal or inconclusive, or in children with underlying bony abnormalities, ^{67}Ga and ^{111}In leukocyte studies provide additional information. The use of combined bone/gallium scintigraphy in the diagnosis of so-called complicating osteomyelitis was first described nearly 30 years ago.[84,85] The uptake mechanisms of gallium and bone seeking tracers are different, and each study, therefore, provides information about different aspects of a particular disease process. Over the years the following standardized

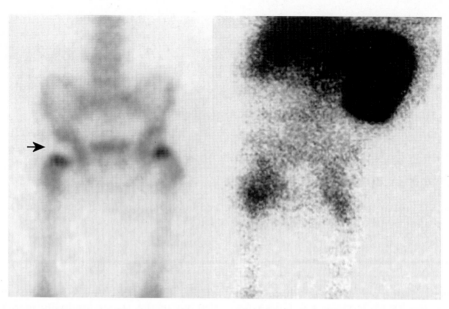

FIGURE 15.16. Bone scan (left) performed on a 3-year-old girl with right hip pain demonstrates absent activity in the right femoral head (arrow), while the labeled leukocyte study (right) performed 24 hours later demonstrates intense activity in the right femoral head and hip joint. Septic arthritis and osteomyelitis were found at surgery. (*Source:* Palestro,[83] with permission of Lippincott Williams & Wilkins.)

criteria for interpreting bone/gallium images have evolved[4,83,86]:

- Bone/gallium imaging is **positive** for osteomyelitis when the distribution of the two tracers is spatially incongruent, *or*, when the distribution is spatially congruent, the relative intensity of uptake of gallium exceeds that of the diphosphonate (Fig. 15.17A).
- Bone/gallium imaging is **negative** for osteomyelitis when the gallium images are normal, regardless of the bone scan findings, *or*, when the distribution of the two tracers is spatially congruent and the relative intensity of uptake of gallium is less than that of the diphosphonate (Fig. 15.17B).
- Bone/gallium imaging is **equivocal** for osteomyelitis when the distribution of the two radiotracers is congruent, both spatially and in terms of intensity (Fig. 15.17C).

Although combined bone/gallium imaging is accurate when the study is clearly positive or negative, the study is frequently equivocal and the approximate overall accuracy ranges between 60% and 80%.[4,83,86] The less than ideal imaging characteristics of gallium and the need for two isotopes with multiple imaging sessions over several days are also disadvantages.

Labeled leukocytes do not usually accumulate at sites of increased bone mineral turnover in the absence of infection and would seem to be ideally suited for diagnosing complicated osteomyelitis. The results reported have been very variable, however. The primary difficulty in the interpretation of labeled leukocyte images is an inability to distinguish labeled leukocyte uptake in infection from uptake in bone marrow.[83,86] The normal distribution of labeled leukocytes includes the liver, the spleen, and the bone marrow, which in adults is limited to the axial and proximal appendicular skeleton. Any focus outside the normal distribution of labeled leukocytes is, therefore, indicative of infection. This "normal" distribution of hematopoietically active marrow, however, is quite variable. Systemic diseases such as sickle

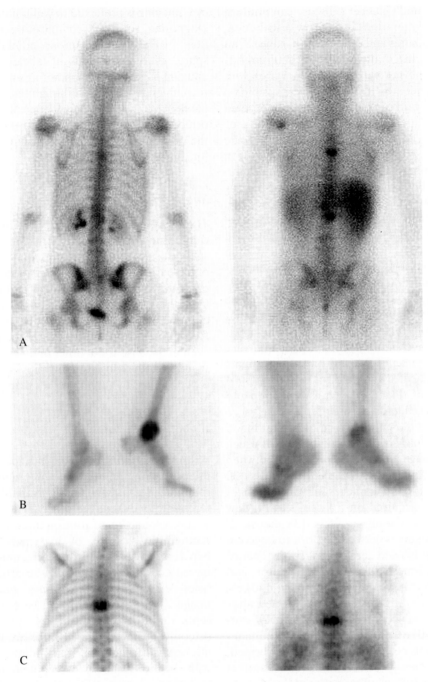

FIGURE 15.17. A: There is increased activity in the midthoracic, lower thoracic, and upper lumbar spine on both the bone (left) and gallium (right) images. Although the spatial distribution of abnormal activity is congruent on both images, the intensity of the abnormal activity on the gallium image is greater than that on the bone image, and the combined study is positive for osteomyelitis. The combined study is also positive for osteomyelitis when the spatial distribution of the two tracers is different (not shown). B: Increased activity is present in the distal left tibia on both the bone (left) and gallium (right) images. The intensity of activity on the gallium image is considerably less than that on the bone image, and the combined study is negative for osteomyelitis. The combined study is also negative for osteomyelitis when the gallium scan is normal, regardless of the findings on the bone scan (not shown). C: Abnormal activity in a midthoracic vertebra is congruent, both spatially and in terms of intensity, on the bone and gallium images, and the combined study is equivocal for infection.

cell disease and Gaucher's disease can produce generalized alterations in marrow distribution, whereas fractures and orthopedic hardware can result in localized alterations. In children, furthermore, the normal distribution varies with age. Consequently, it may not be possible to determine if an area of activity on a labeled leukocyte image reflects infection or marrow.[83,86] Performing complementary bone marrow imaging overcomes this problem. Both labeled leukocytes and sulfur colloid accumulate in the bone marrow; leukocytes also accumulate in infection, but sulfur colloid does not. The combined study is positive for infection when there is uptake on the labeled leukocyte image without corresponding uptake on the sulfur colloid image. Any other pattern is negative for infection (Fig. 15.18).[83,86]

Combined leukocyte/marrow imaging can be performed in various ways. The protocols that follow are offered as general suggestions, albeit ones that have, in our experience, yielded very satisfactory results over the years. Patients should be injected with 0.15 to 0.25 MBq (0.004 to 0.007 mCi)/kg of freshly prepared ^{99m}Tc–sulfur colloid.[13] Using preparations more than 2 hours old may result in persistent blood pool and urinary bladder activity, both of which degrade image quality. The interval between injection and imaging should be at least 30 minutes. Ten-minute images of the region of interest are acquired on a large field of view gamma camera using a 128×128 matrix. If marrow imaging is performed prior to injection of the ^{111}In-labeled leukocytes, a low-energy, high-resolution, parallel-hole collimator and a 15% to 20% window centered on 140 keV should be used. If imaging is performed after injection of labeled cells, a 10% window centered on 140 keV should be used. If simultaneous dual isotope imaging is to be performed, a medium-energy parallel-hole collimator is used, with a 10% window centered on 140 keV, a 5% window centered on 174 keV, and a 10% window centered on 247 keV.[12]

The overall accuracy of combined leukocyte/marrow imaging is approximately 90%, which is superior to the 60% to 80% accuracy of bone/gallium imaging.[83,86,87] Labeled leuko-

cyte imaging is preferred to gallium imaging for diagnosing so-called complicating osteomyelitis.[83,86] The one exception, in adults, is the spine, where the results of labeled leukocyte imaging have been disappointing and gallium is recommended.[12,83,86,88] Although the accuracy of labeled leukocyte imaging in pediatric spinal osteomyelitis is unknown, based on results in the adult population, we use gallium imaging for this indication in children.

Subperiosteal Abscess

The subperiosteal abscess results from extension of infection from the bony cortex into the subperiosteal space with subsequent elevation of the periosteum itself. A subperiosteal abscess presents as an area of hyperperfusion and hyperemia on early images with focal bony photopenia on the delayed bone images. Recognition of this entity is important because, even in the absence of other findings, it strongly suggests underlying osteomyelitis; moreover, it is best treated by surgery rather than antibiotics alone.[89]

Septic Arthritis

Arthritis, or inflammation, of a joint may be infectious or noninfectious in origin, and no radionuclide study currently available can differentiate one from the other. The classic presentation of acute arthritis on three-phase bone scintigraphy consists of hyperperfusion and hyperemia of a joint on early images, with increased activity limited to the articular surfaces of the involved bones on delayed images. This presentation can be seen in both septic and aseptic arthritis. Furthermore, osteomyelitis and acute arthritis are not mutually exclusive, and bone scan findings consistent with septic arthritis can potentially mask underlying osteomyelitis. Neither gallium nor labeled leukocyte imaging is useful for separating infectious from noninfectious arthritis. In the case of leukocyte imaging, positive images have been reported in rheumatoid arthritis, acute gouty arthritis, and pseudogout (Fig. 15.19).[90–93]

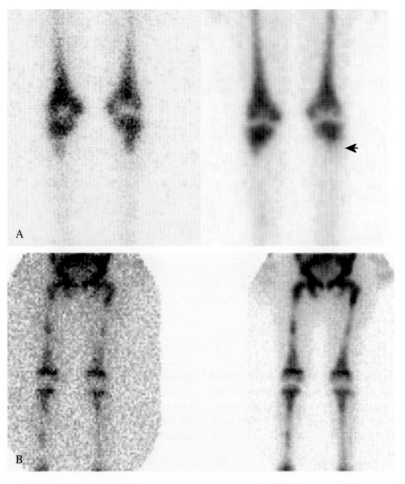

FIGURE 15.18. A: There is irregularly increased labeled leukocyte activity around the knees of a 10-year-old patient with sickle cell disease and lower extremity pain (left). A photopenic defect in the proximal left tibia (arrow) is seen on the marrow image (right) and the combined study is consistent with osteomyelitis of the proximal left tibia. B: Labeled leukocyte (left) and sulfur colloid (right) images of the pelvis and lower extremities, performed on a 3-year-old girl with aplastic anemia and left thigh pain. On the labeled leukocyte image, several foci of activity can be appreciated in the mid-right femur, proximal right tibia, and proximal and mid-left femur. On the basis of the leukocyte image alone, it would be difficult to exclude osteomyelitis. The distribution of activity on the sulfur colloid image is virtually the same, however, and therefore the activity present on the leukocyte image is due to marrow, not infection.

Chronic Recurrent Multifocal Osteomyelitis

Chronic recurrent multifocal osteomyelitis (CRMO) is a rare systemic inflammatory disorder that usually affects children between 5 and 15 years old and is twice as common in girls as in boys.[94] Unlike hematogenous osteomyelitis, the onset of CRMO is insidious. Although there is pain and swelling in the affected area, fever is present in only approximately one third of patients. Most have an elevated erythrocyte sedimentation rate with normal white count and differential.[95] Any part of the skeleton may be affected, although the metaphyses of long bones are the most

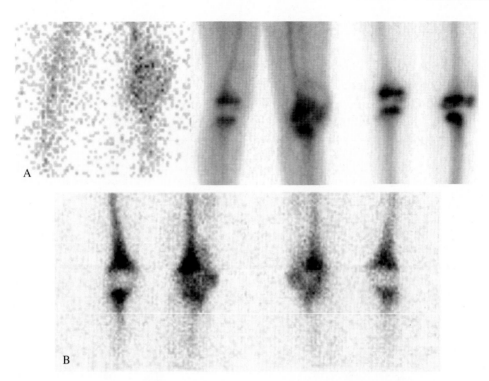

FIGURE 15.19. A: Three-phase bone scan performed on a 9-year-old child with septic arthritis of the left knee. This pattern also can be seen in aseptic arthritis. Increased tracer uptake involving the articular surfaces of the involved bones, moreover, can mask an underlying osteomyelitis. B: The labeled leukocyte study of a 10-year-old child demonstrates increased activity in the left knee joint. This uptake pattern also can be seen in aseptic inflammatory arthritis.

common sites. The medial ends of the clavicles, facial bones, spine, pelvis, and upper extremities are also frequently involved.[74] Although CRMO and infectious osteomyelitis share the common histopathologic feature of chronic inflammation, cultures of the bone lesions in CRMO are sterile. The disease is characterized by intermittent bouts of exacerbations and remissions, over 5 to 8 years, which then gradually resolve over time. Most cases are erroneously diagnosed as septic osteomyelitis initially, but no microorganisms are identified.[75] The diagnosis, based on clinical, imaging, and pathologic findings, is usually established during recurrent episodes. Treatment is symptomatic; steroids and nonsteroidal antiinflammatory drugs may offer some relief.[74] For refractory cases, surgical decortication has been performed. Up to 7% of patients may suffer long-term sequelae, including premature closure of the epiphysis, bone deformities, kyphosis, and thoracic outlet syndrome.[95]

Active lesions are positive on all three phases of the bone scan, though quiescent lesions may be indistinguishable from adjacent normal bone. Scintigraphy facilitates early detection of the global distribution of the lesions and identifies lesions that, with radiographic correlation, may be recognized as characteristic of CRMO. Radionuclide bone imaging also identifies sites suitable for biopsy (Fig. 15.20).[94]

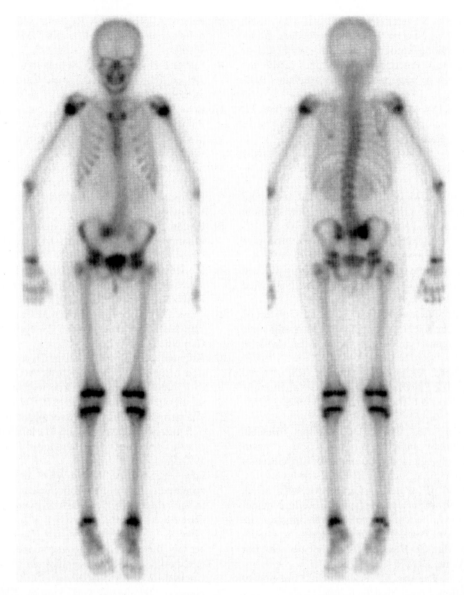

FIGURE 15.20. Anterior and posterior whole-body images from a bone scan performed on an 11-year-old girl with chronic recurrent multifocal osteomyelitis (CRMO). Note the focal areas of increased activity in the right sacroiliac region and in the distal left tibia.

Conclusion

There are now a myriad of radionuclide procedures from which to choose when evaluating the child suspected of harboring infection or inflammation. The practicing nuclear physician, therefore, must be cognizant of the tracers available, as well as the indications for which they are most useful, to maximize the value of radionuclide imaging for diagnosing infection and inflammation in children.

References

1. Scientific Report Number 38, 2005, St. Jude. Children's Research Hospital, Memphis, TN.

2. Donohoe KJ, Henkin RE, Royal HD, et al. Society of Nuclear Medicine procedure guideline for bone scintigraphy. In: Society of Nuclear Medicine Procedure Guidelines Manual. Reston, VA: Society of Nuclear Medicine, 1997: 149–53.

3. Love C, Din AS, Tomas MB, Kalapparambath TP, et al. Radionuclide bone imaging: an illustrative review. RadioGraphics 2003;23:341–58.

4. Palestro CJ. The current role of gallium imaging in infection. Semin Nucl Med 1994;24:128–41.

5. Palestro CJ, Malat J, Collica CJ, et al. Incidental diagnosis of pregnancy on bone and gallium scintigraphy. J Nucl Med 1986;27:370–2.

6. Lopez OL, Maisano ER. Ga-67 uptake post cesarean section. Clin Nucl Med 1984;9:103–4.

7. Desai AG, Intenzo C, Park C, et al. Drug-induced gallium uptake in the breasts. Clin Nucl Med 1987;12:703–4.

8. Vasquez R, Oates E, Sarno RC, et al. Gallium-67 breast uptake in a patient with hypothalamic granuloma (sarcoid). J Nucl Med 1998;19:118–21.

9. Engelstad B, Luks S, Hattner RS. Altered ^{67}Ga citrate distribution in patients with multiple red blood cell transfusions. AJR 1982;139:755–9.

10. Hattner RS, White DL. Gallium-67/stable gadolinium antagonism. MRI contrast agent markedly alters the normal biodistribution of Gallium–67. J Nucl Med 1990;31:1844–46.

11. Seabold JE, Palestro CJ, Brown ML, et al. Society of Nuclear Medicine procedure guideline for gallium scintigraphy in inflammation. In: Society of Nuclear Medicine Procedure Guidelines Manual. Reston, VA: Society of Nuclear Medicine, 1997:75–80.

12. Love C, Palestro CJ. Radionuclide imaging of infection. J Nucl Med Tech 2004;32:47–57.

13. Seabold JE, Forstrom LA, Schauwecker DS, et al. Society of Nuclear Medicine procedure guideline for In-111 leukocyte scintigraphy for suspected infection/inflammation. In: Society of Nuclear Medicine Procedure Guidelines Manual. Reston, VA: Society of Nuclear Medicine, 1997:81–86.

14. Datz FL, Seabold JE, Brown ML, et al. Society of Nuclear Medicine procedure guideline for Tc-99m Exametazime (HMPAO) labeled leukocyte scintigraphy for suspected infection/inflammation. In: Society of Nuclear Medicine Procedure Guidelines Manual. Reston, VA: Society of Nuclear Medicine, 1997:87–92.

15. Palestro CJ, Torres MA. Radionuclide imaging of nonosseous infection. Q J Nucl Med 1999;43:46–60.

16. Ingbar DH. Mechanisms of lung injury. In: Bone RC, ed. Pulmonary and Critical Care Medicine. St. Louis: Mosby, 1998:17–21.

17. Love C, Opoku-Agyemang P, Tomas MB, et al. Pulmonary activity on labeled leukocyte images: physiologic, pathologic, and imaging correlation. RadioGraphics 2002;22:1385–93.

18. Saverymuttu SH, Peters AM, Danpure HJ, et al. Lung transit of [111]Indium-labelled granulocytes: Relationship to labelling techniques. Scand J Haematol 1983;30:151–60.

19. Roddie ME, Peters AM, Danpure HJ, et al. Inflammation: imaging with Tc-99m HMPAO-labeled leukocytes. Radiology 1988;166:767–72.

20. McAfee JG, Samin A. In-111 labeled leukocytes: a review of problems in image interpretation. Radiology 1985;155:221–9.

21. Crass JR, L'Heureux P, Loken M. False-positive ^{111}In-labeled leukocyte scan in cystic fibrosis. Clin Nucl Med 1979;4:291–3.

22. Fineman DS, Palestro CJ, Kim CK, et al. Detection of abnormalities in febrile AIDS patients with In-111–labeled leukocyte and Ga-67 scintigraphy. Radiology 1989;170:677–80.

23. Palestro CJ, Padilla ML, Swyer AJ, et al. Diffuse pulmonary uptake of indium-111 labeled leukocytes in drug-induced pneumonitis. J Nucl Med 1992;33:1175–7.

24. Powe JE, Short A, Sibbald WJ, et al. Pulmonary accumulation of polymorphonuclear leukocytes in the adult respiratory distress syndrome. Crit Care Med 1982;10:712–8.

25. Love C, Tomas MB, Palestro CJ. Pulmonary activity on labeled leukocyte images: patterns of uptake and their significance. Nucl Med Commun 2002;23:559–63.

26. Hangen DH, Segall GM, Harney EW, et al. Kinetics of leukocyte sequestration in the lungs of acutely septic primates: a study using ^{111}In-labeled autologous leukocytes. J Surg Res 1990;48:196.

27. Malmros C, Holst E, Hansson L, et al. Dynamic accumulation of neutrophils in lungs and visceral organs during early abdominal sepsis in the pig. World J Surg 1994;18:811–6.

28. Blomquist S, Malmros C, Martensson L, et al. Absence of lung reactions after complement depletion during dialysis: an experimental study in pigs. Artif Organs 1991;15:397–401.

29. Palestro CJ, Love C, Tronco GG, et al. Fever in the postoperative patient: role of radionuclide

imaging in its diagnosis. RadioGraphics 2000;20: 1649–60.

30. Love C, Palestro CJ. 99mTc-fanolesomab. IDrugs 2003;6:1079–85.

31. Love C, Tomas MB, Tronco GG, et al. Imaging infection and inflammation with [18F]-FDG-PET. Radiographics 2005;25:1357–68.

32. Bell GI, Burant CF, Takeda J, et al. Structure and function of mammalian facilitative sugar transporters. J Biol Chem 1993;268:19161–4.

33. Pauwels EKJ, Ribeiro MJ, Stoot JHMB, et al. FDG accumulation and tumor biology. Nucl Med Biol 1998;25:317–22.

34. Zhuang H, Alavi A. 18-Fluorodeoxyglucose positron emission tomographic imaging in the detection and monitoring of infection and inflammation. Semin Nucl Med 2002;32:47–59.

35. Mochizuki T, Tsukamoto E, Kuge Y, et al. FDG uptake and glucose transporter subtype expressions in experimental tumor and inflammation models. J Nucl Med 2001;42:1551–5.

36. Kubota R, Yamada S, Kubota K, et al. Intra-tumoral distribution of fluorine-18-fluorodeoxyglucose in vivo: high accumulation in macrophages and granulation tissues studied by microautoradiography. J Nucl Med 1992;33: 1972–80.

37. Paik JY, Lee KH, Choe YS, et al. Augmented [18F]-FDG uptake in activated monocytes occurs during the priming process and involves tyrosine kinases and protein kinase C. J Nucl Med 2004;45:124–8.

38. Schelbert HR, Hoh CK, Royal HD, et al. Society of Nuclear Medicine procedure guideline for tumor imaging using F-18 FDG. In: Society of Nuclear Medicine Procedure Guidelines Manual. Reston, VA: Society of Nuclear Medicine, 1997:105–9.

39. Palestro CJ, Goldsmith SJ. The use of gallium and labeled leukocyte scintigraphy in the AIDS patient. Q J Nucl Med 1995;39:221–30.

40. O'Doherty MJ, Barrington SF, Campbell M, et al. PET scanning and the human immuno-deficiency virus-positive patient. J Nucl Med 1997;38:1575–83.

41. Hoffman JM, Waskin HA, Schifter T, et al. FDG-PET in differentiating lymphoma from nonma-lignant central nervous system lesions in patients with AIDS. J Nucl Med 1993;34:567–75.

42. Lorin MI, Feigin RD. Fever without localizing signs and fever of unknown origin. In: Feigin RD, Cherry JD, eds. Textbook of Pediatric Infectious Diseases, 4th ed. Philadelphia: WB Saunders, 1998:820–30.

43. Buonomo C, Treves ST. Gallium scanning in children with fever of unknown origin. Pediatr Radiol 1993;23:307–10.

44. Haentjens M, Piepsz A, Schell-Frederick E, et al. Limitations in the use of indium-111-oxine-labeled leucocytes for the diagnosis of occult infection in children. Pediatr Radiol 1987;17: 139–42.

45. Williamson SL, Williamson MR, Siebert JJ, et al. Indium 111 white blood cell scanning in the pediatric population. Pediatr Radiol 1986;16:493–7.

46. Steele RW, Jones SM, Lowe BA, et al. Usefulness of scanning procedures for diagnosis of fever of unknown origin in children. J Pediatr 1991; 119:526–30.

47. Blockmans D, Knockaert D, Maes A, et al. Clinical value of [18F]-fluoro-deoxyglucose positron emission tomography for patients with fever of unknown origin. Clin Infect Dis 2001;32:191–6.

48. Meller J, Altenvoerde G, Munzel U, et al: Fever of unknown origin: prospective comparison of [18F]FDG imaging with a double-head coincidence camera and gallium-67 citrate SPET. Eur J Nucl Med 2000;27:1617–25.

49. Bleeker-Rovers CP, de Kleijn EMHA, Corstens FHM, et al. Clinical Value of FDG PET in patients with fever of unknown origin and patients suspected of focal infection or inflam-mation. Eur J Nucl Med Mol Imaging 2004;31:29–37.

50. Lorenzen J, Buchert R, Bohuslavizki KH. Value of FDG PET in patients with fever of unknown origin. Nucl Med Commun 2001;22:779–83.

51. Yen RF, Chen YC, Wu YW, et al. Using 18–Fluoro-2–deoxyglucose positron emission tomography in detecting infectious endocardi-tis/endoarteritis. A preliminary report. Acad Radiol 2004;11:316–21.

52. Bleeker-Rovers CP, Bredie SJH, van der Meer JWM, et al. Fluorine-18 fluorodeoxyglucose positron emission tomography in the diagnosis and follow-up of three patients with vasculitis. Am J Med 2004;116:50–3.

53. Blockmans D, Stroobants S, Maes A, et al. Positron emission tomography in giant cell arteritis and polymyalgia rheumatica: evidence for inflammation of the aortic arch. Am J Med 2000;108:246–9.

54. Meller J, Strutz F, Siefker U, et al. Early diagno-sis and follow-up of aortitis with [18F]FDG PET and MRI. Eur J Nucl Med Mol Imaging 2003;30:730–6.

55. Sarosi, Jr GA, Turnage RH. Appendicitis. In: Feldman M, Tschumy WO Jr, Friedman LS,

Sleisenger MH, eds. Sleisenger and Fordtran's Gastrointestinal and Liver Disease, 7th ed. St Louis: WB Saunders, 2002:2089–99.

56. Kipper SL. The role of radiolabeled leukocyte imaging in the management of patients with acute appendicitis. Q J Nucl Med 1999;43:83–92.

57. Rypins EB, Kipper SL. 99mTc-hexamethyl-propyleneamine oxime (Tc-WBC) scan for diagnosing acute appendicitis in children. Am Surg 1997;63:878–81.

58. Kipper SL, Rypins EB, Evans DG, et al. Neutrophil-specific ^{99m}Tc-labeled anti-CD15 monoclonal antibody imaging for diagnosis of equivocal appendicitis. J Nucl Med 2000;41:449–55.

59. Rypins EB, Kipper SL, Weiland F, et al. ^{99m}Tc anti-CD15 monoclonal antibody (LeuTech) imaging improves diagnostic accuracy and clinical management in patients with equivocal presentation of appendicitis. Ann Surg 2002;235:232–9.

60. Ulshen M. Inflammatory bowel disease. In: Behrman RE, Kliegman RM, Arvin AM, eds. Nelson Textbook of Pediatrics, 15th ed. Philadelphia: WB Saunders, 1996:1080–4.

61. Shah DB, Cosgrove M, Rees JIS, et al. The technetium white cell scan as an initial imaging investigation for evaluating suspected childhood inflammatory bowel disease. J Pediatr Gastroenterol Nutr 1997;25:524–8.

62. Alberini JL, Badran A, Freneau E, et al. Technetium-99m HMPAO-labeled leukocyte imaging compared with endoscopy, ultrasonography, and contrast radiology in children with inflammatory bowel disease. J Pediatr Gastoenterol Nutr 2001;32:278–86.

63. Del Rosario MA, Fitzgerald JF, Siddiqui AR, et al. Clinical applications of technetium Tc 99m hexamethyl propylene amine oxime leukocyte scan in children with inflammatory bowel disease. J Pediatr Gastroenterol Nutr 1999;28:63–70.

64. Charron M, Del Rosario JF, Kocoshis S. Comparison of the sensitivity of early versus delayed imaging with Tc-99m HMPAO WBC in children with inflammatory bowel disease. Clin Nucl Med 1998;23:649–53.

65. Bhargava SA, Orenstein SR, Charron M. Technetium-99m hexamethylpropyleneamine-oxime-labeled leukocyte scintigraphy in inflammatory bowel disease in children. J Pediatr 1994;125:213–7.

66. Charron M. Inflammatory bowel disease in pediatric patients. Q J Nucl Med 1997;41:309–20.

67. Charron M, del Rosario FJ, Kocoshis SA. Pediatric inflammatory bowel disease: assessment with scintigraphy with ^{99m}Tc white blood cells. Radiology 1999;212:507–13.

68. Charron M. Pediatric inflammatory bowel disease imaged with Tc-99m white blood cells: The Nuclear Medicine Atlas. Clin Nucl Med 2000;25:708–15.

69. Granquist L, Chapman SC, Hvidsten S, et al. Evaluation of ^{99m}Tc-HMPAO leukocyte scintigraphy in the investigation of pediatric inflammatory bowel disease. J Pediatr 2003;143:48–53.

70. Davison SM, Chapman S, Murphy MS. ^{99m}Tc-HMPAO leucocyte scintigraphy fails to detect Crohn's disease in the proximal gastrointestinal tract. Arch Dis Child 2001;85:43–6.

71. Santiago-Restrepo C, Gimenez CR, McCarthy K. Imaging of osteomyelitis and musculoskeletal soft tissue infections: current concepts. Rheum Dis Clin North Am 2003;29:89–109.

72. Carek PJ, Dickerson LM, Sack JL. Diagnosis and management of osteomyelitis. Am Fam Physician 2001;63:2413–20.

73. Kim MK, Karpas A. Orthopedic emergencies: the limping child. Clin Ped Emerg Med 2002;3:129–37.

74. Krogstad P, Smith AL. Osteomyelitis and septic arthritis. In: Feigin RD, Cherry JD, eds. Textbook of Pediatric Infectious Diseases, 4th ed. Philadelphia: WB Saunders, 1998:683–704.

75. McCarthy JJ, Dormans JP, Kozin SH, et al. Musculoskeletal infections in children: basic treatment principles and recent advancements. J Bone Joint Surg Am 2004;86:850–63.

76. Kleinman PK. A regional approach to osteomyelitis of the lower extremities in children. Radiol Clin North Am 2002;40:1033–59.

77. Schauwecker DS. The scintigraphic diagnosis of osteomyelitis. AJR 1992;158:9–18.

78. Ash JM, Gilday DL. The futility of bone scanning in neonatal osteomyelitis: concise communication. J Nucl Med 1980;21:417–20.

79. Berkowitz ID, Wenzel W. "Normal" technetium bone scans in patients with acute osteomyelitis. Am J Dis Child 1980;134:828–30.

80. Sullivan DC, Rosenfield NS, Ogden J, et al. Problems in the scintigraphic detection of osteomyelitis in children. Radiology 1980;135:731–6.

81. Bressler EL, Conway JJ, Weiss SC. Neonatal osteomyelitis examined by bone scintigraphy. Radiology 1984;152:685–8.

82. Nadel HR, Stilwell ME. Nuclear medicine topics in pediatric musculoskeletal disease: techniques

and applications. Radiol Clin North Am 2001; 39:619–51.

83. Palestro CJ. Musculoskeletal infection. In: Freeman LM, ed. Nuclear Medicine Annual. New York: Raven Press, 1994:91–119.

84. Rosenthall L, Lisbona R, Hernandez M, et al. ^{99m}Tc-PP and ^{67}Ga imaging following insertion of orthopedic devices. Radiology 1979;133:717–21.

85. Lisbona R, Rosenthall L. Observations on the sequential use of 99mTc-phosphate complex and 67Ga imaging in osteomyelitis, cellulitis, and septic arthritis. Radiology 1977;123:123–9.

86. Palestro CJ, Torres MA. Radionuclide diagnosis of orthopedic infections. Semin Nucl Med 1997;27:334–45.

87. Palestro CJ, Roumanas P, Swyer AJ, et al. Diagnosis of musculoskeletal infection using combined In-111 labeled leukocyte and Tc-99m SC marrow imaging. Clin Nucl Med 1992;17:269–73.

88. Palestro CJ, Kim CK, Swyer AJ, et al. Radionuclide diagnosis of vertebral osteomyelitis: indium-111-leukocyte and technetium-99m-methylene diphosphonate bone scintigraphy. J Nucl Med 1991;32:1861–5.

89. Allwright SJ, Miller JH, Gilsanz V. Subperiosteal abscess in children: scintigraphic appearance. Radiology 1991;179:725–9.

90. Coleman RE, Samuelson CO, Bain S. Imaging with Tc-99m MDP and Ga-67 citrate in patient with rheumatoid arthritis and suspected septic arthritis. J Nucl Med 1982;23:479–82.

91. Uno K, Matsui N, Nohira K, et al. Indium-111 leukocyte imaging in patients with rheumatoid arthritis. J Nucl Med 1986;27:339–44.

92. Palestro CJ, Vega A, Kim CK, et al. Appearance of acute gouty arthritis on indium-111-labeled scintigraphy. J Nucl Med 1990;31: 682–5.

93. Palestro CJ, Goldsmith SJ. In-111-labeled leukocyte imaging in a case of pseudogout. Clin Nucl Med 1992;17:366–7.

94. Mortensson W, Edeburn G, Fries M, et al. Chronic recurrent multifocal osteomyelitis in children: a roentgenologic and scintigraphic investigation. Acta Radiol 1988;29:565–70.

95. Schultz C, Holterhus PM, Seidel A, et al. Chronic recurrent multifocal osteomyelitis in children. Pediatr Infect Dis 1999;18:1008–13.

16
Magnification

Royal T. Davis, Robert E. Zimmerman, and S.T. Treves

Magnification is an indispensable technique in pediatric nuclear medicine that is used to improve the overall spatial resolution characteristics of gamma cameras. Magnification scintigraphy is useful in the assessment of diseases of the thyroid, kidney, heart, small bones, and scrotum.[1-7] To achieve magnification, a pinhole collimator or a converging collimator can be used.

Modern gamma cameras exhibit intrinsic spatial resolution (with no collimator) on the order of 3 to 4 mm for technetium-99m (^{99m}Tc). Intrinsic spatial resolution is a measurement of the precision with which an event can be localized by the crystal detector and electronics of the gamma camera. The image of a thin line of radioactivity is used to calculate the line spread function (LSF) (Fig. 16.1). The width of the line spread function measured at 50% of the peak level is a measure of the blurring and hence a measure of the resolution of the gamma camera.[8,9] The result of such a measurement is reported as the full width at half maximum (FWHM). Full width at tenth maximum (FWTM) is a further measure of image resolution related to collimator and camera resolution, scatter, and septal penetration (Fig. 16.1).

Resolution and Sensitivity

In routine use, gamma cameras are fitted with parallel-hole, low-energy collimators. Extrinsic spatial resolution, which is defined as overall system resolution of a gamma camera with col-limator, is in the range of 6 to 9 mm for modern systems. All collimators have a resolution that is a function of hole size, hole length, distance to the patient, and, to a small extent, the type of hole—square, round, or hexagonal.[8]

The resolution of a parallel hole collimator can be expressed by the following equation:

$$R_{par} = \frac{d}{a}(a+b+c)$$

where a, b, c, and d are defined as in Figure 16.2. The sensitivity of a parallel-hole collimator is given by the following equation where K is a geometric constant that depends on the type of hole used in the collimator construction:

$$g_{par} = K^2 \left[\frac{d^2}{a(d+t)} \right]^2$$

Optical Versus Electronic Magnification

There are two types of magnification: optical (collimator) and electronic. These two methods are not equivalent and should not be confused. Optical magnification enlarges the image, and results in better overall system resolution. Electronic magnification enlarges the size of the image without affecting overall system resolution.

Optical magnification is achieved with the pinhole or converging collimator. This results in an image projected on the gamma camera crystal that is larger than that of the object being imaged. Optical magnification leads to spatial distortion since portions of the object at different depths are magnified by different amounts.

The effect of magnification is easily quantified by the following equation. Let:

R_i be the intrinsic FWHM of the gamma camera

R_c be collimator resolution expressed as FWHM

$$M = \frac{\text{image size at the crystal}}{\text{object size}}$$

Then R_s, the system resolution (intrinsic resolution combined with collimator resolution), is given by the equation:

$$R_s = \sqrt{\frac{R_i^2}{M^2} + R_c^2}$$

We see that the effect of the blurring due to the intrinsic camera resolution is reduced by the magnification.

Electronic magnification or zoom can be divided into acquisition zoom and display zoom. Acquisition zoom is achieved by changes in the acquisition amplifier gain. Display zoom is produced by changes in display gain. Neither acquisition zoom nor display zoom can make

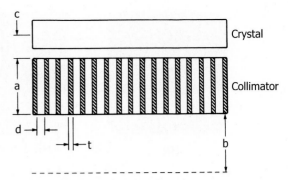

FIGURE 16.2. Parallel-hole collimator. The relevant dimensions are the hole diameter d, the collimator thickness or hole length a, and the distance to the patient b. The gamma ray is stopped in the crystal at distance c, from the back of the collimator. The septal thickness is t. (*Source:* Zimmerman RE. Radionuclide imaging systems. In: Taveras JM, Ferrucci JT, eds. Radiology. Philadelphia: JB Lippincott 1986, with permission.)

up for the intrinsic camera resolution limit as collimator magnification can.

Magnification and Resolution

Collimator magnification has been used since the earliest days of the gamma camera. The first collimator to be used by Anger in his early work with the gamma camera was a pinhole collimator. Converging collimators came into widespread use at the time of the introduction of large field of view (LFOV) cameras in the mid-1970s for imaging small organs.[8,9]

Figure 16.3 shows a comparison between a high-resolution (HR), parallel-hole collimator, the same collimator with acquisition zoom of 1.5, a converging collimator, and a pinhole with 2- and 6-mm inserts. Note that the best resolution is obtained with the small pinhole insert. Also note the more intense center of the converging and pinhole images caused by uneven sensitivity. Figures 16.4 to 16.6 further show the superior properties in clinical imaging for the pinhole collimator.

The resolution of a pinhole collimator is given by

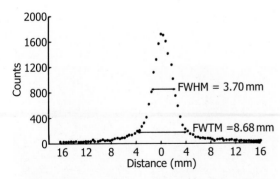

FIGURE 16.1. Line spread function (LSF). The count as a function of distance is known as the line spread function. The full width at half maximum (FWHM) is a measure of image resolution and blurring. The full width at tenth maximum (FWTM) is also a measure of blurring, scatter, and penetration. Typical numbers for camera resolution are given.

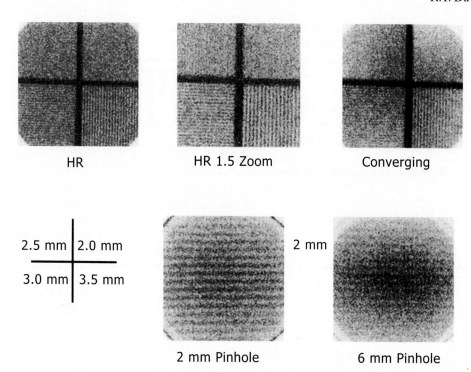

HR   HR 1.5 Zoom   Converging

2 mm Pinhole   6 mm Pinhole

FIGURE 16.3. A comparison of different magnification techniques. All images were acquired on a 256 × 256 matrix. On the top row, three images of a four-quadrant bar pattern are shown. These images have equal counts (500 K). The phantom was in contact with the surface of the collimator, and a sheet source of cobalt 57 was placed behind the bar pattern. The image on the top left was obtained with the high-resolution (HR) collimator and no zoom. The next image was obtained with an acquisition zoom of 1.5, all other factors remaining constant. Note the 2.5-mm bars appear virtually identical for both images, showing that acquisition zoom does not improve resolution. The converging collimator (no zoom) should have a slightly better system resolution than the HR collimator. The two lower images show the dramatic increase in resolution using a 2-mm pinhole. The 6-mm pinhole image shows significantly lower resolution, as expected. The distance to the pinhole in each case is 6 mm, and 150 K counts were collected for each image.

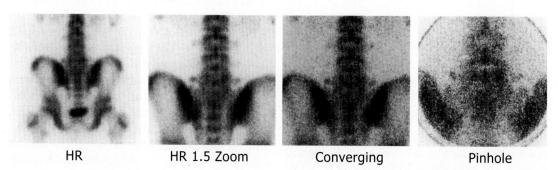

HR   HR 1.5 Zoom   Converging   Pinhole

FIGURE 16.4. A comparison of spine images from the same patient using different planar imaging techniques. The distance to the patient is less than 1 cm for the HR collimator and the converging collimator images. The 2-mm pinhole collimator is 6 cm from the patient. There are 500 K counts in the HR and converging images and 150 K counts in the pinhole images.

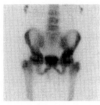
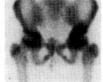
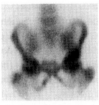
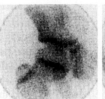
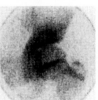

| HR | HR Zoom 1.5 | Converging | Pinhole |

FIGURE 16.5. This is a comparison of images in the evaluation of the hip joint. Note that the best resolution is achieved with the 2-mm pinhole collimator, which more clearly delineates the abnormality found in the left acetabulum.

$$R_{pin} = \frac{d}{a}(a+b)$$

where d is the diameter of the pinhole and a and b are defined as in Figure 16.7.

The magnification of a pinhole collimator is given by the following equation:

$$M_{pin} = \frac{a}{b}$$

Note that the pinhole collimator is capable of minification when b is larger than a.

Resolution of a converging collimator is given by the following equation:

$$R_{conv} = (a+b+c)\frac{d}{a}\frac{1}{\cos\theta}\left[1 - \frac{\left(c+\frac{a}{2}\right)}{f+a+c}\right]$$

Magnification of a converging collimator is given by

$$M_{conv} = \frac{f+a+b}{f-b}$$

Magnification of a converging collimator depends on the focal distance (f), which is defined in Figure 16.8. The collimator and systems resolution, as a function of distance to the patient, are shown in Figures 16.9 and 16.10, respectively.

Sensitivity Versus Object Distance

When selecting a collimator, it is not enough to consider only the spatial resolution; one must

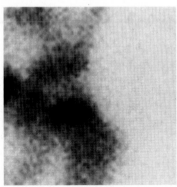
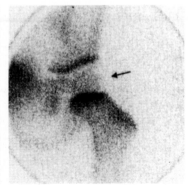

FIGURE 16.6. A comparison between the HR collimator (left) and the 2-mm pinhole collimator (right) for hip imaging. Note the increased clarity of the anatomic features with the 2-mm pinhole view taken at 6 cm from the patient. A display zoom was used for the HR image.

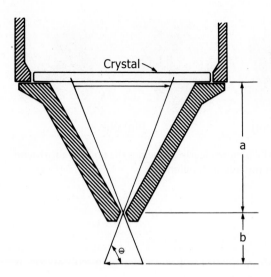

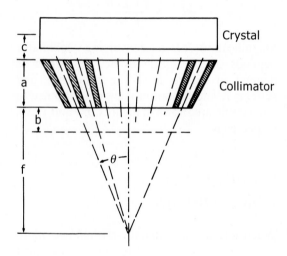

FIGURE 16.7. Pinhole collimator. The relevant dimensions of the pinhole are the diameter of the aperture, the crystal to pinhole distance a, and the distance to the patient b. When $\theta = 90$ degrees, sensitivity is maximum for the pinhole and it drops rapidly as θ decreases. (*Source:* Zimmerman RE. Radionuclide imaging systems. In: Taveras JM, Ferrucci JT, eds. Radiology. Philadelphia: JB Lippincott 1986, with permission.)

FIGURE 16.8. Converging collimator. All the holes in a converging collimator converge at the focal point, which is distance f from the front of the collimator. The other dimensions have a meaning similar to the parallel-hole collimator.

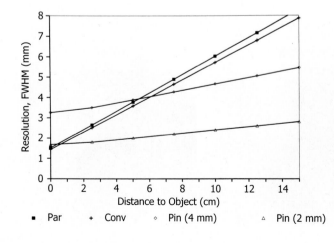

FIGURE 16.9. Collimator resolution versus distance. Note the steady loss of resolution with distance for all collimators, especially the multihole collimators. The multihole collimators are typical low-energy, high-resolution collimators of identical parameters a, b, d, and t. The pinhole has a diameter of 2 and 4mm.

FIGURE 16.10. System resolution versus distance. Note that for this example the parallel-hole collimator is always worse than the converging and that the pinhole has the best system resolution at all distances.

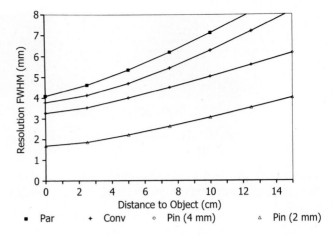

also consider sensitivity. Figure 16.11 shows the sensitivity of collimators versus distance from the object for parallel, converging, and pinhole collimators. The sensitivity of a parallel-hole collimator was described earlier. The sensitivity for a pinhole collimator is given by

$$g_{pin} = \frac{d^2 \sin^3 \theta}{16b^2}$$

Pinhole collimators are supplied with multiple inserts with different hole diameters, d, so that the user has some flexibility regarding resolution/sensitivity trade-offs. Note from the $(\sin^3 \theta)$ factor in the equation that the sensitivity to gamma rays that enter the collimator at increas-

ing angles to the pinhole axis is reduced significantly. This is responsible for the more intense central portion on the pinhole image in Figure 16.3. Also note that the pinhole collimator is capable of very high sensitivity at close distances (Fig. 16.11).

The pinhole is limited by the rapid drop of sensitivity with increasing distance to the patient and by the very pronounced decrease in sensitivity as the edge of the field is approached. This limits its use for quantitative imaging. Finally, the pinhole collimator distorts spatial relationships.

Examples of images using different sized pinholes are shown in Figure 16.12. Figure 16.13

FIGURE 16.11. Sensitivity versus distance. The pinhole sensitivity rapidly decreases with object distance from the collimator. The converging collimator actually increases sensitivity with distance, and the parallel-hole collimator is constant with distance. This example does not take into account attenuation losses, which could be substantial depending on the situation. The effects of off-axis gamma rays is not shown in this graph.

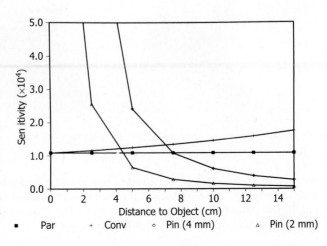

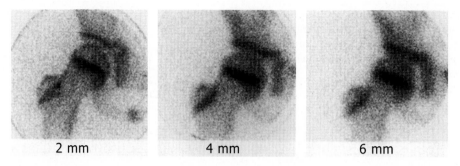

2 mm   4 mm   6 mm

FIGURE 16.12. A comparison among three different pinhole apertures at 6-cm distance from the patient. Note the better definition obtained with the smaller pinhole (2 mm). All images have 150 K counts.

shows the effect of pinhole-to-object distance on the images.

The sensitivity of a converging collimator is given by

$$g_{conv} = K^2 \left[\frac{d^2}{\dfrac{a}{\cos\theta}(d+t)} \right]^2$$

Note that the sensitivity of a converging collimator increases as the distance to the source increases (or as the source approaches the focal point). This is of little practical effect because the patient is always placed as close as possible to the collimator to achieve optimum resolution. However, relative quantitation with such a collimator can be a problem. There is also a slight drop in sensitivity to photons entering the collimator at the edge because the holes there are longer. This effect is seen in Figure 16.3. Distortion of spatial relationships also exists with the converging collimator.

The pinhole collimator has proven to be a most useful adjunct in pediatric nuclear medicine imaging.[10–12] The detail evident when using the pinhole with small structures increases confidence at little increase in imaging time or patient discomfort. Figures 16.14 to 16.18 show some examples of the usefulness of the pinhole

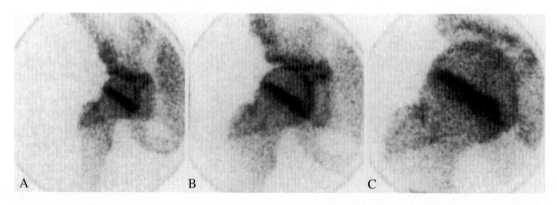

A   B   C

FIGURE 16.13. The effect of distance on 2-mm pinhole imaging. A: The distance to the patient is 12 cm. B: The distance been decreased to 6 cm. C: The distance has been decreased to the point that the collimator is touching the patient. Note the increased detail visible as the distance to the patient is decreased. All images have 150 K counts.

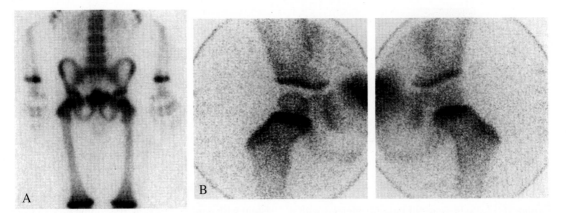

FIGURE 16.14. A 3-year-old patient referred with left hip pain. A: A high-resolution, parallel-hole collimator image for 500K was obtained, followed by pinhole views of both hip joints. B: There was asymmetry of uptake noted on the pinhole.

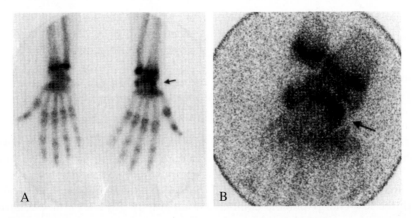

FIGURE 16.15. A 15-year-old soccer player referred for a question of a stress fracture of the right wrist. A: The planar image shows an area of increased uptake corresponding to the radial aspect of the carpal row on the right. B: A pinhole image further delineates the area of interest supporting the findings most consistent with a right scaphoid fracture.

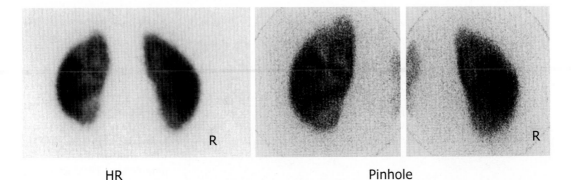

HR   Pinhole

FIGURE 16.16. A 3-year-old patient referred for the evaluation of a renal cortical defect. High-resolution, parallel-hole images and pinhole images were obtained. The pinhole images reveal the left upper pole defect much better than the parallel-hole collimator.

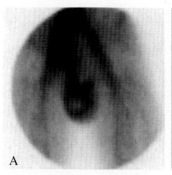 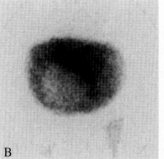 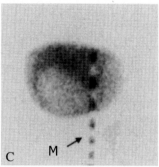

Immediate Static   Pinhole

FIGURE 16.17. A 16-year-old patient referred with a 5-day history of right testicular pain. A: In the immediate image "tissue phase" there is an absence of tracer uptake in the right hemiscrotum surrounded by an area of increased uptake of activity. This is consistent with a missed torsion. B: Pinhole images were obtained showing a decrease of activity centrally in the right hemiscrotum. C: With the use of a flexible cobalt-57 marker over the raphe of the scrotum, the right and left hemiscrotum are delineated.

collimator in clinical practice. Figure 16.18 shows a thyroid imaged with iodine-123 (^{123}I). We have obtained very good thyroid ^{123}I images with the 2-mm pinhole collimator when thyroid uptake is normal or high, using the low-energy pinhole collimator. However, when thyroid uptake is low, penetration of high-energy photons (500 keV and above) distorts the image obtained with the low-energy pinhole collimator. In these cases, a 6-mm pinhole insert works better. High-energy pinhole collimators are more optimal for imaging thyroid ^{123}I.

Pinhole Single Photon Emission Computed Tomography

The use of pinhole imaging has a proven role in pediatric imaging in nuclear medicine as demonstrated in this chapter. Is there a role for pinhole single photon emission computed tomography (SPECT) in pediatric imaging? This is much more problematic. To date there has been little to no commercial support from camera-computer vendors for pinhole SPECT

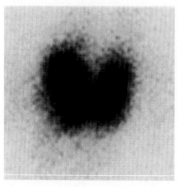 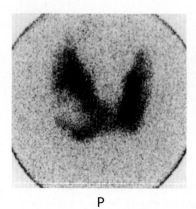

HR   P

FIGURE 16.18. A 12-year-old patient referred for the evaluation of a thyroid nodule. Note that the high-resolution view (HR) when compared to the pinhole view (P) does not clearly delineate the extent of the cold nodule found in the right lobe of the thyroid gland.

imaging. There are several reports in the literature by Bahk and colleagues[13-15] that clearly demonstrate the utility of pinhole SPECT in bone scintigraphy of limbs in adults. This technique does not seem to have been performed by others.

Jaszczak and colleagues[16-21] have investigated pinhole SPECT as applied to high-energy brain imaging and scintimammography. This work has not been performed outside their laboratory. Brain SPECT imaging with a pinhole collimator was performed with therapeutic doses of ^{131}I. This experience is not generally applicable to pediatric imaging. The scintimammography technique may be applicable to pediatric imaging as more conventional isotopes and amounts were used. However, to date, no experience has been reported.

The group at the University of Arizona under Barrett[22,23] has constructed elaborate multi-pinhole SPECT systems that utilize small cameras with each pinhole. Instruments have been built for human brain imaging and small animal imaging using 20 to 24 pinholes. A European group has described its experience with parathyroid pinhole SPECT[24,25] but has provided no technical details.

There is a large and growing literature of pinhole SPECT in small animal imaging.[26-29] Most of this work does not translate directly into imaging of humans, but it is at least conceivable that some pediatric pinhole SPECT imaging can be performed with a well-designed multi-pinhole system that allows a very close approach to limbs or trunk of newborns. Such a system has yet to be designed.

Conclusion

Pinhole magnification scintigraphy continues to be an essential imaging technique within pediatric as well as adult nuclear medicine. Particularly in pediatrics, it continues to provide high-quality images for smaller anatomic areas not easily imaged with a parallel-hole collimator or SPECT. Magnification scintigraphy should be used routinely as a complement to other imaging techniques when evaluating bony abnormalities, renal cortical defects, and thyroid, cardiac, and scrotal pathology.

References

1. Sty JR, Wells RG, Conway JJ. Spine pain in children. Semin Nucl Med 1993;23(4):296–320.
2. Parker JA, Lebowitz R, Mascatello V, et al. Magnification renal scintigraphy in the differential diagnosis of septa of Bertin. Pediatr Radiol 1976;4(3):157–60.
3. Mandell GA, Harcke HT, Hugh J, et al. Detection of talocalcaneal coalitions by magnification bone scintigraphy. J Nucl Med 1990;31(11):1797–801.
4. Sorenson JA, Phelps ME. Physics in Nuclear Medicine, 2nd ed. Orlando: Grune & Stratton, 1987.
5. Rollo FD. Nuclear Medicine Physics, Instrumentation, and Agents. St. Louis: CV Mosby, 1977.
6. Harcke HT, Mandell GA. Scintigraphic evaluation of the growth plate. Semin Nucl Med 1993;23(4):266–73.
7. Connolly LP, Treves ST, Davis RT, et al. Pediatric applications of pinhole magnification imaging. J Nucl Med 1999;40(11):1896–901.
8. Bernier DR. Nuclear Medicine Technology and Techniques, 2nd ed. St. Louis: Mosby, 1989.
9. Early PJ, Sodee DB. Principles and Practice of Nuclear Medicine. St. Louis: Mosby, 1985.
10. Conway JJ. A scintigraphic classification of Legg-Calve-Perthes disease. Semin Nucl Med 1993;23(4):274–95.
11. Gilday DL, Ash JM. Benign bone tumors. Semin Nucl Med 1976;6(1):33–46.
12. Treves ST. Pediatric Nuclear Medicine. New York: Springer-Verlag, 1985.
13. Bahk YW, Chung SK, Park YH, et al. Pinhole SPECT imaging in normal and morbid ankles. J Nucl Med 1998;39(1):130–9.
14. Bahk YW, Kim SH, Chung SK, et al. Dual-head pinhole bone scintigraphy. J Nucl Med 1998;39(8):1444–8.
15. Kim SH, Chung SK, Bahk YW, et al. Whole-body and pinhole bone scintigraphic manifestations of Reiter's syndrome: distribution patterns and early and characteristic signs. Eur J Nucl Med 1999;26(2):163–70.
16. Jaszczak RJ, Li J, Wang H, et al. Pinhole collimation for ultra-high-resolution, small-field-of-view SPECT. Phys Med Biol 1994;39(3):425–37.

17. Tornai MP, Bowsher JE, Jaszczak RJ, et al. Mammotomography with pinhole incomplete circular orbit SPECT. J Nucl Med 2003;44(4): 583–93.
18. Smith MF, Gilland DR, Coleman RE, et al. Quantitative imaging of iodine-131 distributions in brain tumors with pinhole SPECT: a phantom study. J Nucl Med 1998;39(5):856–64.
19. Smith MF, Jaszczak RJ. An analytic model of pinhole aperture penetration for 3D pinhole SPECT image reconstruction. Phys Med Biol 1998;43(4):761–75.
20. Scarfone C, Jaszczak RJ, Li J, et al. Breast tumour imaging using incomplete circular orbit pinhole SPET: a phantom study. Nucl Med Commun 1997;18(11):1077–86.
21. Li J, Jaszczak RJ, Greer KL, et al. A filtered back-projection algorithm for pinhole SPECT with a displaced centre of rotation. Phys Med Biol 1994;39(1):165–76.
22. Rowe RK, Aarsvold JN, Barrett HH, et al. A stationary hemispherical SPECT imager for three-dimensional brain imaging. J Nucl Med 1993; 34(3):474–80.
23. Liu Z, Kastis GA, Stevenson GD, et al. Quantitative analysis of acute myocardial infarct in rat hearts with ischemia-reperfusion using a high-resolution stationary SPECT system. J Nucl Med 2002;43(7):933–9.
24. Profanter C, Gabriel M, Wetscher GJ, et al. Accuracy of preoperative pinhole subtraction single photon emission computed tomography for patients with primary and recurrent hyperparathyroidism in an endemic goiter area. Surg Today 2004;34(6):493–7.
25. Profanter C, Prommegger R, Gabriel M, et al. Comparison of planar scintiscanning and pinhole subtraction SPECT in preoperative imaging of primary hyperparathyroidism in an endemic goiter area. Endocrinologist 2003;13(2): 112–5.
26. Weber DA, Ivanovic M, Franceschi D, et al. Pinhole SPECT: an approach to in vivo high resolution SPECT imaging in small laboratory animals. J Nucl Med 1994;35(2):342–8.
27. Beekman FJ, Vastenhouw B. Design and simulation of a high-resolution stationary SPECT system for small animals. Phys Med Biol 2004;49(19):4579–92.
28. Moore SC, Zimmerman RE, Mahmood A, et al. A triple-detector, multiple-pinhole system for SPECT imaging of rodents. J Nucl Med 2004; 45(5):97P.
29. Schramm NU, Ebel G, Engeland U, et al. High-resolution SPECT using multipinhole collimation. IEEE Trans Nucl Sci 2003;50(3): 315–20.

17
Single Positron Emission Computed Tomography

Frederic H. Fahey and Beth A. Harkness

Single photon emission computed tomography (SPECT) allows the user to obtain a three-dimensional (3D) representation of the patient's in vivo radiopharmaceutical distribution. Planar nuclear imaging leads to a two-dimensional (2D) image of a 3D object. In some cases, it can be difficult to detect or localize a certain feature due to the ambiguity introduced by background activity in the overlying and underlying tissue. Conversely, SPECT allows the 3D object to be represented as a series of thin, tomographic slices. This can lead to a substantial increase in image contrast that can greatly improve the ability to detect small features. Due to the 3D nature of SPECT, it can also greatly improve one's ability to localize these features. In addition, improved contrast can lead to an enhanced quantitative capability that can be of great value for both clinical and research purposes. For all of these reasons, SPECT has become an essential medical imaging modality over the past 30 years.

Although the acquisition and processing of SPECT data is not inherently difficult, it does take attention to detail in order to acquire the highest quality SPECT images. This is particularly true in pediatric SPECT, where the imaging environment may be more challenging and the features being evaluated may be smaller. This chapter briefly reviews the development of SPECT and discusses the basics behind data acquisition, reconstruction, and processing, and the essential components of a suitable quality control program, as well as some practical aspects for acquiring the highest quality images possible in pediatric SPECT.

Single photon emission computed tomography was first reported by Kuhl and Edwards[1] in 1963. They developed a method that acquired the tomographic data using a dedicated rectilinear scanner and reconstructed the data using simple backprojection. The work by Kuhl and Edwards predated that by Hounsfield[2] on computed tomography by 10 years. The Anger gamma camera later became the instrument of choice in nuclear imaging, and, by the late 1970s, prototypes of the rotating gamma camera had been developed by different groups including Keyes et al.[3] at the University of Michigan and Jaszczak et al.[4] at Searle. By 1990, practically all large field of view gamma cameras could also acquire SPECT studies.

Several modifications were necessary to make a conventional gamma camera suitable for performing SPECT. Additional magnetic shielding was placed around phototubes to minimize the effect of the earth's magnetic field on camera response. The gamma camera itself had to be designed to perform at a higher level of uniformity, linearity, and stability. The camera detector had to be mounted onto a gantry that allowed rotation about the patient. A low-attenuation patient table had to be incorporated into the system. The SPECT system had to include a computer that could control the gantry during data acquisition and, subsequently, reconstruct the data into transverse slices. These enhancements not only made the system capable of performing SPECT but

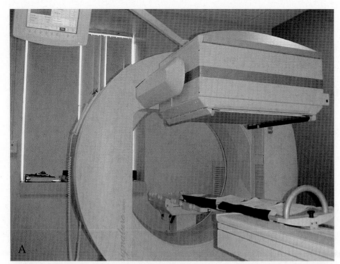

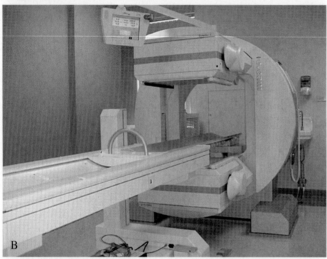

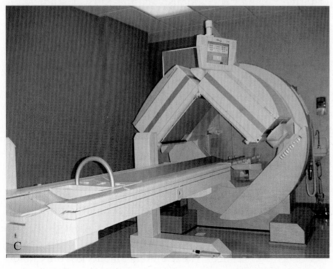

FIGURE 17.1. Rotating gamma camera single photon emission computed tomography (SPECT) modern systems. A: Single-headed SPECT system. B: Dual-headed SPECT system at 180-degree orientation. C: Dual-headed SPECT system at 90-degree orientation.

many of them also led to improvements in image quality for conventional planar nuclear imaging.

Rotating gamma camera SPECT systems were initially developed with a single detector. Multidetector cameras that could perform SPECT with higher sensitivity became readily available in the 1990s. Although both dual- and triple-detector systems were manufactured, the flexibility of the dual-detector gamma cameras led to its popularity. These systems could perform whole-body planar studies as well as SPECT. State-of-the-art single- and dual-detector SPECT systems are shown in Figure 17.1. For cardiac SPECT, there may not be a substantial advantage to acquiring SPECT data over a 360-degree rotation because the heart is in the left anterior portion of the thorax, and thus not many photons will be detected in the right posterior direction. Therefore, in dual-detector systems, the two detectors can be oriented at 90 degrees to each other, as shown in Figure 17.1C. Acquiring cardiac SPECT in this configuration leads to twice the efficiency for 180-degree SPECT relative to a single-detector system.

Basic Concepts

Data Collection

To perform SPECT with a rotating gamma camera, the camera detector is mounted on a gantry, allowing it to rotate about the patient. This is shown in Figure 17.2. During the rotation, the detector surface is parallel to the axis of rotation. The axis of rotation is typically

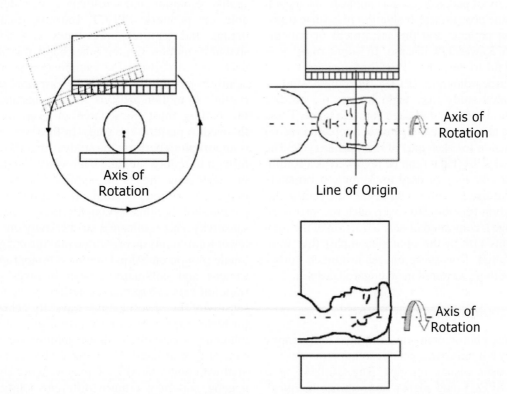

FIGURE 17.2. Data acquisition with a rotating gamma camera SPECT: the geometry of SPECT using a rotating gamma camera. The gamma camera head rotates about the patient, acquiring projection images at a number of viewing angles. The axis of rotation is typically parallel to the long axis of the patient's body. If a gamma ray interacts with the detector, it is assumed to have passed through the collimator on a line parallel to the collimator holes. This line is referred to as the line of origin.

maintained parallel to the long axis of the patient's body. Consider an example of a typical SPECT acquisition. The patient is placed on the imaging table and the camera is placed directly above the patient as in Figure 17.2. The first projection image is acquired in this position for a preset time (e.g., 15 seconds). The camera rotates to its second position, and another projection image is acquired for the same time as the first. This process is repeated until the camera has completely rotated about the patient. In some instances, projections are acquired over a full 360 degrees and in others over 180 degrees. In a typical example, a projection image may be acquired for 15 seconds every 3 degrees for a total of 120 projections over 360 degrees. Such a study acquisition would take about 30 minutes to complete with a single detector camera.

Cardiac SPECT can be of great value in a variety of pediatric cardiac applications including the postsurgical evaluation of cardiac transplant patients and the assessment of patients with Kawasaki's disease. In some cases, it is helpful to gate the SPECT acquisition by the electrocardiogram (ECG). For these studies, a gated study (e.g., eight images per cardiac cycle) is acquired at each rotation angle. These data are processed to provide a separate reconstruction for each part of the cardiac cycle. The gated SPECT data can be reviewed as a continuous cine loop or used to estimate parameters of cardiac function such as the left ventricular ejection fraction. However, each reconstructed image is composed of only a fraction of the total counts (1/8 in the above example) that were acquired. Thus these images are much noisier than those acquired in an ungated fashion.

Resolution and Sensitivity

Single photon emission computed tomography does not improve spatial resolution or sensitivity over planar imaging. The cameras used for SPECT and planar imaging are identical. The best possible spatial resolution (planar or SPECT) is at the collimator surface. In SPECT, the object of interest is often at some depth within the patient and can be from 5 to 25 cm away from the collimator surface, as opposed to

planar imaging, where the camera can sometimes be brought very close to the patient. Noting that the system spatial resolution degrades as the distance from the collimator is increased and that the object-to-collimator distance is usually greater with SPECT than with planar imaging, the spatial resolution in SPECT is actually worse than in planar imaging with the same collimator. Also, the sensitivity is the same for SPECT and planar imaging for a given detector-collimator combination. The advantage of SPECT over planar imaging, therefore, is not improved spatial resolution or sensitivity. Instead, it is the improved image contrast due to the elimination of the ambiguity associated with radioactivity in superimposed layers of tissue. Higher contrast, in turn, improves diagnostic accuracy and increases the potential for greater quantitative accuracy.

A SPECT system with the highest possible spatial resolution and sensitivity is most desirable for pediatric SPECT. Imaging smaller organs and features necessitates very high spatial resolution. On the other hand, it is also necessary to perform the examination as efficiently as possible. Longer studies are more susceptible to motion artifacts. In some instances, the patient must be sedated or even anesthetized to perform the study. In these cases, it is important to perform the study in an efficient fashion to reduce the time over which sedation or anesthesia need be applied. However, improved system spatial resolution with parallel-hole collimators yields lower system sensitivity. This results in a noisier study due to fewer total counts incorporated into the images. Single photon emission computed tomography camera and collimator design involves the trade-off between spatial resolution and system sensitivity by investigating ways to achieve the highest sensitivity for what is considered the minimum acceptable spatial resolution for the clinical task at hand. The clinical tasks associated with pediatric SPECT may be more challenging and may require different solutions than those for SPECT for larger patients. One way to address the need for high sensitivity is to increase the number of camera detectors. The total counts in the study would increase by a factor equal to the number of detectors, presuming one does not alter the injected dose, the imaging time, or the collimator sensitivity. With the multidetector approach, image detail that is not visible in a SPECT study acquired with a single-detector system may be visualized with a multidetector system. Alternatively, one could maintain the same image quality as the single-detector system in a fraction of the time. This approach may be suitable for very busy departments that require higher patient throughput. Lastly, one could choose to sacrifice some of the additional counts for higher spatial resolution by using a more stringent collimator. This approach may be most appropriate in certain pediatric applications where high spatial resolution is necessary for that particular task. This will be discussed in more detail with respect to the appropriate choice of collimators for SPECT imaging.

The introduction of multiple detectors to a SPECT system complicates both the design and quality control of the system. With multidetector SPECT, the underlying assumption is that an image acquired with one detector at a particular angular location is exactly the same as that acquired with the other detectors when they are at the same location. This assumption necessitates that the detectors be accurately mounted to the gantry so that the images from the multiple detectors are registered to each other. Dual- and triple-detector systems have been developed that meet these constraints.

Parallel-Hole Collimators

The choice of collimator is the most important factor in defining tomographic spatial resolution and system sensitivity. The parallel-hole collimator is by far the most commonly used collimator in SPECT. Although any parallel collimator can be used for SPECT, some yield better images than others. In SPECT, it is particularly important that the collimators maintain their spatial resolution for objects that are at some distance from the collimator. As previously discussed, objects of interest are often up to 5 to 25 cm from the collimator during a SPECT study. It is therefore essential that these objects be imaged as well as is practically possible. The tomographic spatial resolu-

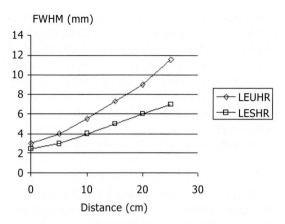

FIGURE 17.3. Collimator spatial resolution at a distance: the system spatial resolution associated with two different collimators—low-energy, ultrahigh resolution (LEUHR) and low-energy, superhigh resolution (LESHR). The spatial resolution is parameterized by the full width at half maximum (FWHM) of the line spread function. The FWHM value decreases with improving spatial resolution. SPECT is typically performed between 5 and 25 cm. The spatial resolution degrades for both collimators with increasing distance. However, the spatial resolution for LESHR does not degrade as quickly due to its longer hole length; thus, LESHR yields excellent spatial resolution at distances associated with SPECT.

tion (as noted by the full width at half maximum, FWHM, of the point spread function) is shown in Figure 17.3 for two different collimators, low-energy, ultrahigh resolution (LEUHR) and low-energy, superhigh resolution (LESHR). It should be noted that a higher FWHM value is associated with poorer spatial resolution. Figure 17.3 shows that the spatial resolution degrades for objects located farther from the collimator face. However, the slope for the graph associated with LESHR is less steep than the one for LEUHR. This indicates that the spatial resolution at depths typical for tomographic imaging is much better for LESHR.

The sensitivity for LESHR is most likely substantially less than that for LEUHR. Higher resolution collimators (i.e., lower FWHM values) typically have lower sensitivities. Therefore, using the LESHR leads to a noisier image than using the LEUHR for the same administered activity and imaging time. For pediatric SPECT, which collimator is most likely to yield the highest quality images? Should one use the higher resolution collimators that provide sharper detail to the images or should one use the higher sensitivity collimators that yield images that are less noisy? This discussion is particularly germane when considering the use of multidetector SPECT where the increased sensitivity could be traded for higher resolution. Muehllehner et al.[5] performed a study that investigated the relationship between sensitivity and resolution. Simulated tomographic images of varying resolution and counts were shown to observers who were asked to select images that were most comparable in image quality. This study indicated that an increase in counts by a factor of 4 was necessary to yield comparable image quality to that obtained with a 2-mm improvement in spatial resolution. For example, an image with 6-mm resolution and 400 K counts was considered to have comparable image quality to an image with 8-mm resolution and 1.6 M counts.

Fahey et al.[6] investigated whether this relationship between spatial resolution and sensitivity was maintained with real SPECT data. A series of phantom images acquired with high-resolution (HR) and ultrahigh-resolution (UHR) collimators were presented to several observers. The collimator spatial resolution of the UHR collimator was determined to be about 2 mm better than that for the HR collimator. However, the sensitivity of the UHR was only about half that of the HR. The HR images were acquired for varying counts, and the observers were asked to select the image from the HR series that was most comparable to a single reference image acquired with the UHR collimator with respect to image quality. These results indicated that a 2-mm improvement in spatial resolution was comparable to an increase in counts by a factor of 2.5 to 3.4. Actual clinical studies of the same patients obtained with both sets of collimators were then presented to the observers. The two studies were acquired for the same time and reconstructed with the same filter. Thus, the UHR studies had 50% of the total counts of the HR studies but demonstrated improved resolu-

tion by approximately 2 mm. The observers were not aware of which images were acquired with which collimator. The observers selected the set of images they preferred with regard to image quality. For liver SPECT studies, the observers always selected the images obtained with the UHR collimator over those using the HR. For brain SPECT studies, the UHR images were preferred in most cases over those with the HR. Other investigators have obtained similar results.[7] To summarize, for parallel-hole collimators, those that maintain their resolution at depths of 15 cm or greater are preferable and higher resolution collimators are preferred over those with higher sensitivity.

Focusing Collimators

For pediatric SPECT, the perfect collimator would be one that provides the highest possible spatial resolution for small objects without sacrificing counts. As previously discussed, improvements in spatial resolution lead to better image quality than do a greater number of counts. In fact, both high resolution and high counts are preferred. Focusing collimators can provide higher spatial resolution without sacrificing counts, particularly for small objects. These collimators magnify the image similarly to using a converging collimator in planar nuclear imaging. When imaging a small object, such as a child, with a large field-of-view camera, it is advantageous to magnify the object to take up as much of the field of view as possible. The improvement in sensitivity for the same spatial resolution is basically given by the magnification factor. In this way, the sensitivity can be improved without degrading the spatial resolution. This approach is particularly suitable for the imaging of smaller organs such as the brain or for smaller patients. Therefore, the use of focused collimators is particularly applicable to pediatric SPECT.

Fan beam collimators have been routinely used for SPECT.[8] These collimators converge in the dimension that corresponds to the x axis of the projection data and are parallel in the y direction (Fig. 17.4). There is magnification of the SPECT projection data in the direction corresponding to the transverse plane. For typical

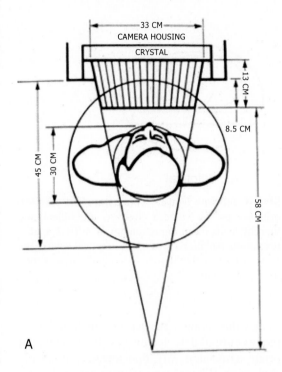

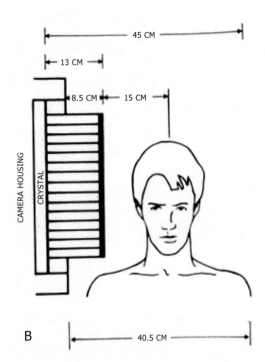

FIGURE 17.4. The geometry associated with the use of fan beam collimators in SPECT. A: This collimator is focused in the transverse, in-plane direction. B: However, its holes are parallel in the axial direction. The sensitivity of this collimator is approximately 50% higher than that of a parallel-hole collimator with the same spatial resolution. (*Source:* Tsui et al.,[8] with permission of the Society for Nuclear Medicine.)

fan beam collimators, the increase in sensitivity is about 50% compared to parallel-hole collimators of comparable spatial resolution. Cone beam collimators have also been used for SPECT, and they can improve the sensitivity by a factor of 2 to 3 relative to parallel-hole collimators for comparable spatial resolution.[9] Using focused collimators for SPECT requires special reconstruction software that tends to be more complicated and thus substantially slower than the software for parallel-hole collimators.

Types of Orbits

Initially, SPECT cameras could perform only circular orbits. However, with a circular orbit, the distance from the camera to the axis of rotation does not change. This distance is often referred to as the "radius of rotation." The cross section through most patients is not circular, and therefore many projection images are acquired with the camera at a distance away from the patient (Fig. 17.5). As discussed previously, the collimator spatial resolution degrades as the distance from the camera to the patient is increased. Thus, acquiring a SPECT scan with any of the projection images at a greater distance than necessary from the patient will lead to a loss in spatial resolution. For this reason, modern SPECT cameras are able to acquire data with either an elliptical or a body-contour orbit. These orbits keep the camera as close to the patient as possible, and the resultant SPECT images have the highest spatial resolution possible.

Tomographic Reconstruction

The acquisition of emission tomography data, be it SPECT or positron emission tomography (PET), consists of acquiring projection data from various viewing angles about the patient.

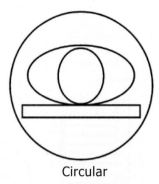
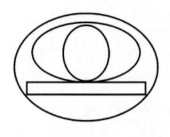

Circular   Elliptical

FIGURE 17.5. Circular and elliptical orbits, two gantry orbits commonly used in SPECT. In the circular orbit configuration, the camera-to-object distance is large in both the anterior and posterior positions, leading to reduced spatial resolution. However, this orbit may still be used for brain SPECT and with focusing collimators. The elliptical orbit keeps the camera close to the object and thereby leads to an improvement in SPECT spatial resolution. An alternative to the elliptical orbit is the body contour orbit that is individually determined for each patient.

In some cases the data are collected over 180 degrees or 360 degrees. The simple viewing of images of different viewing angles gives the observer a three-dimensional sense of the patient. However, with tomographic reconstruction, the projection data can be computer processed or "reconstructed" into tomographic slices through the object. These reconstructed data can be viewed as a series of transverse slices, as slices through the patient in three orthogonal views or presented as 3D renderings.

An imaging configuration is shown in Figure 17.2. In this example, a projection is being acquired with the gamma camera using a parallel-hole collimator. In SPECT using a parallel-hole collimator, a detected photon is assumed to have been emitted from somewhere along the line of origin. Thus, all events detected at a particular location on the gamma camera crystal are referred to as the "ray sum" acquired along that line of response. Single photon emission computed tomography raw data are a series of projection images acquired at various angles about the patient and are characterized by the projection angle at which the data were acquired and the ray sum of detected events at each location at that projection angle.

Consider the cross section through the simple object shown in Figure 17.6. Three projections through the object are also shown.

Each value along a projection is assumed to be the ray sum of detected events along the line of origin associated with that location along the projection. Where along the ray a photon originated cannot be determined, and, thus, the ray sum value is "backprojected" across the entire image along the line of origin. After all of the data have been backprojected, a semblance of the object is generated. However, there are sub-

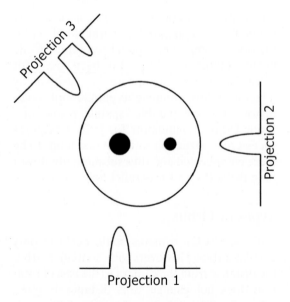

FIGURE 17.6. A simple round object with two smaller features within it, along with three projections (at approximately 0, 90, and 225 degrees, respectively).

stantial streak artifacts associated with this image. With this simple example, the object would still be recognizable, but with a more complicated object the reconstructed image is typically not discernible. This approach to reconstruction is referred to as "simple backprojection."

Images can be considered to consist of signals of varying frequencies that have been added together. The signals with lower frequencies give the image its general shape, and the higher frequencies give the image its sharp edges and fine detail. In a manner similar to that used with audio signals, these frequencies can be "filtered" to modify the appearance of the image. The low frequencies can be removed to enhance the edges in the image, or, alternatively, the high frequencies can be removed to provide a smoother appearance. Removal of the higher frequencies can also be helpful in reducing the high-frequency noise in the image.

The streak artifacts associated with simple backprojection are the result of an uneven sampling of the spatial frequencies during the reconstruction process. Due to the nature of the process, the low spatial frequencies are sampled at a much higher rate than the higher frequencies. To remedy this, a filter is applied that reduces the contribution of the low frequencies and enhances that of the high frequencies. The magnitude of this filter increases linearly with spatial frequency and is thus referred to as the "ramp" filter. Typically, the projections are filtered by the ramp filter and then backprojected. This approach is referred to as "filtered backprojection." With an infinite number of projections consisting of noiseless data, the original object can be reconstructed exactly. However, real SPECT data are noisy, and depending on the magnitude of this noise, the reconstruction will be somewhat less than exact.

A windowing filter is also applied during the reconstruction process, which maintains the ramp filter at lower frequencies but smoothly returns the filter to zero at higher frequencies. The use of this filter reduces both ringing artifacts and quantum noise in the reconstructed image. Windowing filters often used in SPECT include the Butterworth, Hamming, Hanning, and Shepp-Logan filters. The "cut-off" frequency of the windowing filter, that is, the frequency where the filter returns to zero, can be selected depending on the noise content of the underlying data. If the projection data consist of many counts and, thus, have low noise, a high cut-off filter can be used to preserve the fine detail in the reconstructed image, whereas if the projection data are noisy, then a lower cut-off frequency can be used to minimize the noise in the reconstructed image. For example, a higher cut-off frequency typically is used for brain SPECT where the projection data have low noise, whereas a lower cut-off frequency is used with gallium-67 (^{67}Ga) SPECT where the projection data has a high noise level, particularly for the 72-hour image.

In recent years, iterative approaches to tomographic reconstruction have been introduced. This approach is illustrated in Figure 17.7. An initial version of the object is assumed. This may be a uniform image or a filtered backprojection. From this initial image, a series of projections is generated according to a model of SPECT imaging. This model may include such physical aspects of SPECT data acquisition as collimator resolution, scatter, and photon attenuation. These generated projections are compared to the true projections. Variations between the two (either in terms of the difference or the ratio) are backprojected and used to modify the initial image. This modified image is then used to generate a second set of generated projections, and the process is repeated. This can be repeated a number of times until an adequate reconstruction is obtained. Statistical criteria such as maximum entropy or likelihood are used to judge the improvement of the reconstructed image with each iteration. The maximum likelihood expectation maximization (MLEM) algorithm is a popular approach to iterative reconstruction.[10] Iterative reconstruction can potentially improve the accuracy of the reconstruction by incorporating knowledge of the basic physics of SPECT data acquisition and the Poisson statistical nature of radiation detection into the process. However, these methods were traditionally much slower than filtered backprojection. A single iteration took approximately the same time to apply as

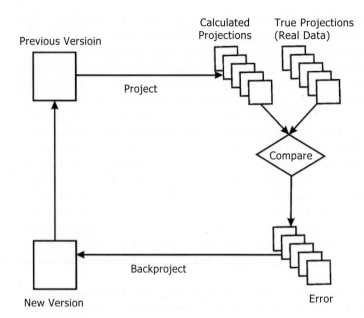

FIGURE 17.7. Iterative reconstruction. The algorithm starts with an initial assumption of the object (previous version). These data are processed to form a series of calculated or estimated projection images. These data are compared to the true projections, that is, the real raw SPECT projection data by taking either the ratio or the difference between the two. The resulting error is backprojected and used to modify the previous version to arrive at a new version. This loop is repeated until the comparison between the calculated and true projections is small. At that point, the reconstructed image should be a good representation of the true object.

filtered backprojection, and sometimes as many as 50 iterations were necessary to achieve an acceptable reconstruction. The development of faster algorithms, such as ordered subset expectation maximization (OSEM),[11] and the availability of faster computers have made the use of iterative reconstruction feasible in routine clinical use. Besides the advantages already discussed, iterative approaches tend to provide reconstructions with less noise and greatly

reduced streak artifacts. Figure 17.8 shows the same SPECT data reconstructed with both filtered backprojection and OSEM.

Attenuation Correction

In abdominal SPECT, a photon emitted from the center of the body is less likely to be detected than one from the periphery because of the higher probability of absorption or scat-

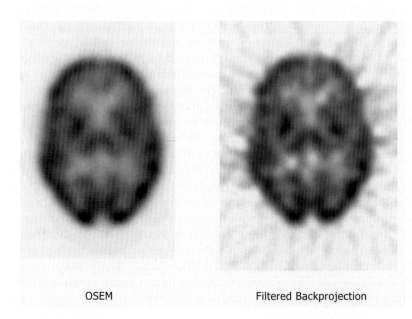

FIGURE 17.8. Iterative ordered subset expectation maximization (OSEM) reconstruction and filtered backprojection of the same brain SPECT data set. Note that the filtered backprojection image appears to be noisier and has notable streak artifacts as compared to the OSEM image.

tering of the photons. Even for a uniformly distributed radiopharmaceutical, the signal from the center of the SPECT study will be less intense than from the periphery. The appearance of the image as well as the ability to quantify the activity distribution will be affected by this photon attenuation effect. Therefore, one must compensate for photon attenuation in order to obtain an appropriate image and to accurately quantify the level of activity. In other words, attenuation correction must be applied to the SPECT study. There are some cases where it is reasonable to assume that the attenuating properties of the surrounding material are uniform. Uniform attenuation correction is typically adequate for brain and abdominal SPECT. However, the tissues of the thorax (e.g., the lung, spine, and heart) have very different attenuation properties. Therefore, uniform attenuation correction is not appropriate in the thorax, and a nonuniform correction is necessary. Both uniform and nonuniform approaches to attenuation correction will be discussed.

Figure 17.9A shows the cross section through the abdomen of a patient. The material in the slice is assumed to have similar attenuating property. In other words, the linear attenuation coefficient, μ, for all the material in the slice is the same. The body outline must be known. Consider a single pixel and the ray that connects that pixel to the body outline. The probability of photons from this pixel traveling along that ray reaching the camera without being attenuated, P, is assumed to be

$$P = e^{-\mu x}$$

where μ is the linear attenuation coefficient for soft tissue at the gamma-ray energy of the radiopharmaceutical, x is the distance along the ray from the pixel to the body outline and e is the base of the natural logarithm. This is referred to as the attenuation factor for this pixel in direction of this ray. The average attenuation factor associated with this pixel is estimated by the average attenuation factor for a number of rays from this pixel to the body outline:

Average Attenuation Factor
$$= 1/n\left(e^{-\mu x1} + e^{-\mu x2} + e^{-\mu x3} + \ldots + e^{-\mu xn}\right)$$

where $x1, x2, x3, \ldots, xn$, are the distances of the n rays from the pixel to the body outline as shown in Figure 17.9A. The reciprocal of the average value is the attenuation correction factor:

Attenuation Correction Factor
$$= 1/(\text{Average Attenuation Factor})$$

In other words, counts originating from this pixel need to be multiplied by this attenuation correction factor to correct for photon attenuation. A correction matrix is generated by calculating an attenuation correction factor for every pixel within the body outline. The reconstructed data of each tomographic slice is multiplied by the attenuation correction matrix for that slice. This postreconstruction attenuation correction method developed by Chang[12] is referred to as the first-order Chang correction for photon attenuation. The Chang correction method works very well for brain and abdominal SPECT. In this approach, the operator must define the body outline (either manually or automatically) for each slice that is to be corrected. The value of μ for the photon energy of technetium-99m (^{99m}Tc) and soft tissue is given in physics tables as $0.15\,\text{cm}^{-1}$, which does not take into account the buildup of Compton-scattered photons that are detected and incorporated into the SPECT image. A lower value for μ, either 0.11 or $0.12\,\text{cm}^{-1}$, is often used to compensate for this inclusion of scattered photons. The use of this slightly reduced value of μ yields a more uniform response.

Although the Chang method works well in the brain and abdomen, it does not work very well for thoracic SPECT and, in particular, for cardiac SPECT. The thorax consists of several very different types of tissues (e.g., lungs, spine, soft tissue) with different attenuating properties. Therefore, a nonuniform attenuation correction must be used in the thorax. The cross section through the thorax of a patient is shown in Figure 17.9B. Again, a single pixel and a ray connecting that pixel to the body outline can be considered, as with the Chang method. However, in this case, photons traveling along this ray traverse different materials that have different linear attenuation coefficients or μ

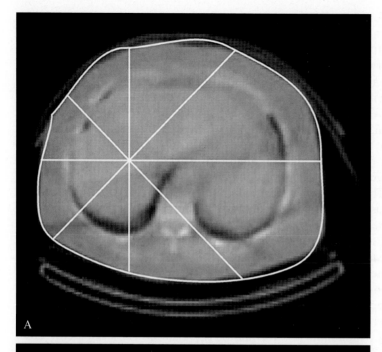

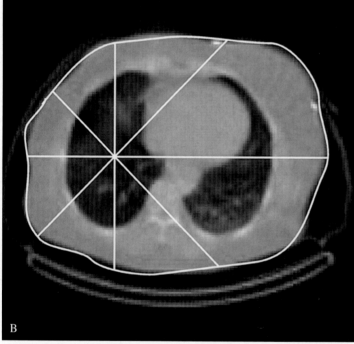

FIGURE 17.9. Uniform and non-uniform attenuation correction. A: A transmission view is shown through the abdomen of a patient. Once the body outline is determined, a series of rays are drawn from the pixel in question to the body outline and the attenuation factor is estimated along each ray. The average attenuation factor is then calculated; this is used to estimate the attenuation correction factor for that pixel. The process is repeated for every pixel within the object to generate an attenuation correction matrix. The initial reconstructed image matrix is multiplied by this correction matrix on a pixel-by-pixel basis to provide the attenuation corrected SPECT study. Note that the assumption of uniform attenuation along each ray is appropriate in the abdomen. B: This figure is similar to that in A, except that it is a slice through the thorax. Note that the assumption of uniform attenuation is not appropriate in this region of the body. Therefore, transmission data must be used to estimate the nonuniform attenuation properties in the thorax and thus to correct appropriately for attenuation correction.

values. Thus, the attenuation factor along this ray is given by

$$A = e^{-\Sigma \mu(x) \Delta x}$$

where $\mu(x)$ is the linear attenuation coefficient associated with the x position along the ray, and Δx is the pixel size along the ray. The symbol Σ represents the sum along the ray. The correction approach has become more complicated compared to the uniform case because one now needs to know the linear attenuation coefficient at every pixel within the body outline. A transmission study of the object is necessary to attain attenuation information for each pixel. The emission data are reconstructed in conjunction with the transmission data to obtain SPECT image data corrected for nonuniform attenuation. The transmission study of the object is acquired with the use of external radioactive sources. Various manufacturers have implemented different approaches to the acquisition of the transmission scan.[13] A scanning, collimated line source, a series of line sources, or a single line source in conjunction with a focusing collimator have been used to acquire this transmission image. The radionuclide gadolinium-153 (^{153}Gd) is often used as the transmission source because it emits a 100-keV gamma ray, and this energy is between the energies of ^{99m}Tc (140 keV) and thallium-201 (^{201}Tl) (80 keV x-rays), the two radionuclides most commonly used for cardiac SPECT. Therefore, it can be used for nonuniform attenuation correction of studies using either isotope.

In recent years, hybrid SPECT/computed tomography (CT) devices have been developed that can be used to acquired the transmission scan. A CT scan is acquired in addition to the SPECT emission study on the same device. Computed tomography inherently provides images of the attenuating properties of the tissues within the slice. The resultant CT image can be used to determine the μ values of the materials within the slice. However, CT is acquired with a continuous spectrum of x-ray energies (mean energy of 50 to 80 keV) yielding slightly different linear attenuation coefficients than those associated with SPECT radiopharmaceuticals. A transformation can be applied to the CT data to correct for this energy difference. The CT scan also needs to be smoothed to a spatial resolution comparable to SPECT to eliminate potential edge artifacts introduced by the process. The CT portion of the hybrid scan can also be used for the anatomic correlation of the function SPECT data.

Software Considerations

The manufacturer of the SPECT system should provide a comprehensive software package for acquisition, reconstruction, quality control, and the display of tomographic images. This should be an integrated package such that the calibration parameters (e.g., uniformity correction, center-of-rotation, and pixel size) need not be entered numerous times. For example, the computer software should also be aware of which collimator is on the camera and automatically make use of this information during acquisition setup and calibration parameter selection.

Acquisition Software

The acquisition software should assure that the acquired, raw data are adequately sampled. One rule of thumb is that the data should be sampled at least twice per the expected spatial resolution in the final tomographic image. For example, if the SPECT spatial resolution is assumed to be 8 mm, the pixel size should be less than 4 mm. This can be achieved by magnifying the acquired data or using a larger acquisition matrix. In other words, a 128×128 matrix with a 500-mm field of view would yield a pixel size of 3.9 mm (500 mm/128 = 3.9 mm). However, a 64×64 matrix with an image magnification (zoom factor) of 2 would also result in the same pixel size (500 mm/2/64 = 3.9 mm).

Body-contour or elliptical orbits should be available on all new cameras as well as circular data acquisition capability. Body-contour orbits are best for imaging in the thorax or abdomen. However, brain imaging is most commonly acquired with circular orbits. In addition, focused collimators, such as the fan beam, often require that the data acquisition be performed using a circular orbit. Many new SPECT systems utilize sensors that automatically contour the orbit to the patient. However, patients, particularly pediatric patients, may move during the acquisition; thus there should be a mechanism to stop the camera if it comes too close to the patient. This is often achieved through the use of touch-sensitive pads on the camera surface.

One needs to be able to acquire the SPECT data as a static, dynamic, or gated study. The SPECT system should be capable of acquiring a series of very rapid SPECT acquisitions, one right after another. This allows one to use the SPECT study to follow the uptake and washout of the radiopharmaceutical in order to evaluate the pharmacokinetics associated with the use of the imaging agent. In addition to dynamic SPECT, gated SPECT studies should also be possible for cardiac SPECT. Modern computer hardware has made it possible to acquire and process the large volumes of data generated during a gated tomographic acquisition.

Reconstruction and Processing Software

Current SPECT systems should be equipped with software for image reconstruction, attenuation correction, and image reorientation. Software that allows one to interactively evaluate the reconstruction filter for various pediatric SPECT procedures is also of great utility. With this application, the operator selects a representative slice to be reconstructed with a variety of filters and cutoff frequencies. Using this tool, the operator can determine the optimum filter and cutoff frequency for the various SPECT procedures for patients of different sizes. For example, a filter that works well for a bone SPECT of a 16-year-old may not be appropriate for a ^{67}Ga SPECT of a 5-year-old. One should also have the option to apply a 2D filter to the projection images prior to reconstruction or to apply an interslice filter during reconstruction. Filtering in the axial direction as well as within the transverse slice improves the quality of the sagittal and coronal images. Modern systems may also have an option for iterative reconstruction. Software for attenuation correction is also essential. The operator should be allowed to vary the attenuation coefficient and define or review the boundaries used for attenuation correction. The algorithm may use a single ellipse as the boundary for correcting all reconstructed images or let one define a different boundary for each slice. This is helpful if the object being corrected varies greatly in size over the range of transverse slices. Using attenuation boundaries that are too large will result in overestimation of the amount of attenuation and overcorrection of the data. Software for applying nonuniform attenuation correction as described previously should also be provided.

There may also be software for registering the functional image data provided by SPECT with the anatomic image data from magnetic resonance imaging (MRI) or CT. One application where image registration has been shown to be clinically useful is in the evaluation of ictal and interictal SPECT images for patients with epilepsy. An ictal, brain SPECT study can be obtained by injecting the radiopharmaceutical during an epileptic seizure, and this could be followed, at a later time, by an interictal SPECT study when the patient is not seizing. These studies can be registered to each other to allow for the determination of the differences between the two scans. Such an analysis can help to better identify the location of the epileptic seizure focus. Image registration is discussed in more detail in Chapter 18.

Software for reorienting the 3D SPECT data should also be available. Such software allows the operator to image the patient in a position that is comfortable for the patient and then reorient the reconstructed images to a standard format for display. This can be of particular utility in pediatric SPECT. In difficult cases or in cases using anesthesia, it may not be possible to maintain the patient in the most proper position during scanning. However, one can then take the data from this challenging study and reorient the data into a proper configuration. It also allows for the display of tomographic slices that are perpendicular to the axes of the organ of interest, rather than to the axis of rotation. This has proven particularly useful in cardiac SPECT.

Cardiac Processing Software

Several different applications have been developed for the processing and display of cardiac SPECT data, and, in particular, gated cardiac SPECT data.[14] These cardiac software applications can further process the data, placing the data in a standard orientation for both review and quantification. Cardiac SPECT data are often acquired during both rest and stress. The rest and stress data can be viewed side by side, making it easier to discern any differences between the two studies. In addition, these data can be displayed in a bull's-eye allowing the review of all of the slices through the myocardium in a single image. Similar bull's-eye displays can also be used to illustrate differences in wall motion or wall thickening during the cardiac cycle. These data could be compared to a database of normal patients to determine which regions of the myocardium are perfused differently than normal. However, the databases typically provided are based on adult data and may not be validated for use with children.

Calibration and Quality Control Software

Calibration of the tomographic system is an important part of the quality control software package. The basic package should include cal-ibrations for field uniformity and center of rotation. Multidetector systems must also be calibrated so that an object at a particular x,y location on one detector is imaged in the same physical location on each of the other detectors.

Another important component of a quality control program that is frequently overlooked is the ability to evaluate the raw, projection data for each study using a sinogram display. The sinogram is generated by taking the same single row out of each projection image and stacking it into a new image (Fig. 17.10). It is called a sinogram because this process performed on the projection data of a point source results in a sine wave. Sinogram displays of the patient data yield useful information about the data acquisition process. Many types of errors may be detected using this type of display, including patient motion and gantry malfunction.

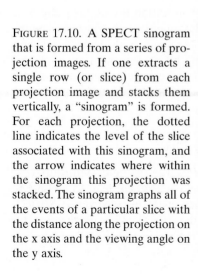
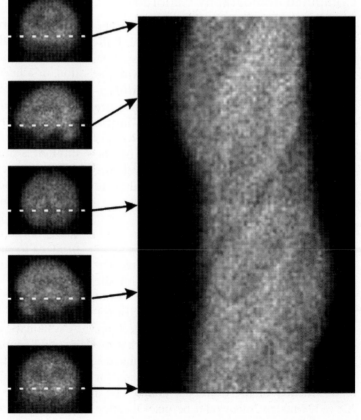

FIGURE 17.10. A SPECT sinogram that is formed from a series of projection images. If one extracts a single row (or slice) from each projection image and stacks them vertically, a "sinogram" is formed. For each projection, the dotted line indicates the level of the slice associated with this sinogram, and the arrow indicates where within the sinogram this projection was stacked. The sinogram graphs all of the events of a particular slice with the distance along the projection on the x axis and the viewing angle on the y axis.

Calibration and Quality Control

Proper calibration and quality control is possibly the most crucial aspect of performing high-quality SPECT imaging.[15] Problems that might not lead to noticeable artifacts in planar nuclear imaging can render a SPECT study unreadable or, worse, lead to a wrong interpretation. This may be of particular import in pediatric SPECT where small losses in resolution can render a pertinent feature undetectable. Calibration and quality control of SPECT is not a difficult process, but it does require attention to detail. This section reviews the principles behind each of the tests and calibrations necessary for high-quality SPECT. The calibrations, acceptance test procedures, and routine quality control procedures are reviewed. In addition, the necessity of evaluating each individual patient study for motion and potential artifacts will be discussed.

Routine Single Photon Emission Computed Tomography Calibrations

In this discussion, a distinction is made between routine calibrations and quality control. Calibrations describe those procedures necessary to provide the reconstruction algorithms with the appropriate information to generate artifact-free SPECT images. These procedures measure or characterize certain aspects of the instrumentation or data acquisition process. Routine calibrations include characterization of the center of rotation, field uniformity, pixel size, and the matching of the heads of a multihead SPECT device.

Center of Rotation

The center of rotation is the point that the computer assigns to the axis of rotation of the camera. Alternatively, it is the point about which the raw projection data of a SPECT study will rotate when viewed as a cine loop. The reconstruction algorithms assume that the axis of rotation of the camera gantry coincides with the center of the image matrix used for reconstruction of the transaxial image. For a 128×128 matrix, this would be pixel location

(63.5, 63.5). The reconstructed image will appear blurred if there is a misalignment between the center of rotation and the center of the reconstructed image matrix. If a point source or a line source is imaged with a small misalignment, the result will be a blurred point. If the misalignment is large, then the point source is reconstructed into a "ring" or "tuning fork" for 360-degree or 180-degree SPECT, respectively. Figure 17.11 shows the effect that center of rotation misalignment has on the reconstruction of point sources and on a ^{99m}Tc–methylene diphosphonate (^{99m}Tc-MDP) bone SPECT. This artifact should not be confused with the concentric ring artifacts associated with nonuniformities. The center-of-rotation rings are centered on the point source or object being imaged, whereas the nonuniformity artifacts are centered at the center of the computer matrix.

For these reasons, the location of the center of rotation in the computer matrix is characterized and the information is incorporated into the reconstruction process. Most rotating gamma camera SPECT systems have a special acquisition program available that will acquire information from either a point source, a collection of point sources in a specific configuration, or a line source for the center of rotation calibration. These data are then incorporated into the reconstruction process. The location of the center of rotation is usually quite stable, not changing over several weeks, and thus this calibration is often performed with the same frequency as the calibration floods. One day or a portion of a day may be set aside for camera calibration on a regular basis. However, if any service work has been performed on either the camera head or the computer, then it would be prudent to update the center of rotation and flood calibrations.

Field Uniformity

A systematic defect in the field uniformity of a rotating gamma camera will lead to a concentric ring artifact in the reconstructed SPECT image.[16–18] These artifacts will be centered at the center of the reconstructed image matrix, for example, located at (63.5, 63.5) for a 128×128

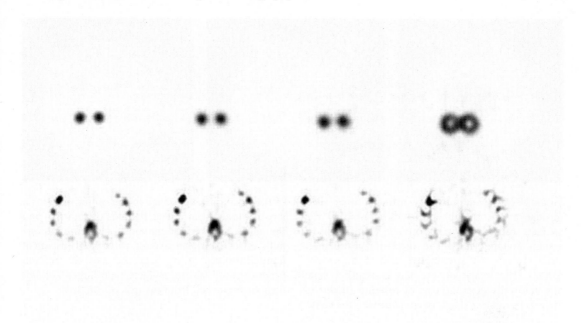

FIGURE 17.11. Artifact from inadequate center of rotation (COR) calibration: the effect an inappropriately specified COR has on SPECT image quality. The top row is a series of point sources and the bottom row is a ^{99m}Tc-MDP bone scan. The first image in each row, far left, represents the data reconstructed with the correct COR. The three images to the right of the first image have the COR specified incorrectly by 1.6, 3.2, and 6.4 mm, respectively. The point sources tend to take on a "donut" appearance with greater COR shifts, and the clinical images become progressively more blurred.

matrix. This is provided the reconstructed image has not been shifted in the matrix to center the organ of interest. The magnitude of the artifact depends on the size and magnitude of the uniformity defect, its distance from the y axis of the two-dimensional camera field of view where the y axis is parallel to the axis of rotation, and the size of the object being imaged (Fig. 17.12). To avoid such artifacts, the field uniformity of the camera is characterized and this information incorporated into either the data acquisition or, less commonly, the reconstruction process. The uniformity correction is obtained by acquiring a very high count flood image, generating a uniformity correction map from this image, and utilizing this map to correct each projection image prior to reconstruction. Correction images should be acquired for each collimator and possibly for

each radioisotope to be used for SPECT. Several manufactures combine a correction map of the collimator with an intrinsic uniformity correction. Because the collimator nonuniformities are stable unless the collimator is damaged, this correction is acquired only once or twice a year. The intrinsic uniformity correction is more likely to vary over time and therefore should be acquired more frequently. Thus, the primary considerations for the acquisition of these uniformity calibration floods are summarized by two questions: how many counts are necessary in these high-count floods and how often should they be acquired?

The number of counts necessary in the calibration flood in order to generate artifact-free SPECT images depends on the noise level in the resultant tomographic images. The reconstruction process treats statistical variations in

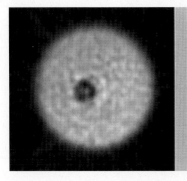 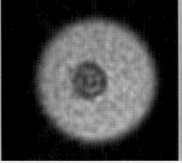 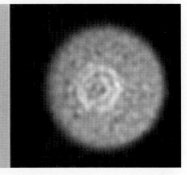

FIGURE 17.12. Nonuniformity artifact: three slices through a uniform phantom with substantial ring artifacts caused by inappropriate calibration for system nonuniformity. The three images demonstrate the effect of size and position of the nonuniformity. The image on the left contains a small nonuniformity near the axis of rotation (note that the axis of rotation does not coincide with the center of the phantom), the image in the center contains a larger nonuniformity near the axis of rotation, and the image on the right contains a larger nonuniformity offset from the axis of rotation. Thus, small nonuniformities at or near the axis of rotation produce more severe artifacts than larger nonuniformities removed from the axis of rotation.

the uniformity calibration exactly like camera nonuniformities. Rogers et al.[18] have shown that it is necessary to acquire images with statistical variations of the pixel values of less than 1% in order to generate artifact-free SPECT images. This requires an average of 10,000 counts per pixel or approximately 30-million- and 120-million-count uniformity correction images in 64×64 and 128×128 matrices, respectively. Most nuclear medicine clinics that acquire a large variety of SPECT studies acquire at least 120-million-count uniformity correction images.

How frequently these floods must be acquired depends on the stability of the system over time and is evaluated during acceptance testing. The underlying assumption is that the nonuniformities present during the SPECT acquisition are the same as those present during the acquisition of the calibration flood. A properly working camera should remain stable for several weeks, and thus the floods should be acquired with that frequency; however, the exact frequency depends on the particular camera. Each manufacturer has a recommended frequency that can be used as a guide. However, the operation of a particular camera may vary, and therefore that camera may need more frequent calibration.

Pixel Size

The image matrix is a map of the area viewed by the gamma camera. Each picture element, or pixel, of the image matrix corresponds to a portion of the camera and as such has a physical size. Most analytic attenuation corrections such as Chang's first-order method require specification of the pixel size.[12] In addition, knowledge of the pixel size can be used to size organs or lesions in the transverse images. On many multihead cameras, the pixel size is set by the manufacturer during the head matching process. However, if it is not set by the manufacturer, it must be measured. Pixel size is typically determined by acquiring an image of two line sources that are a known distance apart. A count histogram is calculated on the image and the number of pixels from peak to peak are determined. The known distance between the two lines (in millimeters) is then divided by the number of pixels between the two peak values to yield the pixel size calibration in mm/pixel.

Head Matching

For a multihead SPECT camera, head matching relates to the registration of the images for the various heads of the device. This requires that an object imaged by one head appear in the same location for the other heads when they are at the same position. This calibration may be performed by the user, but for some cameras it can only be performed by the manufacturer's service representative. This usually entails imaging a standard object (e.g., a special hole mask or a series of point sources in a specific configuration) such that the device can ensure that the objects imaged are in the same location with all heads. If the heads are properly matched, the center of rotation and the pixel size will be the same for all heads, thereby minimizing, but in most cases not alleviating, the necessity for separate calibrations for each head.

Acceptance Testing and Routine Quality Control

Acceptance Testing

When a new SPECT camera is delivered, it is imperative to assess whether the device can perform the tasks necessary for high-quality SPECT. The camera most likely underwent an extensive evaluation at the factory, but it is prudent on the purchaser's part to ensure that the camera performs appropriately after it has been delivered and meets any standards and applications that may be unique to a particular installation. In addition, acceptance testing gives the user a baseline of performance to which future evaluations can be compared. It is highly recommended that a nuclear medicine physicist with experience in SPECT acceptance testing perform these tests. Although many of the tests are straightforward in nature, the interpretation of the results of these tests requires an in-depth knowledge of how the camera performs, how the test was acquired, and how the test may acceptably vary from those performed at the factory. The intention of this section is to give the reader a better understanding of the various tests and what aspects of the SPECT camera are evaluated during acceptance testing.

Acceptance testing for SPECT typically involves inspection of the device, tests of planar

TABLE 17.1. Single photon emission computed tomography (SPECT) camera acceptance tests

Gantry performance
  Controls (performed manually and by computer)
  Angle indicator displays
  Acquisition step-size accuracy
  Timing accuracy (between steps or continuous scan time)
  Motion control including rotation, axial, and table (independence, range, and accuracy)
  Collimators and collimator handling systems
  Emergency procedures and recovery
Planar performance
  Spatial resolution (intrinsic and extrinsic)
  Uniformity (intrinsic and extrinsic)
  Sensitivity (intrinsic and extrinsic)
  Count rate capability and dead time
  Energy resolution
  Multi-window registration
Tomographic performance
  Tomographic uniformity and stability
  Tomographic spatial resolution
  Tomographic lesion contrast

performance, tests of SPECT performance, and finally an evaluation of the software. There are a number of reports that describe the evaluations that can be performed during acceptance testing.[19-23] Based on these reports, a practical protocol for acceptance testing has been developed. The tests associated with this protocol are listed in Table 17.1.

The inspection phase includes evaluation of the mechanical integrity of the rotating SPECT camera among other things. Because the camera is moving during the acquisition, it is important to fully evaluate the safety features of the system, including emergency stops and pressure-sensitive collimator covers. This is of particular importance with pediatric imaging, as the patient is more likely to move during the procedure. Also listed in Table 17.1 are the parameters evaluated as part of the planar evaluations of the camera. The extrinsic measurements (spatial resolution, uniformity, and sensitivity) are performed for each available parallel-hole collimator. These tests would be performed for all gamma cameras, regardless of whether they are SPECT cameras. A SPECT camera must perform well as a planar camera

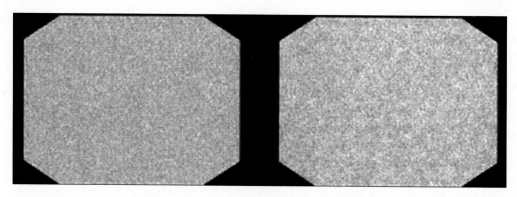

Figure 17.13. Uniformity stability evaluation. These images demonstrate the change in uniformity that can occur with a change in energy. The image on the left is a ^{99m}Tc flood corrected with a ^{99m}Tc uniformity correction matrix. The image on the right is a ^{201}Tl flood corrected with the same ^{99m}Tc uniformity cor- rection matrix. Because the uniformity is different with the ^{201}Tl flood, the correction using a ^{99m}Tc uniformity correction matrix is inadequate. In this cir- cumstance, a separate ^{201}Tl uniformity correction would have to be used to uniformity correct ^{201}Tl data sets.

in order for it to perform well for high-quality SPECT. The planar evaluations for a multi- headed SPECT camera are the same as for a single head unit except that they need to be performed for each head. In addition, it is nec- essary to evaluate the results from the multi- headed camera with respect to consistency of performance between heads. A rule of thumb is that the maximum deviation of the value for each head divided by the mean value should be less than 10%.

Table 17.1 also lists the tomographic mea- surements performed on a new SPECT camera as part of its acceptance testing. Initially, we perform all of the SPECT calibrations required for the camera including uniformity, center of rotation, pixel size, and head matching as described previously. It is prudent to evaluate the stability of field uniformity with respect to rotation, time, and photopeak energy. To evalu- ate the rotational stability, a cobalt-57 (^{57}Co) sheet source is secured to the face of the camera, and a flood image is acquired with the gantry at the 0-degree position. Similar images are acquired for equal time with the gantry at the 90-, 180-, and 270-degree positions. A second image may then again be acquired at the 0-degree position. For temporal stability, high- count flood images are acquired at various times over the span of 1 to 2 weeks. Flood images may also be acquired for various iso-

topes [e.g., ^{201}Tl, ^{99m}Tc, indium-111 (^{111}In), ^{67}Ga] to test the camera's stability with respect to dif- ferent energies. Due to the impracticality of filling liquid flood phantoms with long-lived radionuclides, it is convenient to evaluate only the intrinsic uniformity with different isotopes. In all of these tests, the images are evaluated for systematic differences. In Figure 17.13, the flood image on the left was acquired using a ^{99m}Tc correction matrix for uniformity correc- tion. The image on the right is a ^{201}Tl flood image acquired using the same ^{99m}Tc correction matrix. Because there are changes in the uni- formity with ^{201}Tl, the resultant flood image is not uniform. In this instance, a uniformity cor- rection matrix specifically for ^{201}Tl should be acquired. A simple way to enhance the appear- ance of these differences is to subtract a refer- ence image (e.g., the first image in the series) from the other images in the series.

The tomographic resolution test outlined below evaluates the spatial resolution of a SPECT acquisition compared to that of a planar acquisition. This method is presented due to its simplicity and utility in the clinical setting. A SPECT acquisition is acquired of a line source oriented with its long axis parallel and close to the axis of rotation and a radius of rotation at a set value (15 to 20 cm). The SPECT data are reconstructed with a ramp filter. A planar image is acquired of the line source with a source-to-collimator distance equal to the radius-of-rotation value from the SPECT acquisition. The full width at half maximum (FWHM) values of both line source images are determined and compared. The SPECT resolution should not exceed the planar value by more than 10%. For example, if the planar resolution is 12 mm, the SPECT resolution should be 13.2 mm or less. This is an excellent test to evaluate the adequacy of the center-of-rotation calibration. The National Electrical Manufacturers Association (NEMA) also specifies a method for evaluating SPECT resolution.[23]

Tomographic uniformity and lesion contrast are determined by imaging a cylindrical tomographic phantom with cold spheres. The tomographic spatial resolution can be subjectively evaluated by imaging the phantom with cold rods of different sizes in place. After the phantom study is reconstructed, the uniform portions of the phantom are visually inspected for concentric ring artifacts (Fig. 17.14) indicating inadequate uniformity correction. The cold spheres are also visually evaluated as to their detectability. In addition, the contrast of the lesions can be determined by the formula

$$\text{Contrast} = (B - C_s)/B$$

where C_s is the minimum pixel count over the sphere and B is the average pixel count in a region on a uniform slice.

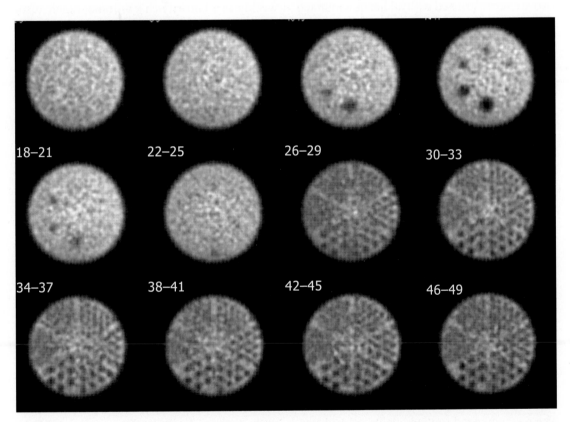

FIGURE 17.14. A SPECT quality control (QC) phantom: a series of reconstructed slices through a cylindrical SPECT QC phantom. The uniform portions of the phantom can be used to look for concentric ring artifacts and thereby evaluate the adequacy of SPECT uniformity correction. The sectors with varying sized rods can be used to evaluate the reconstructed spatial resolution. The cold spheres can be used to evaluate lesion detection and contrast. Thus, by imaging a single phantom, one can evaluate multiple factors associated with SPECT data acquisition and reconstruction.

The multihead cameras require several additional comparisons to be made with respect to the tomographic resolution, contrast, and uniformity measurements. In general, the images should be the same if acquired by a single head of the device rotating over 360 degrees, all heads combined over 360 degrees, or all heads combined with each head rotating through the angle $360/N$ where N is the number of camera heads (e.g., a dual-headed camera rotated over 180 degrees). To maintain comparable count levels, three separate studies are acquired for the line source and the cylindrical phantom: one with a total 360-degree rotation used to reconstruct each head separately, one with a $360/N$ degree rotation for the same time per angle, and one with a 360-degree rotation acquired for $1/N$, the time per angle. The last two are reconstructed with all heads combined. Tomographic spatial resolution, uniformity, and lesion contrast are compared for all of these reconstructions. The comparison of the tomographic resolution for all heads combined to that for a single head is an excellent test of the adequacy of the head matching.

The tomographic software also needs to be evaluated during acceptance testing. This includes the evaluation of standard SPECT software such as that for acquisition, reconstruction, and presentation of the data, as well as the more specialized software such as three-dimensional rendering or the bull's-eye display for myocardial SPECT. Calibration and correction software such as that for uniformity and center-of-rotation calibration and attenuation correction should also be tested. The user should have ensured that this software was available prior to deciding to purchase the camera, so these evaluations are basically to demonstrate that the software performs appropriately on site.

Routine Quality Control

The recommended routine quality control tests are listed in Table 17.2 along with the frequency with which the tests are performed. The floods listed in Table 17.2 are 5 to 10 million count (Met) floods and not the high-count (120 Mct) calibration floods used for SPECT calibration.

TABLE 17.2. Routine quality control of a SPECT camera

Uniformity flood images (daily)*
Bar phantom images (weekly)
Tomographic spatial resolution (quarterly)**
Tomographic uniformity (quarterly)

*These flood images are acquired for 5 to 10 Mct and are only used for quality control. These are not the 120 Mct flood images used for SPECT calibration.
**If center of rotation calibration can only be performed as part of the head-matching calibration, which is typically performed only several times a year, then tomographic resolution should be performed as often as the field uniformity calibration.

These are analogous to the floods performed daily on all gamma cameras. In addition, bar phantom images should be performed at least weekly as a linearity check. Tomographic resolution and uniformity tests as described in the acceptance testing part of this chapter are performed quarterly. If the center-of-rotation calibration is part of the head matching calibration, which may be performed several times a year, then it is suggested that the tomographic resolution test be performed as often as the calibration floods to evaluate the adequacy of the center-of-rotation calibration. Alternatively, one could image a tomographic phantom, with cold rods of several different sizes, to evaluate changes in resolution that could be due to changes in the center of rotation.

Routine Patient Quality Control

It is extremely important to evaluate each patient study for the possible presence of artifacts. Such tools as the sinogram of a selected slice, a summed image of all of the projection data, and a continuous cine loop of the raw projection images can be extremely useful in detecting such problems as patient motion, gantry problems, camera failure, or contamination, as well as such physiologic phenomena as cardiac creep. A display from such a SPECT patient quality control program is shown in Figure 17.15. A particular camera might not have these tools combined in one application, but the individual components are usually available and should be used to evaluate

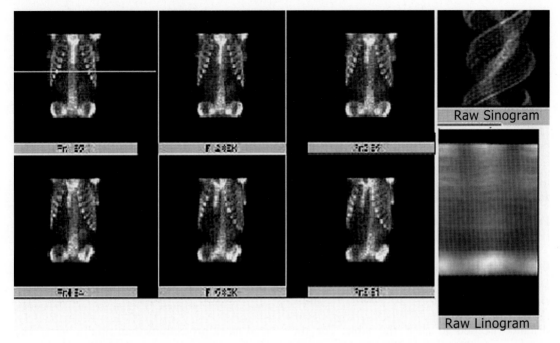

FIGURE 17.15. Display for assessing patient quality control. This figure shows a display from a program used to evaluate the quality of an individual patient SPECT study. The six images on the left represent a portion the projection data. The image in the upper left may be viewed as a continuous cine loop. The image on the upper right is a sinogram generated for the slice at the level of the horizontal line in the cine image. The image on the lower right is a linogram, which is a composite of each projection compressed into a single column of pixels; the columns of data are then stored sequentially into a single image.

SPECT acquisition. In particular, the sinogram display can be used to reveal problems with the data acquisition that may not be readily apparent in the reconstructed images but would compromise the validity of the data. It is also important to review the final reconstructed images for possible artifacts or other technical problems.

Practical Aspects of Rotating SPECT Acquisition

There are many aspects of acquiring a SPECT study that must be considered in order to perform high-quality SPECT. Each parameter affects the final reconstructed image in some manner. Understanding the impact of each will help with determining the optimal method of acquiring a particular SPECT study. This may be particularly true in pediatric SPECT where

acquisition with the highest levels of spatial resolution and sensitivity are essential. Performing the study in the most optimal fashion may be the only way the study can render a clinically useful result.

Radius of Rotation

As stated previously, resolution is dependent on the distance of the object being imaged from the collimator. Thus, keeping the collimator close to the patient is as important a factor in obtaining high-resolution images as the choice of collimator. Figure 17.16 demonstrates that the change in resolution obtained when the radius of rotation is changed from 15 cm to 25 cm is significant. This is particularly important when imaging small children. Young children are significantly smaller than the width of the standard table used for SPECT imaging. Significant resolution can be lost by the large

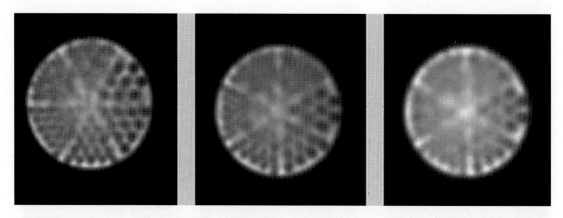

FIGURE 17.16. Effect of radius of rotation. The image on the left was acquired with a radius of rotation of 15 cm, the center image with a radius of 20 cm, and the image on the right with a radius of 25 cm. The difference in image quality is clearly visible. The fourth sector rods are visible (7.9-mm rods) at 15 cm, whereas the rods of the third sector (11.1-mm rods) are barely visible on the periphery at 25 cm.

distance needed to clear the table. For this reason, a special pediatric SPECT pallet should be used when performing SPECT studies on very small children. Extra care should be taken to position the camera as close to the pediatric patient as possible. Because the organs being imaged are smaller, it is very important to use imaging techniques that result in the best overall image resolution. In addition, positioning the pediatric patient with the head out of the gantry and using some form of entertainment to distract the patient from the moving camera can be extremely helpful.

Number of Images to Acquire

The question of how many projection images need to be acquired in SPECT is frequently asked. In simple backprojection, the low-frequency data are seen in the backprojected image as streaks emanating from the center of the images. Filtered backprojection reduces the magnitude of these streaks by filtering these low-frequency components. The radius over which the streak artifacts are eliminated by filtered backprojection is proportional to the number of raw projection images that are acquired and the spatial resolution of the system. This radius should encompass the whole object of interest. Thus large objects need more projections than small objects. The number of projection images that should be acquired over 360 degrees, N_i can be determined by

$$N_i = 2 \cdot \pi \cdot r \cdot \frac{2}{FWHM}$$

where $2\pi r$ is the circumference of the object being imaged, FWHM is the tomographic FWHM at the radius of rotation used for data acquisition, and the factor 2 is for adequate sampling (twice per resolution element). For example, a pediatric patient is having a SPECT dimercaptosuccinic acid (DMSA) renal scan performed. The circumference of the body is 40 cm, and the tomographic FWHM at a radius of rotation of 14.0 cm is 0.9 cm. The number of images to acquire N_i would be

$$N_i = 40 \, cm \cdot \frac{2}{0.9 \, cm} = 88$$

The smaller circumference of a child results in the use of a smaller radius of rotation. A smaller radius of rotation results in better image resolution. Thus, even though the patient is smaller, more images are required because the FWHM decreases along with the circumference. Based on this equation, most acquisitions with current equipment should have at least 90 to 120 images per 360 degrees. If a SPECT camera has

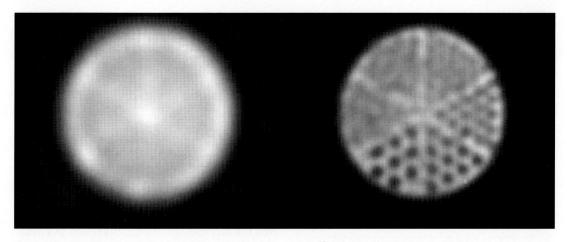

FIGURE 17.17. Effect of matrix size. The image on the right was reconstructed with a 128 × 128 image matrix, whereas the image on the left was reconstructed with a 64 × 64 matrix. The inadequate linear sampling using a matrix with pixels that are too large leads to the loss in spatial resolution. With 128 × 128, the fourth sector rods are visible (7.9-mm rods), whereas none of the sectors are visible with 64 × 64.

either much better or worse resolution, then this number may vary.

Matrix Size

The matrix size used to acquire the projection data plays a large part in the quality of the reconstructed image. The Nyquist theorem states that the highest spatial frequency in the image must be sampled at least twice to be accurately reproduced. In SPECT imaging, this means we need to sample the tomographic FWHM twice. Thus if the tomographic FWHM is 8mm, the pixel size in the projection data should be less than 4mm. Using a pixel size larger than this will result in significant blurring of the reconstructed image (Fig. 17.17). If the pixel size in the 128 × 128 image matrix is 3.56mm, then the projection data could be acquired with this image matrix or its equivalent. An equivalent matrix would be a 64 × 64 matrix with a factor of 2 magnification (zoom). This would also result in a pixel size less than 4 mm. This is particularly useful when imaging pediatric patients. The factor of 2 magnification allows the organ of interest to fill more of the projection image matrix while still providing adequate spatial sampling. The larger image is often easier to interpret.

Step-and-Shoot Versus Continuous Acquisition

First-generation SPECT cameras were single-head devices that rotated a full 360 degrees around the patient to acquire the projection data. The camera would stop and take a picture at each desired projection angle, a technique known a "step and shoot." The step-and-shoot mode is still widely used in current SPECT system.

The time required to step from one image angle to the next in step-and-shoot mode could be as long as 4.5 seconds for these first-generation cameras. No data were acquired during the step time. One method of making use of this dead time was to perform continuous rotation acquisition. In this acquisition mode, the camera would rotate slowly but continuously around the patient. Images were continuously acquired, and each image was the sum of the data acquired over a specified angular interval. If 120 images were to be acquired over 360 degrees, each image would be the sum of the data over 3 degrees. There was no acquisition time lost during the acquisition, but there was a decrease in image resolution because the camera was moving during acquisition, causing motion blur.

TABLE 17.3. Full width at half maximum (FWHM) (mm) at a 14.5-cm radius of rotation

Δ in degrees	Line source position in phantom		
	Center	8.5-cm radial	8.5-cm tangential
Continuous rotation			
6	8.9	8.7	9.0
3	9.0	8.6	6.4
2	8.8	8.3	6.3
1	9.0	8.3	6.0
Step-and-shoot			
6	8.9	7.8	5.6
3	8.9	8.0	5.5
2	9.0	8.0	5.7

We investigated the changes in resolution as a result of continuous rotation acquisition.[24] The tomographic line spread function was measured at the axis of rotation (AOR) and 8.6 cm from the AOR. Step-and-shoot images were acquired with 6-, 3-, and 2-degree steps. Continuous rotation data were acquired and the data stored in 6-, 3-, 2-, and 1-degree integrals. The tomographic line spread functions for the reconstructed images were compared. Continuous rotation had very little effect on the reconstructed resolution at the AOR, but there was a significant difference at 8.6 cm, particularly in the tangential resolution (Table 17.3). Even storing the data in 1-degree integrals with continuous rotation resulted in a loss of resolution in the tangential direction as compared to the step-and-shoot acquisition. The maximum amount of image blurring can be estimated by

$$B_{max} = 2r \left| \cos\left((2 \cdot \theta + \Delta)/2 \right) \cdot \left(\sin \Delta/2 \right) \right|$$

where Δ is the image bin size for continuous rotation and r is the distance of the object being imaged from the AOR. It is apparent from this equation that the amount of blurring is proportional to the distance from the AOR.[25] For higher resolution cameras and cameras with a short stepping time (less than 1 second) like modern SPECT cameras, step-and-shoot is recommended because it provides the highest resolution with little loss in sensitivity. However, for single-head cameras with substantial stepping times and poorer resolution, continuous

acquisition may be a viable alternative, particularly in the pediatric population where the organ of interest is located close to the axis of rotation.

Conclusion

Single photon emission computed tomography with a rotating gamma camera is an essential part of every pediatric nuclear medicine division. Acquiring high-quality SPECT is not difficult but does take attention to detail. Pediatric SPECT requires additional diligence to ensure the highest quality SPECT images possible. Many rotating SPECT cameras may be used for planar as well as SPECT imaging, while cameras with more than two heads are truly dedicated SPECT devices. Regardless of which type of camera is used, the performance must be evaluated for both planar and SPECT imaging. In addition, a straightforward and effective program of quality control and calibration should be established. A camera that is functioning properly, the optimal choice of collimator and acquisition parameters, and careful attention to detail will lead to SPECT images of the highest quality.

References

1. Kuhl DE, Edwards RQ. Image separation radioisotope scanning. Radiology 1963;80:653–61.
2. Hounsfield GN. Computerized transverse axial scanning (tomography). Br J Radiol 1973;46:1016.
3. Keyes JW Jr, Orlandea N, Heetderks WJ, Leonard PF, Rogers WL. The Humongotron—a scintillation-camera transaxial tomograph. J Nucl Med 1977;18:381–7.
4. Jaszczak RJ, Murphy PH, Huard D, et al. Radionuclide emission computed tomography of the head with Tc-99m and a scintillation camera. J Nucl Med 1977;18:373–80.
5. Muehllehner G. Effect of resolution improvement on required count density in ECT imaging: a computed simulation. Phys Med Biol 1985;30:163–73.
6. Fahey FH, Harkness BA, Keyes JW Jr, et al. Sensitivity, resolution and image quality with a

multi-head SPECT camera. J Nucl Med 1992;33: 1859–63.

7. Mueller SP, Polak JF, Kijewski MF, Holman BL. Collimator selection for SPECT brain imaging: the advantage of high resolution. J Nucl Med 1986;27:1729–38.

8. Tsui BM, Gullberg GT, Edgerton ER, Gilland DR, Perry JR, McCartney WH. Design and clinical utility of a fan beam collimator for SPECT imaging of the head. J Nucl Med 1986;27: 810–19, Figure 2.

9. Jaszczak RJ, Greer KL, Coleman RE. SPECT using a specially designed cone beam collimator. J Nucl Med 1988;29:1398–405.

10. Lange K, Carson R. EM reconstruction algorithms for emission and transmission tomography. J Comput Assist Tomogr 1984;8:306–16.

11. Hudson HM, Larkin RS. Accelerated image reconstruction using ordered subsets of projection data. IEEE Trans Med Imaging 1994;13: 601–9.

12. Chang LT. A method for attenuation correction in radionuclide computed tomography. IEEE Trans Nucl Sci 1978;25:638–43.

13. Bailey DL. Transmission scanning in emission tomography. Eur J Nucl Med 1998;25:774–87.

14. Paul AK, Nabi HA. Gated myocardial perfusion SPECT: basic principles, technical aspects, and clinical applications. J Nucl Med Tech 2004;32: 179–87.

15. Graham LS. A rational quality assurance program for SPECT instrumentation. In: Nuclear Medicine Annual 1989. New York: Raven Press, 1989.

16. Greer KL, Coleman RE, Jaszczak RJ. SPECT: a practical guide for users. J Nucl Med Tech 1983;11:61–5.

17. Harkness BA, Rogers WL, Clinthorne NH, Keyes JW Jr. SPECT quality control procedures and artifact identification. J Nucl Med Tech 1983;11:55–60.

18. Rogers WL, Clinthorne NH, Harkness BA, et al. Field-flood requirements for emission computed tomography with an Anger camera. J Nucl Med 1982;23:162–8.

19. American Institute of Physics. American Association of Physicists in Medicine (AAPM) report number 6: scintillation camera acceptance testing and performance evaluation. New York: AIP, 1980.

20. American Institute of Physics. American Association of Physicists in Medicine (AAPM) report number 9: computer-aided scintillation camera acceptance testing. New York: AIP, 1981.

21. American Institute of Physics. American Association of Physicists in Medicine (AAPM) report number 22: rotating scintillation camera SPECT acceptance testing and quality control. New York: AIP, 1988.

22. Mould RF, ed. Quality Control of Nuclear Medicine Instrumentation. London: Hospital Physicists Association, 1983.

23. National Electrical Manufacturers Association. Performance Measurements of Scintillation Cameras: Standards Publication NU1. Washington, DC: NEMA, 2001.

24. Harkness BA, Fahey FH, Keyes JW Jr. Comparison of resolution changes when performing continuous versus step-and-shoot rotation for SPECT data acquisition. Radiology 1988;169(P): 392.

25. Bieszk JA, Hawman EG. Evaluation of SPECT angular sampling effects: Continuous versus step-and-shoot acquisition. J Nucl Med 1987;28: 1308–14.

18
Positron Emission Tomography

Frederic H. Fahey and Ramsey D. Badawi

In the 1960s and 1970s, positron emission tomography (PET) was developed as a research tool, particularly for the investigation of neurophysiology.[1-4] In the 1980s and 1990s, the clinical utility of PET in oncology, neurology, and cardiology was demonstrated.[5-10] The approval of reimbursement by the U.S. Centers for Medicare and Medicaid Services for oncologic PET and the subsequent establishment of regional distribution centers of fluorine-18 (^{18}F)-fluoro-2-deoxy-glucose (FDG) in the late 1990s contributed greatly to the expansion in the clinical use of PET. This expansion led to greater availability of PET for pediatric imaging as well as for adults.[11,12] Pediatric PET has demonstrated utility in neurology as well as oncology, and the application of PET in pediatrics will continue to grow as its clinical potential is further realized and as new positron-emitting radiopharmaceuticals are developed. Several technologic factors, involving both physics and radiopharmaceutical chemistry, have contributed to the popularity of PET. It is substantially easier to develop a PET rather than a single photon emission computed tomography (SPECT) analogue to many naturally occurring, biologically relevant chemicals such as water, oxygen, carbon monoxide, ammonia, glucose, and a whole host of others. Thus PET is well suited to serve a very prominent role in this new and exciting era of molecular medicine.

Unlike SPECT, absorptive collimation is not necessary in PET. As will be discussed, annihilation coincidence detection is used instead to determine the directionality of the detected photons that have been emitted by the radiopharmaceutical. This leads to perhaps a hundredfold increase in photon sensitivity for PET compared to SPECT for the same spatial resolution. This greater sensitivity improves both the image quality and the quantitative capability of PET relative to other forms of nuclear imaging.

Several factors associated with PET data acquisition need to be considered for the optimal application in pediatric imaging. On the one hand, radiation safety concerns require that children be administered smaller amounts of radioactivity. One would also prefer a short acquisition time to minimize patient motion and limit the use of sedation or anesthesia during the imaging session. For these reasons, high sensitivity is extremely important in pediatric PET. On the other hand, the smaller organs and other features of the pediatric patient being imaged put a premium on high spatial resolution. Positron emission tomography data acquisition from a smaller patient can be quite different from a larger, adult patient, and thus conclusions that have been drawn as to the optimal way to acquire PET data for the adult population may not be correct for children. For example, the fraction of photons that have been Compton scattered prior to detection differs for smaller patients, and this may thereby alter how best PET data should be acquired. This chapter reviews the basic aspects of PET in the context of pediatric imaging, and discusses the production of positron-emitting radiopharmaceuticals, the basics of positron emission, annihilation coincidence detection, PET data acquisition, PET instrumentation, image registration, and the radiation safety aspects of the application of pediatric PET.

Positron Emission Tomography Radiopharmaceutical Production

One of major advantages of PET over SPECT is that many of the radionuclides of the elements essential for biology are positron emitters, including carbon-11 (^{11}C), nitrogen-13 (^{13}N), and oxygen-15 (^{15}O). In addition, ^{18}F is very useful as it can often be substituted for hydrogen or a hydroxyl group. Rubidium-82 (^{82}Rb) has also been shown to be useful for myocardial perfusion imaging.[9] These isotopes are listed in Table 18.1 along with their half-lives, mode of production, and positron energies. However, one disadvantage to the use of these nuclides, as seen in Table 18.1, arises from the fact that they have very short half-lives: 2, 10, 20, and 109 minutes for ^{15}O, ^{13}N, ^{11}C, and ^{18}F, respectively. ^{82}Rb has a 1.3-minute half-life, but, as will be discussed, it can be provided through a generator system. Fluorine-18 with its half-life of almost 2 hours can be distributed from regional radiopharmaceutical centers, but the other three radionuclides must be produced on-site in order to have sufficient time to incorporate the radionuclide into a radiopharmaceutical and deliver it to the patient before it has completely vanished via radioactive decay.

The device most commonly used for the production of these isotopes is the cyclotron. Basi-

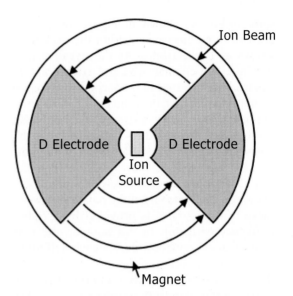

FIGURE 18.1. Cyclotron. The cyclotron provides a method of producing positron-emitting radiopharmaceuticals. Negative hydrogen ions are generated by the ion source. A uniform magnetic field constrains the ions to a spiral orbit. Alternating electric fields between the two D electrodes accelerate the ion beam. Once the beam reaches a sufficient energy, the beam passes through a thin, carbon foil that strips the two electrons from the ions, yielding an energized beam of protons that can be used to irradiate a target of nonradioactive atoms to render them radioactive. For example, a target of ^{18}O can be irradiated by 11 MeV protons to produce ^{18}F.

cally, this device provides a beam of accelerated charged particles (either protons or deuterons) that can impinge upon a target to make the nonradioactive material within the target become radioactive. The cyclotron, as shown in Figure 18.1, has five major components: an ion source, a magnet, a radiofrequency switching circuit, an ion beam extractor, and a target. The ion source provides an electrical discharge across a volume of gas that leads to the production of ions. In most medical cyclotrons, negative hydrogen ions (i.e., a proton with two orbiting electrons) are accelerated. Note that neutral hydrogen consists of a proton with a single orbiting electron. The magnet provides a uniform magnetic field that constrains the movement of the newly generated ions to a

TABLE 18.1. Positron emitting radionuclides

Radionuclide	Half-life (min)	Production mode	Energy (MeV)
^{11}C	20	^{14}N (p,α) ^{11}C	0.96
^{13}N	10	^{16}O (p,α) ^{13}N	1.19
^{15}O	2	^{15}N (p,n) ^{15}O	1.72
^{18}F	110.0	^{18}O (p,n) ^{18}F	0.64
^{82}Rb	1.3	Decay of ^{82}Sr	3.15

spiral orbit. As shown in Figure 18.1, there are two large electrodes within the cyclotron, known as D electrodes. As the negative ions undergo their circular orbit and exit the first D electrode, the voltage of the second electrode is higher than the first; thus, the ions are attracted to it and thereby undergo a small energy boost. As they pass through the second electrode, the polarity of the two electrodes switches and now the first electrode is more positive than the second, and thus the ions receive another boost of energy. The switching of the polarity between these two electrodes is provided by a radio-frequency oscillator. In this manner, the ions receive an energy boost during each half orbit. As the ions attain more energy, the radius of their circular orbit increases and the energized ion beam spirals out. Once sufficient energy has been attained (for example, 11 MeV), the beam is passed through a very thin carbon stripping foil to remove the two electrons from the negative hydrogen ions to provide a beam of 11 MeV protons. This proton beam is aimed at a target of nonradioactive material. For example, if one wishes to produce ^{18}F, a gas target of oxygen gas enriched in the nonradioactive isotope, ^{18}O, is used. With the energetic protons impinging upon them, some of the ^{18}O atoms will absorb a proton, emit a neutron, and thereby be transformed into ^{18}F atoms. This is referred to as a "p-n reaction," symbolically shown as the following:

$$^{18}O \ (p,n) \ ^{18}F$$

Likewise, (p,α) refers to a p-α reaction where a positron is absorbed and an alpha particle is emitted. By using different target materials (as specified in Table 18.1), ^{11}C, ^{13}N, and ^{15}O can likewise be produced.

Once produced, these radionuclides need to be incorporated into the radiopharmaceuticals of interest. By far the most commonly used radiopharmaceutical in clinical PET is ^{18}F-labeled FDG. In general, this radiochemistry is preformed via an automated chemical processing unit. The ^{18}F provided by the cyclotron is mixed with the appropriate reagents and precursors in order to produce a vial of FDG. The use of automated chemical units minimizes the direct contact between the radiochemists and the high levels of radioactivity coming from the cyclotron, and thus reduces the radiation dose received by these individuals. Automated production units have also been developed for other PET radiopharmaceuticals. Quality control must then be performed on the product to ensure the radionuclidic and radiochemical purity as well as the sterility and pyrogenicity of the agent prior to it being administered to the patient.

Certain radionuclides used in PET can be provided via a generator system similar to the molybdenum/technetium generator systems. For example, strontium-82 (^{82}Sr) (25-day half-life) decays to ^{82}Rb (75-second half-life). Therefore, a generator can be produced where ^{82}Sr is chemically bound to a ceramic column. Over time, a fraction of the ^{82}Sr atoms decay to ^{82}Rb. When this column is washed by elution, the ^{82}Rb is removed and can be injected into the patient. Within a few half-lives of the daughter, the activity of the daughter has again built up to a value close to that of the parent. In this manner, a short-lived radionuclide such as ^{82}Rb can be provided every 10 minutes or so. The generator can be used for a period equal to one or two half-lives of the parent. In the case of the ^{82}Sr/^{82}Rb generator, a single generator can provide ^{82}Rb for at least a month. ^{82}Rb has been shown to be a very useful radionuclide for imaging myocardial perfusion.

Positron Emission

Positron emission is analogous to beta-decay and occurs in nuclei that are over-rich in protons. One of the protons in the nucleus converts to a neutron, emitting a positron and a neutrino. Because three bodies are involved, a sample of radionuclide will emit positrons with a range of energies, up to some maximum value (see Table 18.1).

A positron is the antimatter equivalent of an electron; it is identical in every respect to an electron except that it is positively charged. Once emitted, it initially behaves in a similar way to an electron created by nuclear beta-decay; it interacts with electrons (and less fre-

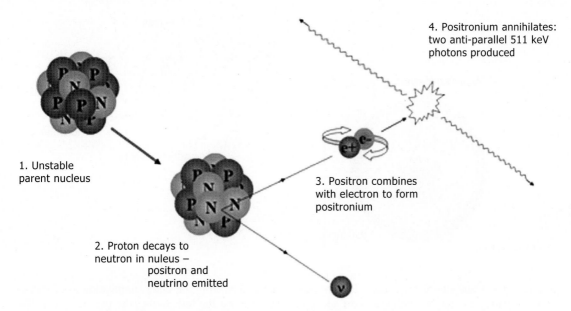

1. Unstable
parent nucleus

2. Proton decays to
neutron in nuleus –
positron and
neutrino emitted

3. Positron combines
with electron to form
positronium

4. Positronium annihilates:
two anti-parallel 511 keV
photons produced

FIGURE 18.2. Positron emission. A radioactive atom emits a positron that travels some distance before interacting with an electron to form "positronium." After a very short time, the positron and the electron annihilate by converting their mass into energy in the form of two 511-keV photons that are emitted at 180 degrees to each other.

quently nuclei) in the local medium, creating ionizations and losing energy until most of its initial momentum is spent. At low energies it can undergo a different kind of interaction with an electron; it can form an orbiting couple called a positronium. This arrangement is short-lived, and annihilation follows rapidly (Fig. 18.2).[13] The vast majority of annihilation events give rise to two photons, each of energy 511 keV. Because the positronium has little momentum (as it can only form at low energies), the two photons are emitted in almost exactly opposite directions; the directional uncertainty is only about 0.5 degrees.

The distance that the positron travels prior to annihilation is dependent on the initial emission energy and the material through which it is traveling. For ^{18}F, the most commonly used positron emitter in PET imaging, the average range in water is less than 1 mm.[14] Thus, the point of annihilation is very close to the point of emission. As a result, an image generated from the distribution of annihilation radiation closely approximates the distribution of radio-nuclide itself.

Imaging Annihilation Radiation

In principle, there is no reason why sources of annihilation radiation cannot be imaged using conventional single-photon imaging methods. However, in practice limiting factors severely constrain the clinical situations in which this can be done effectively. These factors primarily arise from the highly penetrating nature of the 511-keV annihilation photons. First, it is difficult to design a collimator that does not suffer from significant septal penetration while retaining the appropriate balance between photon sensitivity, spatial resolution, and physical weight. Second, good spatial resolution for gamma cameras is achieved by keeping the scintillation crystal relatively thin (usually about 1 to 2.5 cm), and cost is kept down by fabricating the crystal from sodium iodide, which is not very dense. Such detectors have insufficient stopping power at 511 keV, and up to 80% of incident photons pass straight through the crystal without interacting. This approach can only be used in very favorable imaging situations, such as myocardial viability studies.[15]

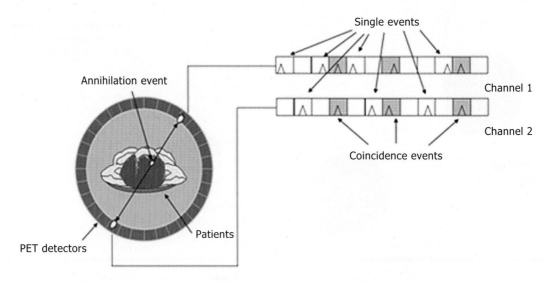

FIGURE 18.3. Coincidence detection. Events that occur in pairs of detectors within a short space of time (within several nanoseconds) are considered to have come from the same annihilation event, which must lie on the line joining the two detectors. This line is referred to as the "line of response" (LOR).

Coincidence Detection

The collimator issue may be addressed using a technique known as "coincidence detection." Two or more detectors are configured so that the positron-emitting object lies between them. As well as measuring the position of arriving annihilation photons, the detectors also measure their time of arrival. Because annihilation events give rise to two photons traveling in opposite directions, if the detectors register two photons within a short time of each other (that is, within a few nanoseconds), the photons are assumed to have arisen from the same annihi-

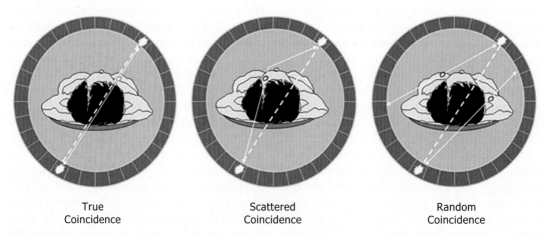

True Coincidence   Scattered Coincidence   Random Coincidence

FIGURE 18.4. Types of coincidence events. If a positron-electron annihilation occurs, and the two 511-keV photons leave the object without interaction and are both detected within the acceptable timing window (within several nanoseconds), this is referred to as a "true coincidence." However, if one of the photons was Compton scattered within the object prior to its detection, this event is referred to as a "scatter coincidence." Lastly, if photons from two unrelated events are detected within the timing window, this is referred to as an "accidental" or "random coincidence." Without correction, scatter and random coincidences degrade the quality of a PET image.

lation event, which must have occurred along a line joining the two detection points (Fig. 18.3). In this way, the direction of photon flight for a detected event may be obtained without the use of a collimator, solving the septal penetration problem and allowing approximately a two order of magnitude increase in the sensitivity of the system to photons compared to the gamma camera.

The coincidence assumption just described is not always good. Sometimes one or both photons undergo a direction-changing Compton scatter interaction in the object prior to detection, giving rise to a scatter coincidence, and sometimes photons from unrelated annihilation events are detected sufficiently close together in time to be registered as coincident, giving rise to an accidental, or random coincidence (Fig. 18.4). In each case the assigned line of response does not intersect the annihilation position(s), leading to compromised spatial localization of the emission site.

Detectors for Annihilation Radiation

Detectors for annihilation radiation should have good stopping power for 511-keV photons and the ability to resolve the time of arrival of incident photons to within at most a few nanoseconds. Additionally, because these detectors are configured without collimators, they must be capable of operating in high photon flux environments. These conditions are not well met by conventional Anger cameras, and a range of specialized detectors has been designed for PET scanners.

The most common design is the block detector,[16] which consists of a small square or rectangular array of scintillation crystals 4 or 5 cm on a side, and 2 or 3 cm deep. The individual crystals are typically 4 to 6 mm on a side. Thus a single detector block may consist of approximately 30 to 70 scintillating elements. The crystal array is frequently fashioned from a single block of crystal, with saw-cuts of different depths to form a light guide. This is then optically coupled to four photomultipliers (Fig. 18.5). An alternative arrangement is to couple individual crystal elements of equal size to a separate light guide, which is in turn coupled to the photomultipliers. A photon interacting in one of the crystals creates a characteristic pattern of light spread between the four photomultipliers, allowing the position to be decoded. The crystal material is chosen first to achieve good stopping power for the high-energy photons, and second to produce fast signals so that dead time is reduced and the detector can operate in a high photon flux.

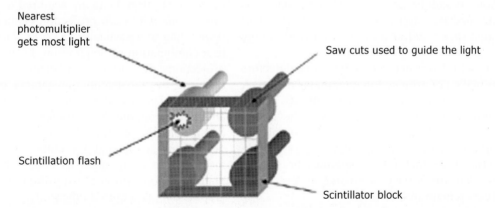

Nearest photomultiplier gets most light

Saw cuts used to guide the light

Scintillation flash

Scintillator block

FIGURE 18.5. Block detector. A high-resolution PET scanner consists of many small radiation detectors. This is accomplished by constructing block detectors where each block consists of a square or rectangular array of small, scintillating elements. The photomultipliers are triggered by the scintillation light flash. The ratio of the photomultiplier signals is used to determine the position of the scintillation event.

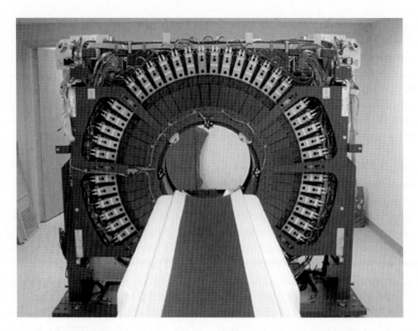

FIGURE 18.6. A state-of-the-art PET scanner with the covers removed. The detector blocks and their associated photomultiplier tube arrays are clearly seen.

Fast signals also allow a short coincidence time window, which results in the acceptance of fewer random coincidences. Typical choices are bismuth germinate (BGO), which has excellent stopping power, or lutetium oxyorthosilicate (LSO), which has good stopping power and excellent signal speed.[17] Another choice is gadolinium silicate (GSO), which has intermediate stopping power but excellent signal speed and also offers improved energy resolution.[18]

In a PET scanner, 200 or 300 block detectors normally are arranged in an annular design. A state-of-the-art PET scanner with its covers removed is shown in Figure 18.6. The use of many small detectors increases the complexity and cost of the scanner, but very significantly increases its high-flux capabilities because if one detector is busy processing an event, the others remain free for use.

Lines of Response and Projections

In a PET scanner, coincidences are detected between pairs of detector elements, and the lines joining such pairs are known as lines of response (LORs). Data are acquired as sets of projections, with each projection element corresponding to a particular LOR, or sometimes to a combination of neighboring LORs. These projections are directly analogous to those acquired by a conventional gamma camera. However, because there are no collimators, and, in general, the detectors form a complete ring around the patient, it is possible to acquire projections at all angles simultaneously. This means there is no need to choose between planar or tomographic acquisition as tomographic data is acquired inherently.

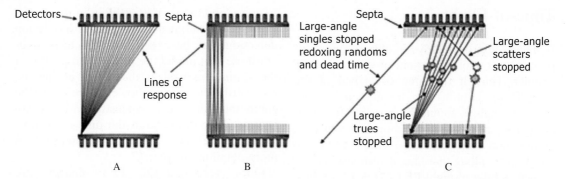

FIGURE 18.7. Two- and three-dimensional acquisition mode. Absorptive septa consisting of either lead or tungsten can be placed between the individual detector rings in order to reduce the interplane scatter and the random coincidences from activity that is outside the axial field of view. However, the use of septa also substantially reduces the sensitivity. Acquiring PET data with septa in place is referred to as 2D mode acquisition. Acquiring without septa is referred to as 3D mode acquisition. A: 3D mode, showing examples of permitted lines of response. B: 2D mode, showing examples of permitted lines of response. C: 2D mode, showing the effects of septa on sensitivity to the various types of coincidence events.

Two- and Three-Dimensional Modes

Even for dedicated PET systems, scatter, random coincidences, and system dead-time due to the high photon flux can cause significant problems. To reduce these effects, many scanners have axial shields or septa that can be positioned in the field of view. In circular systems these take the form of a series of annular rings of tungsten or lead, usually positioned to divide the detector arrays into adjacent rings, each of thickness equal to an individual detector element. These septa are different from collimators because they are not used to determine the flight path of incoming photons, but they do act to significantly reduce the number of scattered and random coincidences and the flux of unpaired or "single" photons that produces dead time. However, they also act to reduce the sensitivity to true coincidences (Fig. 18.7). Operating with septa in place is known as two-dimensional (2D) mode acquisition, whereas operating without septa in place is known as three-dimensional (3D) mode acquisition.

There is a trade-off between the 2D mode and the 3D mode that is dependent on several parameters. These include the size of the object, the amount of activity both within and outside the field of view, the reconstruction method used, and the scanner design. In general, the smaller the object is, and the lower the amount of activity that is in the patient, the fewer the scattered and random coincidences and the less the dead-time for a given amount of activity. Thus more benefit can be obtained from the greater sensitivity of 3D mode.[19,20] Additionally, scanners with detectors constructed of faster scintillator materials with lower stopping power tend to perform better in 3D mode.

For studies of young children in which the body mass and age considerations limit the injected dose, the 3D mode may be preferable.[21] However, caution should be exercised, because systematic errors are usually greater in the 3D mode.[22] These can produce image artifacts and, if the reconstruction techniques are not optimal, reduced spatial resolution. For larger patients, the 2D mode is often preferable, particularly on scanners that utilize BGO detectors.[20]

Time-of-Flight

It takes approximately 3 nanoseconds for photons to traverse the field of view of a PET scanner. Thus, if the time of arrival of the annihilation photons can be measured accurately enough, it should be possible to determine not just the line of response to which an annihilation event should be assigned but also the position along that line of response. This is known as time-of-flight PET (TOF-PET). Prototype TOF-PET scanners were built in the 1980s,[23] but poor electronics and the low stopping power of the fast scintillator material available at the time (barium fluoride, BaF_2) led to an abandonment of the idea. However, the development of fast scintillators with improved stopping power such as LSO and lanthanum bromide (LaBr) has resulted in renewed interest in the technique.[24] It is unlikely that pure TOF-PET scanners will be available in the near future, but there are several efforts currently underway to add time-of-flight information to coincidence detection scanners to improve image quality. Such benefits are likely to be greatest for larger patients.

Tomographic Reconstruction

Until the end of the 20th century, the predominant method of tomographic image reconstruction in PET was filtered backprojection, an analytic technique that produces a faithful representation of the object in the limit of an infinite number of projection angles and with noise-free data. However, when the data are noisy, filtered backprojection produces images with streak artifacts. Today, most image reconstruction techniques are iterative and weight the contribution of individual lines of response by estimates of the statistical certainty of the data associated with them. That is, LORs with more counts in them contribute more heavily toward the final image than do those with fewer. These methods produce images much richer in anatomic information but have the disadvantage that inconsistencies in the data due to noise tend to manifest as blobs in the image, which can sometimes confuse the task of lesion detection. The best reconstruction techniques are those that model the physical properties of the scanner as well as the object during the reconstruction process; however, these can be computationally very expensive and few are commercially available at the time of writing. Tomographic reconstruction is discussed in more detail in Chapter 17.

Once reconstructed, PET images are frequently processed to generate maximum-intensity projections (MIPs). These can be shown in a cine-loop to produce a rotating 3D image of the patient, which can be very useful for an initial survey and for obtaining an overall gestalt of the scan data.

Attenuation Correction

The half-value thickness for 511-keV annihilation photons in soft tissue is approximately 7 cm. That is, a beam of 511-keV photons passing through 7 cm of soft tissue will be attenuated by approximately 50%. At the center of the body, then, a significant fraction of the photons arising from annihilation events will fail to reach the detectors. Even at the surface of the body, those lines of response passing through the body will suffer significant attenuation, but on average the attenuation will be less, as many lines of response pass mostly through air. These differences in average attenuation result in distortions in the reconstructed image if not corrected. In particular, deep structures are poorly visualized, whereas surface features have elevated intensity. For large patients, these effects can be very significant, but even for small patients they are noticeable. Photon attenuation also compromises the ability to obtain quantitative information using PET.

Attenuation distortions are a well-known phenomenon in conventional nuclear medicine, where correction for attenuation effects is non-trivial. However, in PET, the nature of coincidence detection is such that the mathematics of attenuation correction is significantly simplified. The requirement that both annihilation photons be detected means that along a given line of response, the attenuation is only dependent on the total contribution from all the attenuating material along that line of response, because if one photon does not pass through a particular section of the line, the other one must. Thus each line of response can be corrected using a single multiplicative correction factor. Furthermore, this correction factor can be measured simply by determining the attenuation for a positron-emitting source outside of the body.

Until recently, most PET scanners were fitted with extendable positron-emitting rod sources that, once placed in the field of view, could rotate around the body and acquire transmission data to be used for attenuation correction (Fig. 18.8A). The disadvantage of this scheme is that data acquisition is slow, accounting for up to half of the total scanning time. Faster schemes using transmission data acquired using high-energy single-photon emitters such as cesium 137 (^{137}Cs) have been implemented (Fig. 18.8B), but the most popular method in use today is based on x-ray computed tomography (CT) data, which requires the use of a combined PET-CT system (Fig. 18.8C).[25]

Although CT images are based on the transmission of photons through the body, they cannot be used to directly correct for attenuation of 511-keV photons because the average energy of the x-ray CT photons is much lower, at around 70 to 80keV. The CT attenuation factors can be transformed to values appropriate for 511-keV photons, but in general the algorithms used to perform this task do not work well with metallic objects (such as surgical clips or dental prostheses)[26] or with oral or IV contrast agents.[27] The presence of these kinds of material in the field of view can result in focal areas of artifactually high intensity in the PET image that can mimic or mask disease. This problem can be partially overcome by reconstructing the PET data both with and without attenuation correction. The use of negative oral contrast agents such as mannitol and locust bean gum can also be helpful in delineating the gastrointestinal tract without introducing PET artifacts.[28]

Another issue with CT-based attenuation correction relates to patient motion. Voluntary movements of the head can cause misalignment between the emission and transmission data, which result in artifactual asymmetries in the PET images. Lung motion is also an issue because the CT acquisition is fast and acquires a snapshot of lung position, whereas the PET acquisition is slow and images an average of tidal breathing. This mismatch is exacerbated by the use of deep-inspiration breath-hold for the CT, which is not recommended for PET-CT. Best results have been obtained using breath-hold at the end of normal expiration,[29] but this requires careful coaching of the patient and may not always be appropriate in the pediatric setting. In such cases, normal shallow breathing during the CT portion of the study is probably a suitable alternative.

Besides attenuation correction, hybrid PET-CT systems provide other advantages. Positron emission tomography provides outstanding functional images of the patient, but in some cases it can be hard to discern the precise anatomic location of areas of increased activity. The hybrid PET-CT scanner can provide anatomic correlation to the functional data provided by PET. The PET and CT components of these devices are practically separate devices with the two gantries placed back to back with a common patient table. The patient is placed into the CT scanner portion and a helical CT scan is acquired. This acquisition takes less than a minute. The patient table then translates such that the patient is now positioned within the PET scanner, and a PET study is acquired. The patient receives both a CT and a PET scan in a single imaging session. Because the chance of patient motion is reduced, the two image sets are typically well registered to each other, except near the liver/lung boundary, where the effects of lung motion are commonly seen.[30] The use of a PET-CT scanner can greatly reduce the time to scan a patient. The CT scan is acquired in less than 1 minute, whereas the traditional PET transmission scan using rotating, external sources takes 20 to 30 minutes for

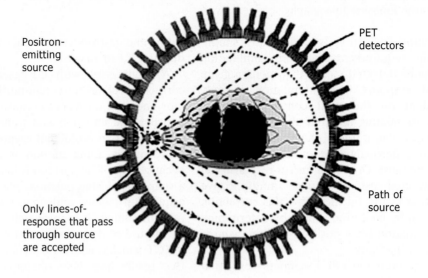

A

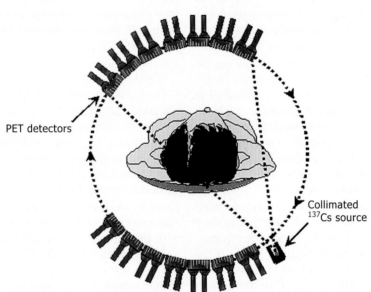

B

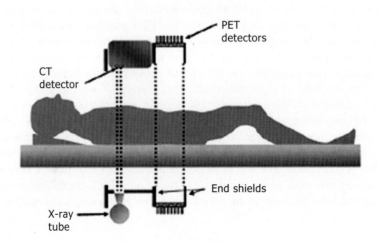

C

FIGURE 18.8. PET attenuation correction. Correction for photon attenuation within the patient improves both the image quality as well as the ability to quantify the PET study. A: A rotating positron emitter rod source can be used to determine attenuation correction factor. A transmission scan is acquired both with and without the patient in place. By dividing the counts obtained without the patient by those with the patient in place, one can determine the attenuation correction factor for each line of response. B: A single photon source such as cesium 137 (^{137}Cs) can be used to determine attenuation correction factor with much improved statistics. C: The CT portion of a combined PET-CT scan can be used for attenuation correction. The photon attenuation information obtained at CT photon energies is transformed to yield attenuation correction factors for 511 keV.

a whole-body PET study. The total scan time for a whole-body study with PET-CT may be 30 to 40 minutes as compared to 60 minutes with the PET-only device. This is of particular interest in pediatric PET because a much shorter acquisition time can greatly reduce the potential for patient motion and minimize the need for sedation or anesthesia. A state-of-the-art hybrid PET-CT scanner with its covers removed is shown in Figure 18.9. In Figure 18.9A, the scanner is viewed from the CT side of the device. The x-ray tube and the detector array are clearly seen. Figure 18.9B shows the PET component, which looks very similar to the scanner shown in Figure 18.6.

Randoms, Scatter, and Dead Time

Random coincidences may be accurately corrected for by using a method known as delayed coincidence channel estimation, or by computing an estimate from the number of single (noncoincidence) events recorded. One of these methods is usually applied by default on most commercial scanners. However, the number of random coincidences is subject to statistical uncertainty, so that the presence of randoms always leads to degradation of the data, even if the bias they introduce is removed. The number of randoms increases with the square of the activity in the field of view. A good rule-of-thumb is to avoid imaging situations where the number of randoms is more than half of the recorded number of all coincidences.

Currently all of the main methods for correction of scattered coincidences are approximate, although adequate for most clinical imaging situations. Problems may arise when imaging large patients in 3D mode, where the fraction of scattered events may become very large. In such circumstances, under- or overcorrection of scatter may lead to artifacts and poor quantification of tracer uptake.[22]

Count losses due to system dead time are significantly greater in PET than they are in single photon imaging due to the absence of the shielding effect of collimators, but in most imaging situations the manufacturers' correction methods are sufficient. However, when system dead time increases, the event position-

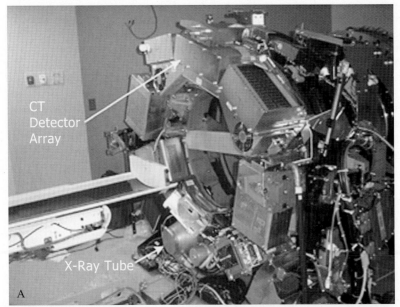

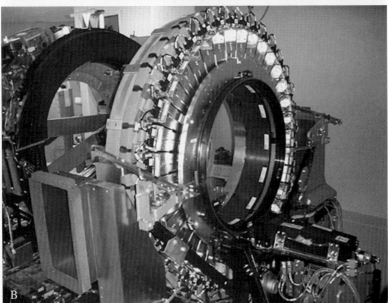

FIGURE 18.9. A state-of-the-art hybrid PET-CT scanner with its covers removed. A: CT component. The x-ray tube and the detector array are marked. B: PET component. Note the resemblance to the scanner shown in Figure 18.6.

ing algorithms used by the detectors also become less accurate, which can result in a decrease in spatial resolution. This is particularly important in systems that use large detectors.[31] Use of 2D mode substantially reduces this problem due to the resultant reduction in the singles rate.

Normalization and Daily Quality Control

A detector failure in a full-ring PET scanner is in general less serious than in a conventional gamma camera because there are so many detectors, and a failed detector does not give rise to ring artifacts because the system is usually nonrotating. Nevertheless, a daily check for detector integrity is highly recommended. This is usually performed using a rotating positron-emitting source and comparing the resulting data against a baseline scan to look for changes. In most commercial systems, this process is automated or semiautomated. In addition to this daily check, the photomultiplier tube gains should be adjusted and a correction matrix for detector nonuniformities generated. This process is known as normalization. It should be performed monthly or quarterly depending on the stability of the system (some manufacturers recommend adjusting tube gains even more frequently). After normalization the scanner should be calibrated against the dose calibrator used to measure patient doses so that the PET data can be reported in kBq/mL, μCi/mL, or other quantitative units.

For combined PET-CT devices, the CT portion also requires a quality control program, including daily air calibrations and checks of image noise and resolution that should be performed at least quarterly. In addition, dose delivery should be checked at least annually. Finally, the alignment between the PET and CT acquisition systems should be checked quarterly and possibly more frequently on mobile systems.

Image Registration

As discussed previously, PET and other nuclear medicine modalities can provide extremely useful images of physiology and function. However, it is not always simple to correlate these functional findings with the underlying anatomy. As described above, one approach is to image the patient on a hybrid scanner that, for example, combines the imaging capability of PET or SPECT with a CT scanner. If the patient does not move between the two acquisitions and because the index distance between the two scanners is known, one can attain very good correlation between the two image sets. However, many centers do not have access to these hybrid scanners, and, in any case, other

registration scenarios present themselves. For example, the most pertinent anatomic image set may be acquired with a different modality than CT, such as magnetic resonance imaging (MRI). Another possibility is that one would like to register several similar studies of the same patient that were acquired either at different times or under different circumstances, for example, PET or SPECT studies performed before and after treatment. In any of these cases, one needs to align or register the image data using a software rather than a hardware approach. There are three basic steps in performing image registration: converting of the image sets to a common image format, determining the transformation required to register one of the image sets with the other, and displaying the results. Each of these steps are reviewed in detail. In this example, it is assumed that one wants to register a PET study to an MRI study.

Although there are a number of intramodality registration applications, in many cases the two image scans will have been acquired on different computer systems using different file formats. To register these two studies, one needs to move these to a common computer platform in the same image format. Institution-wide picture archiving and communication systems (PACSs) using the digital imaging and communications in medicine (DICOM) image standard can greatly facilitate the communication of the image data to a common platform.[32] However, if the data are from an older system or from another institution, it may be necessary to use a hardware approach, such as CDs. There remain aspects of PET and SPECT data acquisition (such as gated SPECT or PET) that are still not supported by the DICOM standard. In such cases, custom-made or third-party software may be needed to convert the data to a common format. A format for this purpose that has gained some acceptance in the nuclear medicine community is the interfile standard.[33]

Once the two image sets are on one computer platform in a common file format, the transformation that relates one of the image sets to the other is determined. In other words, there is a mathematical relationship between the two image sets that, for example, defines the amount one of the sets needs to be "transformed" to match the other. This transformation may be described as rigid or nonrigid. A rigid transformation assumes the two objects are "similar" in the mathematical sense, and the appropriate scaling (i.e., sizing), translation, and rotation will register one of the image sets to the other. In many cases, the pixel size (in millimeters per pixel) is stored in the image header and this information can be used to determine the appropriate scaling between the two scans prior to image registration. For a nonrigid transformation, in addition to scaling, translation, and rotation, there may also be sheering (i.e., different parallel planes being translated by different amounts) and nonlinear warping of one of the image sets to the other. Rigid transformations have been shown to work well in the brain. They may work in some cases in the thorax and abdomen as well. However, in many cases, a nonrigid approach is necessary to obtain adequate registration in the thorax and abdomen. It should be noted, though, that few such nonrigid methodologies have been thoroughly validated for clinical use.

There are a number of different approaches to determining the best transformation for registering the two studies. These approaches include manual, point (or fiducial) matching, surface matching, or voxel matching. In the manual methods, one utilizes tools to translate and rotate one of the image sets relative to the other. These tools allow the image set to be translated in the three Cartesian coordinates (x,y,z) and to rotate the image set about the three Cartesian axes. A viewing tool, such as a merged version of the two images, is used to visually assess how well the two sets are aligned. Depending on the registration task, and with appropriate training, this method can be fast and accurate.[34] However, it does rely on user input and thereby there may be interobserver variability.

In the point matching method, a series of homologous points are identified on the two image sets. These points may be externally applied fiducial markers that are identifiable in the two image sets or a series of easily distinguishable anatomic landmarks. The Procrustes method is one approach to determining the optimal transformation from this series of homologous points.[35,36] The location of each point is defined in x,y,z. If n points are identified in each image set, then two $n \times 3$ matrices are defined. By using singular value decomposition, the transformation that leads to the minimum deviation between the two matrices is determined. This is a statistical method that basically determines the best least squares fit between the two sets of defined points. The minimum number of points necessary for this approach to work correctly is four non-coplanar points. Due to the statistical nature of the method, defining more independent points leads to a better fit. About 10 markers are sufficient for an excellent fit in most cases. This approach requires user intervention. If fiducial markers are to be used, they must be placed in advance of both scans and maintained on the patient through the complete acquisition of both image sets. Practically speaking, this requires the user to know prospectively which studies need to be registered; the two image sets must be acquired in close temporal proximity to each other. If anatomic landmarks are to be used, the image quality of both image sets must be sufficient to define a good number of landmarks. However, if appropriately applied, this approach can provide excellent results.

Pelizzari et al.[37] developed a surface matching method that could be routinely applied retrospectively. This method is sometimes referred to as the "head and hat" approach to image registration. In this approach, the surface of one of the image sets is defined as a series of contours and referred to as the "head." The surface of the other image set is defined as a series of surface points and referred to as the "hat." The transformation is then determined that best fits the hat to the head. Because this approach tries to best fit the two surfaces, it does not work if the object is a sphere, and thus a certain amount of nonsymmetry is required to obtain a good fit. Although this is an automated method, it may require some preprocessing of the data prior to its application.

For example, one needs to define the surfaces with some manual intervention prior to the application of the method. However, this approach has been shown to work well in both the brain and the thorax.[38]

Voxel-based registration methods rely on the values of all of the voxels within the object and not on only a few fiducial markers or anatomic landmarks or surface features of the object. For this reason, these methods tend to be more robust than both the point and surface matching approaches. Voxel-based approaches can be used for both rigid and nonrigid transformations. One of the first widely used, voxel-based methods was the automated image registration (AIR) method developed by Woods et al.[39] In this method, each voxel in one of the image sets is divided by the corresponding voxel in the other image set to form a ratio image. The relative variance (i.e., the variance divided by the mean value) of all of the voxels in the ratio image is determined. The transformation that minimizes this relative voxel variance of the ratio image is considered optimal. This approach has been shown to work well for both intramodality and intermodality registration. Other voxel-based methods have been developed that utilize the statistical concept of "mutual information."[40,41] Mutual information can be considered the amount of information that one image set contains about the other. The optimal transformation is that which maximizes the mutual information between the two image sets. Voxel-based methods using mutual information have been shown to be very robust for a wide variety of image applications and typically do not require any data preprocessing prior to their application.

Many of the developers of image registration techniques have used phantom or simulated data to evaluate the accuracy of their technique. However, it is not clear that such measurements correctly reflect the accuracy of these techniques when used with clinical data. West et al.[42] utilized a series of brain scans of human subjects that were acquired with embedded fiducial markers used to determine the accuracy of a variety of image registration techniques. These fiducial markers were

TABLE 18.2. Accuracy of registration methods

Matching method	Median error (mm)
Point	5.2
Surface	2.9–3.3
Air	2.4
Mutual information	2.0

Source: Data from West et al.[42]

removed from the images, and these were sent to a number of collaborators who were asked to apply some method of image registration to the data sets. These registered data were analyzed using the fiducial markers to determine the accuracy of the various approaches. The results are summarized in Table 18.2. According to this analysis, all approaches were quite accurate. As might be expected, the voxel-based methods were shown to be more accurate than the point or surface matching approaches.

Once the optimal transformation has been determined, the two registered image sets can be displayed for review. This first requires that one of the image sets be resampled according to this transformation. In other words, the transformation is applied to one of the image sets and it is displayed with the same size and orientation and along the same tomographic planes as the other image set. In some instances, this is performed on-the-fly by the image registration software; in other cases, the resampled image set is archived for future display. Most commonly, the image set with the lower, in-plane spatial resolution is resampled to match the anatomic image set. Once resampled, two approaches are commonly used for displaying registered data sets: one is to overlay one of the data sets on top of the other, using different-colored tables for the two data sets; the other is to show the two data sets side by side with a cursor that is mirrored onto both image sets such that it points at homologous locations in the two image sets. Figure 18.10 shows an image display that utilizes both of these approaches.

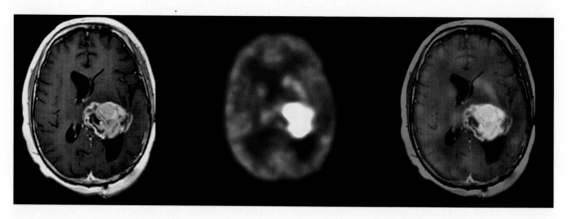

FIGURE 18.10. Display of registered data. Once two image sets have been registered to each other, they can either be displayed side by side or as a fused data set where one of the image sets is overlaid on top of the other in a different color table. Both methods are demonstrated here.

Radiation Safety

The 511-keV photons emitted from positron emitters is of higher energy than that typically used in SPECT and planar nuclear medicine (70 to 360 keV). For these reasons, many of the radiation safety aspects of using positron-emitting agents may be different from those routinely encountered in nuclear medicine. There are also particular issues regarding the use of PET in pediatrics. Technologists and other health professionals may need to be in closer proximity to the patient during the scanning procedure. The parents of the patient may also elect to stay by the patient during the uptake period and imaging procedure; thus one should consider the radiation dose to the parents. There is also the possibility that the patient might receive a higher radiation dose from the use of PET imaging agents as compared to those used for SPECT. Last, the application of PET-CT to pediatrics may lead to a higher radiation dose to the patient due to X-ray exposure from the CT component. All of these aspects of radiation safety as it pertains to application of PET to children are reviewed here.

Table 18.3 lists the gamma exposure rate constants for a number or radionuclides commonly used in nuclear medicine including ^{18}F. This value gives the exposure rate (in mR/h) at a distance of 1 m from a point source of 1 MBq of

this radionuclide. Thus, the exposure rate at 1 m from 1 MBq of ^{18}F is eight times higher than that for 1 MBq of technetium-99m (^{99m}Tc) and more than two times higher than that for iodine-131 (^{131}I). Therefore, one needs to be more cautious when working in PET in order to keep one's exposure as low as reasonably achievable. For the technologist, the highest components of the radiation absorbed dose are received during the preparation and the administration of the radiopharmaceutical to the patient.[43] Therefore, it is prudent on the technologists' part to practice good radiation handling techniques during these portions of the procedure. For example, the radioactivity to be administered should be prepared and assayed behind a lead shield that has been specifically designed for handling PET radiopharmaceuticals. In addition, appropriate PET syringe shields should be used during the injection of the radiopharmaceutical. Also, as in all cases, the technologist needs to consider the dose-reducing factors of distance, time, and shielding throughout the entire procedure.

TABLE 18.3. Exposure rate constant

Radionuclide	mR/h per MBq at 1 m
^{18}F	0.0154
^{99m}Tc	0.00195
^{67}Ga	0.00216
^{123}I	0.00432
^{131}I	0.00589

TABLE 18.4. Effective dose (mSv)

	1-year-old	5-year-old	10-year-old	15-year-old	Adult
Mass (kg)	9.8	19.0	32.0	55.0	70.0
99mTc-MDP (740 MBq)	2.8	2.8	3.7	4.1	4.2
99mTc-HMPAO (740 MBq)	5.1	5.4	5.8	6.4	6.9
67Ga (222 MBq)	19.9	19.9	20.3	22.7	22.2
18F-FDG (389 MBq)	5.2	5.3	6.4	7.6	7.4
(bladder wall for 18F-FDG)	32.1	33.8	49.8	64.2	62.2

Note: Value in parentheses is the administered activity for the 70-kg adult. Pediatric activities are scaled by patient mass. MDP, methylene diphosphonate; HMPAO, hexamethylpropyleneamine oxime. Data from ICRP.[45]

The exposure rate near the adult patient during a PET scan has been shown to be about 15 to 20 mR/h, on the same order as that associated with patients receiving higher activities of 99mTc during such studies as gated cardiac SPECT.[44] Pediatric patients typically receive less activity than adults, and thus the exposure rate near them may be somewhat less. Consider the radiation dose to a parent whose child has received 7 mCi of 18F-FDG. If we assume the child is a point source with no self-shielding (conservative assumptions) and the parent stays 2 m away from the patient for 60 minutes during the uptake phase and 60 minutes during PET imaging, the parent will receive an exposure of less than 1.5 mR. If the parent stays only 1 m from the patient, he or she will receive about 5.5 mR. Therefore, it is considered acceptable to have parents stay with the child during the PET procedure, although it may be prudent to instruct them to stay as far from the patient as they feel comfortable. These levels of exposures can also be considered for health professionals who may need to stay close to the pediatric patient during the procedure. If personnel can stay at least 2 m from the patient, the exposure received during the procedure will most likely be less than 1.5 mR.

Table 18.4 summarizes the radiation dose received by pediatric patients of various ages from 18F-FDG.[45,46] In this table, the effective dose and the dose to the urinary bladder wall are reported. The effective dose is determined from the radiation dose to different organs with each organ weighted by its particular risk for carcinogenesis and genetic effects. Thus, a person who receives an effective dose of 10 mSv has approximately the same risk as a person receiving a uniform, whole-body dose of 10 mSv. The radiation dose to the urinary bladder is presented because this is the organ that receives the highest dose from FDG. In this table, the adult is assumed to receive 389 MBq (10.5 mCi) and the pediatric administered activities are scaled by weight. How do these effective doses compare to those from other nuclear medicine procedures? Table 18.4 also lists the effective doses from a variety of other nuclear medicine procedures. The administered activity of the adult is given in parentheses for each procedure, and, again, the pediatric dose is scaled by weight. It is noted that the effective dose received from FDG is in the range of doses received from other nuclear medicine procedures and less than a third of the effective dose of a gallium-167 (67Ga) scan.

With the development of hybrid PET-CT scanners, there has been concern with the additional radiation dose delivered by the CT portion of the examination, particularly if a diagnostic-quality CT scan is not required and it is only used for attenuation correction or anatomic correlation. Factors that can reduce the radiation dose delivered by CT include the tube voltage (kVp), tube current (mA), the rotation speed, and the pitch. A lower radiation dose is obtained with a lower tube voltage or tube current, faster rotation speed, and greater pitch. A CT dose index was estimated using ionization chamber measurements for a variety of anthropomorphic phantoms of different sizes as a function of tube voltage and current.[47] All measurements were made at the same rotation speed (0.8 second per rotation) and pitch (1.5:1). These results are summarized in Table 18.5. These radiation doses can be compared to

TABLE 18.5. Computed tomography dose as a function of patient size, tube voltage and tube current

Phantom	kVp	CTDI$_{vol}$ (mSv)				
		10 mA	20 mA	40 mA	80 mA	160 mA
Newborn	80	0.42	0.85	1.69	3.39	6.78
Newborn	100	0.80	1.60	3.21	6.41	12.83
Newborn	120	1.26	2.53	5.05	10.10	20.20
Newborn	140	1.77	3.53	7.06	14.13	28.25
1-year-old	80	0.37	0.74	1.47	2.94	5.88
1-year-old	100	0.70	1.40	2.80	5.59	11.19
1-year-old	120	1.11	2.22	4.45	8.89	17.78
1-year-old	140	1.57	3.14	6.28	12.56	25.11
5-year-old	80	0.33	0.66	1.32	2.65	5.30
5-year-old	100	0.64	1.28	2.55	5.10	10.20
5-year-old	120	1.02	2.04	4.08	8.16	16.31
5-year-old	140	1.46	2.91	5.83	11.66	23.32
10-year-old	80	0.30	0.60	1.19	2.38	4.76
10-year-old	100	0.58	1.16	2.32	4.64	9.27
10-year-old	120	0.92	1.84	3.67	7.35	14.69
10-year-old	140	1.32	2.63	5.26	10.52	21.04
Medium adult	80	0.20	0.40	0.80	1.61	3.22
Medium adult	100	0.40	0.79	1.58	3.17	6.33
Medium adult	120	0.64	1.27	2.55	5.10	10.19
Medium adult	140	0.91	1.82	3.65	7.30	14.59

All data were acquired with rotation speed of 0.8 seconds and a 1.5:1 pitch. All data were acquired with 160 mA and linearly scaled for the various tube current values represented in the table.
(*Source:* Data from Fahey et al.[47])

the dose received from the administration of ^{18}F-FDG in Table 18.4. For a diagnostic-quality CT, the dose received from the CT is on the same order or higher than that received from the PET scan. For the same acquisition parameters, the newborn receives approximately twice the radiation dose as the adult. Reducing the tube voltage from 120 to 80 kVp and reducing the tube current from 160 to 10 mA can lower the radiation dose by approximately a factor of 70. It has also been shown that an adequate CT-based attenuation correction for whole-body PET can be obtained with pediatric patients for CT acquisition parameters as low as 80 kVp, 10 mA, 0.5 seconds per rotation, and a pitch of 1.5:1. For larger adult patients, the tube voltage needs to be raised to 120 kVp, with all other parameters remaining the same, to obtain an adequate CT-based attenuation.[47] It is difficult to assess the minimum acquisition parameters necessary for anatomic localization because such a study would be task-specific.

Conclusion

This chapter has reviewed the basics of PET including radiopharmaceutical production, coincidence detection, and instrumentation, with particular emphasis on the impact on its application to pediatric imaging. In addition, tomographic reconstruction, attenuation correction, and image registration were discussed. Last, the radiation safety considerations of the application of PET to children were presented. The clinical application of PET for both adults and children has grown dramatically in the past 10 years. The increased availability of this new and exciting imaging modality, no doubt, will lead to further increase in its use for pediatric imaging. Due to the difference in both the size of the patient and the level of administered activity, optimal protocol parameters for adults may not necessarily apply to children, and care must be taken to ensure that the most appropriate procedures are followed.

References

1. Wrenn FR Jr, Good ML, Handler P. The use of positron emitting radioisotopes for localization of brain tumors. Science 1951;113:525–7.

2. Brownell GL, Sweet WH. Localization of brain tumors with positron emitters. Nucleonics 1953; 11:40–5.

3. Burnham CA, Brownell GL, A multi-crystal positron camera. IEEE Trans Nucl Sci 1972;NS-19:201–5.

4. Ter-Pogossian MM, Phelps ME, Hoffman EJ, Mullani NA. A positron emission transaxial tomograph for nuclear medicine Imaging (PETT). Radiology 1975;114:89–98.

5. Patz EF Jr, Lowe VJ, Hoffman JM et al. Focal pulmonary abnormalities: evaluation with ^{18}F fluorodeoxyglucose PET scanning. Radiology 1993;188:487–90.

6. Newman JS, Francis IR, Kaminski MS, Wahl WL. Imaging of lymphoma with PET with 2–^{18}F-fluoro-2-deoxy-D-glucose: correlation with CT. Radiology 1994;190:111–6.

7. DiChiro G. Positron emission tomography using ^{18}F fluorodeoxyglucose in brain tumors. A powerful diagnostic and prognostic tool. Invest Radiol 1987;22:360–71.

8. Engel J Jr, Brown WJ, Kuhl DE et al. Pathologic findings underlying focal temporal lobe hypometabolism in partial epilepsy. Ann Neurol 1982;12:518–28.

9. Gould KL. Quantitative coronary arteriography and positron emission tomography. Circulation 1988;78:237–45.

10. Schelbert HR. Phelps ME. Positron computed tomography for the in vivo assessment of regional myocardial function. J Mol Cell Cardiol 1984;16:683–93.

11. Snead OC III, Chen LS, Mitchell WG, et al. Usefulness of ^{18}F fluorodeoxyglucose positron emission tomography in pediatric epilepsy surgery. Pediatr Neurol 1996;14:98–107.

12. Shulkin BL, Mitchell DS, Ungar DR, et al. Neoplasms in a pediatric population: 2–^{18}F-fluoro-2-deoxy-D-glucose PET Studies. Radiology 1995;194:495–500.

13. Evans RD. The Atomic Nucleus. New York: Kreiger, 1982.

14. Levin CS, Hoffman EJ. Calculation of positron range and its effect on the fundamental limit of positron emission tomography system resolution. Phys Med Biol 1999;44:781–99.

15. Mabuchi M, Kubo N, Morita K, et al. Value and limitation of myocardial fluorodeoxyglucose single photon emission computed tomography using ultra-high energy collimators for assessing myocardial viability. Nucl Med Comm 2002;23:879–85.

16. Casey ME, Nutt R. A multicrystal 2-dimensional BGO detector system for positron emission tomography. IEEE Trans Nucl Sci 1986;33:460–3.

17. Daghighian F, Shenderov P, Pentlow KS, et al. Evaluation of cerium doped lutetium oxy-orthosilicate (LSO) scintillation crystal for PET. IEEE Trans Nucl Sci 1993;40:1045–7.

18. Surti S, Karp JS, Freifelder R, Liu F. Optimizing the performance of a PET detector using discrete GSO crystals on a continuous lightguide. IEEE Trans Nucl Sci 2000;47:1030–6.

19. Badawi RD, Marsden PK, Cronin BF, et al. Optimization of noise-equivalent count rates in 3D PET. Phys Med Biol 1996;41:1755–76.

20. El Fakhri G, Holdsworth CH, Badawi RD, et al. Impact of acquisition geometry and patient habitus on tumor detectability in whole-body FDG-PET: a channelized hotelling observer study. In: IEEE Nuclear Science Symposium Conference Record. Piscataway, NJ: IEEE, 2002;3:1402–5.

21. Yates RWM, Marsden PK, Badawi RD, et al. Positron emission tomography demonstrates normal distribution of myocardial perfusion following neonatal arterial switch operation. *Pediatr Cardiol* 2000;21:111–8.

22. Holdsworth CH, Badawi RD, Santos PA, et al. Evaluation of a Monte Carlo scatter correction in clinical 3D PET. IEEE Nuclear Science Symposium Conference Record, vol 4. Piscataway, NJ: IEEE, 2003:2540–4.

23. Lewellen TK. Time-of-Flight PET. Semin Nucl Med 1998;28:268–75.

24. Kuhn A, Surti S, Karp JS, et al. Design of a lanthanum bromide detector for time-of-flight PET. IEEE Trans Nucl Sci 2004;51:2550–7.

25. Kinahan PE, Hasegawa BH, Beyer T. X-ray-based attenuation correction for positron emission tomography/computed tomography scanners. Semin Nucl Med 2003;33:166–79.

26. Goerres GW, Burger C, Kamel E, et al. Respiration-induced attenuation artifact at PET/CT: Technical considerations. Radiology 2003;226:906–10.

27. Antoch G, Freudenberg LS, Egelhof T, et al. Focal tracer uptake: a potential artifact in contrast-enhanced dual-modality PET/CT scans. J Nucl Med 2002;43:1339–42.

28. Antoch G, Kuehl H, Kanja J, et al. Dual-modality PET/CT scanning with negative oral

contrast agent to avoid artifacts: introduction and evaluation. Radiology 2004;230: 879–85.

29. Goerres GW, Burger C, Kamel E, et al. Respiration-induced attenuation artifact at PET/CT: technical considerations. Radiology 2003;226: 906–10.

30. Goerres GW, Kamel E, Heidelberg TNH, et al. PET-CT image co-registration in the thorax: influence of respiration. Eur J Nucl Med Mol Imag 2002;29:351–60.

31. Badawi RD, Domigan P, Johnson O, et al. Count-rate dependent event mispositioning and NEC in PET. IEEE Trans Nucl Sci 2004;51: 41–5.

32. National Electrical Manufacturers Association. Digital Imaging and Communications in Medicine: the DICOM Standard. Rosslyn, VA: NEMA, 2004.

33. Todd-Pokropek A, Cradduck TD, Deconinck F. A file format for the exchange of nuclear medicine image data: a specification of Interfile version 3.3. Nucl Med Comm 1992;13:673–99.

34. Habboush IH, Mitchell KD, Mulkern RV, et al. Registration and alignment of three-dimensional images: an interactive visual approach. Radiology. 1996;199:573–8.

35. Marrett S, Evans AC, Collins L, Peters TM. A volume of interest (VOI) atlas for the analysis of neurophysiological image data. Medical Imaging III: Image Processing. SPIE Proc 1989;1092: 467–77.

36. Evans AC, Marrett S, Torrescorzo J, et al. MRI-PET correlation in three dimensions using a volume-of-interest (VOI) atlas. J Cerebr Blood Flow Metab 1991;11:A69–78.

37. Pelizzari CA, Chen GTY, Spelbring DR, et al. Accurate three-dimensional registration of CT, PET and MR images of the brain. Radiology 1989;13:20–6.

38. Yu JN, Fahey FH, Gage HD, et al. Intermodality, retrospective image registration in the thorax. J Nucl Med 1995;36(12):2333–8.

39. Woods RP, Mazziotta JC, Cherry SR. MRI-PET registration with automated algorithm. J Comput Assist Tomogr 1993;17:536–46.

40. Maes F, Collignon A, Vandermeulen D, et al. Multimodality image registration by maximization of mutual information. IEEE Trans Med Imag 1997;16:187–98.

41. Yokoi T, Soma T, Shinohara H, Matsuda H. Accuracy and reproducibility of co-registration techniques based on mutual information and normalized mutual information for MRI and SPECT brain images. Ann Nucl Med 2004;18: 659–67.

42. West J, Fitzpatrick JM, Wang MY, et al. Comparison of retrospective intermodality brain image registration techniques. J Comput Assist Tomogr 1997;21:554–66.

43. Zeff BW, Yester MV. Patient self-attenuation and technologist dose in positron emission tomography. Med Phys 2005;32:861–865.

44. Carey J. Basic radiation protection in nuclear medicine. In: Basic Science of Nuclear Medicine CD. Reston, VA: Society of Nuclear Medicine, 2001.

45. International Commission on Radiation Protection. ICRP Report 80: Radiation dose to patients from radiopharmaceuticals. New York ICRP, 1998:49–110.

46. International Commission on Radiation Protection. ICRP Report 56: Age-dependent doses to members of the public from intake of radionuclides: part 1. New York ICRP, 1989:4.

47. Fahey FH, Palmer MR, Strauss KJ, et al. Dosimetry and image quality associated with low-dose CT-based attenuation correction for pediatric PET (abstract). J Nucl Med 2005;46:470P.

19
Radiation Risk

S. James Adelstein

The practitioner of pediatric nuclear medicine should have some knowledge of radiation effects and the potential hazards that may result from low-level radiation exposures. There are several reasons such information is essential. First, specialists should ensure that the exposure of patients to radiation from diagnostic or therapeutic procedures is not excessive. Although all current radiopharmaceuticals deliver radiation doses within a readily acceptable range, such was not the case 30 years ago when the radionuclides employed were generally longer-lived and emitted significant particulate radiation, e.g., iodine-131, strontium 87. As a result, before 1970 at Children's Hospital Boston, radionuclides were administered only to patients with advanced neoplastic diseases. Today, as new agents are introduced, it is imperative to understand the kinetics of their distribution and the resulting radiation doses delivered to various organs. Moreover, for those who participate in clinical trials, an estimation of the absorbed radiation dose is required by institutional review boards, as is some assessment of the potential hazard.

Second, patients and particularly the parents of young patients are frequently concerned about the radiation risks associated with nuclear medical procedures. It is important to convey these potential risks clearly, placing them in the context of radiologic and other risks as well as the benefits to be gained.

Third, nuclear medical specialists are often asked their advice about the potential harm that may result from nuclear accidents such as those at Three Mile Island and Chernobyl. It serves the practitioner well to respond to such requests in an authoritative and intelligible fashion.

This chapter presents some of the radiobiologic consequences of radiation exposure as well as conclusions from several epidemiologic studies of radiation exposure. How the radiation protection community thinks about low-dose and low-dose-rate exposure is considered. A final section discusses how to explain potential risks to others.

Effects of Radiation Exposure

Radiobiologic Consequences

We are now aware that damage to the genome is the basis for most radiation action on cells; this is the case particularly for late effects—cancer production in somatic cells and mutagenesis in germ cells—although all of the mechanistic details have not been worked out. At the molecular level, ionizing radiation causes base damage, single-strand breaks and double-strand breaks (DSBs) in DNA, and cross-linking between DNA and nuclear proteins. Of particular significance are DSBs, which are susceptible to misrepair. They are induced with radiation doses as small as 1 mGy, and their frequency arises linearly with dose.[1] Molecular damage leads to point mutations, partial and complete gene deletions, disrepair, translocations, and other genetic changes. These changes, in turn, result in inheritable disorders in germ cells and, through the interplay of oncogenes, tumor suppressor genes, and clonal selection, in cellular transformation and carcinogenesis in somatic cells.

Of importance to nuclear medicine is the observation that fractionation of radiation dose or reducing the dose rate decreases the frequency of carcinogenic transformations. Thus a given dose from beta particles or gamma photons, such as that produced by extended radioactive decay, results in a lower transformation frequency than the same dose delivered acutely by x-ray or electron generators.[2]

Chromosomal aberrations are the most obvious of the cytogenetic changes produced by irradiation. Of these changes, chromosome and chromatid breaks and structural rearrangements are the most common. When two breaks are produced in a cell and the ends joined other than in their original sequence, stable and unstable structural anomalies occur. As two electron tracks are generally needed to produce these aberrations, the dose–response relation, taking into account the occasional single track that produces two breaks, is a linear-quadratic one.[3]

Exposure of rodents and other animals to increasing doses of radiation leads to an increased incidence of cancers and genetic abnormalities in offspring. In the case of cancers, the incidence rises with dose to reach a maximum at about 300 to 500 cGy. Decreasing the dose rate or fractionating the dose reduces the incidence of animal cancers—with its obvious relevance to internally deposited radionuclides.[4]

The main source of genetic information about the effects of radiation on the germ cells of mammals comes from experiments with mice. Increasing rates of mutation are found with increasing doses. Again, a reduction in dose rate has a significant effect on mutational frequency. In the male mouse, radiation sensitivity is reduced by a factor of three when the dose rate goes from 100 to 1 cGy per minute, whereas in the female mouse low dose rates produce few if any mutations. From these experiments, the doubling dose (i.e., that quantity of radiation required to double the muta-

tion rate to twice its spontaneous value) is estimated to be approximately 100 cGy.[5] As no direct information on the production of radiation-induced, inheritable human disorders is available, risk estimates are based on mouse experiments. The children of persons exposed acutely to radiation in Hiroshima and Nagasaki have been carefully examined, and no evidence for genetic change above the baseline has been found. Hence, it has been assumed that humans are no more sensitive to inheritable mutations than mice, and, in the case of chronic irradiation, may be considerably less so.[6]

Epidemiologic Studies

In a number of instances, exposure to ionizing radiation has produced cancer in humans. Early radiologists, who performed fluoroscopic examinations with bare hands and high-dose sources, developed skin cancers. Radium-dial painters, who pointed brushes with their tongues, developed sarcomas of the bone. Patients receiving thorium by injection to make the liver opaque to x-rays developed liver tumors. These observations alerted the medical community to the proposition that high-dose exposure could produce human cancer at some later time.

More recent studies have been concerned with quantifying the dose–response relationship in populations exposed to various doses of radiation in the range of 50 to 1000 cGy. These populations include survivors of the atomic bomb detonations in Japan, patients treated by x-rays for ankylosing spondylitis, patients with tuberculosis and thoracoplasties who were followed for long periods with multiple fluoroscopies, patients treated with radiation for mastitis, and children who underwent irradiation of the scalp and thymus with consequent irradiation of the thyroid. In addition, patients given iodine-131 for diagnosis or treatment have been followed. All of these studies have shown an increase in cancer incidence with increasing doses of radiation for a number of organs including bone marrow, breast, thyroid gland, lung, stomach, colon, and ovary. Although among these studies there are some variations in the dose–response relationship, several generalities have emerged[7]:

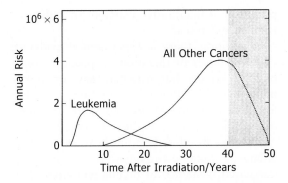

FIGURE 19.1. Nominal risk of cancer mortality versus time following 2 mSv uniform whole-body irradiation. (*Source:* Sinclair WK. Proceedings of the Twentieth Annual Meeting of the National Council on Radiation Protection and Measurements, April 1984. Proceedings No. 6. Bethesda, MD: NCPR, 1985:227, adapted with permission of the National Council on Radiation Protection and Measurements.)

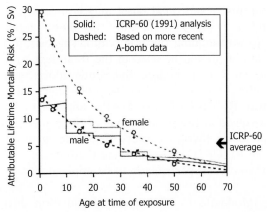

FIGURE 19.2. Estimated lifetime risks of cancer as a function of age at time of exposure based upon life-span study of atomic bomb survivors. (*Source:* Brenner,[9] with permission of Springer-Verlag.)

1. The response of bone marrow differs significantly from that of solid organs. Leukemias appear earlier after exposure than do other cancers; they reach a peak incidence within 5 to 10 years and decline slowly thereafter (Fig. 19.1). Childhood forms, such as acute lymphocytic leukemia, differ from adult forms, such as acute and chronic myelogenous leukemia. The dose–response curve for leukemia has a great deal of structure: at low doses it is relatively shallow; at 100 cGy it rises sharply to reach a peak at 250 cGy, declining thereafter. The decline is thought to result from competition between cell killing and cell transformation. For solid tumors there is a latent period of at least 10 years, and the dose–response curves appear to be approximated by straight lines.[8]

2. Children appear to be more susceptible than adults, perhaps by a factor of three (Fig. 19.2).[9] Moreover, there seems to be an increase in childhood cancers, particularly leukemia, of the same magnitude in children exposed in utero. The incidence of additional cancer cases increases with age in parallel with the increase in cancer of solid organs seen in an unexposed population.

3. Exposure of the thyroid gland to external radiation results in an increased incidence of thyroid nodules and thyroid cancer, as would be expected. Childhood thyroid cancer has increased early and markedly in areas subject to radio-iodine fallout from the Chernobyl nuclear accident (Fig. 19.3).[7] The marked

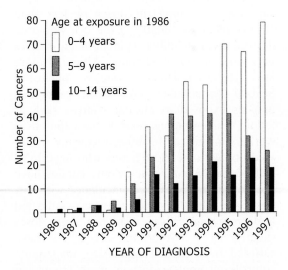

FIGURE 19.3. Increase in childhood thyroid cancers in Belarus after the Chernobyl nuclear power plant accident. (*Source:* Kofler A, Abelin T, Prudyvus I, Averkin Y. Radiation and Thyroid Cancer, 1st ed. Singapore: World Scientific Publishing, 1999, with permission.)

sensitivity and rapid onset may be due to the relative iodine deficiency in these areas. Notwithstanding, this observation suggests that caution should be used in the treatment with iodine-131 of children and young adolescents before the age of 15. The oncogenic pathway RET-RAS-BRAF-MAPK appears to be involved in the pathogenesis of these juvenile papillary thyroid cancers. Rearrangement of the RET/PTC gene following the induction of DSBs seems particularly to be implicated.[10]

Moderate to high doses of radiation also produce developmental defects and functional losses in certain organs. Unlike carcinogenesis and inheritable damage, these responses have a clear threshold above the levels provided by nuclear medical procedures. For this reason they are not described here but can be found in a number of sources.[11,12]

Low-Dose and Low-Dose-Rate Exposure

Most nuclear medical exposures and most nonoccupational accidental radiation exposures are at equivalent doses of less than 10 mSv. Ideally, estimates of the risk would be derived from definitive epidemiologic studies performed in this dose range. Although there are many such studies, none is conclusive. Several populations have been examined: persons exposed to nuclear sources such as fallout from weapons tests, those exposed as workers in nuclear facilities, medically irradiated populations, and persons who have lived in high background areas. Some studies have shown increases in cancer incidence with low doses, and others have not; a few have indicated a decrease in cancer incidence with doses slightly above background levels. All have suffered from small sample size, inadequate controls, incomplete dosimetry, or a range of confounding factors. As the statistical restraints on studies of small populations are so much greater than those on large ones, it is easy to see why these investigations shed little light on the question of a threshold for radiation effects and

provide no quantitative estimate of radiation risks at low doses.[13]

In addition, there is experimental evidence that low doses of radiation do produce some biologic effects, but whether they are detrimental is a matter of contention. Chronic, low-dose exposure (1 mSv per week for mice; 0.8 mSv per day for rats) increases the life span of rodents, an effect that has been ascribed to enhanced immune responsiveness. Similarly, a decreased incidence of thymic lymphoma has been found in mice as a result of chronic, fractionated low-dose total-body x-irradiation.[14] Furthermore, exposure of some cells and organisms to low-dose radiation produces an adaptive response to higher doses of radiation; that is, certain biologic changes occur with less frequency at higher levels of radiation exposure than are found in previously unexposed cells.[15] These changes include survival, chromosome aberrations, and gene mutations. The increased radiation resistance has been ascribed to radical scavenging, stimulated DNA repair mechanisms, or the production of protective stress proteins.

On the other hand, there is now evidence that irradiated cells may produce biologic effects in their unirradiated neighbors, a response called the bystander effect. This phenomenon seems to rely on a transmissible factor(s). Recently, it has been shown in an in vitro cell system that the adaptive response may cancel out the bystander effect, which would make it difficult to predict the importance of the latter at low-dose exposures.[16]

National and international bodies, taking a prudent approach, have adopted the stance that all radiation exposure is potentially harmful, with even the lowest doses producing some damage at the molecular and cellular levels.[3] Thus, considerable effort has been expended in estimating the risks at low doses and low dose rate by extrapolation from moderate- and high-dose epidemiologic data. The principal arguments have focused on the correct form for the dose–response curve (Fig. 19.4). The curve for leukemia, which appears to be of the linear-quadratic form (Fig. 19.4, curve A), agrees with the shape of responses across a wide variety of biologic end points. The initial linear portion of

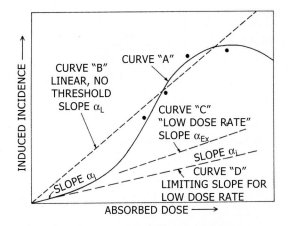

FIGURE 19.4. Incidence versus absorbed dose for low-LET (linear energy transfer) radiation. Solid curved line (A) for high doses and high dose rates is the "true" curve. Linear, no threshold, dashed line (B) was fitted to four indicated experimental points and origin. Slope $\alpha_{1'}$ indicates essentially linear portion of curve A at low dose rates, obtained by extrapolation. Dashed curve (C), marked "low dose rate," slope α_{Ex}, represents experimental data for high doses obtained at low dose rates. This experimental low-dose-rate curve, at very low dose rates, in principle may approach or become indistinguishable from the extension of the solid curve of slope α_1, dashed curve (D) labeled "limiting slope for low dose rate." (*Source:* Adapted from the National Council on Radiation Protection and Measurements, NCRP Report No. 64. Bethesda, MD: NCRP, 1980:7, with permission.)

the dose–response curve is thought to represent the risks at low doses and low dose rates. In the case of solid organs, extrapolation has proved more difficult as the data from higher doses appear to fit a linear curve (Fig. 19.4, curve B). As indicated in Figure 19.4, a linear-quadratic response could still seem linear at high doses. To take into account this possibility and the fact that progressively lowering the dose rate incrementally reduces the slope of the dose–response curve (Fig. 19.4, curves C and D), a dose and dose-rate effectiveness factor has been introduced to approximate the limiting slopes at low dose rate. The value of this factor has been estimated to be 2 to 10, but most agencies have used a value of approximately 2 to be on the conservative side. From all these adjustments, the carcinogenic and inheritable

risk from 10 mSv exposure is estimated at ~5 in 10,000 for adults and about 1 in 1000 for children.

Explaining the Risks to Others

Effective Dose

To estimate the radiation risk from any diagnostic procedure or accidental exposure, it is necessary to relate a dose quantity to a risk quantity. For nuclear medical procedures in which, by design, the dose to different organs varies, it is useful to combine the doses into a single metric that can be used for comparative purposes. This is best done by employing the effective dose (E), the dose to each organ for a given procedure multiplied by a weighting factor and then summed:

$$E = \Sigma \, H_T W_T,$$

where H_T is the dose to organ T, and W_T is the weighting factor for organ T. The weighting factor is proportional to the radiation sensitivity of each organ as determined from epidemiologic studies of carcinogenesis and, in the case of the gonads, from experimental studies of inheritable disorders. Thus the effective dose is a risk surrogate that is corrected for the heterogeneity of absorbed organ doses obtained in most nuclear medical procedures or from accidental exposure to radionuclides. Some representative effective doses from nuclear medical procedures in adults are given in Chapter 20.

It should be appreciated that the effective dose has been calculated for healthy adults and does not take into account either the age or the life expectancy of sick children. It should be used only to compare the radiation risk of one procedure with another and as a basis for comparison with other hazards. Nonetheless, it is possible to estimate the radiation risk from common nuclear medical procedures; for example, that for technetium-99m-disodium [*N*-[*N*-*N*-(mercaptoacetyl)glycyl]-glycinato(2-)-N,N′,N″,S]oxotechnetate(2-) (^{99m}Tc-MAG$_3$) (Table 19.1) has been assessed using the results from Figure 19.2 and Chapter 20.

TABLE 19.1. Assessment of radiation risk from ^{99m}Tc-MAG$_3$

	Administered activity (MBq)	Effective dose (mSv)	Risk (%)	
			Female	Male
Newborn	4.4	1.41	0.04	0.02
5-year-old	55.5	0.78	0.04	0.02
10-year-old	104.0	1.56	0.04	0.01
Adult	370.0	4.44	0.04	0.02

*Note that although the risk per unit of exposure increases with decreasing age, the scaling of administered activity with body surface area evens out the relative risk.

Institutional Review Boards

The institutional review process that is required before new or experimental procedures are introduced is greatly facilitated by having a uniform radiation risk standard with which the new procedures may be compared. Of course, review boards are also interested in the relative benefit and effectiveness of the new procedure in relation to its hazard; introduction of the procedure to the clinic, after all, is based on efficacy. In pediatric nuclear medicine, these questions are especially important as many new procedures and agents are first tested in adult patients and then extended to children on a trial basis. We have found that a good comparison is with equivalent doses from well-established radiologic and nuclear medical procedures. (Keep in mind that the background equivalent dose, excepting radon exposure, is about 1 mSv per year.) Some representative equivalent doses are chest radiograph, 0.5 mSv; mammogram, 5 mSv; dental radiograph, 6 mSv. For computed tomography (CT) scans, estimates have been made of the risks as a function of age (Fig. 19.5).

Patients and Their Families

When providing information to patients who are to undergo a diagnostic nuclear medical procedure or to those inadvertently exposed to radiation releases, as well as to their families, the goal should be to reduce anxiety by conveying a realistic and comprehensible estimate of the projected harm. This is not always an easy task. As described above, the long-term

consequences of radiation exposure are frightening in their potential prospect: cancers and genetic defects. Moreover, the perception of risk is often contextual with the fear of radiation exposure from a nuclear accident being greater than that from medical and natural sources.[17]

There are several ways to facilitate the discussion of these matters with patients. First, the time course for the late effects of radiation can be described with the help of a diagram such as that shown in Figure 19.1. The risk of leukemia starts after a latent period of 2 years, peaks at 6 to 7 years, and is generally exhausted after 25 years. The risk of a solid tumor begins after 10

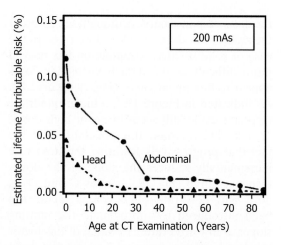

FIGURE 19.5. Estimated lifetime attributable cancer risk, as a function of age at examination, for a single computed tomography (CT) examination. (*Source:* Brenner,[9] with permission of Springer-Verlag.)

years and may peak after 40 years. The time-integrated risk of a 5-mSv exposure in children is 1 in 10,000 for leukemia (0.01%) and 4 in 10,000 for a fatal solid tumor (0.04%). One way of expressing this risk is to compare it with the ordinary risk of dying of cancer—a probability of approximately 20%. The incremental risks are small and are outweighed by the benefits.

A similar approach can be taken for inheritable genetic risks. It is important to convey that the uncertainty is greater in this instance because estimates are based on animal data, although we are fairly certain that humans are less sensitive than mice. In humans the probability of an offspring having a genetic abnormality, which includes genetic and chromosomal diseases as well as constitutional diseases and anomalies, is about 6%. Following a radiation exposure of 5 mSv, there is an additional probability of 0.0002%, so the total probability becomes 6.0002%, hardly a significant increment.[18]

Another approach is to compare these risks to other hazards of everyday living (e.g., accidents). With an average fatal accident rate of 6 per 10,000 per year, over a 50-year period this risk is approximately 3%, or the equivalent of an exposure to 600 mSv or 120 average nuclear medical procedures. Fatal accidents also provide a useful spectrum of risks: on an annual basis, motor vehicle accidents account for 3 per 10,000; drowning accounts for 3 per 100,000; air travel, 9 per million; and lightning, 5 per 10 million. The analogy, however, can be faulted as these accidents are generally immediately fatal in comparison with the long-term consequences of radiation exposure. In contrast, the frightening aspects of radiation risk are the uncertainty of outcome and relatively long period of latency.

Low levels of exposure, in the range of 10 mSv, can be contrasted with some natural exposures. For example, living in a high background area (Kerala, India, for 1 year; Yangjiang County, Guangdong Province, China, for 5 years; or Denver for 12 years) or working regularly in certain trades (nuclear fuel-cycle plant for 2 years) exposes one to increments of radiation of this magnitude. Where epidemiologic studies have been performed, they have failed to show any increase in cancer incidence over the general variability seen in the disease from region to region.

Conclusion

Practitioners of pediatric nuclear medicine should have a firm understanding of the risks of radiation, particularly for low doses and low dose rates. We have an obligation to look at the absorbed doses from new procedures with these risks in mind and to convey the risks to institutional review boards in a fashion that compares them with the risks of other medical tests. We must be able to present these risks to patients and their families in a manner that allows them to appreciate the hazards and benefits in a realistic way and in relation to the risks of other activities.

References

1. Rothkamm K, Löbrich M. Evidence for a lack of DNA double-strand break repair in human cells exposed to very low x-ray doses. Proc Natl Acad Sci USA 2003;100:5057–62.
2. Dale RG. Dose-rate effects in targeted radiotherapy. Phys Med Biol 1996;41:1871–84.
3. National Council on Radiation Protection and Measurements. Evaluation of the linear-nonthreshold dose-response model for ionizing radiation. NCRP Report No. 136. Bethesda, MD: National Council on Radiation Protection and Measurements, 2001.
4. Ullrich RL, Storer JB. Influence of γ irradiation on the development of neoplastic disease in mice. III. Dose-rate effects. Radiat Res 1979;80:325–42.
5. United Nations Scientific Committee on the Effects of Atomic Radiation. Hereditary effects of radiation, UNSCEAR 2001 Report to the General Assembly with scientific annex. New York: United Nations, 2001.
6. Asakawa J, Kuick R, Kodaira M, et al. A genome scanning approach to assess the genetic effects of radiation in mice and humans. Radiat Res 2004;161:380–90.
7. United Nations Scientific Committee on the Effects of Atomic Radiation. Sources and effects of ionizing radiations. UNSCEAR 2000 Report to the General Assembly with scientific

annexes, vol. II: effects. New York: United Nations, 2000.

8. Preston DL, Shimizu Y, Pierce DA, et al. Studies of mortality of atomic bomb survivors. Report 13: solid cancer and noncancer disease mortality: 1950–1997. Radiat Res 2003;160:381–407.

9. Brenner DJ. Estimating cancer risks from pediatric CT: going from the qualitative to the quantitative. Pediatr Radiol 2002;32:228–31.

10. Fagin JA. Editorial: challenging dogma in thyroid cancer molecular genetics–role of RET/PTC and BRAF in tumor initiation. J Clin Endocrinol Metab 2004;89:4264–6.

11. Schull WJ, Otake M. Cognitive function and prenatal exposure to ionizing radiation. Teratology 1999;59:222–6.

12. Adelstein SJ. Administered radionuclides in pregnancy. Teratology 1999;59:236–9.

13. Brenner DJ, Doll R, Goodhead DT, et al. Cancer risks attributable to low doses of ionizing radiation: assessing what we really know. Proc Natl Acad Sci USA 2003;100:13761–6.

14. Ishii K, Hosoi Y, Yamada S, et al. Decreased incidence of thymic lymphoma in AKR mice as a result of chronic, fractionated low-dose total-body X irradiation. Radiat Res 1996;146:582–5.

15. Johansson L. Hormesis: an update of the present position. Eur J Nucl Med Mol Imaging 2003;30:921–33.

16. Mitchell SA, Marino SA, Brenner DJ, et al. Bystander effect and adaptive response in C3H 10T$\frac{1}{2}$ cells. Int J Radiat Biol 2004;80:465–72.

17. Adelstein SJ. Uncertainty and relative risks of radiation exposure. JAMA 1987;258:655–7.

18. Sankaranarayanan K. Estimation of the hereditary risks of exposure to ionizing radiation: history, current status, and emerging perspectives. Health Phys 2001;80:363–9.

20
Internal Dosimetry

Michael G. Stabin

The science of internal dosimetry is a specialty within the general field of health physics. A working definition of health physics might be "the protection of people and their environment from the harmful effects of radiation while allowing its beneficial applications." In any application involving the use of ionizing radiation, the risks of its use must be balanced against its benefits. In medical uses of radiation, the benefits are immediately obvious and are directly received by the person who is exposed to the risk. This makes the balancing process considerably easier than, for example, in the use of nuclear power, where a small number of people incur a risk so that a broad region can receive a benefit. The evaluation of this balance, however, cannot occur without some quantification of the risks. Internal dosimetry calculations provide estimates of the amount of radiation that is absorbed by different organs or organ systems. The assignment of a risk to a given radiation dose estimate is not a clear-cut procedure, but without the absorbed dose estimate it cannot be attempted.

This chapter outlines the basic concepts inherent in current dose calculations, describes the calculation framework, and provide dose estimates for a number of radiopharmaceuticals in use in pediatric nuclear medicine today. A more extensive discussion of these concepts may be found in other sources.[1,2]

Basic Concepts

To define the task of calculating internal doses, we must define the quantities we wish to estimate. The principal quantity of interest in internal dosimetry is the *absorbed dose*, or the *equivalent dose*. Absorbed dose (D) is defined as follows[3]:

$$D = \frac{d\varepsilon}{dm} \tag{1}$$

where $d\varepsilon$ is the mean energy imparted by ionizing radiation to matter of mass dm. The units of absorbed dose are typically erg/g or J/kg. The special units are rad, equal to 100 erg/g, and with the advent of SI units, the gray (Gy), equal to 1.0 J/kg (1 J/kg = 100 rad = 10^4 erg/g). The equivalent dose (H) is the absorbed dose multiplied by a *radiation weighting factor* w_R[4] [formerly called *quality factor* (Q)], the latter accounting for the effectiveness of different types of radiation in causing biologic effects:

$$H = D \times w_R \tag{2}$$

Because the radiation weighting factor is in principle dimensionless, the pure units of this quantity are the same as absorbed dose (i.e., erg/g or J/kg). However, to note the difference, the special units have unique names, specifically, the rem and sievert (Sv). Values for the

TABLE 20.1. Currently recommended radiation weighting factors

Alpha particles	20
Beta particles (+/−)	1
Gamma rays	1
X-rays	1

radiation weighting factor have changed as new information about radiation effectiveness has become available. Current values, recommended by the International Commission on Radiological Protection (ICRP), are given in Table 20.1. The quantity equivalent dose was originally derived for use in radiation protection programs. The development of the effective dose equivalent (to be defined later) by the ICRP in 1977[5] allowed nonuniform internal doses to be expressed as an equivalent whole-body dose. This, at least in principle, would permit direct comparison of different procedures, including nuclear medicine and radiology, and use with risk factors based on whole-body exposure. The use in medicine was suggested and supported by the ICRP,[6,7] although this was not its original intended application. The international scientific community, with the possible exception of the Medical Internal Radiation Dose (MIRD) Committee,[8] has accepted this concept for diagnostic nuclear medicine applications (it has *no* applicability to situations involving radionuclide therapy).

Calculation Framework

A generic equation for the absorbed dose in any target organ can be given as follows:

$$D = \frac{k\tilde{A}\sum_i n_i E_i \phi_i}{m} \qquad (3)$$

D = absorbed dose in a target organ (rad or Gy)
$\tilde{A}$ = cumulated activity (sum of all nuclear transitions that occurred) in a source organ (μCi-hr or MBq-s)
n = number of radiations with energy E emitted per nuclear transition
E = energy per radiation (MeV)

i = the number of radiations in a radionuclide's decay scheme
ϕ = absorbed fraction (fraction of radiation energy absorbed in the target)
m = mass of target region (g or kg)
k = proportionality constant (rad-g/μCi-hr-MeV or Gy-kg/MBq-sec-MeV)

The dose equation historically used by the MIRD system is as follows:

$$D = \tilde{A} \cdot S = A_0 \cdot \tau \cdot S \qquad (4)$$

where $\tilde{A}$ is defined as above, τ is the residence time [which is equal to $\tilde{A}/A_0$, the cumulated activity divided by the patient's administered activity (A_0)], and S is given by

$$S = \frac{k\sum_i n_i E_i \phi_i}{m} \qquad (5)$$

The cumulated activity in the equation above is the integral of the time-activity curve (i.e., $\tilde{A} = \int A(t)\,dt$, usually from time zero to infinity). Much confusion has arisen over another concept developed by the MIRD Committee, namely that of "residence time." The MIRD definition of "residence time" is

$$D = A_0 \tau S \qquad (6)$$

$$\tau = \tilde{A}/A_0 \qquad (7)$$

where A_0 is the initial activity *administered*. The time zero intercept of an organ's time-activity curve generally represents the fraction of A_0 initially associated with that organ, but it is not A_0 as given in these equations. So, however the cumulated activity for an organ is determined, this quantity divided by the initial activity administered gives the residence time (in units of time, e.g., μCi-hr/μCi ≡ hr). An alternate formulation was proposed by Stabin and Siegel and was used in the development of data for the RADAR Internet Web site[9] and OLINDA/EXM personal computer software[10] (which was designed to replace the widely used MIRDOSE code[11]):

$$D = N \times DF \qquad (8)$$

where N is the number of disintegrations that occur in a source organ and DF is as follows:

$$DF = \frac{k \sum_i n_i E_i \phi_i}{m} \qquad (9)$$

The DF is mathematically the same as an S value as defined in the MIRD system. The number of disintegrations is the integral of a time-activity curve for a source region. The integral of this function has units of activity × time, for example Bq-s (a Bq is one disintegration per second). We could also use non-SI units for the number of disintegrations (e.g., μCi-hr, 1 μCi-hr is equivalent to 1.33×10^8 disintegrations). If we give the total number of disintegrations that occur in a source region, we will get the total dose to all target regions. If we give the number of disintegrations that occur in a source region per unit activity administered, we define N in units of (for example) Bq-s per Bq administered, and N will have units of Bq-s/Bq.

The effective dose equivalent (EDE, often designated H_e) is calculated as the *sum* of the products of the dose equivalents calculated and their appropriate tissue weighting factors (not to be confused with radiation weighting factors, as used in Eq. 2). The weighting factors recommended in ICRP 26 in the original definition of the EDE, which were updated in ICRP 60, are shown in Table 20.2. With the update in tissue weighting factors, the ICRP also changed the name slightly to *effective dose* and used the symbol E. By equation, the E or H_e is

$$E \text{ or } H_e = \sum_T w_T H_T \qquad (10)$$

where w_T is the weighting factor for tissue T and H_T is the calculated dose equivalent for tissue T. The weighting factor assigned to "Remainder" organs in Table 20.2 follows different rules for the E or H_e, as described by the ICRP in the appropriate documents. The effective dose supersedes the effective dose equivalent and should be used as much as possible. Some U.S. regulations that have not been updated still call for reporting of the effective dose equivalent, so the weighting factors are still shown in this chapter (and H_e is still calculated, for this purpose and for historical comparison, in the OLINDA/EXM code). Although this quantity and the weighting

TABLE 20.2. Tissue weighting factors recommended in International Commission on Radiological Protection ICRP 30 and ICRP 60 for calculation of the effective dose equivalent

Organ	Weighting factor	
	ICRP 30	ICRP 60
Gonads	0.25	0.20
Red marrow	0.12	0.12
Colon	—	0.12
Lungs	0.12	0.12
Stomach	—	0.12
Bladder (urinary)	—	0.05
Breasts	0.15	0.05
Liver	—	0.05
Esophagus	—	0.05
Thyroid	0.03	0.05
Skin	—	0.01
Bone surfaces	0.03	0.01
Remainder	0.30	0.05

factors employed to calculate it were developed for working adults, the application to nuclear medicine procedures for pediatric as well as adult populations was advanced by the ICRP, as was discussed previously. The weighting factors, therefore, are assigned to all age groups for the calculation of effective dose equivalent in the following tables. Because of the nonuniformity of organ doses resulting from internal exposures, the E or H_e is a better quantity to use in evaluating overall risk of a procedure or comparing procedures (for *populations*, not *individuals*) than the so-called total-body dose.[12] Use of the E or H_e cannot and should not replace consideration of individual organ absorbed doses. Reporting of the effective dose alone can be as misleading as reporting of the total-body dose.

Sources of Data for the Equation

Physical Factors

We first address the factors in the equation that deal with the physics aspects of dosimetry calculations. All of these factors are contained in the S value or DF value, as defined above. The factor k in Eq. 3 is determined from first principles, once the units of the equation are chosen. The energy of decay of a nuclide and the fraction of time that energy occurs are quantities easily found in several references. Some recent references of this type include the MIRD Radionuclide Data and Decay Schemes,[13] ICRP Publication 38,[14] and the RADAR decay data database.[15]

Organ masses have traditionally been derived from compilations of such data that have appeared in various forms in the literature. The earliest comprehensive reference for these data was the document ICRP 23,[16] which gave estimates (Table 20.3) of many of these values for the reference adult male worker. This work was supplemented by the research of Cristy and Eckerman,[17] which gave estimates of many organ parameters (Table 20.4) for children of various ages and adults. Younger members of the series are taken to represent either sex, whereas the 70-kg phantom is taken to represent the adult male or large adult female. All members of the series have both male and female organs.

These anatomic models are also used to estimate the absorbed fractions of energy (ϕ) from organs to themselves and from one region to the next. This feat is accomplished through use of various Monte Carlo codes that simulate the transport and absorption of radiation within these phantoms, log the events, and report the fractional distribution of photon energy in all regions of the phantom from energy originating in one region. For beta particles (plus or minus) and other electrons (as well as alpha particles, if applicable), all of the emitted energy is usually assumed to be absorbed where it is emitted, and the absorbed fraction is set to 1.0 for the source organ and 0.0 for all other organs. In fact, Eq. 4 needs to be generalized to account for different source organs irradiating the various target organs of interest:

$$D_{r_k} = \sum_h \tilde{A}_h \times S(r_k \leftarrow r_h)$$
$$= \sum_h \tilde{A}_h \times \frac{k \sum_i n_i E_i \phi_i(r_k \leftarrow r_h)}{m_{r_k}} \quad (11)$$

where r_h represents a source region and r_k represents a target region, and other terms are defined as in Eq. 3. The absorbed fraction $\phi_i(r_k \leftarrow r_h)$ [or sometimes $\phi_i(r_k \leftarrow r_h)/m$, called the *specific absorbed fraction*, usually designated as $\Phi_i(r_k \leftarrow r_h)$] is estimated by the Monte Carlo codes.

Kinetic Data

Time-activity data (to determine values of $\tilde{A}$ or N) must be derived from direct measurements on human subjects or animals or obtained from literature sources. The proper analysis of time-activity data is an important key to calculating radiation dose estimates. Generally speaking, the uncertainties in the biologic data are far greater than any uncertainties in the physical parameters (such as energy per decay, absorbed fraction, or even organ mass). The dose esti-

TABLE 20.3. Masses of source regions (G) in reference adult male worker

Adrenals	14
Gastrointestinal tract:	
LLI contents	135
LLI wall	160
SI contents and wall	1,040
Stomach contents	250
Stomach wall	150
ULI contents	220
ULI wall	210
Kidneys	310
Liver	1,800
Lungs	1,000
Ovaries	11
Pancreas	100
Remaining tissue	48,000
Skin	2,600
Spleen	180
Testes	35
Thymus	20
Thyroid	20
Urinary bladder contents	200
Urinary bladder wall	45
Uterus	80
Whole body	70,000

LLI, lower large intestine; SI, small intestine; ULI, upper large intestine.

Table 20.4. Masses of source regions in the Cristy and Eckerman phantom series

Phantom: Total phantom weight (kg)	Newborn 3.4	Age 1 9.8	Age 5 19	Age 10 32	Age 15 55–58	Adult 70
	Mass (g) of organ in each phantom					
Adrenals	5.83	3.52	5.27	7.22	10.5	16.3
Brain	352	884	1,260	1,360	1,410	1,420
Breasts, including skin	0.205	1.1	2.17	3.65	407	403
Breasts, excluding skin	0.107	0.732	1.51	2.6	361	351
Gallbladder contents	2.12	4.81	19.7	38.5	49	55.7
Gallbladder wall	0.408	0.91	3.73	7.28	9.27	10.5
Gastrointestinal tract:						
LLI contents	6.98	18.3	36.6	61.7	109	143
LLI wall	7.98	20.6	41.4	70	127	167
SI contents and wall	52.9	138	275	465	838	1,100
Stomach contents	10.6	36.2	75.1	133	195	260
Stomach wall	6.41	21.8	49.1	85.1	118	158
ULI contents	11.2	28.7	57.9	97.5	176	232
ULI wall	10.5	27.8	55.2	93.4	168	220
Heart contents	36.5	72.7	134	219	347	454
Heart wall	25.4	50.6	92.8	151	241	316
Kidneys	22.9	62.9	116	173	248	299
Liver	121	292	584	887	1,400	1,910
Lungs	50.6	143	290	453	651	1,000
Ovaries	0.328	0.714	1.73	3.13	10.5	8.71
Pancreas	2.8	10.3	23.6	30	64.9	94.3
Remaining tissue	2,360	6,400	13,300	23,100	40,000	51,800
Skeleton						
Active marrow	47	150	320	610	1,050	1,120
Cortical bone	0	299	875	1,580	3,220	4,000
Trabecular bone	140	200	219	396	806	1,000
Skin	118	271	538	888	2,150	3,010
Spleen	9.11	25.5	48.3	77.4	123	183
Testes	0.843	1.21	1.63	1.89	15.5	39.1
Thymus	11.3	22.9	29.6	31.4	28.4	20.9
Thyroid	1.29	1.78	3.45	7.93	12.4	20.7
Urinary bladder contents	12.4	32.9	64.7	103	160	211
Urinary bladder wall	2.88	7.7	14.5	23.2	35.9	47.6
Uterus	3.85	1.45	2.7	4.16	79	79
Whole body	3,600	9,720	19,800	33,200	56,800	73,700

LLI, lower large intestine; SI, small intestine; ULI, upper large intestine.

mates given in this chapter (Table 20.5) are taken, except where noted otherwise, from the extensive work done by the ICRP Task Group on Radiopharmaceuticals.[18,19] The ICRP used the Cristy and Eckerman phantom series and its own compilations of biokinetic data from a number of sources to develop the dose estimates. The reader is referred to these ICRP documents for listings of doses to individual organs. The ICRP is currently recalculating many of the values in Publication 53 to reflect newer models and the more recent tissue weighting factors. These data may become available in electronic form as well. The dose estimates in Table 20.5, and much additional information on kinetic models, organ doses, and other parameters, are also available in electronic form on the RADAR Web site.

Table 20.5. Effective doses to various age groups from different radiopharmaceuticals

	Adult		15 years old		10 years old		5 years old		1 year old		Reference
	mSv/MBq	rem/mCi	mSv/MBq	rem/mCi	mSv/MBq	rem/mCi	mSv/MBq	rem/mCi	mSv/MBq	rem/mCi	
[18]F-fluorodeoxyglucose	0.016	0.059	0.021	0.078	0.031	0.11	0.049	0.18	0.091	0.34	20
[6]Ga citrate	0.10	0.37	0.13	0.481	0.20	0.74	0.33	1.22	0.64	2.37	
[123]I sodium iodide (0% uptake)	0.013	0.0481	0.016	0.059	0.024	0.089	0.037	0.137	0.037	0.137	
[123]I sodium iodide (5% uptake)	0.038	0.141	0.053	0.196	0.08	0.296	0.15	0.555	0.29	1.07	
[123]I sodium iodide (15% uptake)	0.075	0.278	0.11	0.407	0.17	0.629	0.35	1.30	0.65	2.41	
[123]I sodium iodide (25% uptake)	0.11	0.407	0.17	0.629	0.26	0.962	0.54	2.00	1.0	3.7	
[123]I sodium iodide (35% uptake)	0.15	0.555	0.23	0.851	0.35	1.30	0.74	2.74	1.4	5.18	
[123]I sodium iodide (45% uptake)	0.19	0.703	0.29	1.07	0.44	1.628	0.94	3.48	1.8	6.66	
[123]I sodium iodide (55% uptake)	0.23	0.851	0.35	1.295	0.53	1.961	1.1	4.07	2.1	7.77	
[111]In pentetreotide, also known as OctreoScan	0.054	0.200	0.071	0.263	0.10	0.37	0.16	0.592	0.28	1.04	
[111]In white blood cells	0.638	2.36	0.836	3.09	1.24	4.59	1.91	7.07	3.38	12.5	21
[99m]Tc-disofenin, also know as HIDA (iminodiacetic acid)	0.017	0.063	0.021	0.078	0.029	0.107	0.045	0.167	0.10	0.37	
^{99m}Tc-DMSA (dimercaptosuccinic acid), also known as Succimer	0.0088	0.0326	0.011	0.041	0.015	0.056	0.021	0.078	0.037	0.137	
[99m]Tc-exametazime, also known as Ceretec and HMPAO	0.0093	0.0344	0.011	0.041	0.017	0.063	0.027	0.10	0.049	0.181	

99mTc-macroaggregated albumin (MAA)	0.011	0.0407	0.016	0.059	0.023	0.085	0.034	0.126	0.063	0.233
99m-medronate, also know as 99mTc-methylene diphosphonate (MDP)	0.0057	0.0211	0.007	0.026	0.011	0.041	0.014	0.052	0.027	0.10
99mTc-mertiatide, also know as MAG$_3$	0.0070	0.0259	0.009	0.033	0.012	0.044	0.012	0.044	0.022	0.081
99mTc-bicisate, also known as ECD and Neurolite	0.011	0.0407	0.014	0.052	0.021	0.078	0.032	0.118	0.06	0.222
99mTc-pentetatem also know as 99mTc-DTPA	0.0049	0.0181	0.0062	0.023	0.0082	0.030	0.0090	0.033	0.016	0.059
99mTc-pyrophosphate	0.0057	0.0211	0.0070	0.026	0.011	0.041	0.014	0.052	0.027	0.10
99mTc-red blood cells	0.0070	0.0259	0.0089	0.033	0.014	0.052	0.021	0.078	0.039	0.144
99mTc-sestamibi, also know as Cardiolite (rest)	0.0090	0.0333	0.012	0.044	0.018	0.067	0.028	0.104	0.053	0.196
99mTc-sestamibi, also know as Cardiolite (stress)	0.0079	0.0292	0.010	0.037	0.016	0.059	0.023	0.085	0.045	0.167
99mTc-sodium pertechnetate	0.013	0.0481	0.017	0.063	0.026	0.096	0.042	0.155	0.079	0.292
99mTc-sulfur colloid	0.0094	0.0348	0.012	0.044	0.018	0.067	0.028	0.104	0.050	0.185
99mTc-tetrofosmin, also know as Myoview (rest)	0.0076	0.0281	0.0096	0.036	0.013	0.048	0.022	0.081	0.043	0.159
99mTc-tetrofosmin, also know as Myoview (stress)	0.0070	0.0259	0.0082	0.030	0.012	0.044	0.018	0.067	0.035	0.13
201Tl-thallous chloride	0.16	0.592	0.26	0.962	0.97	3.59	1.3	4.81	2.0	7.4

22

References

1. Loevinger R, Budinger T, Watson E. MIRD Primer for Absorbed Dose Calculations. New York: Society of Nuclear Medicine, 1988.
2. Stabin MG, Siegel JA. Physical models and dose factors for use in internal dose assessment. Health Physics 2003;85(3):294–310.
3. International Commission on Radiation Units and Measurements. Report 33: Radiation Quantities and Units, ICRU 33. International Commission on Radiation Units and Measurements. Washington, 1980.
4. International Commission on Radiological Protection. 1990 Recommendations of the International Commission on Radiological Protection. ICRP Publication 60. New York: Pergamon Press, 1991.
5. International Commission on Radiological Protection. Recommendations of the International Commission on Radiological Protection. ICRP Publication 26. New York: Pergamon Press, 1977.
6. International Commission on Radiological Protection. Radiation dose to patients from radiopharmaceuticals. ICRP Publication 53. New York: Pergamon Press, 1988.
7. International Commission on Radiological Protection. Protection of the patient in nuclear medicine. ICRP Publication 52. New York: Pergamon Press, 1987.
8. Poston J. Application of the effective dose equivalent to nuclear medicine patients. J Nucl Med 1993;34(4):714–6.
9. Stabin M, Siegel J, Hunt J, Sparks R, Lipsztein J, Eckerman K. RADAR—the radiation dose assessment resource. An online source of dose information for nuclear medicine and occupational radiation safety. J Nucl Med 2001;42(5):243P.
10. Stabin MG, Sparks RB. MIRDOSE4 does not exist. J Nucl Med 1999;40(5, suppl):309P.
11. Stabin MG. MIRDOSE: personal computer software for internal dose assessment in nuclear medicine. J Nucl Med 1996;37(3):538–6.
12. Toohey RE, Stabin MG. Comparative analysis of dosimetry parameters for nuclear medicine. In: Stelson A, Stabin M, Sparks R, eds. Sixth International Radiopharmaceutical Dosimetry Symposium, held May 7–10, 1996, in Gatlinburg, TN. Gatlinburg, TN: Oak Ridge Associated Universities, 1999:532–51.
13. Weber D, Eckerman K, Dillman LT, Ryman J. MIRD: Radionuclide Data and Decay Schemes. New York: Society of Nuclear Medicine, 1989.
14. International Commission on Radiological Protection. Radionuclide Transformations: Energy and Intensity of Emissions. New York: Pergamon Press, 1983.
15. Stabin MG, da Luz CQPL. New decay data for internal and external dose assessment. Health Phys 2002;83(4):471–5.
16. International Commission on Radiological Protection. Report of the task group on reference man. ICRP Publication 23. New York: Pergamon Press, 1975.
17. Cristy M, Eckerman K. Specific absorbed fractions of energy at various ages from internal photons sources. ORNL/TM-8381 V1–V7. Oak Ridge, TN: Oak Ridge National Laboratory, 1987.
18. International Commission on Radiological Protection. Radiation Dose to Patients from Radiopharmaceuticals. ICRP Publication 53. New York: Pergamon Press, 1988.
19. International Commission on Radiological Protection. Radiation Dose to Patients from Radiopharmaceuticals. ICRP Publication 80. Supplement to ICRP Publication 53. New York: Pergamon Press, 1998.
20. Hays MT, Watson EE, Thomas SR, Stabin M. MIRD Dose estimate report No. 19: radiation absorbed dose estimates from 18F-FDG. J Nucl Med 2002;43:210–4.
21. Radiation Internal Dose Information Center, Oak Ridge, TN. Personal communication, 2001.
22. Thomas SR, Stabin MG, Castronovo FP. Radiation-absorbed dose from 201TI-201 thallous chloride. J Nucl Med 2005;46:502–8.

Index